Anatomy and Physiology for Midwives

Third Edition

Jane Coad BSc PhD PGCEA

Associate Professor in Human Nutrition, Massey University, New Zealand

with

Melvyn Dunstall BSc MSc PGCEA RM RGN

Lecturer/Practitioner in Midwifery, Frimley Park Hospital NHS Foundation Trust;
Supervisor of Midwives

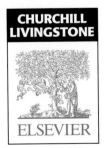

CHURCHILL
LIVINGSTONE

ELSEVIER

Edinburgh   London   New York   Oxford   Philadelphia   St Louis   Sydney   Toronto   2011

First edition 2001
Second edition 2005
Third edition 2011

ISBN 9780702034893

British Library Cataloguing in Publication Data
A catalogue record for this book is available from the British Library

Library of Congress Cataloging in Publication Data
A catalog record for this book is available from the Library of Congress

Notices
Knowledge and best practice in this field are constantly changing. As new research and experience broaden our understanding, changes in research methods, professional practices, or medical treatment may become necessary.

Practitioners and researchers must always rely on their own experience and knowledge in evaluating and using any information, methods, compounds, or experiments described herein. In using such information or methods they should be mindful of their own safety and the safety of others, including parties for whom they have a professional responsibility.

With respect to any drug or pharmaceutical products identified, readers are advised to check the most current information provided (i) on procedures featured or (ii) by the manufacturer of each product to be administered, to verify the recommended dose or formula, the method and duration of administration, and contraindications. It is the responsibility of practitioners, relying on their own experience and knowledge of their patients, to make diagnoses, to determine dosages and the best treatment for each individual patient, and to take all appropriate safety precautions.

To the fullest extent of the law, neither the Publisher nor the authors, contributors, or editors, assume any liability for any injury and/or damage to persons or property as a matter of products liability, negligence or otherwise, or from any use or operation of any methods, products, instructions, or ideas contained in the material herein.

ELSEVIER your source for books,
journals and multimedia
in the health sciences
www.elsevierhealth.com

Working together to grow
libraries in developing countries
www.elsevier.com | www.bookaid.org | www.sabre.org
ELSEVIER BOOK AID International Sabre Foundation

The
Publisher's
policy is to use
**paper manufactured
from sustainable forests**

Printed in China

Contents

Preface

Many of the most magical aspects of physiology are associated with reproduction, from before conception, through fetal development and maternal responses to the growing fetus, to the signalling and progression of labour, continued development of the neonate, optimized by maternal behaviour and lactation and the mother's subsequent return to fertility. Reproductive physiology continues to be a fast-moving field as recent advances in fertility treatment, postnatal care of premature infants and the implications of HIV and other viral infections such as influenza make evident.

Midwives are expected to understand in depth the science underpinning midwifery practice but have often had little background in this exciting field. Midwives also often find themselves to be bombarded with questions from interested, fascinated, and increasingly well-informed prospective parents due to information availability via the Internet. This book aims to support students and practising midwives wanting more detailed scientific knowledge that can be applied within the practice setting.

The book provides a thorough review of anatomy and physiology applicable to midwifery from first principles through to current research. It acknowledges the importance of the research basis and aims to integrate theory and practice.

The chapters are organized such that learning objectives lead into the body of the chapter. Case studies provide the reader with the opportunity to reflect on the implications for practice. Wherever possible, information is provided as illustrations. At the end of each chapter, key points are provided and the applications of the scientific content to practice are summarized. Each chapter is comprehensively referenced and has a list of annotated recommendations for further reading.

Chapter 1 begins by introducing the reader to the basic unit of structure, the cell, and describes the relationship between cellular structure and function. It provides an introduction to the major tissue types and physiological systems found within the body and reviews the principles of regulation and maintenance of homeostatic systems.

Chapter 2 focuses on the reproductive and urinary systems of the human. The basic anatomy and physiology of the urinary system are explored in the first part of this chapter. The female reproductive tract and the organs associated with it are then described, relating both their structure and function specifically to childbirth. The last part of this chapter focuses on the male reproductive organs and the process of spermatogenesis.

Chapter 3 introduces the principles of endocrinology, laying the foundation for the understanding of changes that occur in pregnancy. It describes the different types of hormones, how and where they are produced, and their modes of action.

Chapter 4 covers the endocrine control and regulation of reproductive cycles. Ovarian function and follicular development lead on to gamete formation within the female and consideration is given as to why this is so dramatically different to spermatogenesis within the male. One of the essential roles of reproductive cycles is that the coordination of oogenesis and the cyclical changes within the endometrium occur to optimize fertilization and implantation. Thus the menstrual cycle is described in depth in this chapter. Some of the hormonal causes of infertility are discussed as is the endocrine manipulation to achieve contraception. The chapter concludes with a brief description of the physiological changes at puberty and menopause.

Chapter 5 integrates the concepts introduced in the first four chapters by focusing on how sexual differentiation is achieved and the biological basis for the differences in reproductive physiology and behaviour in women and men. This chapter leads on to the next two chapters. Chapter 6 describes how sexual bimorphism facilitates fertilization, very early development and implantation of the zygote and the maternal physiological responses that allow successful fertilization and implantation. The principles and techniques used in artificial fertilization are briefly described. Chapter 7 introduces the science of genetics, highlighting an essential component of the human reproductive strategy: that of how genetic mixing and thus variation within the species is achieved. An introduction to the aetiology and types of genetic disease and how these may be detected within the clinical situation are discussed. The basic concepts of genetic testing and screening are also included.

Chapter 8 presents the development and function of the placenta and its interaction with maternal physiology. It also discusses some of the causes and effects of placental pathology. Following this, Chapter 9 provides a comprehensive overview of the development of the embryo and its physiological systems. The factors that promote and influence fetal growth are also discussed in this chapter.

Chapter 10 brings the reader back to maternal physiology by introducing and giving an overview of immunological issues and principles related to pregnancy. The maternal acceptance of the fetus and its implications are discussed, as are the effects of pregnancy upon the maternal immune system. A section is included on the interaction of the maternal and fetal immune systems, using some clinical conditions as examples of these interactions. The neonate's vulnerability to infection is described in relation to midwifery care together with the principles of immunization. Finally, the specific effects of the human immunodeficiency virus (HIV) and the influenzia virus in pregnancy are considered.

One of the most striking aspects of reproductive physiology is the physiological changes that occur within the pregnant female. Chapter 11 explores why these changes occur and how they are orchestrated in order to facilitate an optimal outcome of pregnancy. These changes are related to how the woman experiences pregnancy and the signs, symptoms and discomforts she might encounter. Following on from this, Chapter 12 provides a brief overview of nutrition and nutritional requirements in pregnancy. This lays the basis for exploring how maternal nutrition and health can influence pregnancy outcomes not only for the mother but also for the fetus, both *in utero* and potentially throughout life.

Chapter 13 specifically explores the physiology of parturition and how the maternal physiology is altered to facilitate this. Current theories and evidence relating to the timing and initiation of labour in humans are discussed. An overview is provided of pain physiology related to labour and how this is affected by pain-relieving interventions. This chapter includes a section that explores the effects of labour upon the fetal physiology.

Following birth, the physiological changes that occur during pregnancy are dramatically and efficiently reversed and so the puerperium is the subject of Chapter 14. Alongside the maternal postnatal changes, the neonate has to quickly adapt to extrauterine life and so Chapter 15 focuses on the transition to neonatal life, including how these changes are assessed.

The final chapter, Chapter 16, highlights the physiology of lactation and how this meets the unique requirements of the neonate not only from a nutritional perspective but also from an immunological basis and a developmental basis. It is essential that midwives understand the physiological aspects of lactation in order to promote breastfeeding, as the evidence is overwhelming that successful breastfeeding can positively influence the health and well-being, both physically and mentally, of the infant for the rest of its life.

The demand for this book came primarily from our students, including preregistration students, midwives returning to practice and those following postregistration study. Enthusiastic questions, demands for explanation and an evident relish for understanding the theory related to practice stimulated the birth and continued development of the book resulting in this third edition. We hope that readers will continue to enquire about and enjoy this exciting field so that they can successfully utilize scientific knowledge in the ongoing development and promotion of effective midwifery practice.

Jane Coad
Melvyn Dunstall

Acknowledgements

It is now over a decade since we first began working on this book and, as in the previous editions, we would like, once again, to thank our patient families and friends who again provided us with the encouragement and support to complete the third edition of this book. We'd also like to thank all our colleagues at Massey University in New Zealand, Frimley Park Hospital NHS Foundation Trust and the Faculty of Health and Medical Sciences at the University of Surrey for their continued help, support and guidance in the development of this latest edition. Our midwifery and physiology students and other readers of the book have continued to ask questions and demand answers and their views and opinions have, once again, shaped the development of this latest edition and so we continue to be indebted to them all. Within the clinical situation, there is now an even greater need for evidence-based practice and students and practitioners demand a knowledge base that will support this. Finally, we continue to owe much to the production team at Elsevier, especially Mairi McCubbin, Fiona Conn and Cheryl Brant. We would like to thank them all for their help, guidance and continuing patience in supporting us complete the third edition.

Abbreviations

ABP	androgen-binding protein		DHA	docosahexaenoic acid
ACTH	adrenocorticotrophic hormone (corticotrophin)		DHEAS	dehydroepiandrosterone sulphate
ADH	antidiuretic hormone		5α-DHT	5α-dihydrotestosterone
AFP	alpha-fetoprotein		DIC	disseminated intravascular coagulation
AIDS	acquired immune deficiency (immunodeficiency) syndrome		DIT	diet-induced thermogenesis
AMH	anti Müllerian hormone, also known as Müllerian-inhibiting substance, MIS or Müllerian-inhibiting hormone, MIH		DNA	deoxyribonucleic acid
ANP	atrial natriuretic peptide		DVT	deep vein thrombosis
APC	antigen-presenting cell		E_1	oestrone
ATP	adenosine triphosphate		E_2	oestradiol-17β
AV	arteriovenous		E_3	oestriol
AVN	atrioventricular node		ECG	electrocardiogram
BAT	brown adipose tissue		ED	erectile dysfunction
BMI	body mass index		ED-PAF	embryo-derived platelet-activating factor
BMR	basal metabolic rate		EDRF	endothelium-derived relaxing factor
BPD	biparietal diameter		EGF	epidermal growth factor
CaH	congenital adrenal hyperplasia		ER	endoplasmic reticulum
CAM	calcium-binding protein (calmodulin)		ERPC	evacuation of retained products of conception
cAMP	cyclic adenosine monophosphate		FBM	fetal breathing movement
CAP	contraction-associated protein		FGM	female genital mutilation
CBP	corticosteroid-binding protein		FHR	fetal heart rate
CCK	cholecystokinin		FHV	fetal heart variability
CCT	controlled cord traction		FIL	factor inhibitor of lactation
CD	cluster of differentiation		FISH	fluorescent in situ hybridization
CDH	congenital dislocation of the hips		FPU	fetal–placental unit
cGMP	cyclic guanosine monophosphate		FSH	follicle-stimulating hormone
CMV	cytomegalovirus		GALT	gut-associated lymphoid tissue
CNS	central nervous system		GFR	glomerular filtration rate
CoA	coenzyme A		GH	growth hormone
COC	combined oral contraceptive		GI	glycaemic index
COX	cyclo-oxygenase		GIFT	gamete intrafallopian transfer
CRH	corticotrophin-releasing hormone		GIP	gastric inhibitory peptide
CRH-BP	corticotrophin-releasing hormone-binding protein		GL	greatest length
			GLUT	glucose-transport protein
			GM-CSF	granulocyte–macrophage colony-stimulating factor
CRL	crown–rump length		GnRH	gonadotrophin-releasing hormone
CSF	cytostatic factor		GP	general practitioner
CVS	chorionic villus sampling		Hb	haemoglobin
D&C	dilatation and curettage		hCG	human chorionic gonadotrophin
			HDL	high-density lipoprotein
			HDNB	haemorrhagic disease of the newborn

HELLP	haemolysis, elevated liver enzymes and low platelet counts	PESA	percutaneous epididymal sperm aspiration
HFEA	Human Fertilisation & Embryology Authority	PGC	primordial germ cell
HIV	human immunodeficiency virus	PGD	preimplantation genetic diagnosis
HLA	human leukocyte antigen	PGH	placental growth hormone
hMG	human menopausal gonadotrophin	PGDH	prostaglandin dehydrogenase
HPA	hypothalamic–pituitary–adrenal	Pi	inorganic phosphate
hPL	human placental lactogen	PID	pelvic inflammatory disease
HPV	human papillomavirus	PKU	phenylketonuria
HRT	hormone replacement therapy	PLA$_2$	phospholipase A$_2$
ICSI	intracytoplasmic sperm injection	PLC	phospholipase C
IDDM	insulin-dependent diabetes mellitus	PMDD	premenstrual dysphoric disorder
Ig	immunoglobulin	PMS	premenstrual syndrome
IGF	insulin-like growth factor	PPH	postpartum haemorrhage
IGF-BP	insulin-like growth factor binding protein	PRL	prolactin
IL	interleukin	PROM	premature rupture of the membranes
IU/i.u.	international units	PSA	prostate specific antigen
IUGR	intrauterine growth retardation	PUFA	polyunsaturated fatty acid
IVF	in vitro fertilization	RAS	renin–angiotensin system
kDa	kilodalton	RDI	recommended dietary intake
LBW	low birth weight	RDS	respiratory distress syndrome
LC-PUFA	long-chain polyunsaturated fatty acid	REM	rapid eye movement
LDL	low-density lipoprotein	RER	rough endoplasmic reticulum
LH	luteinizing hormone	RNA	ribonucleic acid
LHRH	luteinizing hormone releasing hormone	rRNA	ribosomal ribonucleic acid
LIF	leukaemia-inhibitory factor	RSA	recurrent spontaneous abortion
LSCS	lower-segment caesarean section	SAN	sinoatrial node
LUS	lower uterine segment	SER	smooth endoplasmic reticulum
MCV	mean blood cell volume	SGA	small for gestational age
MESA	microepidermal sperm aspiration	sIg	surface immunoglobulin
MHC	major histocompatibility complex	SLE	systemic lupus erythematosus
MIS	Müllerian-inhibiting substance (also known as Müllerian-inhibiting hormone, MIH)	SNP	single nucleotide polymorphism
		SRY	sex determining region on the Y chromosome
MLCK	myosin light-chain kinase	STD	sexual transmitted disease
mRNA	messenger ribonucleic acid	SUZI	subzonal sperm injection
MRSA	methicillin-resistant *Staphylococcus aureus*	T$_3$	tri-iodothyronine
MSH	melanocyte-stimulating hormone	T$_4$	thyroxine
MSU	midstream specimen of urine	TB	tuberculosis
mtDNA	mitochondrial DNA	TBG	thyroxin-binding globulin
NIDDM	non-insulin-dependent diabetes mellitus	TBP	thyroid-binding protein
NK cell	natural killer cell	TEF	thermic effect of food
NO	nitric oxide	TENS	transcutaneous electrical nerve stimulation
NPN	non-protein nitrogen	TGF	transforming growth factor
NPU	net protein utilization	T$_h$ cells	T helper cells
NPY	neuropeptide Y	TNF	tumour necrosis factor
NSAID	non-steroidal anti-inflammatory drug	tRNA	transfer ribonucleic acid
NSP	non-starch polysaccharide	TSH	thyroid-stimulating hormone
NST	non-shivering thermogenesis	TxA$_2$	thromboxane A$_2$
NT	nuchal translucency	U-LGL	uterine large granular leukocytes
NTD	neural tube defect	UVR	ultraviolet radiation
NVP	nausea and vomiting in pregnancy	UTI	urinary tract infection
PE	pulmonary embolism	VIP	vasoactive intestinal peptide
PCOS	polycystic ovary syndrome	VLDL	very-low-density lipoprotein
PDE	phosphodiesterase	WHI	Women's Health Initiative (studies on HRT)
PDZ	partial zona dissection	ZIFT	zygote intrafallopian transfer
		ZP	zona pellucida

Chapter | 1 |

Introduction to physiology

INTRODUCTION

Physiology is the biological science which explores how living organisms are able to function in order to survive and reproduce. Physiology investigates the relationship between the structure and function of body systems. The physiological systems are complex structures, which serve a particular function such as blood circulation or respiration. Organs are made up of cells organized into different tissue types such as nerve tissue or muscle tissue. The physiological systems communicate and interact with each other. A key concept of physiology is that life is only possible within some tightly regulated conditions such as temperature and ion concentration. Homeostasis describes an organism's ability to control its internal environment and maintain a stable condition; this allows the organisms to adjust to, and survive in, a broad range of environments. This book focuses on human reproductive function. This chapter aims to provide an illustrated introduction to, and an overview of, some of the basic physiological concepts referred to and developed in subsequent chapters, with specific references to reproduction. (For more details, readers are recommended to look at the list of further reading at the end of the chapter.)

Chapter case study

Zara is a 29-year-old primipara who presents herself at the midwife's clinic, which is held at her GP's surgery, giving a history of a positive pregnancy test.
- If Zara had accessed pre-conceptual care what advice do you think she should have been given in her preparation for pregnancy?
- What information would be available in Zara's medical records that would be useful to the midwife in her initial assessment of Zara's pregnancy?
- How could this information be used by the midwife to inform Zara of the physiological changes that have started to occur in her body?

THE CELL

The cell is the fundamental unit of structure and function of all living organisms. The evolution of multicellular organisms has led to the differentiation of cells, which means that different cells have evolved to perform specific functions and processes that contribute to the well-being of the organism as a whole. Differentiated cells form tissues, which combine with other tissues to form organs, which are linked together in physiological systems (Fig. 1.1). However, although cells can be highly specialized, they all share common features of the single cellular organisms from which we evolved. A typical human cell is about 10 μm in diameter. The largest human cell is the oocyte (see Chapter 6); it can just be seen with the naked eye. The follicular cells surrounding the oocyte have a more typical human cell size. The sperm cell is one of the smallest human cells. Smaller cells and organelles can be visualized by light and electron microscopy.

Cell structure

Most cells contain cytoplasm and are bound by a plasma membrane. Within them are various structures, called organelles (see Table 1.1), and a specialized part of the cell, called the nucleus (Fig. 1.2). The fluid surrounding the organelles is called cytosol.

CELLS AND TISSUES

Although about 200 types of cells with different structures can be identified within the body, cells can be grouped together in functional categories (Table 1.2). The study of the physical characteristics of cells is called histology (see Box 1.1). There are four types of tissue: epithelial tissue, muscle, connective tissue and neural tissue.

Epithelial tissue

Epithelial cells line the internal and external surfaces of body organs (Fig. 1.3), forming the outer layer of the skin, the mucous membranes, the lining of the lungs, gut, reproductive and urinary tracts, and also the endocrine and exocrine glands. Epithelial cells are often 'polarized' and have different characteristics on their apical (top) surface and their basal surface (which is in contact with the basement membrane). Epithelial cells are relatively undifferentiated and tend to undergo frequent mitotic divisions (see Chapter 7). This is because they are often exposed to wear and tear and so replacement epithelial cells are generated from a basal layer where cell division takes place. Epithelial cells form a barrier, which allows secretion

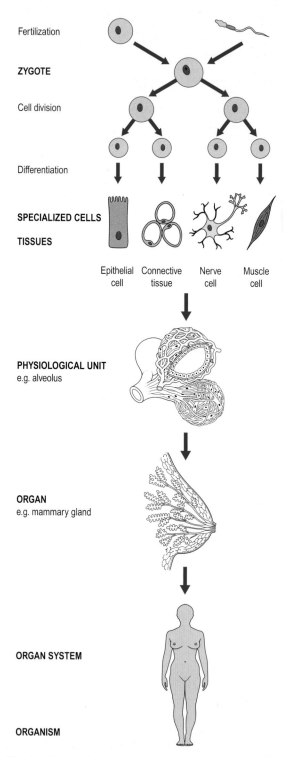

Fig. 1.1 Physiological systems: levels of organization of cells, tissues, organs and physiological systems, using breast tissue as an example.

Table 1.1 Cell components

CELL COMPONENT	STRUCTURE	FUNCTION
Cell membrane	The cell membrane is composed of a phospholipid bilayer embedded with various protein structures such as hormone receptors, ion channels and antigen markers	The membrane acts as a differential permeable membrane between the cell and its immediate environment
The nucleus	The nucleus is bound by a membrane, similar to the plasma membrane of the cell; this contains openings referred to as nuclear pores, which allow the movement of substances in and out of the nucleus	The nucleus contains deoxyribonucleic acid (DNA), the genetic instruction for the organism. Most of the time, the DNA is organized as chromatin threads; these condense into chromosomes prior to cell division. The nucleus stores and replicates DNA, which is expressed to synthesize proteins via a second type of nucleic acid, ribonucleic acid (RNA). These proteins determine the structure and function of the cell
Endoplasmic reticulum	This is a system of membranes, enclosing a space, which is continuous with the nuclear membrane. Endoplasmic reticulum (ER) exists as rough (granular) endoplasmic reticulum (RER) and smooth (agranular) endoplasmic reticulum (SER)	RER appears rough because of the attached ribosomes. RER is involved in protein packaging. SER is involved in lipid and steroid synthesis and the regulation of intracellular calcium levels
Mitochondria	Spherical or elongated rod-like structures surrounded by a folded inner membrane and a smooth outer membrane. There are more mitochondria in cells that are metabolically active and have a high energy requirement	Chemical processes involved in the formation of adenosine triphosphate (ATP). The cristae (inner membrane folds) are the site of oxidative phosphorylation and the electron transfer chain of aerobic respiration. Krebs (tricarboxylic acid or TCA) cycle and the oxidation of fatty acids take place within the matrix. Mitochondria contain mitochondrial DNA, which is maternally inherited and contains the genes for mitochondrial proteins
Golgi apparatus (complex)	A series of flattened curved membranous sacs	Modifies proteins from the RER and sorts them into secretory vesicles
Lysosomes	Spherical or oval organelles enclosed by a single membrane	Enclose acidic fluid containing digestive enzymes which act as a 'cellular stomach' breaking down cellular debris
Peroxisomes	Similar structure to lysosomes	Destroy reactive oxygen species and protect cell
Cytoskeleton	Filamentous network	Involved in maintaining cell shape and motility

and absorption of substances from one compartment to another. The skin is a specialized epithelial layer. The basal layer produces cells that are enriched with the protein keratin. The outer layers of skin cells are dead and so lack cytoplasm; it is these keratinized dead cells that provide the barrier function of the skin. Epithelial cells are classified by shape (cuboidal or columnar) and the number of layers. If there is a single layer of cells, the epithelium is described as simple; if there is more than one layer of cells (such as skin), it is stratified. Pseudostratified cells are a single layer of cells that appear to consist of more than one layer. Glands are derived from epithelial tissue.

Muscle tissue

Muscle cells contain contractile elements, so the cells can generate the mechanical force required for movement of

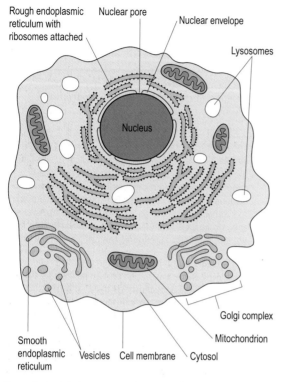

Rough endoplasmic reticulum with ribosomes attached

Nuclear pore

Nuclear envelope

Lysosomes

Nucleus

Golgi complex

Mitochondrion

Smooth endoplasmic reticulum

Vesicles

Cell membrane

Cytosol

Fig. 1.2 A typical cell.

Box 1.1 **Histology**

The study of tissue structure is described as histology. The functions of tissues are reflected in the microscopic structure of the cells of which the tissue is composed. For example, cells that are metabolically active contain many mitochondria, whereas cells that produce hormones or enzymes, for instance, will contain a large proportion of ER. Specific tissues and cellular structures are often identified by the application of various chemicals that stain particular tissues. Histology is important in diagnosing cancer, as the cancerous tissue often has histological characteristics different from those of the tissue in which the cancer has developed. Malignant cancerous tumours have highly differentiated cells, which means they often appear different from the normal tissue cells from which they arose; they often have a simpler structure and are usually prolific in their division rate. These cells are less likely to adhere to neighbouring cells as normal cells do, so they are shed into the circulatory system and carried to other parts of the body where they seed more tumours (secondary tumours or metastases). Benign tumours usually have undifferentiated cells, which may closely resemble the cells of the tissue from which they arose and tend only to grow in the one position. Although cancers in pregnancy are rare, many cancerous cells may respond to oestrogen (sometimes referred to as oestrogen dependent); therefore, cancer growth during pregnancy can be quite rapid.

Table 1.2 Functional classification of cells

CELL GROUP	EPITHELIAL CELLS	SUPPORT CELLS	CONTRACTILE CELLS	NERVE CELLS	GERM CELLS	BLOOD CELLS	IMMUNE CELLS	HORMONE-SECRETING CELLS
Example	Lining gut and blood vessels Covering skin	Fibrous support tissue, cartilage, bone	Muscle	Brain	Spermatozoa Ova	Circulating 1. red cells 2. white cells 3. platelets	Lymphoid tissues, nodes and spleen	Islets, thyroid adrenal
Function	Barrier; absorption; secretion	Organize and maintain body structure	Movement	Direct cell communication	Reproduction	1. Oxygen transport 2. Defence	Defence	Indirect cell communication
Special features	Tightly bound together by cell junctions	Produce and interact with extracellular matrix material	Contractile proteins	Release chemical messengers directly on to other cells	Haploid (i.e. half-normal chromosome number)	1. Proteins bind oxygen 2. Proteins destroy bacteria 3. Blood clotting	Recognize and destroy foreign material	Secrete chemical messengers into blood

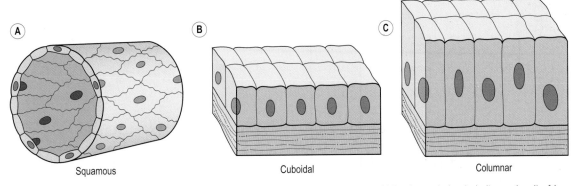

Fig. 1.3 Types of epithelial cell: (A) squamous epithelium provides a smooth lining of blood vessels (endothelium, alveoli of lung and glomeruli of kidney); (B) cuboidal epithelium is often found on absorptive surfaces such as in kidney tubules; (C) columnar epithelium is often associated with secretory and absorptive tissues and may have microvilli, as in the gut; it may also be ciliated, as in the upper airways. (Reproduced with permission from Brooker, 1998.)

the body or substances within the body (Fig. 1.4) or change shape and size. Muscle tissue is formed from the mesodermal layer of the embryo (see Chapter 9). There are three types of muscle tissue: skeletal, cardiac and smooth muscle. Skeletal muscle may be attached to bones

and controls movement of the skeleton. Skeletal muscle can also be attached to the skin, for instance the muscles of the face involved with expression. Contraction of skeletal muscle is usually under voluntary or conscious control. Skeletal muscle is often described as 'striated' because of the striped appearance of the sarcomeres of the muscle observed under the light microscope. Skeletal muscle fibres can be subdivided into slow and fast twitch fibres. Fast twitch fibres contract more strongly but they tire easily, whereas slow twitch fibres can contract for prolonged periods.

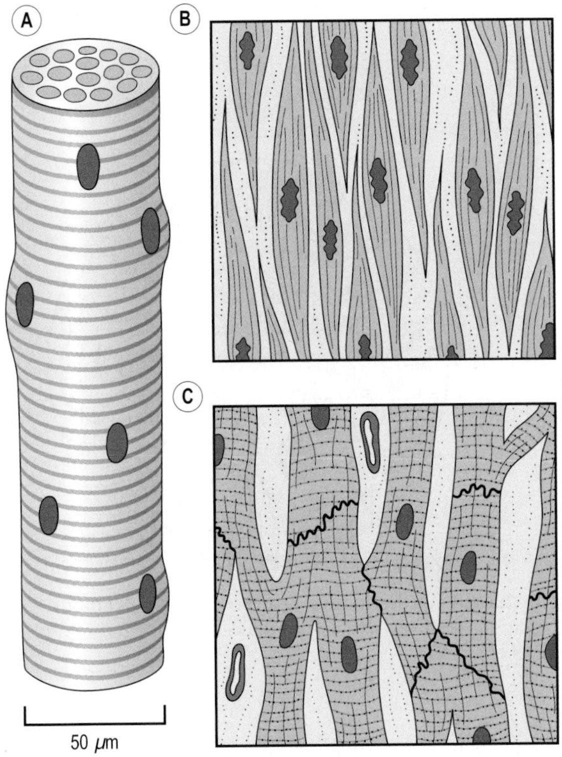

Cardiac muscle is only found in the heart; it has some structural similarity with skeletal muscle. Smooth muscle and cardiac muscle are usually under involuntary control (meaning there is no conscious awareness of the control). Smooth muscle surrounds many of the 'tubes' in the body, maintaining the function of several body systems. Smooth muscle cells are linked by gap junctions, and muscle contraction is relatively slow. Blood pressure is maintained by the contraction of a smooth muscle layer in the walls of the blood vessels. If the smooth muscle constricts, described as 'vasoconstriction', the internal lumen of the vessel will decrease and blood pressure will increase. 'Vasodilatation' is the opposite condition: the smooth muscle relaxes and the lumen diameter increases, so blood pressure falls. Organized synchronized waves of smooth muscle contraction, for instance in the gut, renal system and uterine tubes, generate peristaltic waves; these produce unidirectional movement of the contents within the lumen of the tube (Fig. 1.5).

Connective tissue

Connective tissue functions to connect, anchor and support body structures (Fig. 1.6). Connective tissue cells often produce an extracellular matrix composed of

Fig. 1.4 Muscle: (A) skeletal muscle; (B) smooth muscle; (C) cardiac muscle. (Adapted with permission from Brooker, 1998.)

50 μm

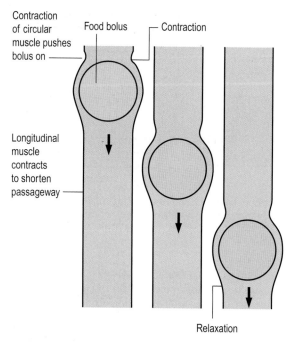

Contraction of circular muscle pushes bolus on

Food bolus

Contraction

Longitudinal muscle contracts to shorten passageway

Relaxation

Fig. 1.5 Peristaltic waves: peristalsis is achieved through the interaction of both longitudinal and circular smooth muscle fibres found in vessels with patent lumen. The peristaltic waves are responsible for (usually) unidirectional movement of the contents within the lumen. (Reproduced with permission from Brooker, 1998.)

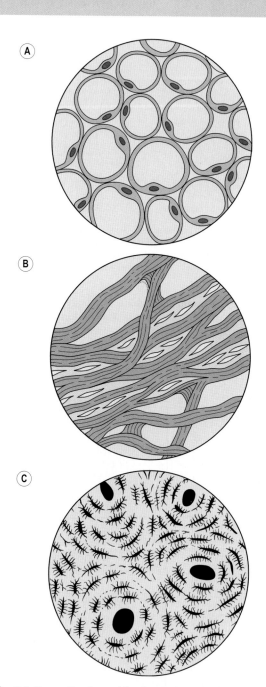

Fig. 1.6 Connective tissue: (A) adipose tissue; (B) fibrous tissue; (C) compact bone. (Reproduced with permission from Brooker, 1998.)

proteins in a ground substance of sugars, proteins and minerals. Bone is a type of connective tissue, whereas collagen is an example of an extracellular matrix. Adipose tissue is composed of specialized cells that store fat for future energy requirements and have an endocrine role. Adipose tissue also acts as an insulating layer to conserve body heat loss and so contributes to the maintenance of the homeothermic status of the organism. Fibrous tissue is an example of dense connective tissue. It is a tough tissue that forms ligaments, tendons and protective membranes.

Neural tissue

Neurons are cells that are specialized to initiate and conduct electrical signals (Fig. 1.7). Neurons require the presence of glial cells for nourishment and support; glial cells are also involved in the propagation of the electrical impulses in the neurons. As neurons are so highly specialized, they do not usually undergo further mitotic divisions once developed. Therefore, in the fetal and early neonatal period, the number of neurons produced far exceeds the level required for normal neurological function. To survive and function, neurons need regular stimulation. Throughout life, millions of neurons become dysfunctional and die.

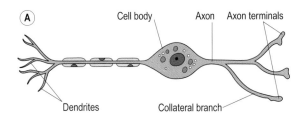

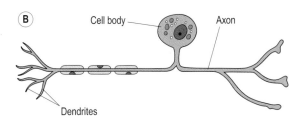

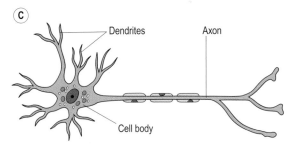

Fig. 1.7 Types of neuron: (A) bipolar; (B) unipolar; (C) multipolar.

THE STRUCTURAL ORGANIZATION OF THE BODY

The body's organization can be understood by considering each component organ system separately (see below). However, these systems all work together, as a whole. Together the systems provide nutrients and oxygen for the cells and the excretion of waste products (Fig. 1.8). Movement is controlled and the temperature is maintained. Survival until reproductive function is completed has allowed the species to multiply. Cells are bathed in extracellular fluid, which can be differentiated into the interstitial fluid surrounding the tissue cells and the plasma within the blood vessels.

Homeostasis

Homeostasis is the term used to describe the processes of the various physiological systems that maintain the constancy of the internal environment. Multicellular animals are able to maintain an internal stability that is essential for the optimal functioning of all body systems, whereas simple unicellular

organisms tend to inhabit stable environments or have adapted to overcome fluctuations in the environment, for instance by forming spores during dry periods. Unicellular organisms rely on basic nutrients being present in the environment to allow cell growth and reproduction.

The evolution of multicellular organisms and the development of motility meant that these animals were able to move within the environment to seek out the conditions that suited them best and so optimize their ability to reproduce. Mammals have developed homeostasis to a high degree. Motility, together with the homeostatic challenge of counteracting fluctuations in the external environment, places a huge energy burden upon these individuals. This increased energy requirement is above the basal metabolic rate, which is the rate of energy required to maintain essential functioning only.

Homeostasis can be considered to have three main components:

- chemostasis: the maintenance of electrolytes and pH balance
- haemostasis: the maintenance of an adequate circulatory system facilitating the passage of nutrients and oxygen into and waste products out of the organism
- thermostasis: the maintenance of a constant internal temperature.

Homeostasis is regulated by the nervous system, the endocrine system and behavioural factors that are dependent on conscious or subconscious action by the organism. A homeostatic control system requires monitoring a variable, detecting changes and generating responses which will restore the composition of the internal environment (Fig. 1.9). (This type of system, involving a process called negative feedback, is dealt with in more detail under Hormonal regulation in Chapter 3, p. 64.)

Thermoregulation

Temperature regulation is one example of homeostasis (Fig. 1.10). Enzymes regulating biochemical changes, and physiological and metabolic functions, have optimal activity within a narrow temperature range. Outside this physiological temperature range, the protein structure of the enzyme begins to denature, so the configuration (shape) of the enzyme distorts, which affects its functional activity. A warm-blooded (homeothermic) animal is well prepared to react quickly and efficiently to changes within the environment, unlike a cold-blooded (poikilothermic) animal, which depends upon the ambient temperature of the environment.

The nervous system

The nervous system coordinates body functions. It monitors physiological processes by processing input from the senses, integrating them and initiating responses or

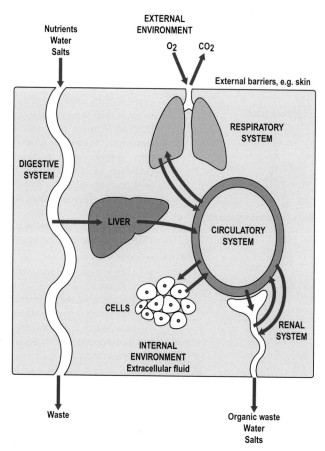

Fig. 1.8 Organization of the body.

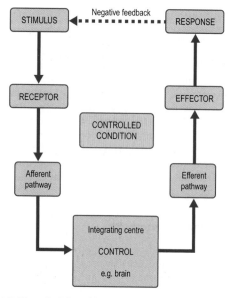

Fig. 1.9 The principles of homeostasis.

motor output. The nervous system is an organization of millions of neurons, or nerve cells, and glial cells, which support and regulate the composition of the nervous system. It is composed of the brain, the spinal cord (in the centre of the vertebral column) and the neurons throughout the body. The skull and the vertebral column protect the brain and the spinal cord. The brain and spinal cord form the central nervous system (CNS) and the remainder is the peripheral nervous system (Fig. 1.11). Neurons usually consist of a cell body and dendrites (extensions) and an axon or nerve fibre, which carries information from the cell body to or from the CNS. They are of different sizes; some neurons have axon projections over 1 m in length. A nerve is a collection of axons running alongside each other over the same distance. A ganglion is a collection of cell bodies of neurons within the peripheral nervous system. Ganglions are located in dorsal (back) or ventral (front) branches of the spinal cord. The spinal cord and spinal nerves are organized on a segmental basis; this corresponds to the embryonic origin of the dermatomes (see Chapter 9). Cranial nerves carry information between the brain and

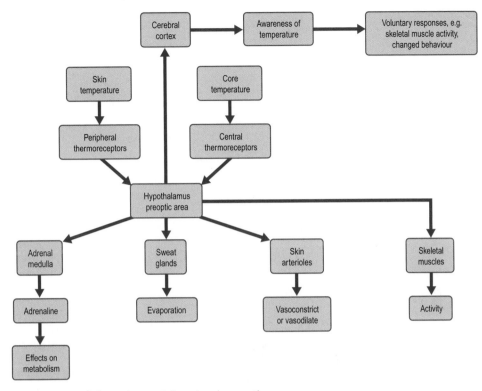

Fig. 1.10 Temperature regulation: a homeostatic system in operation.

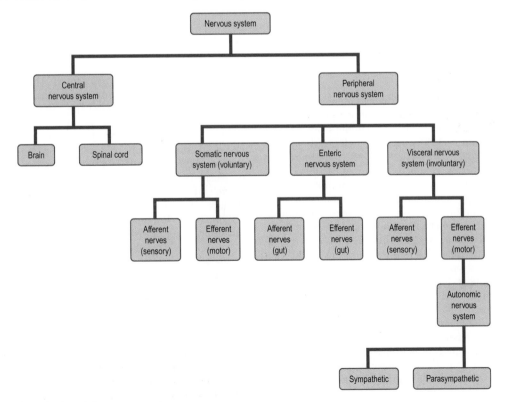

Fig. 1.11 Organization of the nervous system.

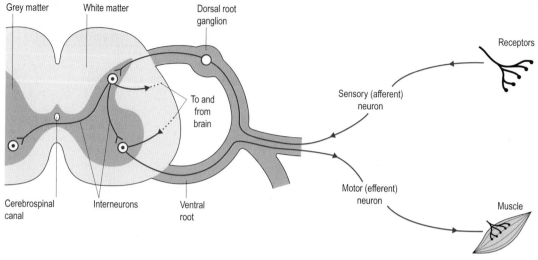

Fig. 1.12 Afferent and efferent neurons.

regions of the head. Neurons that carry information towards the brain, entering the dorsal roots of the spinal cord, are sensory or afferent neurons. Neurons carrying information from the CNS to the skeletal muscles, and leaving the spinal cord at the ventral roots, are motor or efferent neurons (Fig. 1.12). Neurons that carry information between a sensory neuron and the CNS (or between the CNS and a motor neuron) are known as interneurons.

The action potential

Neurons carry information or nerve impulses by changing the electrical charge along their axon length so the transmembrane polarity changes rapidly from negative to positive and back. This change in electrical charge is termed an 'action potential'. When the impulse reaches the axon, specific channels known as 'sodium gates' open, allowing the movement of extracellular sodium ions across the concentration gradient into the axon. As the sodium ions carry a positive charge, the immediate local area around the sodium gate inside of the axon becomes electrically positive compared with the immediate area outside and so the membrane becomes temporarily depolarized. At the height of the action potential (about 1 ms) the sodium channels close and the membrane becomes leaky to potassium ions; these move out of the axon down the electrochemical gradient. The result is restoration of the membrane potential, described as 'repolarization'. That segment of the axon then enters a refractory period when no further action potential can be produced. However, depolarization in one small segment of the neuron leads to depolarization

in the next segment; the rapid movement of the altered electrical activity is therefore propagated along the length of the neuron.

The action potential moves along the axon. The information detected at the periphery triggers activity at the neuron receptor and the action potential travels along the axon to the synapse, a junction with another neuron. There is a gap between two neurons at the synapse. Information transmission across this gap is by chemicals called neurotransmitters. These are released from the first neuron, travel across the synapse and trigger an action potential in the second neuron. The connection between a stimulating neuron and a muscle is called a neuromuscular junction. Action potentials move faster in axons of greater diameter, and if the axon is insulated by a myelin sheath. Myelin sheaths surround the nerve for short lengths punctuated by the nodes of Ranvier. Action potentials in myelinated nerves are not propagated as waves but move by saltatory conduction whereby they 'hop' along the nerve in a fast and efficient manner. Multiple sclerosis is due to breakdown of the myelin sheath, limiting the normal conduction of action potentials along nerves.

The somatic and autonomic nervous systems

The somatic nervous system controls muscles that change position. These muscles are called skeletal or voluntary muscles as they are controlled voluntarily, whereas smooth muscle and cardiac muscle are controlled involuntarily by the autonomic nervous system (ANS). The ANS controls the internal functions of the body such as circulation, respiration, digestion and metabolism.

Table 1.3 The autonomic nervous system

	SYMPATHETIC DIVISION	PARASYMPATHETIC DIVISION
Characteristics	Preganglionic outflow originates in thoracolumbar portion of spinal cord Chain of ganglia Postganglionic fibres distributed throughout body Divergence of pathways, so system as a whole is usually stimulated. 'Fear, fight and flight'	Preganglionic outflow originates in midbrain, hindbrain and sacral portions of spinal cord Terminal ganglia near or in effector organs Postganglionic fibres mainly associated with head and viscera Little divergence, so limited parts of the system are stimulated 'Resting and digesting'
Examples of effect	Eye: dilation of pupil Cardiovascular system: increased heart rate and increased strength of myocardial contraction, vasoconstriction of peripheral vessels and increased blood pressure Lungs: dilation of bronchioles Bladder: increased muscle tone Uterus: contraction in pregnant woman; relaxation in non-pregnant woman Penis: ejaculation	Eye: constriction of pupil Cardiovascular system: decreased heart rate and vasodilation of peripheral vessels and decreased blood pressure Lungs: constriction of bronchioles Bladder: increased contraction Penis: vasodilation and erection

Traditionally, the ANS has been divided into the sympathetic and parasympathetic systems (Table 1.3); these two branches of the ANS are described as working in tandem, either synergistically or antagonistically. The sympathetic nervous system controls the responses and provision of energy required for stressful situations; it is often known as the fear–fight–flight system. Effects of the sympathetic system include increased heart rate and blood pressure, pupillary and bronchial dilation, increased skeletal muscle blood flow (at the expense of blood flow to other tissues), increased glycogenolysis and lipolysis to increase energy provision and other responses that facilitate fight or escape and heightened awareness to threatening situations. The sympathetic system operates in conjunction with the endocrine system, facilitating the release of adrenaline, which augments the manifesting fear–fight–flight reflexes. Conversely, the parasympathetic branch of the ANS is more influential in periods of rest and inactivity and favours rest, increased digestive activity and restoration. Effects of parasympathetic nervous activity include increased blood flow to the gut and skin, stimulated salivary gland secretion and peristalsis, and slowing of the heart rate. In the ANS, two neurons carry information from the CNS to the target organ; these are described as autonomic ganglia. There is a further division of the ANS called the enteric nervous system, which affects smooth muscle and secretion in the gut.

The brain

The brain is the centre of the nervous system; it is the most complex organ and is not fully understood. The vertebrate brain develops from three anterior bulges of the neural tube (see Chapter 9), which are the brain stem, the cerebellum and the cerebrum. The brain stem is formed of the medulla oblongata (which controls autonomic functions), the pons (which relays information to and from the higher centres of the brain) and the midbrain (which integrates sensory information). The brain stem is an evolutionarily older structure which regulates essential automatic and integrative functions; it is often called the 'lower brain' and is particularly important in maintaining homeostasis, coordinating movement. The cerebellum coordinates and error-checks motor activities and perceptual and cognitive factors.

The most highly evolved structure of the brain is the cerebrum. The outer layer of the brain is the grey matter of the cerebral cortex, which is divided into the left and right hemisphere (Fig. 1.13). The fibres that connect these hemispheres are the corpus callosum, the largest white matter structure. Different regions of the cortex are associated with different functions; they can be illustrated in a figure known as the 'sensory homunculus' (Fig. 1.14). The reticular formation acts as a sensory filter and is concerned with states of waking and alertness. The hypothalamus is involved in motivation and regulation and integration of many metabolic and autonomic processes. The hypothalamus controls body temperature, hunger and thirst, and circadian cycles and links the nervous and endocrine systems. The cerebellum is mainly concerned with coordination of movement and repetitive performance of previously learned tasks.

The digestive system

As animals grew larger, they could not rely upon obtaining nutrients through diffusion and random contact with the environment; they became hunters and grazers.

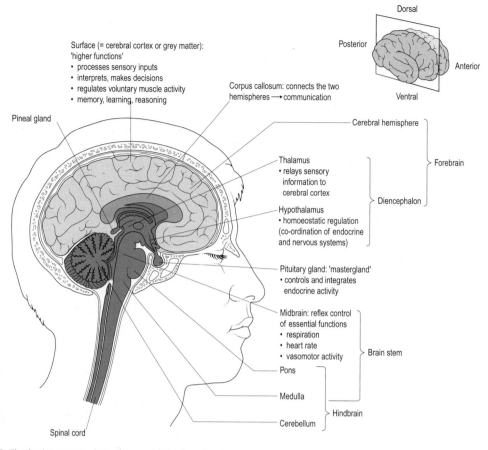

Dorsal

Posterior

Anterior

Ventral

Surface (= cerebral cortex or grey matter): 'higher functions'
• processes sensory inputs
• interprets, makes decisions
• regulates voluntary muscle activity
• memory, learning, reasoning

Corpus callosum: connects the two hemispheres ⟶ communication

Pineal gland

Cerebral hemisphere

Thalamus
• relays sensory information to cerebral cortex

Forebrain

Diencephalon

Hypothalamus
• homoeostatic regulation (co-ordination of endocrine and nervous systems)

Pituitary gland: 'mastergland'
• controls and integrates endocrine activity

Midbrain: reflex control of essential functions
• respiration
• heart rate
• vasomotor activity

Brain stem

Pons

Medulla

Hindbrain

Spinal cord

Cerebellum

Fig. 1.13 The brain: an overview of some of the functional areas.

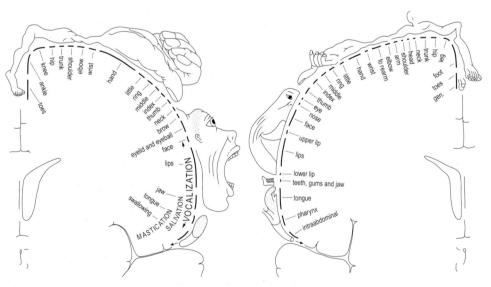

Fig. 1.14 The 'homunculus': a representation of the (A) motor and (B) sensory areas of the brain illustrating the proportion of brain tissue dedicated to these areas. (Reproduced with permission from Brooker, 1998.)

12

As they evolved, they became able to feed intermittently. They could do this because they had developed the ability to digest (break down) large organic macromolecules into smaller molecules through the action of digestive enzymes. They were able to store and digest food slowly. Mechanisms for food storage, such as the deposition of fat within adipose tissue, enabled periods of food shortage to be overcome. The ability to synthesize new tissue with energy expenditure is termed anabolism. When tissue is broken down there is a reverse process termed catabolism; this usually results in the production of energy and waste products, which require excretion.

The gastrointestinal tract, or gut, is a long tube that runs from mouth to anus (Table 1.4) in which food is digested and absorbed, to extract energy and nutrients; the remaining waste is expelled. Food enters the mouth; here it is masticated (mechanically broken down, thus increasing its surface area) and lubricated and enzymes are added before it is passed through the oesophagus to the stomach. The stomach is a bag-like swollen structure where the first major digestive processes occur. Hydrochloric acid secreted into the stomach maintains a pH of about 2; this has an important role in destroying microorganisms. There is some protein breakdown in the stomach and the food is mixed well. The mixed food, or chyme, then moves into the duodenum where most of the digestion and absorption take place. Digestive enzymes and bicarbonate ions (which neutralize the acidic pH) are produced from the pancreatic exocrine tissue and secreted into the duodenum. Bile salt secretion is important for the digestion of fats. The small intestine is a major site of absorption and has a very large surface area provided by finger-like projections called villi (Fig. 1.15). Tiny projections or microvilli on the surface of the individual epithelial cells further increase the surface area. The net result is a surface area of about 300 m^2. The epithelial cells lining

Table 1.4 The digestive system	
REGION OF GASTROINTESTINAL SYSTEM	**MAIN DIGESTIVE EVENTS**
Mouth	• Taste • Mechanical digestion (chewing, mastication) • Food moistened and lubricated, to facilitate passage down oesophagus • Starch digestion (amylase)
Oesophagus	• Peristalsis enables transfer of food bolus to stomach • Buccal amylase activity continues

Stomach	• Stores, mixes, dissolves, releases food
	• Hydrochloric acid (HCl)
	  – lowers pH to 2
	  – kills microbes
	  – denatures proteins
	  – converts pepsinogen to pepsin
	• Mucus: protects gastric lining
	• Pepsin: protein digestion

Pancreas	• Enzyme production: digestion • Bicarbonate: neutralizes pH
Liver	• Bile production
Gall bladder	• Bile concentration and coordinated release facilitating emulsification of fats
Small intestine	• Digestion and absorption of most nutrients
Large intestine	• Passage of undigested matter • Absorption of water and vitamins • Provides environment for commensal symbiotic bacteria
Rectum	• Storage of undigested matter • Defecation

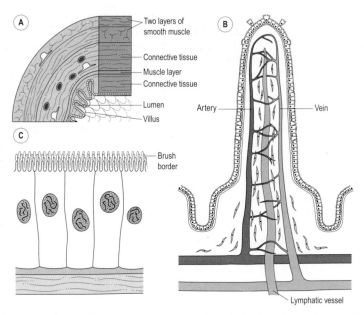

Fig. 1.15 Structure of the small intestinal villi: (A) transverse section through the intestinal wall; (B) a villus; (C) details of the epithelium. (Reproduced with permission from Saffrey and Stewart, 1997.)

the absorptive surfaces of the gastrointestinal system have membrane-bound enzymes, for further digestion of the food molecules, and specific transport mechanisms for absorbing different molecules into the bloodstream.

Cells of the mucosa that lines the gut have a very rapid turnover; the entire cell lining is renewed every 4 or 5 days. Therefore, agents that inhibit cell division such as radiation and chemotherapy drugs compromise the epithelium and total surface area. The absorbed nutrients pass from the capillaries of the small intestine into the hepatic portal vein and the liver. The wall of the gut is lined with smooth muscle, which undergoes synchronous contraction, generating waves of peristaltic movement propelling the food along the gut. The control of the smooth muscle is via the enteric nervous system.

The large intestine is important in the maintenance of fluid and iron balance and the absorption of vitamins. It is colonized and inhabited by bacteria, many of which synthesize vitamins, including vitamin B_{12}, vitamin K, thiamin and riboflavin, which can be absorbed across the gut wall. Motility of food through the gut is increased if there are more undigested non-starch polysaccharides (fibre) present. Some breakdown of these polysaccharides occurs by bacterial action, which can produce gas (flatus): nitrogen, carbon dioxide, hydrogen, methane and hydrogen sulphide.

Secretion and motility of the gut are controlled by nervous stimulation (Fig. 1.16). There are three phases

or stages of nervous control. The cephalic phase is stimulated by the smell, taste and sight of food, which increase motility and hydrochloric acid secretion. When food reaches the stomach it causes distension, increased acidity and increased peptide formation, which stimulate the gastric phase of control. The hormone gastrin is released, which stimulates secretion of acid and affects the lower regions of the gut. The third phase of control is the intestinal phase, which is stimulated by food within the intestine. The intestinal phase causes the reflex inhibition of gastric secretion.

The digestive system interacts with the immune system; effectively, the lining of the digestive system is an exterior surface of the body in contact with potentially pathogenic microorganisms. Most of the body's immune cells (about 70%) are located at the digestive system mucosal interface as individual cells and forming the gut-associated lymphoid tissue (GALT) which surveys and protects the digestive system. In addition, the digestive system provides the habitat for trillions of microorganisms (10^{13}–10^{14} microbes, about 10–100 times the total number of human cells, with a biomass of at least 1 kg). Most of these microorganisms reside in the colon and provide a repository of functional genes that make a significant contribution to host processes such as protecting against pathogens, interacting with the immune system, promoting gut development and synthesizing essential nutrients such as vitamins.

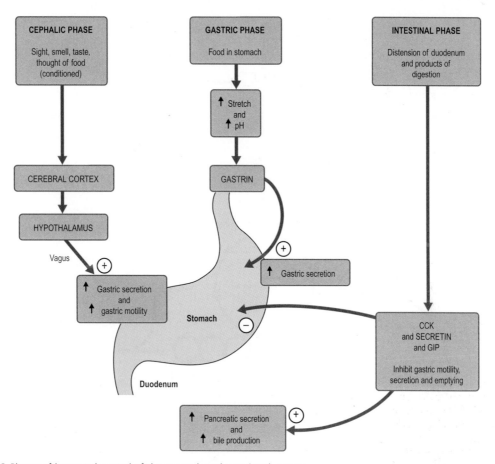

Fig. 1.16 Phases of hormonal control of the stomach and associated organs.

The respiratory system

Respiration is the exchange of gases between the environment and the body. Respiration is essential for the functioning of all living organisms. There are two types: aerobic and anaerobic. In aerobic respiration, organic molecules from ingested food are oxidized to produce energy (Fig. 1.17). Anaerobic respiration is when energy is produced in the absence of oxygen. This form of respiration is relatively inefficient compared with aerobic respiration.

Anaerobic respiration is common among single-celled organisms. Large animals, such as humans, can produce some energy anaerobically, for instance in times of acute stress and rapid muscle activity when oxygen demand exceeds oxygen provision. However, anaerobic respiration results in the rapid accumulation of toxic metabolites. In simple organisms, these may simply diffuse out of the cell into the environment, but for large animals this rapid excretion cannot be achieved and so anaerobic processes are self-limiting. Asphyxia is the term that describes irreversible damage to cells due to the build-up of these toxins (see Box 15.1 for a description of 'Fetal asphyxia').

Aerobic respiration is an extension of anaerobic respiration. The metabolites, produced under anaerobic processes such as glycolysis, are further broken down producing carbon dioxide, water and significantly more energy. Aerobic respiration requires the presence of oxygen and mitochondria, the sites of the enzymes involved in these biochemical pathways. Cells require a continuous source of oxygen for metabolism.

The respiratory system consists of the lungs, the branching airways, the gaseous exchange membranes, the rib cage and respiratory muscles. Ventilation is the mechanical activity that moves gases in and out of the lungs; the movements of the intercostal muscles and diaphragm allow filling and emptying of the lungs (Fig. 1.18). An adult at rest will inspire about 250 mL of oxygen and expire about 200 mL of carbon dioxide every minute. The respiratory tract provides a very large surface area that, while optimizing gas exchange, is vulnerable as it is constantly exposed to microorganisms. An important function of the respiratory system is to defend itself and prevent pathogens gaining access to the body.

15

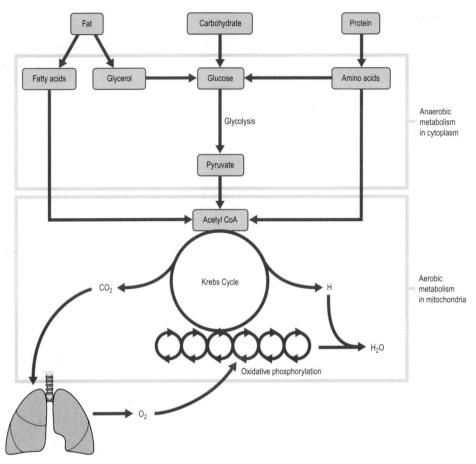

Fig. 1.17 A summary of metabolism: substrate molecules (such as glucose from food) are oxidized (using respiratory oxygen), producing carbon dioxide (expired) and energy in the form of ATP.

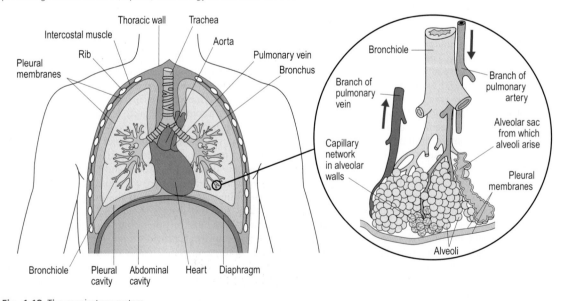

Fig. 1.18 The respiratory system.

Gas exchange occurs across the capillary membranes of the alveoli, which are very thin and therefore have a very low diffusion distance. Oxygen from the inspired air diffuses into the capillaries where it binds temporarily to haemoglobin in the red blood cells. The binding of oxygen and haemoglobin can be described by the oxygen–haemoglobin dissociation curve (Fig. 1.19). Haemoglobin has a high affinity for oxygen at higher concentrations and its binding sites are saturated with oxygen in the alveoli. At low concentrations of oxygen, haemoglobin has a low affinity for oxygen so it releases oxygen at the tissues. Binding of oxygen to haemoglobin is altered by carbon dioxide, pH, temperature and the glycolytic intermediate 2,3-bisphosphoglycerate (also known as 2,3-diphosphoglycerate). These alter the shape of the haemoglobin molecule, which affects its oxygen-binding sites. Substances that reduce haemoglobin–oxygen affinity increase the release of oxygen (so the curve is shifted towards the right).

Carbon dioxide diffuses from the tissues into the capillaries. It is taken up by the red blood cells where it reacts with water to form carbonic acid. This reaction is catalyzed by the enzyme carbonic anhydrase in the red blood cell. Carbonic acid is unstable and dissociates to bicarbonate and hydrogen ions (Fig. 1.20); the bicarbonate diffuses out of the red blood cell into the plasma.

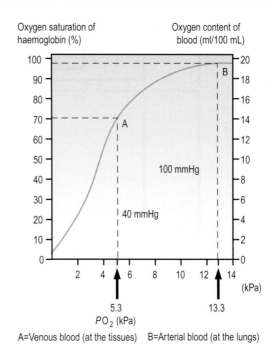

Fig. 1.19 The oxygen–haemoglobin dissociation curve. (Reproduced with permission from Brooker, 1998.)

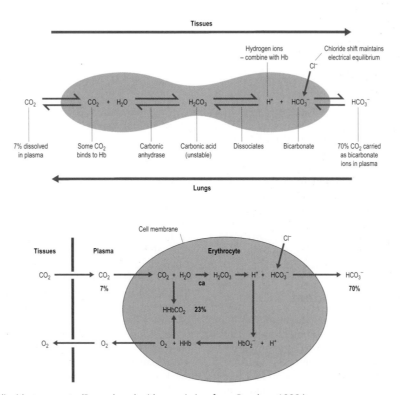

Fig. 1.20 Carbon dioxide transport. (Reproduced with permission from Brooker, 1998.)

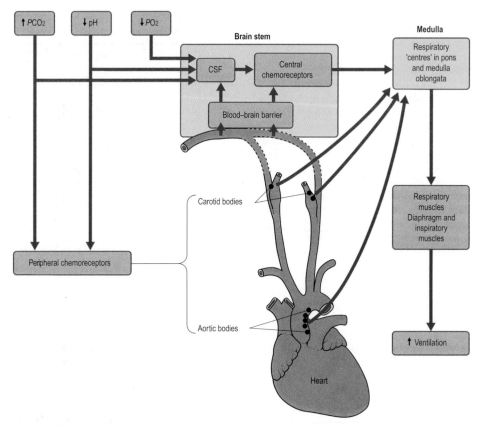

Fig. 1.21 Chemoreceptor control of respiration: the regulation of ventilation is achieved via peripheral and central chemoreceptors, which sample the blood, and then via a neuronal pathway influencing the rate and depth of breathing. CSF, cerebrospinal fluid.

The respiratory control centre, in the medulla oblongata of the brain stem, affects the activity of the inspiratory and expiratory neurons that control the respiratory muscles, which contract to allow inspiration and expiration. The respiratory centre receives information from stretch receptors in the lungs and from the peripheral and central chemoreceptors that monitor the pH and oxygen content of the blood (Fig. 1.21).

There is homeostatic regulation of acid–base balance to maintain pH within narrow parameters at around 7.3 (Fig. 1.22). This regulation involves both the respiratory and the renal systems (see Chapter 2).

The cardiovascular system

The cardiovascular system includes the heart, the blood vessels and the blood. The blood is pumped around a network of blood vessels (Fig. 1.23). Arteries transport blood away from the heart and have thick muscular walls. Veins carry blood towards the heart; they function as a capacitance system. Capillaries link the arterial and venous systems and allow exchange of substances between the blood and the tissues.

The heart functions as a double pump, pumping blood to the tissues of the body and the lungs (Fig. 1.24). Blood from the right side of the heart enters the pulmonary circulation to the capillaries surrounding the alveoli of the lungs where the blood is oxygenated. Oxygenated blood returns to the left side of the heart in the pulmonary veins. The oxygenated blood is then pumped from the left side of the heart around the body. The pulmonary circulation takes blood from the right side of the heart, to the lungs, and back to the left side of the heart. The systemic circulation is the circulation of blood around the body from the left side of the heart to the tissues and back to the right side of the heart. There are two circulatory routes which do not fit the general pattern of double circulation. The portal blood blow from the hypothalamus to the anterior pituitary gland (see Chapter 3) is one of these. The other is associated with the gut. The deoxygenated blood from the digestive system drains into the portal vein which goes to the liver, allowing the liver to take up absorbed

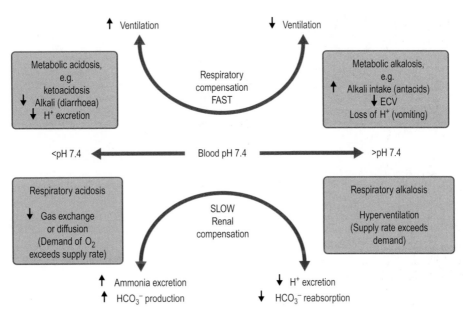

Fig. 1.22 Acid–base balance.

nutrients (and neutralize any absorbed toxins). From the liver, blood drains to the hepatic portal veins into the inferior vena cava and from there to the heart.

The coronary circulation is the circulation of blood within the vessels of the heart. Blood flow to the brain is via a circular arrangement of vessels (the circle of Willis); this ensures that there will always be sufficient oxygen and nutrients, albeit at the expense of other parts of the body when the circulatory system is under stress. The blood–brain barrier protects the brain against the entry of some harmful substances, such as toxins.

The adult heart beats about 70 times a minute at rest, forcing blood from the ventricles into the pulmonary artery and the aorta. The increased volume of blood entering the blood system causes a fluctuating increase in blood pressure. Blood pressure can be measured using a sphygmomanometer to record pressure within an artery and a stethoscope to hear the turbulence of blood within the blood vessels (Fig. 1.25). The amount of blood that leaves the heart per minute is described as the cardiac output. This is the volume of blood ejected from the ventricles each time the heart beats multiplied by the number of beats per minute (Fig. 1.26). The amount of oxygen that reaches the cells of the tissue depends on the proportion of the cardiac output the tissue receives.

The heart's internal pacemaker, the sinoatrial node (SAN), sets the heart rate. The SAN spontaneously depolarizes and triggers a wave of electrical activity, which stimulates the heart muscle to contract (Fig. 1.27). The SAN is innervated by both parasympathetic and sympathetic nerves. Receptors throughout the body respond to changes in blood pressure and respiratory gas level. These baroreceptors and chemoreceptors transmit information to afferent nerves in the medulla of the brain (the brain stem) that control efferent nerves to the heart, lungs and blood vessels (Fig. 1.28).

The total capacity of blood vessels in the body exceeds the volume of the blood. To maintain homeostasis and tissue requirements, the cardiovascular system is carefully regulated to ensure optimal oxygenation of the tissues. The control of blood flow is regulated by alteration of the diameter of the blood vessels, which changes peripheral resistance. The diameter of the blood vessels is altered by the activity of sympathetic nerves that innervate the smooth muscle in the vessel walls. Increased sympathetic activity, or increased adrenergic stimulation, increases vasoconstriction, reducing blood flow and increasing peripheral resistance. Decreased sympathetic activity causes vasodilation, which increases blood flow and reduces peripheral resistance. Blood vessel diameter is also controlled locally by tissue metabolites. This autoregulation increases blood flow to metabolically active tissues.

Blood

Blood is a suspension of cells in plasma (see Table 1.2). Blood cells are all derived from stem cells in the bone marrow. The majority (>99%) of cells are red blood cells (or erythrocytes). Red blood cells contain haemoglobin, which binds to oxygen. Iron, folic acid and vitamin B_{12} are required for the production of erythrocytes.

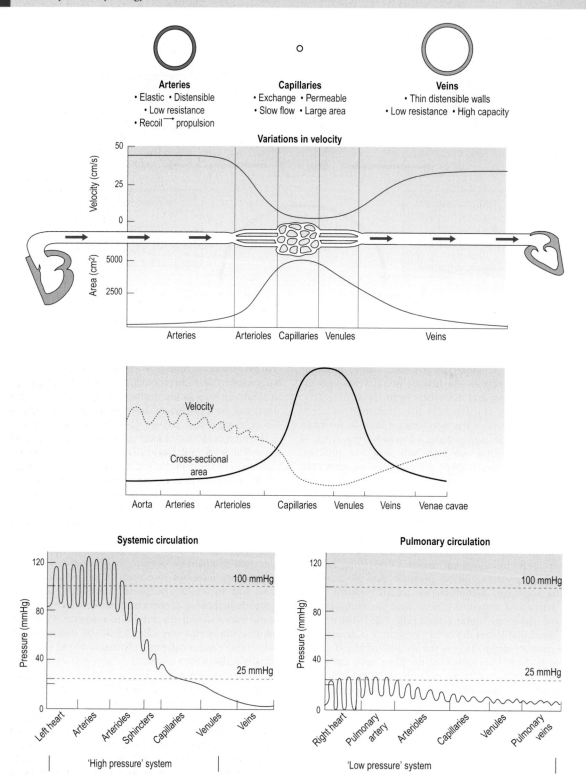

Arteries
- Elastic • Distensible
- Low resistance
- Recoil → propulsion

Capillaries
- Exchange • Permeable
- Slow flow • Large area

Veins
- Thin distensible walls
- Low resistance • High capacity

Variations in velocity

Velocity (cm/s)

Area (cm²)

Arteries   Arterioles Capillaries Venules   Veins

Velocity

Cross-sectional area

Aorta   Arteries   Arterioles   Capillaries   Venules   Veins   Venae cavae

Systemic circulation

Pressure (mmHg)

100 mmHg

25 mmHg

Left heart   Arteries   Arterioles   Sphincters   Capillaries   Venules   Veins

'High pressure' system

Pulmonary circulation

Pressure (mmHg)

100 mmHg

25 mmHg

Right heart   Pulmonary artery   Arterioles   Capillaries   Venules   Pulmonary veins

'Low pressure' system

Fig. 1.23 Blood vessels: the major role of arteries is in the generation of elastic recoil, which propels the blood around the body. The capillaries are involved in gas exchange and the veins act as capacitance vessels returning blood to the heart.

Fig. 1.24 Interior of the heart to show layers, chambers and valves. (Reproduced with permission from Brooker, 1998.)

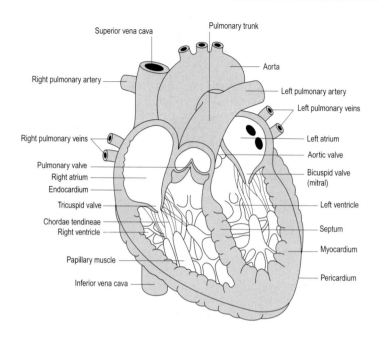

Fig. 1.25 Blood pressure measurement. (Reproduced with permission from Brooker, 1998.)

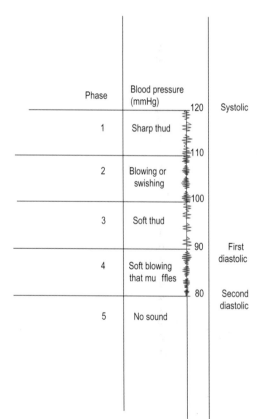

Phase	Blood pressure (mmHg)	
		120 Systolic
1	Sharp thud	
		110
2	Blowing or swishing	
		100
3	Soft thud	
		90 First diastolic
4	Soft blowing that mu ffles	
		80 Second diastolic
5	No sound	

The kidneys produce a hormone, erythropoietin, in response to low oxygen levels, which stimulates an increase in the production of red blood cells from the bone marrow. Leukocytes, or white blood cells, include polymorphonuclear granulocytes (neutrophils, eosinophils and basophils) and the agranular monocytes and lymphocytes. The role of white blood cells is the defence of the body (see Chapter 10). Platelets are cellular fragments of megakaryocytes, which are an essential component of the blood-clotting mechanism (Fig. 1.29). Plasma contains proteins (albumin, globulins and some clotting factors, such as fibrinogen), nutrients, hormones, waste products and ions.

The lymphatic system

The lymphatic system is part of the circulatory system and consists of a network of thin branching vessels, lymph nodes and lymphatic fluid (Fig. 1.30). It collects the interstitial fluid from cells and returns it to the blood. Lymph vessels have one-way valves like veins and depend on the movement of skeletal muscle to propel the fluid which moves slowly under low pressure. The lymphatic system transports lymphocytes and is important in defending the body against microorganisms (see Chapter 10). Lymph nodes in the lymphatic system are lymphocyte-filled and act as collecting filters for viruses and bacteria which are then destroyed. Lymphatic vessels are present in the lining of the digestive tract and transport digested lipids to the thoracic duct and into the venous circulation.

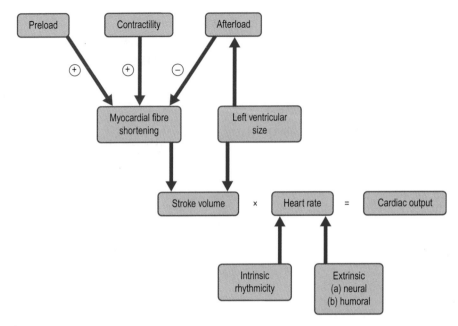

Fig. 1.26 Cardiac output.

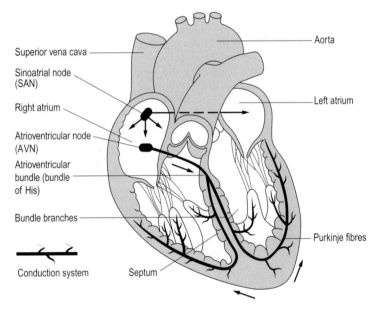

Fig. 1.27 Sinoatrial node (SAN) depolarization: the conduction pathway of the heart enables the organ's coordinated and rhythmic beating.

METABOLISM

Energy production and storage

Cells have a continuous requirement for energy and adenosine triphosphate (ATP). The energy from ATP drives virtually all the body processes but there is very little ATP present at any one time, just enough to provide energy requirements for only a few minutes. Every organ requires energy but some, such as muscles, have a very variable energy requirement. Meals provide fuel from food components, which are oxidized to provide ATP and heat. However, the intake of food is irregular and does not coordinate with the requirement for energy. The energy substrates from a meal are usually absorbed within 3 h;

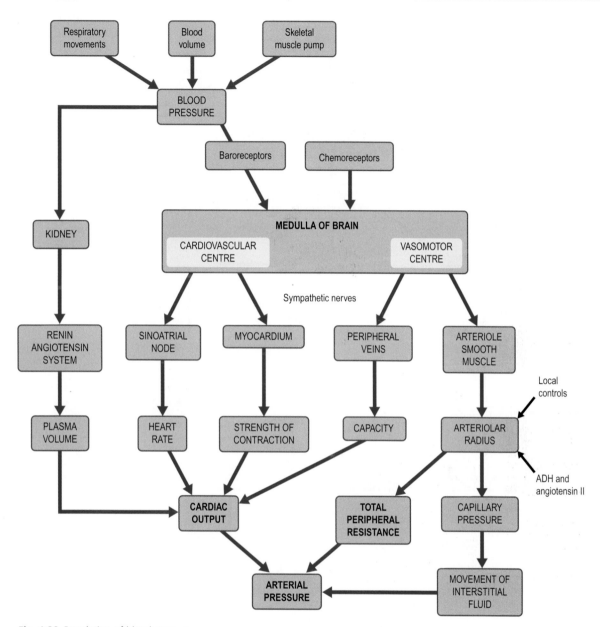

Fig. 1.28 Regulation of blood pressure.

as the next meal can be hours away, animals have evolved successful methods of storing energy substrates.

The main storage forms of energy are glycogen in the liver and skeletal muscle and triacylglycerides in adipose tissue. Carbohydrates are the major fuels for the brain and nervous tissue. Oxidation of glucose occurs in several stages (Fig. 1.31). Glycolysis takes place in the cell cytosol and produces a little ATP anaerobically. If oxygen is present, there is further oxidation through the Krebs cycle and oxidative phosphorylation (the electron transfer chain). This increased efficiency of ATP production takes place in cells that have mitochondria and adequate provision of oxygen. In tissues lacking mitochondria, such as red blood cells, or those with insufficient oxygen, such as active muscle, there is a build-up of the key intermediate pyruvate. Pyruvate can be converted into lactate and oxidized by the heart and kidneys or converted to glucose by the liver and kidneys.

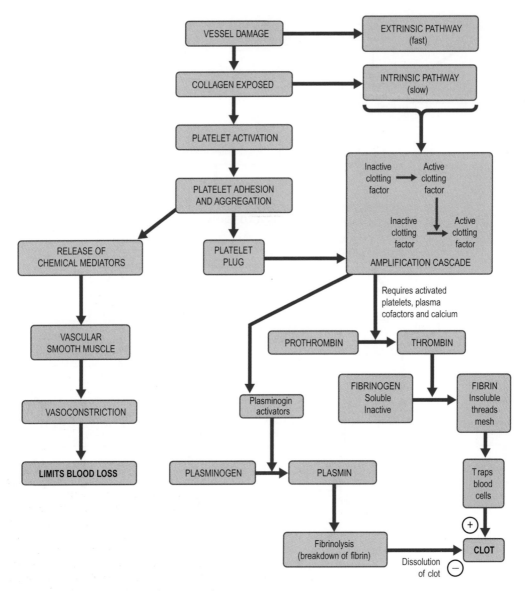

Fig. 1.29 Haemostasis: the blood coagulation cascade.

About 500 g of the glucose polymer, glycogen, is stored: 100 g in the liver, which can release the glucose when required (by glycogenolysis), and 400 g in the skeletal muscles, which is available for use by the muscle. Triacylglycerides are stored in virtually unlimited amounts, as observed in obesity. As they do not mix with water, the storage form is very calorie dense and efficient. Triacylglycerides are composed of three fatty acids bound to a glycerol backbone. The glycerol can be converted into glucose, thereby providing a substrate for the brain to oxidize for energy. Fatty acids are released with free glycerol from the adipose tissue and can be oxidized by the liver, muscles and kidneys. Fatty acids cannot cross the blood–brain barrier and cannot be converted to glucose so they provide little substrate for the brain. Ketone bodies are water-soluble derivatives of fatty acids formed by the liver during starvation or prolonged severe exercise. When sufficient concentrations of ketone bodies accumulate, the brain and kidney use them to generate ATP. Certain amino acids are also ketogenic, and can be converted into ketone bodies. Overproduction of ketone bodies, as in uncontrolled diabetes, overwhelms the buffering capacity of the body and can cause life-threatening acidosis.

There is no reserve storage form of protein independent of function. Protein can be metabolized to provide energy but at the expense of the breakdown of structural and functional

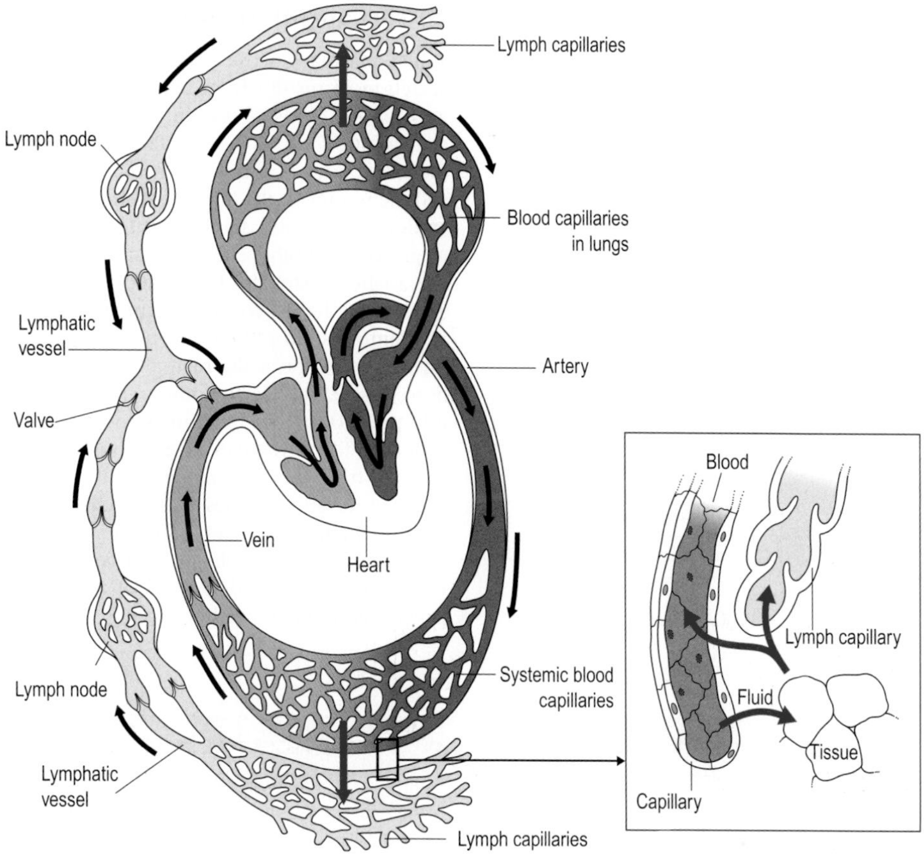

Fig. 1.30 The lymphatic system.

components of the body. The use of protein as a fuel potentially damages the body, so it is used only as a 'last resort' when the protein is broken down and the amino acids are converted into components of the glycolytic pathway to produce energy. However, proteins constitute a large proportion of body structure and therefore can provide a substantial source of energy when other supplies have been exhausted. Protein in excess of requirements can be irreversibly converted into glucose or triacylglycerides.

The brain consumes about a quarter of the body's daily energy production when the body is at rest. The brain's requirement for fuel drives energy metabolism. The main fuel storage form of the body is triacylglycerides, but the brain cannot use fatty acids directly. Although the brain can oxidize ketone bodies, derived from fatty acids, for 80% of its energy requirements, 20% must come from glucose. Glucose comes from the diet or from glycogenolysis or gluconeogenesis in the liver. Other cells therefore utilize other substrates in preference to glucose. The hierarchy of fuel use means that the brain utilizes ketone bodies when they are available, or glucose. Muscle has a major reserve of protein and glycogen. Muscle spares brain fuel by preferentially oxidizing fatty acids, thus sparing ketone bodies

and glucose for the brain. The glycogen stored in the muscle is specifically available for muscle use.

The external environment is continually fluctuating and energy requirements are constantly changing. However, the body maintains homeostasis or internal stability by ensuring a constant level of amino acids and glucose in the blood, despite intermittent high loads following a meal. The level of ATP within cells is kept relatively constant although the rate of usage is variable; for instance, activity increases energy requirement of a muscle by up to 20 times. Cellular energy requirement is regulated very sensitively; metabolic pathways that predominate after a meal (called the absorptive state) are different from those between meals (the postabsorptive state) (Fig. 1.32). Dominance of the pathways is via changed enzyme activity and altered uptake of substrates, controlled by hormones. Interconversion from one metabolic step to the next is regulated by substrate activation, where the substance stimulates its own use, and product inhibition, where the product prevents the reaction from continuing. Enzymes catalysing the same reaction may exist as isoenzymes in different types of tissue, having different affinities for their substrates. This means that different concentrations of substrate are required for the biochemical pathway to progress.

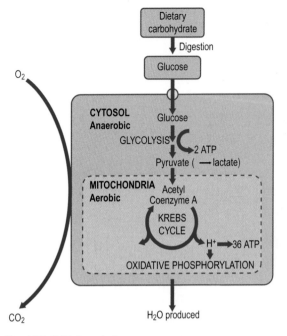

Fig. 1.31 Oxidation of glucose.

Blood sugar regulation

When plasma glucose concentration rises after a meal, secretion of insulin from pancreatic β-cells is stimulated and plasma levels of insulin increase. Insulin triggers the translocation of vesicles containing the insulin-sensitive glucose transporter, GLUT4, from intracellular sites to the cell membrane of the insulin-sensitive tissues, skeletal and cardiac muscle and adipocytes. This increases the uptake of glucose and other substrates into the cell and promotes the anabolic (storage) biochemical pathways (Fig. 1.33). Tissues that have a constant requirement for glucose, such as brain cells, do not have insulin-sensitive glucose transport but do express the high-affinity transporter, GLUT3, as well as GLUT1. Under conditions of low glucose, pancreatic production of glucagon is increased, which acts to mobilize tissue reserves of metabolic fuels. Adrenaline, secreted from the adrenal medulla in response to sympathetic innervation, causes a rapid mobilization of fuels for 'fight or flight' (see p. 11). Adrenaline stimulates glucose production from muscle glycogen and increases lipolysis in adipose tissue so that levels of fatty acids increase to provide additional metabolic fuel.

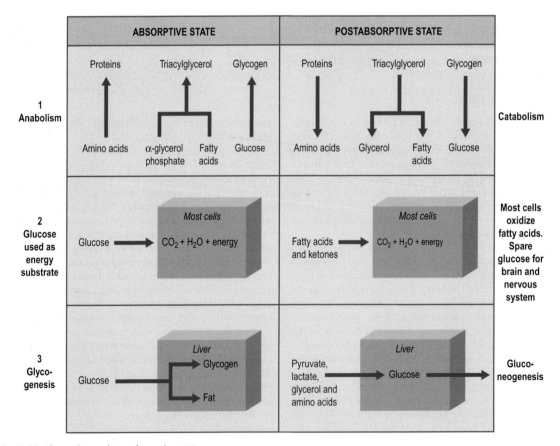

Fig. 1.32 Absorptive and postabsorptive states.

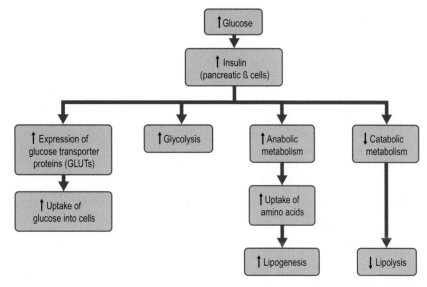

Fig. 1.33 The effects of insulin.

Physiological observations to assess maternal well-being

In order to assess well-being during pregnancy, practitioners must consider how physiological parameters are altered in pregnant women and when these altered parameters become abnormal in relation to pregnancy, but observations to assess well-being cannot be considered in isolation. It is important to monitor respiratory rate as well as blood pressure, pulse and temperature. A rising respiratory rate can be an early indicator of respiratory distress. Ideally respiratory rate should be counted without informing the woman so that she is not conscious of her breathing as being conscious of it is likely to affect the respiratory rate. Tachypnoea (rapid breathing) is a significant clinical feature which should not be dismissed as being caused by anxiety or stress, or related to pain. If tachypnoea is present with a rapid pulse and a fall in blood pressure, then the maternal condition might be deteriorating because of cardiovascular problems, such as haemorrhage or sepsis. It is common for oxygen saturation to be monitored to assess respiratory function; however, oxygen saturation is often maintained in the presence of tachypnoea (98% +) and a fall in oxygen saturation is therefore a late indicator of advanced maternal distress.

A raised temperature is a significant indicator of sepsis; however, if sepsis is severe, body temperature measured orally or in the axilla may be misleadingly low because of peripheral vascular shutdown caused by toxicity. Thus, an abnormally low temperature can also indicate sepsis. In such cases, core temperate should be measured, for example by use of a rectal probe. The greater the difference between core and peripheral temperature, the more likely it is that sepsis is severe.

If the pulse rate is higher (beats per minute) than the systolic blood pressure (measured in millimetres of mercury, mmHg) this also indicates serious deterioration in the well-being of the woman.

Blood pressure is lower and pulse rate is faster in pregnancy, so direct comparisons to non-pregnant values are not valid. Whenever possible, midwives should access pre-pregnancy observations, for example, from well women clinic records, family planning clinics, GP notes, etc., thus providing a reference point when assessing normal physiological changes in pregnancy. As computerized single patient records are developed, access to this information will be easier and faster. Women who do not have lower blood pressure in the first trimester than their pre-pregnant parameter are at greater risk of hypertensive problems in pregnancy and in later life or may have underlying renal problems.

Blood pressure must be measured using a cuff appropriate to the size of the woman's arm. If automated machines are being used to measure blood pressure, blood pressure should be measured manually at least once to confirm that the electronic measurement is valid.

Women should have direct access to midwives as soon as pregnancy is confirmed so that pregnancy care can be planned to meet their individual needs.

Key points

- Cells have different anatomical structures, which are related to their physiological functions.
- Cells are organized together to form tissues, which are organized into organs and the physiological systems of the body.
- The role of the physiological systems is to provide internal stability or homeostasis, which will ensure that the cells' variable but essential requirements for energy are met by an adequate supply of oxygen and nutrients.
- As the enzymes that regulate cellular activity have a protein structure, they are affected by fluctuations in pH and temperature, so homeostasis has to maintain optimum temperature and acid–base balance as well.

Application to practice

The basic physiology described in this chapter relates to the non-pregnant state. During pregnancy there are many physiological changes, which are explored through the rest of the book. A basic knowledge of physiology is essential so that the complexities of the physiological changes in pregnancy can be understood and explained as required. This knowledge is also essential for the midwife to be able to monitor the development of pregnancy effectively.

ANNOTATED FURTHER READING

Alberts B, Bray D, Lewis J, et al: *Molecular biology of the cell*, ed 5, New York, 2008, Garland.

A beautifully written and well-illustrated text on molecular and cellular biology which is accessible, easy to read and up to date; the cell biologist's 'bible'.

Berne RM, Levy NM: *Physiology*, ed 6, St Louis, 2008, Mosby.

A comprehensive illustrated textbook, which emphasizes physiological concepts and basic principles.

Koeppen BM, Stanton B: *Renal physiology*, ed 4, 2006, Mosby.

Provides a useful reference to the area of renal physiology.

Salway J: *Metabolism at a glance*, ed 3, Oxford, 2003, Blackwell.

A large-format book which provides a comprehensive review of basic human metabolism, including inborn errors of metabolism and clinical aspects of metabolism. Metabolic pathways are summarized as segments with a clear diagrammatic pathway map on one page and an outline of the metabolism on the facing page.

Salway J: *Medical biochemistry at a glance*, ed 2, Oxford, 2006, Wiley Blackwell.

A useful overview of human biochemistry which provides a synopsis using detailed flow-charts and explanatory diagrams.

Tortora GJ, Derrickson BH: *Principles of anatomy and physiology*, ed 13, New York, 2011, Harper Collins.

A clear, illustrated 2-volume textbook (with CD-ROM) providing an in-depth overview of physiology and anatomy. It is targeted at students in health professions and includes clinical applications and study outlines.

Ward JPT, Linden R: *Physiology at a glance*, ed 2, Oxford, 2008, Wiley Blackwell.

Another of the 'at-a-glance' series of books which provides clear illustrated and bullet-point summaries of the role of physiological systems.

Widmaier EP, Raff H, Strang KT: *Vander's Human physiology*, ed 12, New York, 2010, McGraw-Hill.

An updated version of the classical textbook which provides a useful guide to the principles of human physiology using clear diagrams and flow-charts; the new edition includes more clinical applications.

REFERENCES

Brooker CG: *Human structure and function*, ed 2, St Louis, 1998, Mosby, pp 15, 30, 32, 33, 88, 207, 211, 228, 277, 279, 296, 372, 383.

Saffrey J, Stewart M, editors: *Maintaining the whole. SK220 Human biology and health, book 3*, Milton Keynes, 1997, Open University Press, p 65.

Chapter | 2 |

The reproductive and urinary systems

LEARNING OBJECTIVES

- To describe the structure and function of the urinary system.
- To compare the structure of the female and male reproductive systems.
- To identify differences between the male and female reproductive tracts in relation to reproduction and adaptations to facilitate childbirth.

INTRODUCTION

This chapter reviews the basic anatomy of human reproductive and urinary systems. The human urinary system differs only slightly between the male and female, mostly in relation to the structure of the external genitalia. The function of the urinary system is also essentially the same in men and women. However, the renal system can be severely stressed by pregnancy, mostly because of its close proximity to the reproductive organs and the major changes in fluid balance resulting in fluid retention during pregnancy. The midwife needs to know the basics of normal renal physiology in order to understand the changes that take place in the renal system during pregnancy and how these may affect the general condition of the woman. For example, not only are the regulation and retention of fluid altered in pregnancy but also excretion of glucose and other substances is affected by these changes. Drug excretion via the kidneys may also be affected, so long-term medication may need to be changed as pregnancy progresses. The effectiveness of medication may be reduced and altered drug dosage may also be required. (Specific changes in the renal system in pregnancy are covered in Chapter 11.)

Chapter case study

Zara, during the booking appointment, is asked by the midwife to provide a mid stream specimen of urine to screen for infection. The midwife notes that the specimen appears cloudy although Zara does not have any other signs of a urinary tract infection.
- Are there any reasons apart from infection that could explain the cloudiness of the specimen?
- If the culture of the specimen proves positive, how will this be managed and what advice should the midwife give to Zara?
- If the analysis of the specimen showed a bacteraemia of group B haemolytic streptococcus what would be the significance of this, how should it be managed and what are the possible future consequences for Zara and her baby?

THE URINARY SYSTEM

The urinary system is composed of two kidneys, which produce urine, two ureters running from the kidneys to the bladder, which collects and stores the urine, and a urethra from which urine is discharged to the exterior (Fig. 2.1). The uroepithelium which lines the renal pelvis, ureters and bladder is not just a passive impermeable barrier; it can modulate the composition of urine and also transmit information about pressure and composition of the urine to the underlying nervous and muscular tissue (Khandelwal et al., 2009).

The kidneys

The kidneys have a broad range of other functions (see Box 2.1) as well as producing urine. The kidneys are

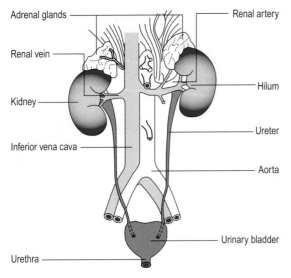

Fig. 2.1 The urinary system. (Reproduced with permission from Brooker, 1998.)

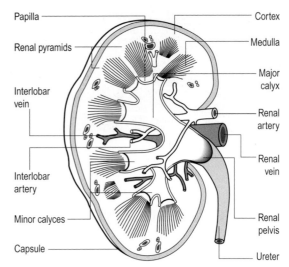

Fig. 2.2 The structure of the kidney (longitudinal section). (Reproduced with permission from Brooker, 1998.)

Box 2.1 **Functions of the kidney**

- Regulation of water balance
- Regulation of pH (acid-base balance) and inorganic ion balance (sodium, potassium and calcium)
- Excretion of metabolic and nitrogenous waste products (urea from protein, uric acid from nucleic acids, creatinine from muscle creatine and haemoglobin breakdown products)
- Hormone secretion (erythropoietin, renin, 1,25-dihydroxyvitamin D3 (1,25-dihydroxycholecalciferol, also called calcitriol) and prostaglandins)
- Removal of toxic chemicals (drugs, pesticides and food additives)
- Regulation of blood pressure (renin–angiotensin system)
- Control of formation of red blood cells (via erythropoietin)
- Vitamin D activation and calcium balance
- Gluconeogenesis (formation of glucose from amino acids and other precursors)

---

situated upon the posterior wall of the abdominal cavity, one on either side of the vertebral column at the level of the thoracic and lumbar vertebrae (just below the rib cage). The right kidney is slightly lower than the left owing to its relationship to the liver. Each kidney is about 10 cm long, 6.5 cm wide and about 3 cm thick (about the size of a clenched fist). Each kidney weighs about 100 grams (a small proportion of the total body mass), but they receive about 25% of the cardiac output (which per

unit of tissue is about eight times higher than the blood flow to muscles undergoing heavy exercise). The renal blood supply arises from the aorta via the renal arteries and returns to the inferior vena cava via the renal veins. Each kidney is enclosed by a thick fibrous capsule and has two distinct layers: the reddish-brown cortex, which has a rich blood supply, and the inner medulla, within which the structural and functional units of the kidney, the nephrons, are found (Fig. 2.2).

The nephron

Each kidney has approximately a million nephrons (though the number declines with increasing age), each of which is about 3 cm long. The nephron is a tubule that is closed at one end and opens into the collecting duct at the other. The nephron has six distinct regions, each of which is adapted to a specific function (Fig. 2.3). There are two types of nephron. Most nephrons (85–90%) are cortical nephrons; these have short loops of Henle and are mainly concerned with the control of plasma volume during normal conditions. The juxtamedullary nephrons, which have longer loops of Henle extending into the renal medulla, facilitate increased water retention (and thus the production of hyperosmotic or concentrated urine) when the availability of water is restricted.

The renal corpuscle comprises the Bowman's capsule, a blind-ended tube, and the glomerulus, a coiled arrangement of capillaries around which the Bowman's capsule is invaginated. The glomerulus provides a large area of capillary vessels from which substances can leave, crossing the specialized flattened epithelial cells to enter the

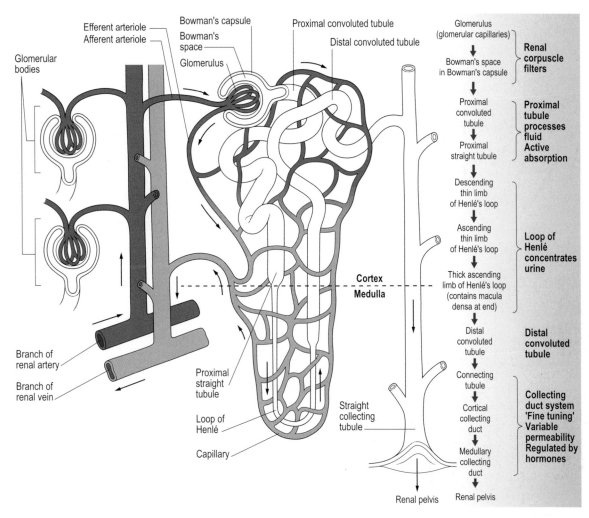

Fig. 2.3 The nephron and double capillary arrangement. The panel on the right shows the functions of the regions of the nephron.

capsule of the nephron. There is a double capillary arrangement (see Fig. 2.3) whereby afferent arterioles supply the glomerular capillaries and efferent arterioles lead from the glomerulus to a second capillary bed supplying the rest of the nephron. Differential vasoconstriction of the afferent and efferent arterioles maintains a constant blood pressure within the glomerulus, which results in a constant rate of filtration. Urine production relies on three steps: simple filtration, selective reabsorption and secretion (Fig. 2.4).

Filtration

Filtration is a non-selective passive process that occurs through the semipermeable walls of the glomerulus and glomerular capsule. All substances with a molecular mass of less than 68 kilodaltons (kDa) are forced out of the glomerular capillaries into the Bowman's capsule. Therefore, water and small molecules such as glucose, amino acids and vitamins enter the nephron whereas blood cells, plasma proteins and other large molecules are usually retained in the blood. The content of the Bowman's capsule is referred to as the 'glomerular filtrate' and the rate at which this is formed is referred to as the 'glomerular filtration rate' (GFR). The kidneys form about 180 L of dilute filtrate each day (a GFR of about 125 mL/min). Most of it is selectively reabsorbed so the final volume of urine produced is about 1–1.5 L/day.

Box 2.2 describes an example of disrupted renal function in pregnancy that is detected by abnormal urine composition.

Fig. 2.4 Urine production.

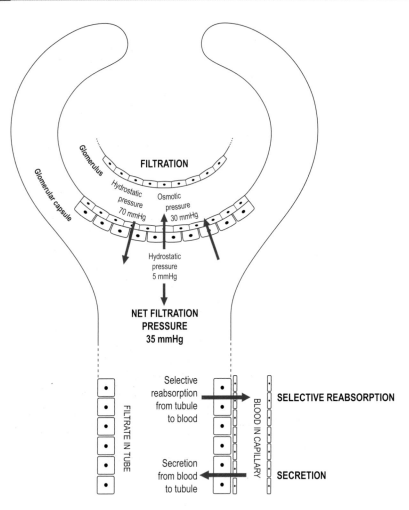

Box 2.2 **Hypertension in pregnancy**

Hypertensive disorders in pregnancy can disrupt renal function. The detectable presence of protein within the urine (proteinuria) may indicate that larger molecules than normal are being forced into the Bowman's capsule. This is caused by the increased blood pressure resulting in abnormal ultrafiltration. Women who have a degree of renal damage prior to pregnancy are less likely to be able to adapt to the pregnancy-induced physiological changes as effectively as women with normal renal function. These women tend to develop high blood pressure during early pregnancy and so do not normally demonstrate such a marked physiological reduction in blood pressure parameters, putting both the mother and fetus at risk.

Selective reabsorption

Substances from the glomerular filtrate are reabsorbed from the rest of the nephron into the surrounding capillaries. The proximal convoluted tubule (PCT in Fig. 2.6) is the widest and longest part of the whole nephron (approximately 1.4 cm long). The epithelial cells lining the nephron contain a large number of mitochondria to provide energy for facilitating active transport as most of the reabsorption of the glomerular filtrate takes place here. Some substances, such as glucose and amino acids, are completely reabsorbed and are not normally present in urine. Reabsorption of waste products is largely incomplete, so, for instance, a large proportion of urea is excreted. The reabsorption of other substances is under the regulation of several hormones. Antidiuretic hormone

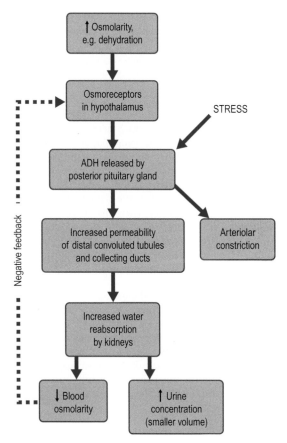

Fig. 2.5 The action of ADH.

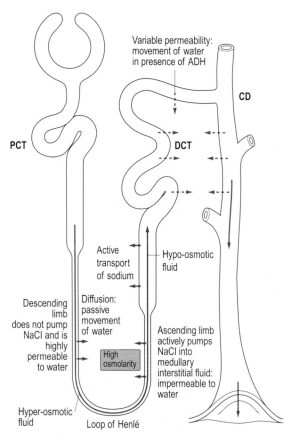

Fig. 2.6 Formation of concentrated urine.

(ADH) controls the insertion of aquaporins, pore-forming membrane proteins, into the walls of the distal convoluted tubule (DCT in Fig. 2.6) and collecting ducts (CD in Fig. 2.6), which allows water to leave the filtrate, thus producing less urine (Fig. 2.5). The formation of concentrated urine is facilitated by the physical arrangement of the loop of Henle and its surrounding capillaries, which create and maintain the conditions for the reabsorption of water by osmosis (Fig. 2.6, Box 2.3). Calcitonin increases calcium excretion and parathyroid hormone enhances reabsorption of calcium from renal tubules. Aldosterone affects the reabsorption of sodium (Fig. 2.7). Atrial natriuretic peptide (ANP) inhibits NaCl reabsorption in the DCT and cortical collecting duct of the nephron. ANP also increases the GFR by dilating the afferent glomerular arterioles and constricting the efferent glomerular arteriole, thus increasing NaCl excretion.

Secretion

Some waste products may be actively transported directly into the tubules from the surrounding blood capillaries. These include hydrogen and potassium ions, creatinine,

Box 2.3 **Hypertonic urine**

The evolution of the mammalian kidney has enabled mammals to become highly adapted to terrestrial living. The kidney aids water conservation by producing urine that is able to be concentrated far more than the internal body fluid environment. The scarcer water is within the environment, the longer the nephron to conserve water.

toxins and drugs. The cells of the renal tubules synthesize some substances, such as ammonia ions and peptides, which can be secreted into the filtrate.

The ureters

The ureters, which are tubes about 25–30 cm long and 3 mm in diameter, transport the urine from the kidneys to the bladder. From each kidney the collecting ducts open into the renal pelvis, which leads to the ureter. The walls of the renal pelvis have smooth muscle, which has

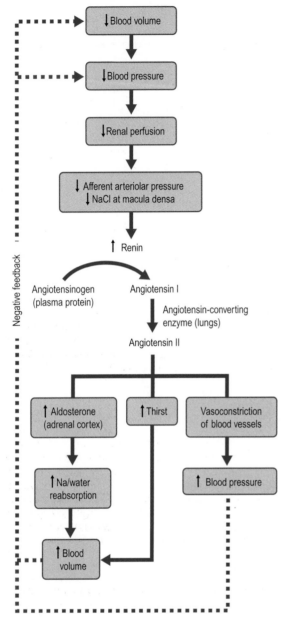

Fig. 2.7 Aldosterone regulation of sodium (Na) excretion.

area called the trigone which has its apex at the urethral opening. As urine accumulates in the bladder, the ureters are compressed, effectively forming a valve (the vesicoureteral valve), which prevents urinary reflux.

The bladder

The bladder is a distensible hollow organ, also composed of smooth muscle, which acts as a reservoir for urine. It is intermittently emptied under conscious control. Stretch receptors within the muscle and trigone provide the signals that indicate that the bladder is full. The normal capacity of the bladder is approximately 700–800 mL; however, the natural desire to void urine becomes conscious when the level of urine in the bladder reaches approximately 300 mL. Inflammation in the trigone region caused by infection and or trauma often results in a frequent and urgent desire to void urine but on voiding only small amounts of urine are passed.

As the bladder lies below the uterus, its capacity is compromised by the growing uterus in early pregnancy. Later on, once the pregnant uterus has become an abdominal organ, the pressure on the bladder is relieved. Finally, at the end of pregnancy, bladder capacity is again compromised as the presenting part of the fetus engages, occupying space within the true pelvic cavity and thus restricting the space available to the bladder.

The urethra

Urine is voided via the urethra. The female urethra is considerably shorter and straighter than the male urethra: only 4 cm in length compared with about 20 cm. This anatomical difference predisposes women towards an increased incidence of ascending urinary tract infections (UTIs). Thus, a colony count of more than 100 000 bacterial cells per millilitre of urine is considered to be pathologically significant and is often referred to as bacteraemia. There are small mucus-secreting glands in the urethra that help to protect the epithelium from the corrosive urine. The upper internal sphincter, at the exit from the bladder, is composed of smooth muscle and is under autonomic control. The external sphincter is composed of skeletal muscle and is under voluntary control. The urethra in the man has a dual role as the route for urine and the delivery of spermatozoa, via coitus. Structural differences related to the development of the external genitalia are covered in Chapter 5. Trauma to the pelvic floor during childbirth may result in neurological damage affecting the function of the internal sphincter resulting in urgency of micturition. Urgency to void is increased by the degree of weakness in the sphincter and the amount of urine held in the bladder. Treatment options range from a variety of surgical procedures to drug treatment such as anti-cholinergic drugs (NCCWCH, 2006).

intrinsic activity (i.e. not controlled by nerves), generating peristaltic waves of contraction every 10 s. These waves of contraction propel urine along the ureters to the bladder. Each ureter is also lined with smooth muscle and transitional epithelium; the lumen has a star-shaped cross-section.

The ureters lie upon the posterior abdominal wall outside the peritoneal cavity, entering the bladder at an oblique angle, one at each side of the base of the specialized muscle

Urine

Urine has a specific gravity of 1.010–1.030 and is usually acidic. The volume and final concentration of urea and solutes depend on fluid intake. Sleep and muscular activity also inhibit urine production. The amber colour is due to urobilin, the bile pigment. Urine has a characteristic smell, which is not unpleasant when fresh. Odour or cloudiness generally indicates a bacterial infection (Box 2.4).

Control of micturition

Micturition (urination) is a coordinated response that is due to the contraction of the muscular wall of the bladder, reflex relaxation of the internal sphincter of the urethra and voluntary relaxation of the external sphincter (Fig. 2.8). It is assisted by increased pressure in the pelvic cavity as the diaphragm is lowered and the abdominal muscles contract. Over-distension of the bladder is painful and can cause involuntary relaxation of the external sphincter resulting in urgency of micturition, incontinence and overflow. The tone of this sphincter is also affected by psychological stimuli (such as waking or getting ready to leave the house) and external stimuli (such as the sound of water or the feel of the lavatory seat). Any factor that raises the intraabdominal and intravesicular pressures (such as laughter or coughing) in excess of the urethral closing pressure can result in stress incontinence.

Accumulation of urine increases bladder wall tension, stimulating the stretch receptors of the bladder, which relay parasympathetic sensory impulses to the brain, generating awareness. However, there is conscious descending inhibition of the reflex bladder contraction and relaxation of the external sphincter. Entry of urine into the urethra irritates and stimulates stretch receptors, augmenting the sensory pathways as the bladder fills. Micturition is postponed until a socially acceptable time and place. This inhibition of the spinal reflex and contraction of the external sphincter is learned. Infants tend to develop bladder control when they are about 2 years old. Irritation of the bladder or urethra, for instance as a result of infection, can also initiate the desire to urinate regardless of the bladder capacity.

Normal physiological control of micturition requires an intact nerve supply to the urinary tract, normal muscle tone (of bladder, urethral sphincters and pelvic floor muscles), absence of any obstruction to flow, normal bladder capacity and, finally, the absence of psychological factors that may inhibit the micturition cycle (such as embarrassment and discomfort).

THE FEMALE REPRODUCTIVE TRACT

The main features of the female reproductive tract distinguishing it from the male are that the female reproductive organs are internal and in the non-pregnant state are situated within the true pelvic cavity. The female reproductive tract consists of two ovaries, two uterine (fallopian) tubes, the uterus and cervix, the vagina and external genitalia. The female reproductive system undergoes considerable changes throughout life from childhood through reproductive life (see Box 2.5) to the menopause. Superimposed on these changes are the effects of the menstrual cycle (see Chapter 3). Prevention of infection in the female reproductive tract is essential; the cervix, endometrium and uterine tubes all produce natural antimicrobial secretions with production peaking about the time when implantation would occur (King et al., 2007).

The ovaries

The ovaries are dull-white almond-shaped bodies, approximately 4 cm long. They lie posteriorly and laterally relative to the body of the uterus and below the uterine tubes. They are anchored by the ovarian ligaments and attached to the posterior layer of the broad ligament, a fold within the peritoneum that extends from the uterus (Fig. 2.9). The blood supply to the ovary is via the ovarian artery, which runs alongside the ovarian ligament, and the ovarian branch of the uterine artery

---

Box 2.4 Urinary tract infections (UTIs)

Pregnancy further increases the risk of UTIs in pregnancy and so routine culture and sensitivity test to detect bacteraemia is a common practice. Some women with bacteraemia may be asymptomatic, for example, group B haemolytic streptococcus. If group B streptococcus is present within the urine, antibiotic therapy is recommended (Royal College of Obstetricians and Gynaecologists, 2006) as this represents a high bacterial load which could put the neonate at risk of infection following birth (see Chapter 10).

Box 2.5 Changes to the genital tract at puberty

- Hair appears on mons veneris and subcutaneous fat accumulates
- Secretory glands mature and become active
- Labia majora and minora become pigmented with melanin
- Enlargement of the clitoris occurs
- Vaginal epithelium thickens and becomes responsive to oestrogen
- Vaginal pH decreases as lactobacilli metabolize glycogen from cell secretions
- Uterus grows and cervix doubles in length

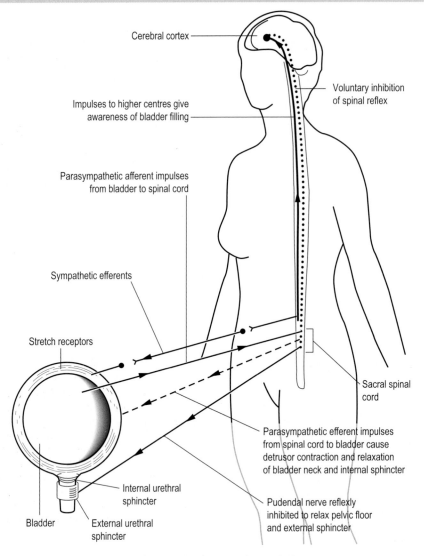

Cerebral cortex

Voluntary inhibition
of spinal reflex

Impulses to higher centres give
awareness of bladder filling

Parasympathetic afferent impulses
from bladder to spinal cord

Sympathetic efferents

Stretch receptors

Sacral spinal
cord

Parasympathetic efferent impulses
from spinal cord to bladder cause
detrusor contraction and relaxation
of bladder neck and internal sphincter

Internal urethral
sphincter

Pudendal nerve reflexly
inhibited to relax pelvic floor
and external sphincter

Bladder   External urethral
sphincter

Fig. 2.8 Control of micturition. (Reproduced with permission from Brooker, 1998.)

(see Fig. 2.12). This dual blood supply is important in maintaining reproductive function; if the ovary becomes twisted, for instance because it is displaced by a tumour or cystic growth, the ovarian ligament may occlude the blood supply from the ovarian artery. This torsion of the ovary can cause ischaemia of the tissues and intense pain.

The ovaries are composed of two distinct layers: the outer layer is the cortex and the inner section is referred to as the medulla. The ovary is contained within a sheath of connective tissue, the tunica albuginea. The cortex contains the developing follicles that contain the primary oocytes and is also responsible for the production of the female steroid hormones oestrogen and progesterone (see Chapters 4 and 5). The medulla is composed primarily of connective tissue and blood vessels and provides precursors

to facilitate steroid production within the cortex. The ovary has two main functions: to produce fertilizable oocytes which can undergo full development and to secrete the steroid hormones which prepare the reproductive tract for fertilization and to establish and support the pregnancy.

The long-held belief that all oocytes in adults are formed in the fetal and perinatal period (prenatal 'total endowment') has been challenged (Bukovsky et al., 2009) as studies of oogenesis have demonstrated that follicular renewal continues through much of female reproductive life and oocyte renewal probably only totally ceases at the onset of natural menopause. This has important clinical significance particularly for the many young women rendered infertile by chemotherapy.

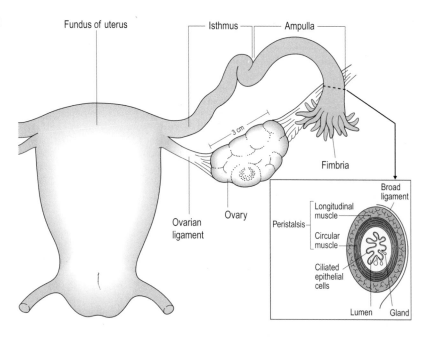

Fig. 2.9 Position of the ovary, and ovarian and broad ligaments. (Reproduced with permission from Sweet, 1996.)

The uterine (fallopian) tubes

The uterine tubes (also known as the fallopian tubes or oviducts) are approximately 12 cm long and have walls of smooth muscle lined with ciliated epithelial and secretory cells. The uterine tubes are mobile and not fixed to the ovaries. The distal end of the uterine tube has specialized structures called fimbriae, which surround the opening into the tube. The fimbriae lie in close proximity to the ovary and, at ovulation, assist the entry of the ovum into the uterine tube by a wafting action, which facilitates movement of the interperitoneal fluid. The lining of the uterine tubes lies in many folds (called plicae) and is composed of ciliated columnar epithelial cells interspersed with goblet cells that secrete pyruvate to nourish the ovum. The cilia facilitate the movement of the ovum down the uterine tube; this is augmented by coordinated peristaltic contractions of the smooth muscle. The distal end of the uterine tube has a slightly wider area, called the ampulla, where fertilization of the ovum by the sperm usually occurs.

If both uterine tubes are completely blocked, fertilization is prevented as the sperm are unable to access the ovum. If one uterine tube is patent or only partially blocked then sperm may encounter and fertilize an ovum within the peritoneal cavity. However, if a fertilized ovum enters a partially or totally blocked uterine tube its passage to the uterus will be impeded and so the pregnancy may develop within the uterine tube or peritoneal cavity (see Case Study 2.1 and Box 2.6). Infection of the genital tract with Chlamydia trachomatis is becoming more common and can often be asymptomatic (Carey and Beagley, 2010). Undetected or multiple infections can lead to pelvic inflammatory disease which is the main cause of ectopic pregnancy and tubal infertility. Although the prime site of chlamydial infection is the columnar epithelial cells of the cervix, the infection can quickly ascend to the upper reproductive tract probably by attaching to sperm or by being transported in the flow of fluids. Infection leads to production of proinflammatory cytokines which interact with the infected woman's immune system (see Chapter 10) causing inflammation and tissue destruction. The incidence of infection is increasing because the organism is developing antibiotic resistance and the development of effective vaccines in very early stages.

The uterus

The functions of the uterus are to prepare to receive the fertilized ovum, to provide a suitable environment for growth and development of the fetus and to assist in the expulsion of the fetus, placenta and membranes at delivery. In the non-pregnant state the pear-shaped uterus is situated

 Case study 2.1

Julie, during the booking appointment, informs the midwife that she had previously suffered an ectopic pregnancy with her last pregnancy, which was treated conservatively with methotrexate. What does the midwife need to do to ensure that Julie's pregnancy is progressing normally? What are the signs and symptoms of an ectopic pregnancy; and when are they most likely to become apparent?

Box 2.6 **Ectopic pregnancy**

An ectopic pregnancy is one that implants in the uterine tubes or, more rarely, the cervix, ovaries or abdomen. It is relatively common as it occurs in about 1% of all pregnancies and although the fatality rate is much reduced, ectopic pregnancy still remains a significant cause of maternal morbidity and mortality (Raine-Fenning and Hopkisson, 2009). It is usually confirmed by an ultrasound scan revealing an empty uterine cavity and a positive pregnancy test. Raised human chorionic gonadotrophin (hCG) levels confirm pregnancy but levels are lower in ectopic pregnancy than in uterine pregnancy. The term 'pregnancy of unknown location' (PUL) is used to describe a pregnancy where there is a positive pregnancy test but no intra- or extra-uterine pregnancy can be visualized on an ultrasound scan (Kirk and Bourne, 2009). In these cases, it is recommended that serial hCG measurements be made to monitor whether the PUL is failing (the hCG ratio is used to compare initial hCG levels with those 48 h later) and also that serum progesterone measurements are made to predict the likely outcome (higher levels are associated with pregnancies subsequently demonstrated to be viable).

The usual first warning sign of an ectopic pregnancy is abdominal pain at around 8 weeks' gestation which may present with symptoms mimicking gastrointestinal disease (misdiagnosis of ectopic pregnancy as gastroenteritis is associated with maternal mortality). Ectopic pregnancy should be suspected in all women of childbearing age who present with fainting or sudden unexpected collapse (Neilson, 2007); no form of contraception is 100% effective, so pregnancy should not be excluded in women who use contraception. If the uterine tube ruptures, the woman may become clinically shocked owing to excessive bleeding into the peritoneal cavity. The growing fetus can be surgically removed together with the damaged uterine tube if necessary (this is referred to as a salpingectomy). Occasionally, an abdominal pregnancy may ensue if implantation occurs on the peritoneum. The pregnancies rarely go to term; however, delivery of live infants via abdominal surgery has been documented. This phenomenon underpins scientific interest enabling men to have babies through a process of peritoneal implantation. The main causes of tubal blockage are infection (usually due to pelvic inflammatory disease), the formation of scar tissue from surgery or trauma and congenital malformation. High levels of steroid hormones can also affect cilia movement. If a tubal pregnancy is diagnosed early before trauma occurs, it can be treated by the intramuscular administration of the drug methotrexate. Methotrexate is a chemotherapeutic drug which inhibits folic acid metabolism (by inhibiting difolate reductase so DNA synthesis ceases) thus targeting rapidly dividing tissue such as the trophoblast; the embryo is eventually reabsorbed. Methotrexate has side effects on mucosal surfaces as they also have a fast rate of cell division and can cause conjunctivitis, gastrointestinal disturbances and stomatitis (inflammation of the mucous membranes in the mouth). Women may experience some degree of abdominal pain because of tubal miscarriage; it can be difficult to distinguish this from tubal rupture. Although the uterine tube is saved, the risk of another ectopic pregnancy is high. As the rate of sexually-transmitted disease is increasing and there are more assisted conceptions, the rate of ectopic pregnancy is expected to increase (Raine-Fenning and Hopkisson, 2009).

within the true pelvic cavity. It is described as being anteverted (tilted forwards) and anteflexed (curved forward), situated in a superior position to the urinary bladder (Fig. 2.10). A uterus in an abnormal position, such as a retroverted uterus, is not in an optimal position to expand in pregnancy and surgical intervention may be required to adjust its position to allow the pregnancy to proceed. The anatomical position of the uterus is maintained by the uterine ligaments, which are important in supporting the weight of the uterus, particularly during contractions (Fig. 2.11). Its blood supply is shown in Fig. 2.12.

The non-pregnant uterus weighs approximately 50 g with a cavity of approximately 10 mL and is composed of three layers (Fig. 2.13). The inner layer of the uterus is the endometrium. This layer is markedly different in the body of the uterus compared with the cervix. The cells of the endometrium are ciliated and the entire cell layer undergoes considerable growth changes during the menstrual cycle; the superficial decidual layers are shed in menstruation at the end of the cycle (see Chapter 4). The vascular connective tissue, or stroma, contains many glands that secrete alkaline mucus into the uterine cavity.

The middle layer is composed of smooth muscle, called the myometrium, which is arranged in three muscle layers (see Box 2.7). In the non-pregnant state, these layers are not very distinctive.

Box 2.7 **The uterine muscle layers**

1. *Inner layer*: fibres in the longitudinal plane that run from the anterior cervix, up over the fundus and back to the posterior edge of the cervix
2. *Middle layer*: interlaced spiral fibres concentrated in, and originating from, the fundal region of the uterus and getting less dense approaching the cervical region; the circular arrangement of the fibres is accentuated at the junctions with the uterine tubes and the cervix (internal os), thus providing closures to the expanding pregnant uterus
3. *Outer layer*: combination of longitudinal and circular fibres

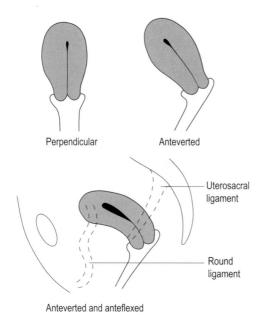

Fig. 2.10 The anteverted and anteflexed position of the non-pregnant uterus. (Reproduced with permission from Sweet, 1996.)

The uterus has an outer layer of peritoneum that drapes over the uterus anteriorly to form a fold between the uterus and bladder, and over the uterine tubes to cover the myometrium. This is referred to as the perimetrium; it forms the broad ligament, thus maintaining the anatomical position of the uterus. The body of the uterus is about 5 cm in both length and width (excluding the dimensions of the cervix).

Arterial blood to the uterus is supplied by left and right uterine arteries which branch along their length giving rise to arcuate arteries which penetrate the myometrium.

Branches of the arcuate arteries anastomose freely ensuring that the blood supply to the uterus is robust. Radial arteries branching from the arcuate arteries supply the tissue towards the lumen of the uterus. The radical arteries branch at the myometrial-endometrial boundary into the basal arteries that supply the myometrium and continue as spiral arteries. The spiral arteries are tightly coiled in the basal layer of the uterine lining but markedly narrow as they near the uterine lumen and divide into smaller straighter branches before terminating in capillary beds under the uterine surface and surrounding the uterine glands. The walls of the spiral and radical arteries are rich in smooth muscle and are innervated by the autonomic nervous system, so they are responsive to adrenergic stimuli, particularly the segments of the spiral arteries close to the myometrial-endometrial junction. These parts of the spiral arteries may spontaneously constrict before menstruation, and may induce menstruation (Burton et al., 2009).

The uterus is innervated by both parasympathetic nerves (arising from the second, third and fourth sacral segments) and sympathetic nerves via the presacral nerve (branching from the aortic plexus) and branches from the lumbar sympathetic chain. Both types of innervation to the uterus are via the Lee–Frankenhäuser plexus, which is situated in the lower region of the pouch of Douglas.

The cervix

The cervix is the neck of the uterus at the top of the vagina. It has an important role in protecting the uterus from infection and undergoes important changes preceding labour (see Chapter 13). The isthmus, an indistinct layer of tissue that forms the lower uterine segment in pregnancy (see Chapter 13), separates the body of the uterus and the cervix. The cervix is about 2.5 cm in length and is composed of dense collagenous circular fibres. The cervix is spindle-shaped with an os (smooth muscle

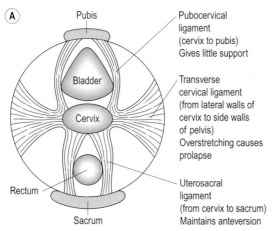

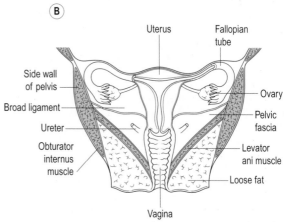

Fig. 2.11 The uterine ligaments ((A) transverse and (B) coronal sections). (Reproduced with permission from Sweet, 1996.)

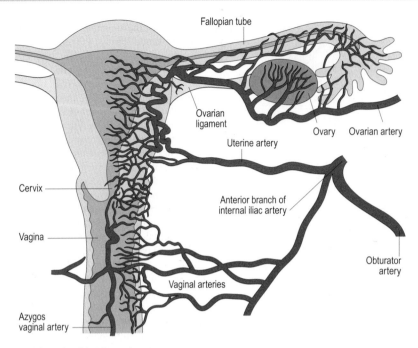

Fig. 2.12 The uterine and ovarian blood supply.

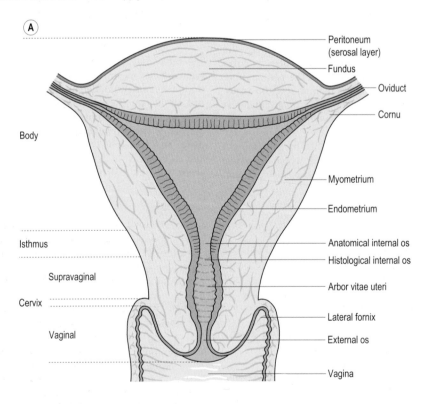

Fig. 2.13 Structure of (A) the non-pregnant uterus and (B) endometrium. (B reproduced with permission from Brooker, 1998.)

Continued

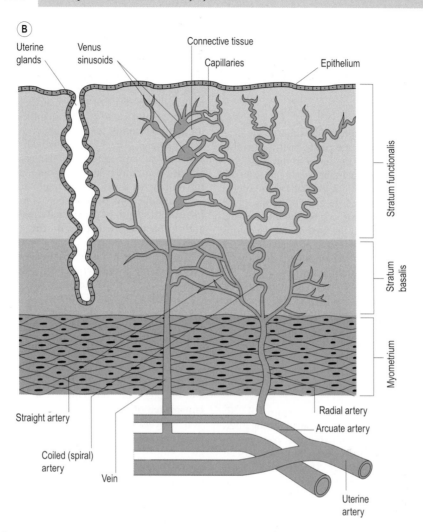

Fig. 2.13, cont'd

arrangement forming a constriction) at the top and bottom. The internal os forms the inner opening of the cervix at the junction with the body of the uterus. The external os is located at the bottom of the cervical canal where it projects into the vagina. Two different types of cell meet at this junction: the columnar cells of the cervical canal and the squamous epithelial cells of the outer cervix. Abnormal precancerous cells are most likely to arise at this junction. Cervical cancer is one of the more common cancers affecting women of reproductive age. One of the risk factors for cervical cancer is the presence of antibodies to certain strains of human papilloma virus (HPV). HPV itself is benign but it is thought to trigger changes in the cells of the cervix such as cervical dysplasia. HPV is one of the most common sexually transmitted diseases and is thought to infect the majority of sexually active women. Vaccination of girls and young women (usually aged 9–25 years) against certain types of high-risk HPV has recently been introduced in many countries to reduce the incidence of cervical cancer, some genital cancers and genital warts and also reduce the need for colposcopy-based surgical treatments (RCOG, 2007). The Pap smear (named after Georgios Papanikolaou) is a cervical swab which samples cells and allows checking for precancerous changes but many women who develop cervical cancer have never had a cervical smear. The shape of the spatula used to take cell samples during a cervical smear accommodates the curve of the external part of the cervix. About 5–7% of cervical smears identify abnormal results such as dysplasia indicating the need for increased vigilance and further examination. The lining of the cervix does not undergo cyclical changes in growth rate although glandular activity changes. The inner tissue lies in folds that appear branched, giving it the name arbor vitae. These folds allow dilatation during delivery.

The vagina

The vagina is a distensible fibromuscular tube, about 8–10 cm long, situated within the true pelvic cavity, extending through the pelvic floor from the cervix to the vulva. The vagina is described as a potential tube because its walls are in contact but easily separated, but the walls of the vagina are not uniform. The distal and the proximal parts of the vagina have different embryonic origins; the distal vagina forms an integrated entity with the urethra and the clitoris (O'Connell et al., 2008). The cervix protrudes into the vagina, normally pointing to the posterior wall of the vagina because of the anteverted and anteflexed position of the uterus. The spaces between the cervix and the upper portion of the vaginal wall are referred to as the anterior, lateral and posterior fornices (singular: fornix). The vagina has three main functions: the facilitation of coitus, as a passage for the release of the menses and as the route for the baby to be born, commonly referred to as the birth canal. It also helps to support the uterus and prevent ascending infection through the release of antibacterial secretions favouring the growth of commensal bacteria.

The vagina is lined by a layer of moist epithelial cells folded into ridges (called rugae) that distend during intercourse and childbirth, thus facilitating the stretching of the vagina. There is also a lining of smooth muscle, which maintains the tone of the vagina. The opening of the vaginal canal, the introitus, is protected by the external genitalia. The introitus lies below the urethral opening, which is situated below the clitoris (see Fig. 2.14). The vagina does not have glands but is maintained in a moist state by secretions from the cervical glands and transudate of fluid from the blood vessels that lie below the vaginal lining.

The external genitalia

The external genitalia (also known as the vulva) are those structures that can be seen (Fig. 2.14). Most of the structures are well innervated; therefore, they are very sensitive and are a source of sexual arousal responses. The external genitalia are well vascularized, which means they bleed easily if subjected to trauma but also heal rapidly.

The mons veneris (or mons pubis) is a pad of subcutaneous fat covered by skin lying over the pubic bone; it provides support to the clitoris and urethra and functions as a cushion during intercourse. At puberty it becomes covered with a triangular area of pubic hair, which is coarse and curly because of the unusually oblique hair follicles. The labia majora (singular: labium majus) are two fatty folds of tissue extending from the mons veneris in which the round ligaments terminate. The labia majora narrow where they come together between the vagina and anus. The outer surface is covered in pubic hair; the inner surface is rich in sebaceous and sweat glands. The labia majora enclose and protect the urogenital cleft. The labia minora are two smaller longitudinal fleshy folds of tissue; they are erectile and very vascular. They are pigmented, hairless and have some sweat and sebaceous glands. The labia minora enclose the clitoris anteriorly and unite posteriorly at the fourchette, which is commonly torn at the first delivery. The functions of the labia minora are probably to increase the depth of the vaginal canal during intercourse and to increase retention of the ejaculate following intercourse.

The clitoris is a highly sensitive erectile body that is about 2.5 cm long exteriorly but projects internally for up to 9 cm forming the body and root of the clitoris (O'Connell et al., 2008) before diving into two arms, the crura, which extend around to the interior of the labia majora. The external part of the clitoris, the clitoral glans, is covered and protected by a fold of skin called the clitoral hood, or prepuce which is homologous with the foreskin in males. The erectile bodies, analogous to the spongy tissue structures of the penis, become erect and engorged on stimulation. The clitoris is an important source of sexual arousal, generating reflex lubrication responses from the surrounding tissue. When the labia are held open, the vestibule (the area from the glans clitoris to the fourchette) can be seen. It contains the external orifice of the urethra and the vaginal introitus. The urinary orifice or meatus lies about 2.5 cm below the clitoris and is a characteristic vertical slit with prominent margins formed by a horseshoe shaped arrangement of the erectile tissue of the bulbs of the clitoris (O'Connell et al., 2008). It is important to clearly identify the urinary orifice in women requiring catheterization of the bladder. To each side, slightly behind the urinary meatus, are the dimple-like exits of the Skene's ducts, which produce mucus and are useful landmarks for the urinary orifice. The Skene's ducts are the source of the urethral secretions that are produced in states of sexual arousal; these secretions may have an antimicrobial function (Moalem and Reidenberg, 2009) and contain components such as 'prostate' specific antigen (PSA; Zaviacic and Ablin, 2000) at similar levels to those found in male seminal fluid.

The vaginal introitus is almost closed in children but in adult women is extremely elastic; it can stretch to allow the passage of the baby's head and subsequently return to a small size of about 3 cm. The vaginal introitus is partly occluded by the protective hymen, which is probably most important in preventing ascending infection before puberty when the pH of the vagina is less acidic. Once ruptured, the skin tags are referred to as hymen

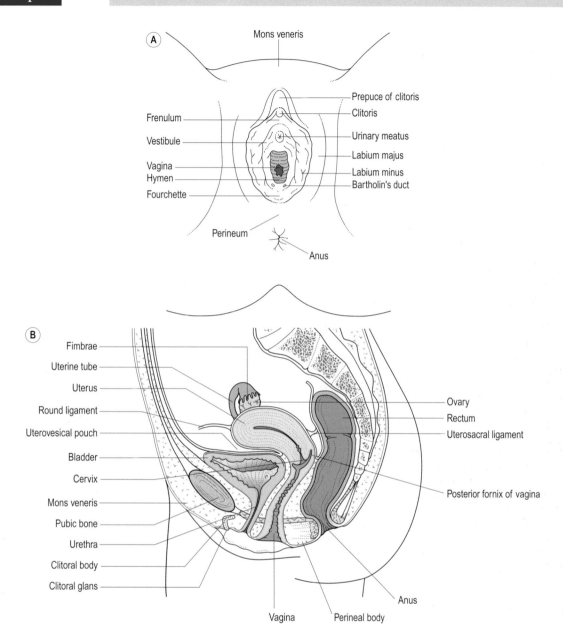

Fig. 2.14 The (A) female external genitalia and (B) female internal reproductive organs.

remnants. The appearance of an intact hymen can have important significance in some societies as it is considered to indicate virginal status. The Bartholin's glands lie posteriorly, each side of the vagina. These mucus-producing glands are the size and shape of haricot beans and, unless inflamed, cannot normally be seen. Their rate of secretion increases with the erection of the clitoris. The vestibular bulb posterior to the vagina is also formed of erectile spongy tissue.

Box 2.8 describes an example of problems caused by mutilation of the external genitalia.

The pelvic floor

The pelvic floor is composed primarily of the muscle fibres of the levator ani and soft tissues suspended within the outlet of the pelvis, forming a sling-like sheet of tissue that encloses and supports the pelvic contents (Box 2.9). In women, the

Box 2.8 Female genital mutilation (FGM; 'female circumcision' or 'cutting')

Many ethnic groups, particularly those of Muslim origin in North Africa, Indonesia and other countries, regard female genital mutilation as essential to moderate sexual desire or to increase hygiene. It is important to note that pressure for women to undergo FGM may be considerable and that many women who have undergone FGM consider it normal practice and could be offended by the term 'mutilation'. The surgery, performed in infancy, early childhood or puberty, may involve removal of the prepuce of the clitoris, removal of the labia minora and clitoris or removal of most of the labia and clitoris. The procedures may be carried out without anaesthetics and under unclean conditions such as using thorns to form stitches of the vaginal walls which increase the risks of infection, scarring and infertility. Genital mutilation may be accompanied by infibulation, the surgical closure of the labia majora (apart from a small opening for urine and menses) to ensure chastity. Although the practices are unacceptable and illegal in Western Europe, they may be undertaken illicitly or girls may be mutilated in other countries. At delivery, the urogenital tissue is extremely vulnerable to trauma, which can be minimized by anterior and mediolateral episiotomy incision. Failure to deliver vaginally may result in rejection of the woman from her family. Infibulation will require surgical division to facilitate vaginal birth and although there may be pressure from the woman and her family to have the infibulation restored, this is illegal in many countries. Following division of infibulations, the introitus is restored by the suturing of the skin edges on the same side together.

main characteristic distinguishing it from that of the pelvic floor of the man is that there are three openings instead of two. As well as the anal canal and urethra, the woman also has a vaginal opening. This is why women are much more likely to suffer from pelvic inflammatory disease (PID) as there is a direct route from the external environment via the genital tract, uterine cavity and uterine tubes to the internal pelvic cavity lined by the peritoneum.

Pelvic shape and adaptation

The pelvis is a girdle composed of a number of bones held together by ligaments and cartilaginous and fused joints (Fig. 2.16). The dimensions of the inlet, cavity and outlet affect the passage of the fetus. This means that the fetus has to negotiate the pelvic cavity by undergoing a rotational manoeuvre. The sling-like arrangement of the gutter-shaped pelvic floor muscles means that the fetus is forced to rotate in a forward position. This arrangement has evolved because of humans adopting an upright stance.

The female pelvis is wider and shallower than the male pelvis. Each half of the pelvis is known as the innominate bone, which is composed of ilium, ischium and pubic. Traditionally, pelvic morphology has distinguished four major categories (Fig. 2.17). In practice, there is a wide variation in pelvic form combining features from all four of the categories. There are also recognized abnormalities of the pelvis including justominor pelvis (normal shape but overall dimensions smaller than normal), Nägele's pelvis (asymmetrical due to abnormal bone formation on one side) and Robert's pelvis (similar to Nägele's pelvis but the abnormal bone formation is bilateral). Pelvic shape can also be affected by disease, for example rachitic pelvis due to rickets, which is an extreme form of the platypelloid pelvis. The shape of the pelvis affects the mechanism of labour (see Chapter 13); abnormal pelvic shape is associated with problems at delivery as the rotation of the presenting part may be suboptimal.

THE MALE REPRODUCTIVE TRACT

The male reproductive tract comprises a number of structures that permit gamete formation to occur below body temperature and provide conditions that allow sperm maturation and ejection (Fig. 2.18).

The testes

The testes are suspended within the scrotal sac or scrotum. Optimal spermatogenesis in humans is achieved 2–3°C below the body's core temperature. There are a number of mechanisms to regulate the temperature of the testes. The testes are suspended outside the abdominal cavity but can be retracted upwards towards the warmth of the body by contraction of the cremaster muscle which covers the testes. This muscle will also reflexly raise the testes towards the body if the inner thigh is stroked or scratched; this cremaster reflex is used as a neurological test. The pigmented skin of the scrotum lies in rugae (folds), which increase the surface area. The scrotum is well vascularized but has no insulating hair or subcutaneous fat. It is lined by dartos muscle, which contracts in response to cold. Blood flow to the testes allows heat to be transferred from the descending testicular arteries to the ascending pampiniform venous plexus forming a countercurrent heat-exchange mechanism, which helps to maintain the lower temperature of the testes relative to the body.

The testes are a pair of glandular organs, analogous to the ovaries, that produce gametes (spermatozoa) and male sex hormones. Within the scrotum, the testes are surrounded by a thick fibrous capsule called the tunica albuginea, which penetrates internally dividing the testes into lobules. Each testis has about 200 lobules, each containing about three seminiferous tubules, about 0.2 mm in diameter and up to 70 cm long (Fig. 2.19). The seminiferous tubules are the site of spermatogenesis (sperm production). Within

Box 2.9 Functions and characteristics of the pelvic floor

- Its muscles are arranged in two layers: superficial and deep (see Fig. 2.15)
- It supports and maintains the anatomical position of the internal female reproductive organs
- It provides voluntary muscle control for micturition and defecation

- It facilitates birth by resisting descent of the descending presenting part, so forcing the fetus to rotate forward in the presence of strong regular uterine contractions. The human pelvic floor plays an essential role in delivery as the fetus would not otherwise be able to rotate to negotiate its passage through the pelvic girdle because of the morphology of the pelvis influenced by the evolution of our upright stance

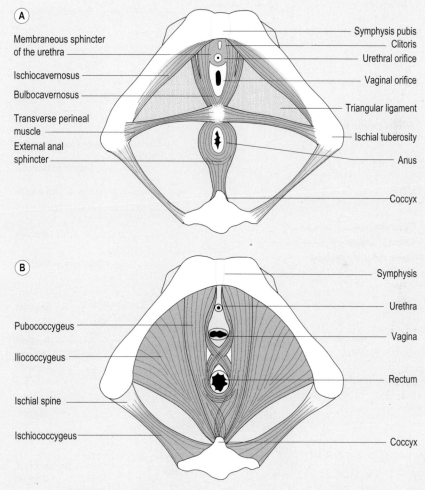

Fig. 2.15 (A) The superficial pelvic floor muscles; (B) the deep pelvic floor muscles. (Reproduced with permission from Bennett and Brown, 1999.)

the tubules are spermatogenic cells (germ cells) and their supporting Sertoli cells which cordon off the spermatogenic cells and the developing sperm into distinct compartments. Between the tubules are the interstitial cells of Leydig, which produce testosterone.

The sperm produced from the seminiferous tubules are stored in the epididymis where they are concentrated, becoming mature and motile. The epididymis is a comma-shaped convoluted tube, about 6 cm long, leading into the vas deferens. The vas deferens provides the conduit for sperm delivery

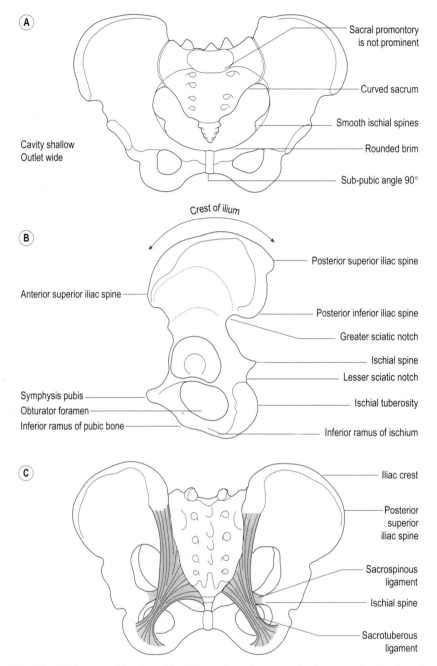

Fig. 2.16 The pelvic girdle: (A) the normal female pelvis; (B) innominate bone showing important landmarks; (C) posterior view of the pelvis to show ligaments. (Reproduced with permission from Bennett and Brown, 1999.)

during emission and ejaculation. It is a thick-walled tube leading from the tail of the epididymis to the ejaculatory duct. The vas deferens dilates into a storage reservoir, or ampulla, just before it joins with the exit of the seminal vesicle to form the ejaculatory duct. Just as infection or trauma can cause blockage of the uterine tubes, the male reproductive capacity can be also affected by blockage, of the epididymis or vas deferens for instance, impeding the passage of spermatozoa. The vas deferens, blood vessels and cremaster muscle lie closely together forming the spermatic cord.

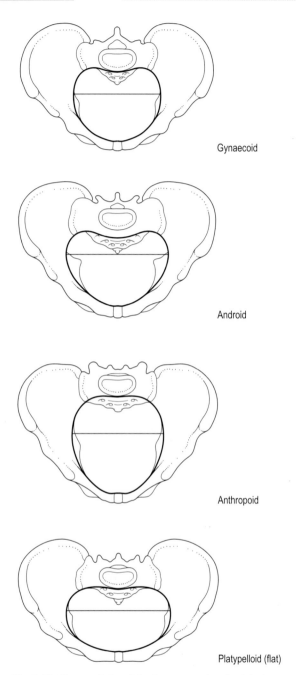

Gynaecoid

Android

Anthropoid

Platypelloid (flat)

Fig. 2.17 Characteristics of the four categories of pelvic shape.

The seminal vesicles are two pyramid-shaped membranous sacs, about 4 cm long, lying between the base of the bladder and the rectum. They produce semen, a fructose-rich viscous fluid, which facilitates sperm transport and nourishment. The fluid component of semen is principally produced by the seminal vesicles and prostate gland. Secretory activity of the seminal vesicles depends

on the level of testosterone. The ejaculatory ducts begin at the base of the prostate gland and terminate in the single prostatic urethra. These muscular ducts carry sperm and seminal fluid through the prostate gland. The prostate gland is a walnut-sized exocrine gland lying just below the neck of the bladder, between the rectum and pubic bone. It is a compound gland, formed of about 20–40 smaller glandular units each with its own exit into the ejaculatory duct. Prostatic fluid is a thin lubricating secretion that mixes with the sperm and seminal fluid. The prostatic gland can be palpated through the rectal wall. In elderly men, the prostate gland may undergo hypertrophy causing benign prostatic hyperplasia which can compress the urethra and impede micturition. Prostatitis or inflammation of the prostate gland can affect men of all ages. Prostatic carcinoma is one of the most common cancers affecting elderly men in developed countries; it is a major cause of death if it is not detected early. Prior to ejaculation, the bulbourethral glands (or Cowper's glands) secrete clear lubricating fluid into the urethra just below the prostate gland.

The penis carries the urethra, which provides a shared passage for sperm and urine, and allows intromission: the delivery of sperm into the vagina. Unlike other mammalian species, the human penis does not have an erectile bone and relies entirely on engorgement to achieve erection; it also cannot be withdrawn into the groin. Humans have one of the largest penis:body size ratios. The penis has three columns of erectile tissue: two lateral corpora cavernosa and a ventromedial corpus spongiosum (Fig. 2.20). The corpus spongiosum contains the urethra and does not engorge as much as the corpora cavernosa. This prevents trauma to the urethra and generates an appropriate angle for intromission. The expanded cone-shaped end of the corpus spongiosum forms the glans penis where the urethra opens. The penis is covered with a fold of skin or prepuce (foreskin), which can be retracted in an adult and older child to expose the glans. The foreskin attaches to the underside of the penis at a small fold of tissue called the frenum. The prepuce and shaft skin are not attached to underlying tissue so they are free to glide along the shaft of the penis, which reduces friction, abrasion and loss of lubricating fluid during intercourse. On the underside of the penis, there is a small ridge called the raphe which runs from the opening of the urethra across the scrotum to the perineum (between the scrotum and anus). The spongy bodies of the penis become distended with blood during an erection (see Chapter 6).

GAMETOGENESIS

The process of gametogenesis is achieved through a specialized form of cellular division called meiosis (Fig. 2.21). The stages of meiosis are reviewed in Chapter 7. Gametogenesis is remarkably different in the male

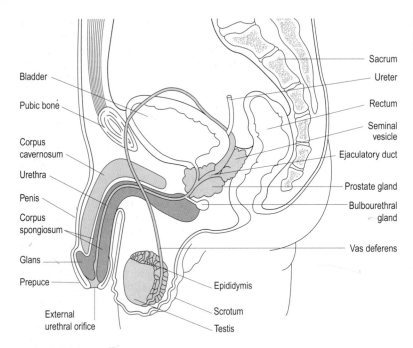

Fig. 2.18 The male reproductive system. (Reproduced with permission from Brooker, 1998.)

Bladder

Pubic bone

Corpus cavernosum

Urethra

Penis

Corpus spongiosum

Glans

Prepuce

External urethral orifice

Sacrum

Ureter

Rectum

Seminal vesicle

Ejaculatory duct

Prostate gland

Bulbourethral gland

Vas deferens

Epididymis

Scrotum

Testis

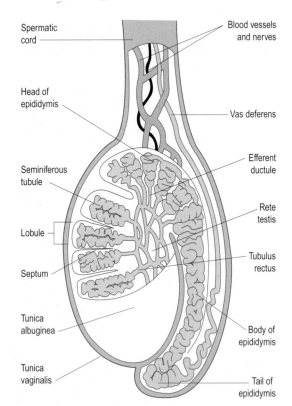

Spermatic cord

Head of epididymis

Seminiferous tubule

Lobule

Septum

Tunica albuginea

Tunica vaginalis

Blood vessels and nerves

Vas deferens

Efferent ductule

Rete testis

Tubulus rectus

Body of epididymis

Tail of epididymis

Fig. 2.19 The structure of the testis and ducts conveying sperm from the seminiferous tubules to the urethra. (Reproduced with permission from Brooker, 1998.)

and female reproductive systems, both representing adaptation of the process of meiosis to facilitate reproduction. Gametes are specialized sex cells that contain half the genetic material (and, therefore, half the number of chromosomes) of the normal cell content. Their fusion, referred to as fertilization, is described in detail in Chapter 6.

The production of spermatozoa begins at puberty in the male and results in the continual production of millions of sperm. Spermatozoa have completed all the meiotic divisions prior to ejaculation and fusion with the oocyte. In this sense, they are true gametes containing the haploid number of chromosomes. (These terms are explained in Chapter 4.)

The differences between male and female gamete formation have evolved with the development of sexual reproduction and internal fertilization. Oocytes are relatively protected within the abdominal cavity and so it is not necessary for a large number to be produced. Movement of oocytes is passive, influenced by the structure of the uterine tube. Sperm, in contrast, must become highly motile in order to travel along the female reproductive tract. Many are lost and, of the millions contained within the ejaculate, only a few hundred will make it to the vicinity of the oocyte. In addition, sperm have to survive transplantation into the female reproductive tract which is effectively equivalent to a foreign host in order to perform their physiological role of fertilizing the oocyte. Thus, they have to be adapted to evade the innate immune defence mechanisms which protect the female reproductive tract such as the complement (see Chapter 10) which is present in the secretions; both sperm and seminal fluid have complement regulators which enhance sperm survival (Harris et al., 2006).

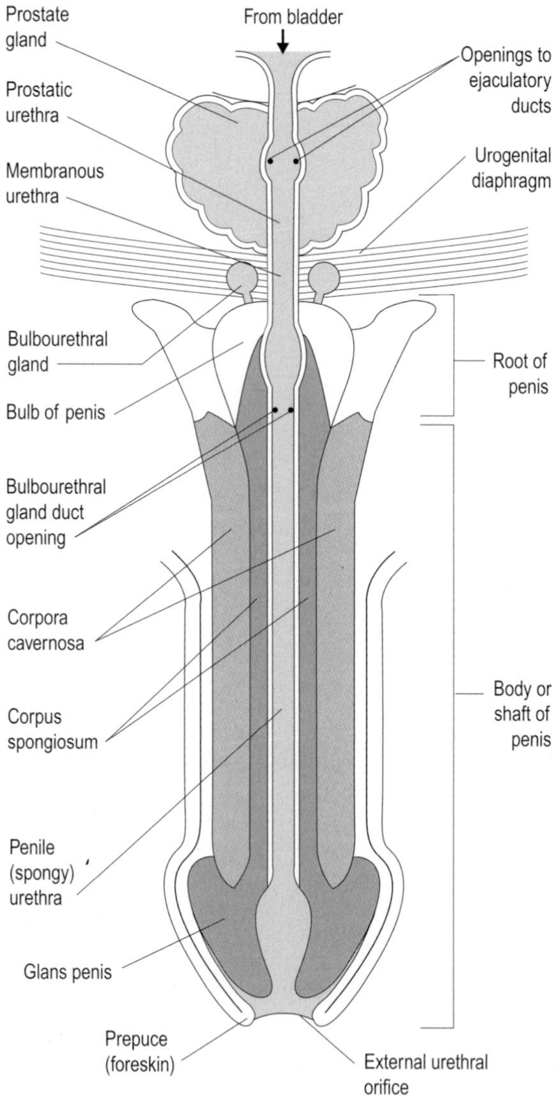

Fig. 2.20 Internal structure of the penis.

Spermatogenesis

Spermatogenesis begins at puberty and continues into senescence, albeit less efficiently. It is a complex process, well-organized temporally and spatially, which takes place in the epithelium of the seminiferous tubules; groups of cells progress in clearly defined stages of cell division within a particular tubule, which is described as a 'spermatogenic wave'. There are three processes involved in spermatogenesis: (1) the renewal of the stem cells and the formation and expansion of undifferentiated progenitor germ cells (spermatogonia) around the inner circumference of the seminiferous tubule, which divide and replicate by a process called mitosis (see Chapter 4), forming many spermatogonia (Fig. 2.22);

(2) the reduction of the number of chromosomes in each progenitor cell by meiosis; and (3) the differentiation of the haploid cells into spermatozoa (spermiogenesis). Each spermatogonium first divides into two diploid primary spermatocytes. The primary spermatocytes then undergo meiosis producing two genetically diverse secondary spermatocytes and then, after the second meiotic division, four haploid spermatids. For each cell undergoing meiosis, therefore, four gametes are produced. The round spermatids undergo spermiogenesis (nuclear and cytoplasmic changes) producing the characteristic morphology (shape) of a spermatozoon. As meiosis progresses, the immature sperm are supported within Sertoli cells (Griswold, 1998), which then release the sperm into the lumen of the seminiferous tubule by degrading the cell-cell junctions (Hogarth and Griswold, 2010). Sertoli synthesize and secrete a number of glycoproteins involved in Sertoli-germ cell interactions including bioprotective proteins, proteases and protease inhibitors involved in tissue remodelling processes, glycoproteins that form the basement membrane and other regulatory glycoproteins (Box 2.10).

The spermatozoa are stored in the epididymis, where they mature acquiring both motility and the capability for fertilization, for 2 weeks and may stay for up to 6 months. The shortest time between the initial meiosis and ejaculation is about 10 weeks, which is therefore the critical preconception period in men. Spermatogenesis is regulated by gonaodotrophins and steroid hormones, the interaction of these hormones with the somatic cells of the testis (Leydig and Sertoli cells) and by vitamin A (Hogarth and Griswold, 2010). It is affected by temperature, malnutrition, alcohol, cottonseed oil (a potential source of contraception), some drugs and heavy metals.

Steroidogenesis

The interstitial cells of Leydig interspersed between the seminiferous tubules produce 90% of the circulating testosterone (the remainder has an adrenal origin). Testosterone is responsible for male secondary sex characteristics (see Chapter 3) and, together with follicle-stimulating hormone (FSH), controls production of sperm. Testosterone production is stimulated by luteinizing hormone (LH) from the pituitary gland (Fig. 2.23). Testosterone binds to androgen-binding protein (ABP) in the seminiferous tubules, which means that testosterone levels within the tubule can be very high while maintaining a concentration gradient that drives diffusion from outside to inside. Testosterone exerts a negative feedback mechanism on the hypothalamic–pituitary axis in a manner analogous to the feedback control by oestrogen in the female cycle (see Chapter 4). FSH stimulates the production of ABP by the Sertoli cells. Inhibin produced from the Sertoli cells inhibits FSH production. Illness and stress affect male reproductive capacity probably via the hypothalamic–pituitary axis.

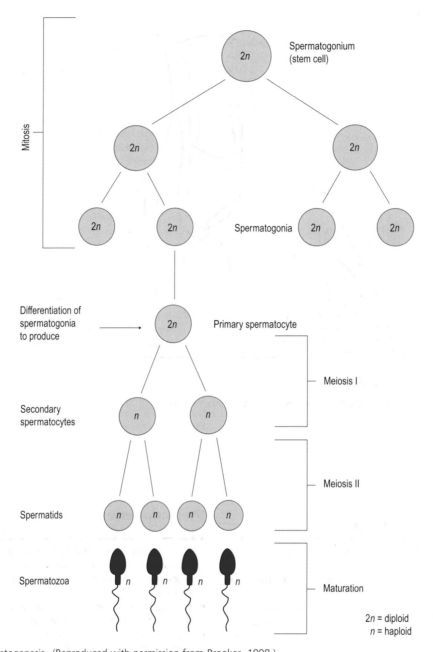

Fig. 2.21 Gametogenesis. (Reproduced with permission from Brooker, 1998.)

Control of gametogenesis

The controls of gametogenesis and steroidogenesis in the man and woman have some similarities. The hypothalamus regulates reproduction by secreting gonadotrophin-releasing hormone (GnRH; see Fig. 2.23). This stimulates both FSH and LH production from the anterior pituitary gland. FSH stimulates gametogenesis: spermatogenesis in men and follicular development in women. Luteinizing hormone plays a pivotal role in steroidogenesis: increasing testosterone production from the Leydig cells in men and stimulating the increases in progesterone and oestrogen secretion in the second half of the menstrual cycle in women (see Chapter 4).

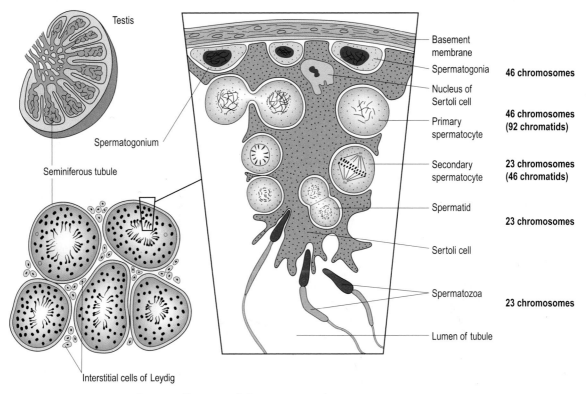

Fig. 2.22 Spermatogenesis, showing cell stages and chromosome numbers.

Box 2.10 **The role of Sertoli cells**

- Support ('nurse') spermatogenic cells and move them inwards
- Provide nutrients to spermatocytes and spermatids (hence their former name of 'nurse cells')
- Secrete fluid to aid release of sperm into lumen
- Act as a barrier between sperm-producing areas and lumen, forming environmentally distinct compartments of the seminiferous epithelium
- Engulf and digest cellular debris left from spermiogenesis
- Produce inhibin and activins, which regulate follicle-stimulating hormone (FSH) secretion
- Produce androgen-binding protein (ABP, also known as testosterone binding globulin), which increases seminiferous tubule testosterone concentration and thereby spermiogenesis
- Produce aromatase which converts testosterone to oestradiol, a step essential in the induction of spermatogenesis (note that this enzyme is also produced by adipose tissue which is one of the reasons why obesity in men is associated with altered sex hormone profiles)
- Produce anti Müllerian-inhibiting hormone, which affects sexual differentiation (see Chapter 5)
- Produce glial cell line-derived neurotrophic factor (GNDF), a small protein which regulates kidney development and spermatogenesis
- Produce Ets-related molecule (*ERM*), a member of the Ets transcription factor family essential for spermatogonium stem cell maintenance and self-renewal
- Synthesis and secrete several proteins found in serum including the iron and copper binding proteins, transferrin and ceruloplasmin, which seem to be involved spermatogenesis (Gupta, 2005)

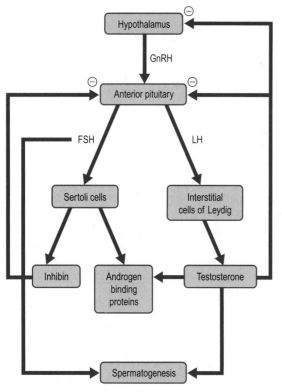

Fig. 2.23 Production of testosterone.

- The female reproductive system produces female gametes, receives male gametes, and provides the optimum environment for fertilization, implantation and nurture of the fetus. It remains quiescent in pregnancy and generates the forces required for delivery at the end of gestation. The system is quickly restored to a fertile state at the end of pregnancy.
- Gametogenesis begins with mitosis of the primordial germ cells followed by meiosis, which reduces the chromosome number and creates infinite variation in the genetic complement of the gametes.
- The male gonads produce gametes from the seminiferous tubules and testosterone from the Leydig cells. Gametogenesis has a relatively short time-span in the man.
- The hypothalamus regulates reproduction by secreting gonadotrophin-releasing hormone (GnRH), which stimulates production of FSH and LH from the anterior pituitary, which in turn have effects on the gonads. The sex steroids produced by the gonads exert negative feedback inhibition at the hypothalamic–pituitary axis.

Application to practice

Why is an in-depth knowledge of the female genitalia required by the midwife and how will this knowledge affect the decisions made by the midwife within practice?

You might consider what the midwife needs to know in order to suture the peritoneum, to catheterize a woman during labour or to recognize the sex of a baby at birth (see Chapter 5). There are many signs and 'symptoms' in pregnancy that are indicative of changes occurring within the renal system; knowledge of this will help the midwife to explain these fully to the woman.

During routine antenatal check-ups, the midwife routinely performs urinalysis. Are you able to explain the significance of the findings as a whole or do you think it is appropriate that midwives just observe for evidence of proteinuria?

The hormones of pregnancy affect muscle tone and relax ligaments, so bladder control is often less effective in pregnancy and these effects may continue after pregnancy. In such cases, muscle tone can be improved by encouraging pelvic floor exercises to promote optimal continence following childbirth. Displacement of the pelvic organs resulting in anterior and posterior prolapses becomes increasingly common as the parity due to the loss of effective muscle tone and ligament support is higher, and so pelvic floor exercises should be encouraged to minimize these problems.

Application to practice

Women with pre-existing renal disease need careful monitoring and maternity care should include expert renal care. For some women, underlying renal disease may only become apparent in pregnancy when a woman fails to have the normal expected physiological fall in blood pressure in the first trimester and subsequently develops hypertension during the pregnancy. The earlier the hypertension develops, the higher is the risk for long-term problems for the mother. The fetus is also at increased risk of severe intrauterine growth retardation.

Women who have had a kidney transplant may become pregnant; however, the risk to the pregnancy must be carefully managed against the risk of reducing or modifying anti-rejection medication. It is important to consider that the anatomical placement of the donor kidney is usually much lower in the abdominal cavity. This is particularly important should the woman require surgical intervention for delivery to ensure that the donor kidney is not damaged during the procedure.

ANNOTATED FURTHER READING

Braddy CM, Files JA: Female genital mutilation: cultural awareness and clinical considerations, *J Midwifery Womens Health* 52:158–163, 2007.

A review, written for health professionals, which describes the cultural background surrounding the practice of FGM, the different types of procedures used and the complications.

Johnson MH: *Essential reproduction*, ed 6, Oxford, 2007, Blackwell Science.

An integrated and well-organized research-based textbook that explores comparative reproductive physiology of mammals, including anatomy, physiology, endocrinology, genetics and behavioural studies.

Leeson S: Abnormal cervical smears: a practical guide, *Obstet Gyn Reproduc Med* 18:163–167, 2008.

A clear description of the colposcopy (the diagnostic procedures for detecting abnormalities of the cervix and vagina) illustrated with case studies, together with consideration of the issues associated with the examination, treatment and quality control.

O'Connell HE, Eizenberg N, Rahman M, et al: The anatomy of the distal vagina: towards unity, *J Sex Med* 5:1883–1891, 2008.

A comprehensive, objective and unambiguous factual presentation of female sexual anatomy which is clearly-presented and well-illustrated.

Raynor MD, Morgan M: Female genital mutilation: unveiled and deconstructed. In Fraser D, editor: *2000 Professional studies for midwifery practice*, Edinburgh, 2000, Churchill Livingstone.

This chapter gives an excellent overview of female genital mutilation, the different classifications and prevalence and explores racial, ethnic and cultural aspects of this phenomenon. Guidance is provided for the midwifery care of women who have undergone mutilation and the health problems related to these practices.

Royal College of Obstetrics and Gynaecology (RCOG): *The management of tubal pregnancies (clinical guideline 21)*, London, 2004, RCOG.

This guideline provides a detailed account of methotrexate in the non-surgical management of ectopic pregnancy.

Stoker J: Anorectal and pelvic floor anatomy, *Best Pract Res Clin Gastroenterol* 23:463–475, 2009.

This well-illustrated review provides detailed descriptions of the layers of the pelvic floor based on magnetic resonance imaging (MRI).

Thomas R, Stanley B, Horton-Szar D: *Crash course: renal and urinary systems*, ed 3, St Louis, 2007, Mosby.

This well-illustrated book provides a useful reference text for students requiring more details of the renal and urinary systems.

Tilly JL, Telfer EE: Purification of germline stem cells from adult mammalian ovaries: a step closer towards control of the female biological clock? *Mol Hum Reprod* 15:393–398, 2009.

An interesting commentary about the evidence suggesting mammals retain the capacity to generate oocytes throughout adulthood.

Readers are recommended also to read chapters on the renal and reproductive systems in a physiology textbook, such as those listed at the end of the previous chapter.

REFERENCES

Bennett VR, Brown LK: *Myles' textbook for midwives*, ed 13, Edinburgh, 1999, Churchill Livingstone, pp 940, 941, 942, 949.

Bogin B: *Patterns of human growth*, ed 2, Cambridge, 1999, Cambridge University Press.

Brooker CG: *Human structure and function*, ed 2, St Louis, 1998, Mosby, pp 344, 345, 363, 470, 471, 473, 476, 483.

Bukovsky A, Caudle MR, Virant-Klun I, et al: Immune physiology and oogenesis in fetal and adult humans, ovarian infertility, and totipotency of adult ovarian stem cells, *Birth Defects Res C Embryo Today* 87:64–89, 2009.

Burton GJ, Woods AW, Jauniaux E, Kingdom JC: Rheological and physiological consequences of conversion of the maternal spiral arteries for uteroplacental blood flow during human pregnancy, *Placenta* 30:473–482, 2009.

Carey AJ, Beagley KW: Chlamydia trachomatis, a hidden epidemic: effects on female reproduction and options for treatment, *Am J Reprod Immunol* 63:576–586, 2010.

Griswold MD: The central role of Sertoli cells in spermatogenesis, *Semin Cell Dev Biol* 9:411–416, 1998.

Gupta GS: *Proteomics of Spermatogenesis*, 2005, New York, Springer.

Harris CL, Mizuno M, Morgan BP: Complement and complement regulators in the male reproductive system, *Mol Immunol* 43:57–67, 2006.

Hogarth CA, Griswold MD: The key role of vitamin A in spermatogenesis, *J Clin Invest* 120:956–962, 2010.

Khandelwal P, Abraham SN, Apodaca G: Cell biology and physiology of the uroepithelium, *Am J Physiol Renal Physiol* 297:F1477–F1501, 2009.

King AE, Kelly RW, Sallenave JM, et al: Innate immune defences in the human uterus during pregnancy, *Placenta* 28:1099–1106, 2007.

Kirk E, Bourne T: Pregnancy of unknown location, *Obstet Gyn Reproduc Med* 19:80–83, 2009.

Moalem S, Reidenberg JS: Does female ejaculation serve an antimicrobial purpose? *Med Hypotheses* 73:1069–1071, 2009.

NCCWCH: *Urine incontinence: the management of urinary incontinence in women*, 2006, London, National Institute for Health and Clinical Excellence.

Neilson J: Early pregnancy deaths. In Lewis G, editor: *Saving mother's lives: reviewing maternal deaths to make motherhood safer 2003–2005. The seventh report of Confidential Enquiries into Maternal Deaths in the United Kingdom, London*, 2007. Available from:www.cemach.org.

Royal College of Obstetricians and Gynaecologists: *Prevention of group B streptococcus (GBS) infection in newborn babies*, London, 2006, RCOG (amended 2007).

O'Connell HE, Eizenberg N, Rahman M, et al: The anatomy of the distal vagina: towards unity, *J Sex Med* 5:1883–1891, 2008.

Raine-Fenning N, Hopkisson J: Management of ectopic pregnancy: a clinical approach, *Obstet Gyn Reproduct Med* 19:19–25, 2009.

RCOG Royal College of Obstetricians and Gynaecologists (Scientific Advisory Committee): *The Changing Role of the Gynaecologist in the Management of Women with Cancer (Opinion Paper 10)*, 2007.

Sweet B: *Mayes' midwifery*, ed 12, London, 1996, Baillière Tindall, p 29.

Zaviacic M, Ablin RJ: The female prostate and prostate-specific antigen. Immunohistochemical localization, implications of this prostate marker in women and reasons for using the term "prostate" in the human female, *Histol Histopathol* 15:131–142, 2000.

Chapter | 3 |

Endocrinology

- To introduce the terminology used within endocrinology.
- To define the different types of hormones, their functions, main sites of production and mechanism of effects.
- To describe the role of the sex steroids.
- To relate endocrinology to the physiological process of reproduction.

INTRODUCTION

This chapter presents an overview of endocrinology and summarizes the role of hormones in the regulation of human physiology. Throughout the chapter, links to reproductive physiology will be highlighted and referenced to other chapters in the book where the relevant interactions will be described more specifically.

The endocrine system, in conjunction with the nervous system, coordinates, regulates and adjusts the internal physiology in response to changes in the external environment. The nervous system tends to react in situations where an immediate response is required, whereas the endocrine system is involved in sustaining body functions over a longer period (Table 3.1). For example, shivering is induced by neuromuscular activity to counteract a drop in the environmental temperature, whereas many body cycles, such as the menstrual cycle, are almost entirely orchestrated through hormonal systems. However, the two systems interact with each other and so some rapid responses have a hormonal component. For instance, the release of adrenaline, the fear–fight–flight reflex and hormonal release are often regulated by a neuronal pathway via the hypothalamus.

The advantage of the endocrine system over the nervous system is that it can instigate a much more diffuse response in all body tissues at about the same time and coordinate integrated responses.

Chapter case study

Zara is now just 6 weeks pregnant. She feels concerned about feeling increasingly nauseated, especially late in the evening; she actually vomited last night. Zara rings you, as her midwife, the next day expressing her concern, especially as her sister has told her that this is not the typical morning sickness of pregnancy.
- What explanations could you give Zara to the likely cause of her nausea and what advice should you give her to help her cope with her nausea?
- How is nausea and vomiting of pregnancy differentiated from hyperemesis gravidarum?
- What are the possible complications of hyperemesis and what specific treatment is required to minimize complications?

  Later on in her pregnancy, Zara has a routine appointment at about 26 weeks gestation with her midwife who undertakes routine urinalysis and discovers that Zara has glucosuria.
- What are the possible causes for this, what further investigations need to be undertaken and what advice and treatment may be required?

WHAT IS ENDOCRINOLOGY?

The endocrine system originally appeared to be a relatively simple system of discrete glands (Fig. 3.1) that secreted chemical messengers, or hormones, into the

Table 3.1 Characteristics of the nervous and endocrine systems

	NERVOUS SYSTEM	ENDOCRINE SYSTEM
Source of signal	Brain	Endocrine gland
Signal	Neurotransmitter and action potential	Hormone
Usual route	Efferent nerve	Blood
Response rate	Fast	Slow
Specificity	Specific	Diffuse
Target	Single	Multiple
Type of effect	Immediate effect	Long-term control and integration

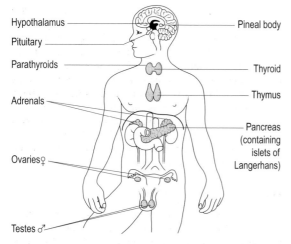

Hypothalamus — Pineal body
Pituitary
Parathyroids — Thyroid
— Thymus
Adrenals
— Pancreas (containing islets of Langerhans)
Ovaries♀
Testes♂

Fig. 3.1 The endocrine glands. (Reproduced with permission from Brooker, 1998.)

blood where they would be carried to specific target cells at a distant site, inducing a reaction. However, it is now clear that the endocrine system is more complex. Some hormones are secreted into ducts and not into blood; for instance, androgens are secreted into the seminiferous tubules. Some organs that have other functions also produce hormones. For instance, the atrium of the heart produces atrial natriuretic peptide (ANP), which inhibits reabsorption of sodium chloride in the kidneys and hence affects blood pressure. Some hormones are produced by several different glands, for instance somatostatin, which is produced by the hypothalamus, pancreas, stomach

and intestine. Although the trophoblast is the prime site of human chorionic gonadotrophin (hCG) production, it can also be produced by other tissues, albeit in very low concentrations (Iles and Chard, 1991). The placenta appears to be capable of synthesizing a very broad range of hormones and releasing factors that interact with both maternal and fetal physiology. Some substances such as noradrenaline can act as both hormone and neurotransmitter depending on their mode of delivery and whether they are released from a gland or from a nerve. The hypothalamus produces neurohormones that are important in the interaction between the endocrine and nervous systems.

Overall, the endocrine system (in partnership with the neural system) has the following functions:

- coordinates the homeostatic balance
- regulates various physiological systems such as the digestive system and reproductive system
- facilitates differentiation of the sexes in the embryonic stage and the manifestation of the secondary sexual characteristics at puberty
- modifies and induces behavioural changes within the individual.

THE EVOLUTION OF ENDOCRINOLOGY

The evolution of the endocrine system has its rudiments within the activity of single-cell (unicellular) organisms. The unicellular organisms developed the ability to be attracted to chemicals, described as a chemotactic response, or to chemicals that were vital for the functioning of the organism, described as a chemotrophic response. Equally, these organisms developed the ability to recognize noxious chemicals (toxins) and were thus able to avoid them. The cell reacting to chemical signals interacting with receptor sites upon the cell membrane and within the cytoplasm led to the development of active mobility.

As multicellular organisms developed, the group of unicellular organisms that were the prototypes of multicellular organisms evolved chemical communication as an extension of the chemotrophic response. As multicellular evolution progressed further, the cells became more differentiated and specialized. Regulation therefore became the function of more specialized types of cells. This is reflected in the developmental sequence of a fetus, beginning with the division of a single cell (see Chapter 7). With each successive division, the resulting cells are slightly different from the original zygote cell (although differentiation during the initial divisions may be induced by the presence of maternally derived factors within the cytoplasm of the zygote). Although this differentiation is primarily under genetic control, it is achieved through a process of induction from chemical signals produced by one cell type that influence the division of other neighbouring cells. The altered gene expression of the dividing cells results in a changed morphology and developmental pathway.

As organisms became larger and more complex, cell-to-cell communication became more complicated. It evolved in two ways: the endocrine system (of chemical transmission via the circulating blood system) and the neural system (via transmission of an action potential; see Chapter 1). Under the traditional approach to biological science, the endocrine and neural systems were always considered in isolation; however, they are now considered to be extensions of the same system that are highly interactive. Many endocrine responses are initiated by a neuronal influence. Many neurotransmitters and neuromodulators have also been found to be endocrine hormones.

CLASSIFICATION OF HORMONES

Hormones regulate metabolism, activate or inhibit the immune system, stimulate or inhibit growth, induce or suppress apoptosis (see below) and prepare the body to respond (such as fleeing or fighting) or undergo transition to a new stage of life such as puberty, pregnancy or the menopause. Hormones are produced by almost every organ and type of tissue; they function as cellular messengers. The action of hormones depends on the responses of the target cells and the pattern of hormonal secretion. Endocrine means 'secreted inwards' and is applied to hormones that fit the classical description of being secreted into the bloodstream and having an effect at a distant target. There are also exocrine hormones, which are 'secreted outwards' into ducts. These include hormones that are secreted into the vas deferens and uterine tubes.

A number of hormones have a local or paracrine effect, diffusing short distances to act on neighbouring cells or cells separated only by an intracellular space. Examples of a paracrine response are the effects of testosterone and anti-Müllerian hormone (AMH; also known as Müllerian-inhibiting hormone or substance, MIH or MIS) on sexual differentiation (see Chapter 5). If the hormone produced acts upon the same cell that produced it, it is described as autocrine. For example, an autocrine hormone may induce cellular division or signal the programmed death of the cell (apoptosis). If it affects adjacent cells and has a very localized action, it is described as a juxtacrine hormone. Therefore, the effect of a hormone depends on how and where it is secreted, the mode of transport (e.g. whether it is soluble or carried by a binding protein) and how quickly it is metabolized or inactivated.

Neuroendocrine hormones are synthesized in specialized neurons, and their effects can also be paracrine in nature (these are usually described as neurotransmitters and neuromodulators). Oxytocin is an example of a neuroendocrine hormone. It is released from the posterior lobe of the pituitary gland and influences the contractility of the myometrium (see Chapter 13) and myoepithelial cells in the breast (see Chapter 16). In these respects, oxytocin has an endocrine effect, but in many mammals it also modifies female behaviour by inducing parental behaviour in the presence of the sex steroids (Insel, 1992). Oxytocin is thought to influence the successful transition to parenthood in different ways; maternal behavioural changes tending to influence affectionate behaviour and emotional bonding and paternal parenting behaviour tending to affect play and social interaction with their infants (Gordon et al., 2010).

A pheromone is a hormone produced by an individual that induces a response, usually social, within another member of the same species. Releaser pheromones stimulate rapid behavioural responses such as attracting potential mates. Primer pheromones act via the olfactory and neuroendocrine system to produce delayed responses which are usually developmental. Receptors for pheromones are found on the vomeronasal organ close to the nasal cavity of mammals, which use pheromones to indicate identity of kin or family territory. It is controversial as to whether the human vomeronasal organ retains a function; some scientists think it is involved in social behaviour such as pair bonding, parental attachment, sexual attraction and synchrony of menstrual cycles (Halpern and Martinez-Marcos, 2003). The synchronization of menstrual cycles within a group of women, responses between lactating women and their offspring and female responses to non-odorants in male perspiration are suggested to be examples of pheromone effects in humans (Bhutta, 2007).

Secretion of hormones is influenced by a number of factors, including the nervous system, hormone-binding proteins, plasma concentrations of nutrients and ions, environmental changes and other hormones, such as stimulating and releasing hormones.

Hormone structure

Hormones can be classified according to their structure (see Table 3.2). Steroid hormones and eicosanoids (the prostaglandin family of hormones) are lipids. The other classes are protein and peptide hormones and monoamines.

Steroid hormones

The steroid group of hormones consists of the sex steroids (progestagens, androgens and oestrogens), the glucocorticoids, mineralocorticoids, thyroid hormones and 1,25-dihydroxyvitamin D_3. Steroid hormones are derived from cholesterol which is synthesized from acetate (Fig. 3.2). As well as being the precursor for the steroid hormones, cholesterol is also an important structural component of cell membranes, providing rigidity.

The first and common step in the biosynthesis of sex steroids is the formation of pregnenolone, which is rate-limiting, and therefore important in controlling production of sex steroids. Pregnenolone is produced on the

Table 3.2 Classification of hormones and examples

Lipid hormones	Steroid hormones	Sex steroids, e.g. androgens, oestrogens and progestagens
		Glucocorticoids, e.g. cortisol
		Mineralocorticoids, e.g. aldosterone
		Thyroid hormones; 1,25-Dihydrovitamin D_3
	Eicosanoids	Prostaglandins
		Leukotrienes
Protein hormones	Gonadotrophic glycoproteins	Follicle-stimulating hormone (FSH)
		Luteinizing hormone (LH)
		Human chorionic gonadotrophin (hCG)
		Thyroid-stimulating hormone (TSH)
	Somatotrophic polypeptides	Prolactin (PRL)
		Human placental lactogen (hPL)
		Growth hormone (GH)
	Cytokines	Insulin
		Activins and inhibins
		Anti-Müllerian hormone (AMH)
		Interferons
		Growth factors
Small peptides		Gonadotrophin-releasing hormone (GnRH)
		Oxytocin (OXY)
		Antidiuretic hormone (ADH or vasopressin)
		β-Endorphin
		Vasoactive intestinal peptide (VIP)
Monoamines	Catecholamines	Adrenaline, noradrenaline and dopamine
		Melatonin
		Dopamine

Adapted from Johnson and Everitt, 1995.

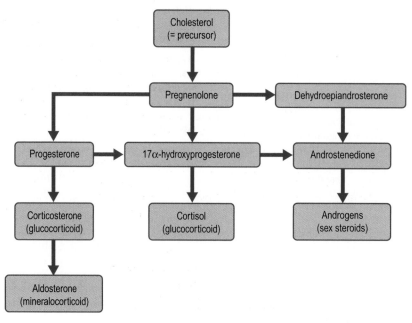

Fig. 3.2 Steroid hormone production.

inner mitochondrial membrane whereas the next stages take place in the smooth endoplasmic reticulum (SER).

The three classes of sex steroids are structurally related, which offers the opportunity for interconversion. This means that a genetic defect in one of the steps can result not only in a deficiency of the normal amount of the product but also in an excess of another sex steroid. For instance, a genetic deficiency of the enzyme that converts 17α-hydroxyprogesterone to the precursor of cortisol results in increased levels of 17α-hydroxyprogesterone, which is converted into androstenedione and then into androgens. The unusually high level of androgens can cause masculinization of the female fetus. These structural similarities mean that the steroid hormones can affect the activity of other steroid hormones by exerting agonistic and antagonistic properties at the receptor level (see below). However, the effects of the hormones vary depending on their structure (see Table 3.3).

The main role of androgens is in the development and maintenance of masculine characteristics and fertility. Similarly, the dominant role of oestrogens is in development and maintenance of feminine characteristics and fertility.

The key role for progesterone is the preparation for pregnancy and its maintenance. However, all the steroid hormones are produced in men and women but with varying profiles; therefore, for instance, men produce more androgens than women but also produce some oestrogen. Although androgens are primarily associated with the development and maintenance of male sex characteristics, they also affect sexual behaviour in women (Johnson, 2007).

As steroid hormones are lipid-soluble, they are able to diffuse freely across the cell membrane and have their effect within the target cell. In the cytoplasm, the steroid hormones may be altered. The receptor sites for thyroid hormone and the sex steroids are within the nucleus. Specific receptors for the other steroid hormones are within the cytoplasm; binding usually results in cleavage of smaller 'heat-shock' proteins from the receptors. Steroid hormones exert their effect by altering ribonucleic acid (RNA) synthesis and subsequent protein synthesis (Box 3.1). The steroid-receptor ligand binds to specific segments of DNA, steroid response elements (SRE) in promoter regions of the gene in that section of DNA, affecting the rate of transcription and gene expression. Protein synthesis can be increased

Table 3.3 Biological activity and effects of the sex steroids

SEX STEROID	FAMILY MEMBERS (AND APPROXIMATE BIOLOGICAL ACTIVITY)	MAIN EFFECTS
Androgens	5α-dihydrotestosterone (100%) Testosterone (50%) Androstenedione (8%) Dehydroepiandrosterone (4%)	Differentiation of male embryo Secondary sex characteristics Spermatogenesis Male secondary sex characteristics Sexual and aggressive behaviour Growth promoting, protein anabolism, ossification and erythropoiesis
Oestrogens	Oestradiol-17β (E_2) (100%) Oestriol (E_3) (10%) Oestrone (E_1) (1%)	Female secondary sex characteristics Prepares uterus for ovulation and fertilization Vascular effects – increased blood flow, neovascularization Growth-promoting effects on endometrium and breasts Primes endometrium for progesterone action Mildly anabolic Increases calcification of bones May be associated with sexual behaviour
Progestagens	Progesterone (100%) 17α-hydroxyprogesterone 20α-hydroxyprogesterone (5%)	Prepares uterus for pregnancy Maintains pregnancy (17α-OHP) (40–70%) Stimulates glandular growth of breasts (but suppresses milk secretion) Affects sodium and water excretion Mildly catabolic Relaxes smooth muscle tone Affects appetite and thirst, metabolic rate, sensitivity to carbon dioxide

Adapted from Johnson and Everitt, 1995.

(or decreased) within 30 min, and the effects of steroid hormones are therefore relatively slow in action compared with those of protein hormones. The term 'anabolic steroids' describes the effect of steroid hormones in influencing new tissue growth.

The other class of lipid hormones is the eicosanoids (prostaglandins and leukotrienes) which have an important role in reproduction. Eicosanoids are formed from an arachidonic acid precursor, generated by the activity of either phospholipase C or phospholipase A_2 (Fig. 3.3). Arachidonic acid production appears to be the rate-limiting step. Phospholipase A_2 is present in an inactive form in lysosomes in cells that are released if the cell membranes become unstable. Most tissues of the body including the myometrium, cervix, ovary, placenta and fetal membranes synthesize prostaglandins. They have a short half-life and are metabolized quickly. They have an important role in amplifying signals at the onset of labour (see Chapter 13). Leukotrienes are also synthesized from arachidonic acid by the enzyme 5-lipoxygenase in leukocytes and macrophages.

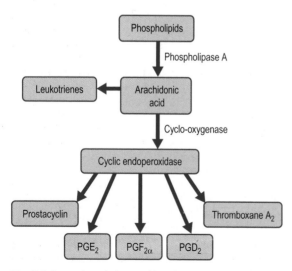

Fig. 3.3 Formation of eicosanoids.

They are involved in inflammatory reactions particularly in asthma and allergy and also seem to be important in pregnancy.

Protein, peptide and monoamine hormones

Protein and peptide hormones bind to receptors located on or within the cell membrane. They initiate plasma membrane depolarization and a cascade of second-messenger systems and chemical changes within the cytoplasm, generating a faster response than steroid hormones. They primarily affect the functioning of the cell by stimulation or inhibition. Their action is initiated through the activation of G-proteins located within the cell cytoplasm, which initiate various chemical reactions (Box 3.2). G-proteins may open ion channels or stimulate phosphorylation of internal proteins, thus generating the signalling cascade. Many peptide hormones function as neurotransmitters in the brain. The monoamine hormones are derivatives of the amino acids tryptophan and tyrosine.

Gonadotrophic glycoproteins

This group includes TSH (thyroid stimulating hormone), FSH, LH and hCG, all of which are structurally similar. Their structure is a globular protein which is a heterodimer formed of two polypeptide chains, a common alpha subunit and a unique beta subunit. The beta subunit has unique carbohydrate side-chains that bestow stability and biological activity. hCG is produced by the placental tissue (the cytotrophoblasts produce the alpha subunit and the syncytiotrophoblast produces the beta subunit), whereas the other gonadotrophic glycoproteins are produced by the anterior pituitary gland.

Somatomammotrophic polypeptides

This group of hormones includes prolactin (PRL), human placental lactogen (hPL; also known as human placental somatomammotrophin) and growth hormone (GH);

GH is also known as somatotrophin, which has marked effects on tissue growth including the breasts. Their structure is a single polypeptide chain. PRL and hPL are involved with lactation. GH has a role in puberty including breast development. Although PRL and GH are pituitary hormones, the placenta also produces them in addition to hPL. However, the activity of the placental hormones is often not exactly the same as that of the pituitary hormones. For instance, placental GH has a higher affinity for the PRL receptor than has pituitary GH. The somatomammotrophic polypeptide hormones affect growth including angiogenesis, functioning of the immune system and metabolism.

Cytokines

Cytokines are small polypeptide chains. There is a large number of cytokines including inhibin, activin, epidermal growth factors and AMH (see Chapters 5 and 13 and Box 3.3). Cytokines have a broad range of activity. They are usually made in a variety of cell types rather than in a specific gland. Cytokines act on many different cell types, often interacting with and modulating each other's responses. Several cytokines have similar and overlapping functions. They usually have paracrine activity and often modulate or mediate the actions of other types of hormone.

Box 3.3 **Anti-Müllerian hormone**

A good example of the range of activity demonstrated by cytokines is AMH which has long been known for its role in promoting regression of the Müllerian ducts in the male embryo (see Chapter 5). The female embryo does not produce AMH, so the Müllerian ducts develop into female internal genitalia. AMH is secreted from the Sertoli cells of the testes and continues to be produced in male children but declines throughout adulthood. Women produce AMH, from the granulosa cells of the ovary, from puberty onwards; the role of AMH in the ovary is to limit excessive follicular recruitment by FSH, so it controls the number of primary follicles formed. It seems that puberty is preceded by a rise in AMH in girls and by a fall in AMH in boys. The changing levels of AMH also affect brain development via AMH receptors and are thought to mediate gender-specific behaviour. In women, AMH seems to be one of the best markers for ovarian reserve (the number of remaining follicles in the ovaries) and can be used to predict menopause and also the likely effectiveness of assisted reproductive technologies (Broekmans et al., 2008). Synthetic AMH is potentially a therapy for rapidly proliferating cancer cells and endometriosis as it inhibits not only growth and development of Müllerian ducts but also other tissues which express AMH receptors; as it has little known toxicity, it appears to be a suitable adjunct to other treatment and has an effect on some drug-resistant tumours (MacLaughlin and Donahoe, 2010).

Cytokines act by binding to their specific receptors on the cell membrane; typically, these receptors are also tyrosine kinase (enzymes that transfer a phosphate group to a tyrosine residue of protein which then regulates the activity of other enzymes).

Small peptide hormones

This group of hormones includes gonadotrophin (GnRH), a decapeptide (i.e. a chain of 10 amino acids) from the hypothalamus, and other releasing hormones, oxytocin, antidiuretic hormone (ADH; also known as vasopressin), β-endorphin (described in Chapter 13) and vasoactive intestinal peptide (VIP). Most of these small peptide hormones are initially produced in the form of pre-prohormones (large inactive polypeptide precursors). The pre-prohormone is then processed in the endoplasmic reticulum to form a prohormone. The processing may involve glycosylation (addition of polysaccharides) or removal of the N-terminal signal sequence. Prohormones often contain redundant amino acid residues that were required to direct the folding of the molecule into its active configuration but then have no further function. Endopeptidases cleave the prohormone, thereby producing the mature functional form of the hormone just before it is released from the cell. Some of the 'pro'-fragments of the prohormones also exert a biological effect. The identification of secondary sites of hormone production, such as GnRH being produced in the placenta and ovary and oxytocin being produced in the testes and uterus, suggests that these small peptide hormones have diverse roles and may function as neurotransmitters (Johnson, 2007).

Monoamine hormones

This group includes catecholamines (dopamine, adrenaline and noradrenaline) and melatonin, all of which are derived from tyrosine (an amino acid) and may have a role in neuroendocrine control mechanisms. The medulla of the adrenal gland is a modified sympathetic ganglion; its cell bodies release adrenaline and noradrenaline (in the ratio 4:1) into the blood. Its effects, therefore, augment sympathetic nervous system activity. Dopamine is synthesized from tyrosine and then can be sequentially modified to form noradrenaline and then adrenaline. Dopamine released from the hypothalamus affects prolactin secretion (see Chapter 16). Melatonin, from the pineal gland, may have a role in seasonal and environmental influences on reproductive capability, which are particularly important in species other than humans.

HORMONE TRANSPORT

Peptide and protein hormones are water-soluble and are carried dissolved in the blood, whereas steroid hormones circulate bound to plasma proteins. When hormones are secreted into the blood supply, a large proportion become protein-bound, leaving only a small proportion free (unbound and able to access the target cell) and physiologically active. There are many types of hormone-binding proteins, all of which are colloidal in nature. Some hormones bind with great affinity to specific proteins. Other proteins may bind to numerous different hormones with different affinity rates that may be affected by the concentration of the hormone. Therefore, the amount of hormone present may affect its activity. For instance, oxytocin at high concentrations binds to ADH (or vasopressin) receptors within the renal tubule. During labour, levels of oxytocin do not normally rise until the end of the first stage. However, exogenous oxytocin can be administered to augment uterine contractions. If the administration of oxytocin is high and prolonged, however, water retention can occur because oxytocin also stimulates the ADH receptors. This overlap in the biological activity of hormones is described as promiscuity.

HORMONAL REGULATION

One of the most important functions of the endocrine system is maintenance of the internal environment. This 'steady' state is described as homeostasis (see Chapter 1). Homeostatic mechanisms buffer changes within the external environmental conditions. For example, mammals have evolved to be homeothermic (warm-blooded) so that the chemical processes essential for physiological function proceed under optimal conditions of temperature. Fluctuations in temperature are monitored and the homeostatic mechanisms ensure that body temperature is held within narrowly defined limits. Homeostasis is achieved through the integration of the neural system with the endocrine system, commonly referred to as feedback systems.

As mentioned above, hormonal release is often instigated by neurological stimulation. Hormone release may also be stimulated by another hormone. Factors that facilitate the release of hormones are referred to as positive influences and factors that inhibit the release of hormones are termed negative influences. The negative feedback tends to slow down a process and maintain stability whereas positive feedback tends to speed up a process and generate rapid change.

Positive feedback

Positive feedback describes a specialized chain of events involving one or more hormones in which there is a cycle of positive effects, greatly amplifying the original signal (Fig. 3.4). An example of positive feedback is the maintained production of PRL secretion from the anterior pituitary gland during lactation. Suckling of the infant stimulates PRL secretion, which maintains lactation.

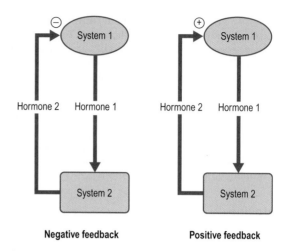

Fig. 3.4 Negative and positive feedback.

If suckling decreases or stops then the amount of stimulation decreases and PRL production is reduced. Other examples of positive feedback include coagulation of blood and the hormonal control of parturition.

Negative feedback

Negative feedback describes a similar specialized chain of events involving one or more hormones, except that here there is a cycle of negative influence (Fig. 3.4). An example of negative feedback is that the anterior lobe of the pituitary gland produces TSH, which stimulates the thyroid gland to produce thyroid hormone. TSH production is, however, inhibited by the presence of thyroid hormone, the downstream production of the pathway.

Activation and deactivation

Hormones may be released by the presence of a certain stimulus. For example, insulin release depends on plasma glucose levels. Many specific metabolic pathways are activated by the build-up of specific metabolites within the internal environment. Similarly, some hormones may be inhibited by the presence of a signal. This may be another hormone, such as adrenaline, neurological, such as light stimulation inhibiting melatonin release from the pineal gland, or chemical, such as insulin inhibiting the release of glucagon.

HORMONE ACTION

Hormones have their effects by interacting with a specific receptor. The receptor structure corresponds to the structure of the hormone (or 'ligand') so that the two fit together in a way which is often described as being a lock and a key. The interaction of the hormone and its receptor triggers the intercellular steps resulting in the consequences of the hormone action. The effects of hormones depend on a number of factors including affinity of the hormone for the receptor, agonist–antagonist effects, receptor number and hormone levels. Receptor number is important in the selection of the dominant follicle (see Chapter 4) and the increased sensitivity of the uterus to oxytocin in early labour (see Chapter 13). A lack of receptor expression can cause abnormal development, such as testicular feminization in the absence of androgen receptors (see Chapter 5). Genetic variations in the structure of receptors, for instance caused by single nucleotide polymorphisms, can influence the binding of the hormone to its receptor and affect an individual's sensitivity and responses to the hormone (Johnson, 2007). Hormone levels are affected by local circulation, stability, metabolism and excretion. Many hormones are inactivated within the blood, liver and their specific target cells. The breakdown of hormones is achieved by the action of various enzymes.

Hormone secretion may fluctuate with time. For instance, secretion of testosterone and prolactin exhibit circadian rhythms (characteristic pattern of changes during a 24-h period), whereas GnRH, FSH, LH and PRL are released in a pulsatile fashion. A continuous infusion of these hormones would diminish their response as the constant occupancy of the receptors uncouples them from the second-messenger system, effectively exhausting the cell. A high blood flow increases dissipation of hormones and is likely to increase a systemic endocrine response but decreases paracrine response.

Levels and metabolism of binding proteins will also affect the activity of hormones. The protein-bound hormone complex renders the bound hormone inactive but also protects the hormone from enzymatic degradation. Hormone turnover may be affected by multiple sites of production. Different tissues may have different feedback mechanisms controlling hormone production. Replicating hormone production occurs physiologically from the placental cells, but also pathologically from tumours. Hormones and their metabolites may be excreted via the kidney during the formation of urine. As the rate of excretion of many hormones is proportional to the rate of secretion, excretion rate indicates secretion rate. Generally, peptide hormones are readily metabolized by blood enzymes and are easily excreted, so their half-life in the blood is short compared with that of protein-bound steroid hormones.

Levels of hormones may change within the tissues themselves as hormones can be converted to a form with a higher biological activity. For instance, the enzyme 5α-reductase in many of the target tissues for testosterone converts testosterone to 5α-dihydrotestosterone, which has twice the biological activity. A deficiency of this enzyme can cause poor development of the male external

---

Box 3.4 5α-Reductase deficiency

In the Dominican Republic, there is an increased incidence of an autosomal recessive condition resulting in 5α-reductase deficiency (Imperato-McGinley et al., 1986). 5α-Reductase is the enzyme that converts testosterone to the more biologically active 5α-dihydrotestosterone within the target cell. The lack of enzyme means that there is a diminished response to testosterone during fetal sexual development (see Chapter 5), so an affected baby may have small and ambiguous genitalia, appearing female at birth (testicular feminization). However, at puberty the surge in testosterone production is adequate to stimulate the cells; therefore, the child then develops male external genitalia. This condition is known as 'Guevodoces' (penis-at-twelve).

---

genitalia (see Box 3.4). The target cell may metabolize a hormone. Peptide hormones are endocytosed and catabolized and the receptors are recycled.

Agonist and antagonist effects

An agonist is a ligand or substance that binds to a receptor on the cell membrane or within the cytoplasm and activates a response. An antagonist also binds to the receptor often partially and does not therefore activate it, thus blocking or inhibiting the normal physiological response of the receptor. By occupying the receptor site, a competitive antagonist blocks the action of the specific hormone (agonist) that normally binds to the site; antagonists can also be non-competitive. A partial agonist activates a receptor to a lesser degree and elicits a smaller physiological response. The physiological overlap of oxytocin and ADH is an example of an agonist effect. The molecular structures of oxytocin and ADH are similar. Oxytocin can elicit the same biological response as ADH because it can bind to the same receptor sites. Therefore, oxytocin is agonistic to the ADH receptor and may be described as an ADH agonist. Progesterone acts as a glucocorticoid agonist and affects metabolism (see Chapter 11).

A number of natural and environmental chemicals can mimic the effects of hormones and act as antagonists or agonists. These are detailed in Box 3.5.

ENDOCRINE GLANDS, HORMONES AND REPRODUCTION

Hormones can influence the ability of the target cell to respond by regulating the number of hormone receptors. Prolonged exposure to a low concentration of hormone may increase the number of receptors expressed by the cell (described as 'up-regulation'). Conversely, prolonged

Box 3.5 **Environmental influences on hormonal expression**

A number of environmental chemicals, such as phthalates (plasticizers) and PCBs (polychlorinated biphenyls), exert hormone-like effects. The chemicals may mimic or antagonize endogenous hormones, disrupt synthesis and metabolism of endogenous hormones and/or affect receptor expression. These oestrogenic contaminants were initially linked to abnormal sexual development in wild animals and fish but effects on humans, such as reproductive abnormalities in male fetuses and effects on male fertility, are also under investigation. The pesticide DDT has been associated with reduced sperm counts and decreased libido. Chemicals used in plastics have been demonstrated to have oestrogenic properties. Degradation of alkylphenols used in detergents releases oestrogenic compounds. These environmental chemicals have been implicated in the increased incidence of testicular cancer, hypospadias (incomplete fusion of the urogenital folds of the penis), cryptorchidism (undescended testicles), breast cancer and endometriosis. It has also been suggested that fetal development, particularly of reproductive organs, may be affected by exposure to these compounds. The protective effect of phytoestrogens (see Chapter 4) may be related to interaction with environmental contaminants. Phytoestrogens, such as genestein from soy protein, may affect the length of the menstrual cycle and have similar protective effects on cardiovascular health and bone mineralization as endogenous oestrogen.

exposure to a high concentration of hormone might decrease the number of receptors for that hormone (described as 'down-regulation'). For instance, the expression of oxytocin receptors is down-regulated on prolonged exposure to oxytocin; this may explain the lack of response to exogenous oxytocin in induction of labour (see Chapter 13). Hormones can also affect receptors for other hormones, increasing or decreasing their effectiveness. When one hormone has to be present for another to have its full effect, it is described as permissive.

The endocrine glands and their main functions are summarized in Table 3.4.

The pituitary gland

The pituitary gland is a pea-sized gland at the base of the brain which is connected to the hypothalamus via the tuberoinfundibular pathway. It is often likened to a 'master' gland as it secretes hormones which regulate a broad range of body activities including trophic hormones which regulate other target endocrine glands. The pituitary gland has two main lobes, the anterior lobe (or adenohypophysis) and the posterior lobe (or neurohypophysis) (Fig. 3.5). The anterior lobe originates from the primitive oral cavity,

whereas the posterior lobe is a projection of the hypothalamus. The anterior lobe produces hormones such as LH and FSH that regulate gametogenesis and steroidogenesis by the gonads (see Chapter 4). The maintenance of lactation is achieved through the production of PRL (see Chapter 16). The anterior lobe also produces PRL, TSH, GH, adrenocorticotrophic hormone (ACTH) and endorphins. The posterior lobe of the pituitary gland does not produce hormones but stores and secretes oxytocin and ADH, the latter being also known as vasopressin. The tiny intermediate lobe of the human pituitary gland, which is almost indistinguishable from the anterior pituitary, produces melanocyte-stimulating hormone (MSH).

The thyroid gland

The thyroid gland is butterfly-shaped and is the largest endocrine gland. It lies in front of the trachea, posterior to the larynx, and produces thyroid hormones. Thyroid hormones affect all tissues in the body and regulate metabolic rate, growth, brain development and function. The thyroid hormones, which contain iodide, are thyroxine (T_4) which is circulated and converted to the active form, and triiodothyronine (T_3) within the target tissues. Essentially T_4 is the prohormone and T_3 is 5–10 times more active than T_4. During pregnancy, the fetus initially utilizes maternally derived thyroxine, so the maternal thyroid gland hypertrophies (increases in size) to compensate for this. This is achieved by the thyrotrophic effect of hCG and a placentally derived hormone called human chorionic thyrotrophin. Thyroid hormones are essential for development and maturation of the fetal brain. Maternal thyroid gland activity is stimulated by oestrogens and hCG; the changes contribute to glucose provision for the fetus. The increase in thyroid activity increases the basal metabolic rate of the pregnant woman, resulting in an increase of maternal and fetal oxygen consumption. The parafollicular cells of the thyroid gland produce calcitonin, which is involved in the metabolism of calcium and phosphorus, in response to hypercalaemia. Calcitonin promotes the uptake of calcium by bone; levels increase in pregnancy and it is suggested that this may protect the maternal skeleton from excessive bone resorption. Hyperthyroidism is an overactive thyroid gland and hypothyroidism is an underactive thyroid gland; both conditions can affect fertility and treatment of either condition can be affected by pregnancy.

The parathyroid glands

There are about four parathyroid glands, closely associated with the thyroid gland, that produce parathyroid hormone to maintain calcium homeostasis. Parathyroid hormone levels increase in response to a fall in serum calcium; it causes a decrease in urinary calcium excretion, increased

Table 3.4 The endocrine system

ENDOCRINE GLAND	MAIN FUNCTION(S)
Hypothalamus	Regulates homeostasis Controls pituitary function Integrates nervous and endocrine systems
Pituitary	'Master gland' Stimulates other endocrine glands
Pineal body	Produces melatonin during nocturnal period Involved in biological rhythms and body 'clock'
Thyroid	Affects metabolism and growth
Parathyroid glands	Maintenance of calcium homeostasis
Thymus	Development of immune system
Adrenal glands	Medulla: 　Secretion of catecholamines (adrenaline and noradrenaline) Cortex: 　Secretion of corticosteroids 　—glucocorticoids affect metabolism and responses to stress 　—mineralocorticoids affect electrolyte and fluid homeostasis Sex steroids
Pancreas	Insulin and glucagon control cellular uptake of glucose and regulate cellular metabolism affecting blood glucose Somatostatin: growth hormone-inhibiting hormone
Gonads (testes or ovaries)	Produce sex steroids that affect reproductive cycles and gamete formation
Kidney	Erythrocyte production stimulated by erythropoietin
Heart	Atrial natriuretic peptide lowers blood pressure
Adipose tissue	Appetite suppressed by leptin Affects steroid hormone metabolism

mobilization of calcium from bone and, indirectly, causes an increase in calcium absorption (via an increase in vitamin D). Although parathyroid hormone is the primary regulator of 1,25-dihydroxyvitamin D synthesis in the non-pregnant state, it may not be particularly important in pregnancy as levels do not change much in pregnancy, and women without functioning parathyroid glands still have a raised level of circulating 1,25-dihydroxyvitamin D during pregnancy (Fig. 3.6).

The adrenal glands

The adrenal glands are triangle-shaped glands situated on top of the kidneys that regulate the response to stress by synthesizing corticosteroids (from the cortex of the gland) and catecholamines (from the medulla of the gland). Glucocorticoids, such as corticosterone and cortisol, are involved in the regulation of carbohydrate metabolism, the body's responses to stress and the regulation of the immune system. Carbohydrate metabolism is altered during pregnancy but it would appear that the fetal–maternal interaction concerning carbohydrate metabolism is mediated through the action of other hormones (see Chapter 11). Corticotrophin-releasing hormone (CRH) from the hypothalamus controls the release of ACTH from the anterior pituitary which regulates the production of hormones from the adrenal cortex; this is described as the hypothalamic–pituitary–adrenal axis. In pregnancy, maternal CRH levels increase dramatically, predominantly as a result of placental production. Placental CRH also enters the fetal circulation and may play a role in fetal organ maturation and also parturition. During pregnancy, ACTH levels double and cortisol levels increase. The adrenal glands also produce steroid hormones and mineralocorticoids such as aldosterone, which are principally involved in the regulation of the electrolyte balance of the body (see Chapter 2). Aldosterone levels increase in pregnancy as a response to increased renin and angiotensin II levels.

The gonads

The gonads are responsible for the production of the sex steroids. In men, the testes predominantly produce testosterone. In women, the ovary produces oestrogens and progesterone. The endocrine cells of the gonads lack the enzymes to produce mineralocorticoids and glucocorticoids. The gonadal function of the regulation of reproduction is discussed in Chapter 4.

FETAL ENDOCRINOLOGY

Many of the endocrine and metabolic changes of pregnancy are results of hormonal signals originating from fetal–placental unit (FPU), which is a major site of protein and steroid hormone production and secretion. The interactions of neuronal and hormonal factors mediated by the FPU are critical in directing the initiation and maintenance of pregnancy, maternal adaptations to pregnancy, fetal growth and development, coordination of the timing of parturition

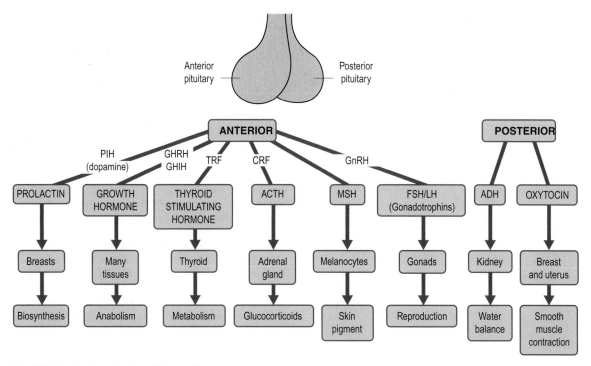

Fig. 3.5 The pituitary gland and its secretions.

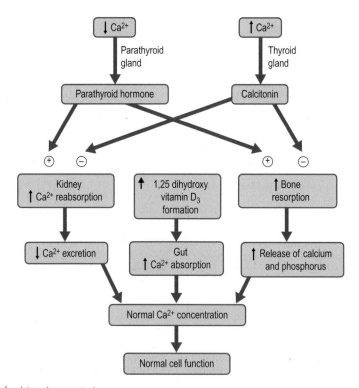

Fig. 3.6 Maintenance of calcium homeostasis.

and preparation for lactation. Production of oestradiol involves cooperation between the maternal and fetoplacental systems (see Chapter 11). The fetal endocrine system is also involved in the differentiation and development of the sexes (see Chapter 5).

Key points

- The endocrine system and the nervous system interact and are involved in communication and maintenance of the internal environment.
- The classic description of a hormone as a substance released from a gland and transported in the blood to its target organ(s) cannot be applied to all hormones.
- Hormones can be classified structurally as monoamine, protein, peptide or lipid (steroid) hormones.
- Steroid hormones are produced from cholesterol precursors and include mineralocorticoids (such as aldosterone), glucocorticoids (such as cortisol) and sex steroids (oestrogen, progesterone and testosterone).
- Steroid hormones circulate bound to plasma proteins and exert their effect by altering protein synthesis in their target cells.
- Peptide hormones and catecholamines circulate in the plasma and affect signal transduction in their target cells.
- Hormonal effects are modulated by binding proteins, receptor expression, hormone metabolism and agonist–antagonist effects.
- Testosterone and oestrogen are responsible for the development and maintenance of sexual characteristics and fertility. Progesterone is involved in preparation for and maintenance of pregnancy.

Application to practice

During pregnancy, apart from the growth of the fetus, there is much tissue growth and development within the mother that is controlled by the action of hormonal changes within the maternal system and interactions with hormones produced by the fetal–placental complex.

Throughout the entire antenatal, perinatal and postnatal periods, the midwife should be able to observe these physiological changes and use them to form an assessment of the progression and well-being of the pregnant woman and fetus.

Gestational diabetes results from a reduced capacity to increase insulin production to compensate for the increase of glucose orchestrated by placental hormones and, in severe cases insulin therapy may be required to minimize the risks to the fetus, for example macrosomia. Women with type one diabetes may require significantly more insulin during pregnancy to compensate for the pregnancy induced hyperglycaemia.

Other endocrine disorders are also complicated by pregnancy, for example, hypothyroidism resulting in an increase in the amount of thyroxine required as the pregnancy progresses.

ANNOTATED FURTHER READING

Holt RIG, Hanley NA: *Essential endocrinology and diabetes*, Oxford, 2006, Wiley Blackwell.

An excellent textbook which is supported by introductory chapter summaries, integrated case studies and clear diagrams.

Carlson NR: *Physiology of behaviour*, ed 9, New York, 2009, Pearson Education.

An interesting and comprehensive exploration of how physiological processes regulate and influence the behaviour and psychology of an organism; this textbook

describes sexual behaviour in depth, relating it to endocrine and neurological interactions.

Greenstein B, Wood D: *Endocrinology at a glance*, ed 2, Oxford, 2006, Wiley Blackwell.

Introduces the study of endocrinology in a clear, precise and easy-to-understand way.

Johnson MH: *Essential reproduction*, ed 6, Oxford, 2007, Blackwell Science.

An integrated and well-organized research-based textbook that explores

comparative reproductive physiology of mammals, including anatomy, physiology, endocrinology, genetics and behavioural studies.

Finlayson A, Horton-Szar D: *Crash course: endocrine and reproductive systems*, ed 3, London, 2007, Mosby.

This book provides essential information for students who need to have a basic understanding of the endocrine and reproductive systems.

REFERENCES

Bhutta MF: Sex and the nose: human pheromonal responses, *J R Soc Med* 100:268–274, 2007.

Broekmans FJ, Visser JA, Laven JS, et al: Anti-Mullerian hormone and ovarian dysfunction, *Trends Endocrinol Metab* 19:340–347, 2008.

Brooker CG: *Human structure and function*, ed 2, St Louis, 1998, Mosby.

Gordon I, Zagoory-Sharon O, Leckman JF, et al: Oxytocin and the

Development of Parenting in Humans, *Biol Psychiatry* 2010.

Halpern M, Martinez-Marcos A: Structure and function of the vomeronasal system: an update. *Progress Neurobiol.* 70:245–318, 2003.

Iles RK, Chard T: Human chorionic gonadotrophin expression by bladder cancers: biology and clinical potential, *J Urol* 145:453, 1991.

Imperato-McGinley J, Gautier T, Peterson RE, et al: The prevalence of 5-alpha-reductase deficiency in children with ambiguous genitalia in the Dominican Republic, *J Urol* 136:867–873, 1986.

Insel TR: Oxytocin—a neuropeptide for affiliation: evidence from behavioral, receptor autoradiographic and comparative studies.

Psychoneuroendocrinology 17:3–35, 1992.

Johnson MH: *Essential reproduction*, ed 6, Oxford, 2007, Blackwell.

MacLaughlin DT, Donahoe PK: Mullerian inhibiting substance/ anti-Mullerian hormone: a potential therapeutic agent for human ovarian and other cancers. *Future Oncol* 6:391–405, 2010.

Chapter | 4 |

Reproductive cycles

INTRODUCTION

The function of the ovaries is to release female gametes or ova (singular: ovum or 'egg'; see Box 4.1) and to produce the steroid hormones oestrogen and progesterone. Relatively few oocytes (immature ova) are produced during a woman's reproductive life compared with the number of male gametes (spermatozoa). The ovarian follicles produce all the oocytes, steroid hormones and inhibin (a cytokine which inhibits synthesis and secretion of FSH). The cyclical pattern of hormone release has cyclical effects on the whole body, and behaviour, of the woman. The effects are particularly pronounced on the genital tract, facilitating its functions in gamete transport and the implantation and

development of the conceptus. The first part of the cycle, the follicular phase, is dominated by the release of oestrogen produced by the developing follicles (Fig. 4.1). This oestrogen-dominant phase prepares the woman for ovulation, receipt of the sperm and fertilization of the oocyte. In the second half of the cycle, the luteal phase, the effects of progesterone are dominant. The physiological changes in this phase of the cycle prepare the woman's body for pregnancy and promote implantation and nurture of the conceptus should fertilization be successful. Progesterone is secreted from the corpus luteum; thus, this phase of the cycle is known as the luteal phase.

	Chapter case study

Zara is now 12 weeks pregnant and has just attended the midwives' clinic to arrange her 12-week nuchal fold scan at her local maternity unit. Zara is quite excited because not only is her twin sister pregnant but her husband's sister and two of her best friends as well are pregnant and all the babies are due within the same 2 weeks. They, and their partners, had all been working abroad together doing voluntary work over a period of 1 year and had lived together in shared accommodation.

They had helped build and set up an orphanage for children whose parents had died from AIDS-related illnesses in an African country, and had only returned home a week before Zara's pregnancy was confirmed.

- What possible explanation could account for all five of the women conceiving together?
- What environmental factors could have influenced the menstrual cycles of the women and what possible physiological mechanisms may have resulted in the group apparently ovulating simultaneously?

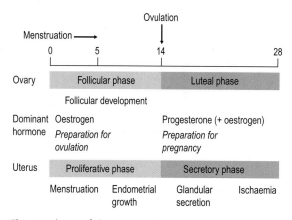

Fig. 4.1 Phases of the menstrual cycle.

Box 4.1 **Note about terminology**

Although the terms are often used interchangeably, the term 'oocyte' refers to the developing gamete within the ovary, whereas the term 'ovum' (plural ova) refers to the gamete after ovulation had occurred. Oogenesis refers to the process of formation (mitotic division) of oocytes from oogonia (formed from the primordial germ cells). The primary oocyte is an oocyte which has undergone mitosis and entered meiosis (which is arrested in the 7th month of gestation). By the time the female infant is born, all of her oogonia are primary oocytes in meiotic arrest. The secondary oocyte is formed (together with the first polar body) when the first meiotic division is completed just before ovulation. So the ovum is the egg after the second meiotic division, when the second polar body is extruded. As fertilization triggers the completion of the second meiotic division, the newly-ovulated female gamete does not stay an 'ovum' very long as the sperm has already penetrated the ovum; once the chromosomes from the egg and sperm are united, the fertilized ovum is correctly known as an embryo. The one-celled embryo is also referred to as a zygote. At the 16-cell stage, the embryo is called a morula (Latin for mulberry). When the fluid-filled cavity (blastocoele) forms in the embryo separating the trophoblast cells from the inner cell mass, the embryo is called a blastocyst.

Ovulatory cycles usually have a duration of 24–32 days; the follicular phase is 10–14 days and the luteal phase between 12 and 15 days. Longer cycles usually have a prolonged follicular phase and delayed ovulation.

THE FOLLICULAR PHASE

Developmental stages

The stages of cell division leading to the production of the female gamete begin early in fetal life. The process is halted until puberty when ovulation begins, and then halted again until fertilization. The developing egg is called an oocyte; it differentiates into a mature haploid ovum (or egg). Although dramatic progress in the development of an oocyte takes place during the follicular phase, the development of the follicle begins about 3 months prior to the menstrual cycle in which it is released at ovulation (Fig. 4.2). Folliculogenesis begins with the recruitment of primordial follicles from the ovarian pool; the signals which initiate recruitment are unknown. At the beginning of the cycle, a number of primary follicles are recruited to undergo initial development, stimulated by luteinizing hormone (LH). These secondary follicles express follicle-stimulating hormone (FSH) receptors. One follicle is selected to continue development as the dominant follicle. It is this follicle that releases the ovum at ovulation. The remnants of the follicle then become the corpus luteum.

In the female fetus, the primordial germ cells migrate to the ovary at 21 days postfertilization and become oogonia. They proliferate by mitotic division and then differentiate into primary oocytes; by 20 weeks of gestation, in each ovary, there are about 10 million primary oocytes ready to enter meiotic division (see Chapter 5). The oocytes degenerate throughout fetal life so the female neonate is born with a finite number of 250 000–500 000 oocytes; this is all the oocytes she will ever have. Degeneration of the oocytes continues throughout postnatal life; there are fewer than 200 000 oocytes left at puberty and numbers continue to fall. However, if one assumes a reproductive life of about 35–40 years, the maximum number of ova released from the ovaries will be no more than a few hundred. Although it was thought that the oocytes number was established during fetal development, it is now suggested that some ovarian oogonia still unassociated with follicular cells persist from the fetal period and can undergo mitosis thus acting as a stem cell population of oocytes in postnatal life (Johnson et al., 2004).

Arrested meiosis

Meiosis is a specialized cell division involved in the production of gametes (see Chapter 7, p. 149, for a detailed description). In it, the number of chromosomes is reduced from 46 (known as the diploid number) to 23 (the haploid number). In the first part of meiosis, the DNA replicates, so each chromosome is composed of two chromatids. The homologous chromosomes pair up along their long axes and crossing over occurs so the chromosomes exchange genetic material. In humans, two or three exchanges of DNA occur per chromosome pair ensuring that the combination of genes will be unique (Box 4.2). This is achieved by areas of fusion (called chiasmata) forming between adjacent chromosomes (see Chapter 7). The oocyte remains arrested in the prophase stage of division I of meiosis for a number of years until sexual maturity (Fig. 4.3). During this time, the primary

Fig. 4.2 Ovarian follicles. (Reproduced with permission from Brooker, 1998.)

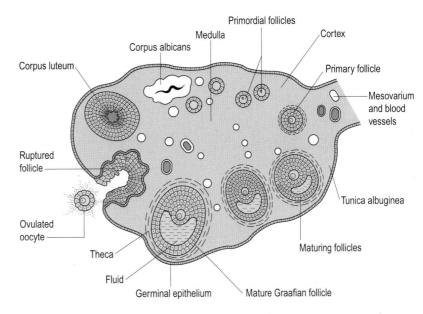

Box 4.2 **Gamete formation**

- Cell proliferation (mitosis)
- Genetic reshuffling and reduction (meiosis)
- Packaging of chromosomes
- Gamete maturation

---

oocytes synthesize the extracellular matrix and the secretory vesicles. Arrested meiosis provides a specialized mechanism to allow the oocyte to grow while it contains duplicate copies of chromosomes and, therefore, twice as much DNA is available to direct synthesis of RNA as in a somatic cell. The hormones of puberty release the oocyte from the first meiotic block; this process is called oocyte maturation. The oocyte resumes division I of meiosis. The chromosomes re-condense, the nuclear envelope breaks down and the meiotic spindle forms. The chromosomes then segregate into the two daughter nuclei. The cytoplasm divides asymmetrically to form a large secondary oocyte and a small polar body, each of which contains 23 chromosomes as pairs of chromatids. Meiotic division then arrests for a second time, so the oocyte released at ovulation has still not completed meiosis. Activation of the oocyte and release from the second meiotic block occurs at fertilization. In the second meiotic division, the sister chromatids finally segregate into two nuclei and the cytoplasm again divides asymmetrically, this forming the mature ovum and a second polar body, each with 23 chromosomes. Because both divisions of the cytoplasm are asymmetrical, the ovum is large. Effectively, the polar bodies are small packages of cytoplasm which contain discarded chromosomes. During *in vitro* fertilization (IVF),

observing the presence of the second polar body indicates that fertilization has occurred (see Chapter 6).

In the female, mitosis of the gametes stops in the fetal period, whereas in the male, mitotic division of gametogenesis begins at puberty and continues until senescence (see Box 4.3). The termination of mitosis in the female, and entry into meiosis, is under the control of protein complexes, maturation-promoting factor (MPF) and cytostatic factor (CSF), which regulate the oocyte's progression through meiosis (Dale et al., 1999). MPF phosphorylates multiple proteins involved in chromosome condensation and the breakdown of the nuclear envelope. The hormones of puberty increase MPF activity at the exit of the first meiotic block. It is hypothesized that the second meiotic block occurs because the maturing oocyte accumulates CSF which inhibits cell division. Oocyte activation and the release from the second meiotic block are thought to be triggered by a component of the sperm that enters the oocyte at fertilization and causes CSF degradation.

Both premature arrest at the end of oocyte maturation and parthenogenic release from meiotic arrest are thought to cause infertility. As women age, the extended duration of arrested meiosis, which may last for over 50 years, probably results in the meiotic spindles (see Fig. 7.11, p. 153) becoming increasingly fragile; this leads to an increased rate of abnormalities such as Down's syndrome and failed implantation.

Primordial follicles

Development of a mature female gamete depends on complex interactions between the developing gamete and the surrounding cells forming the outer layers of the follicle. Mitosis is completed during fetal development.

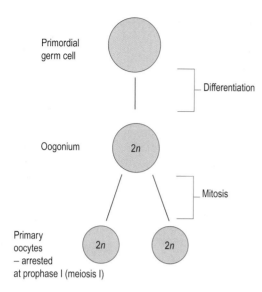

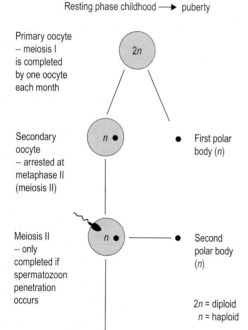

NB Polar bodies eventually degenerate within the ovum

Fig. 4.3 Arrest of oocyte meiosis. (Reproduced with permission from Brooker, 1998.)

Box 4.3 **Oogenesis compared with spermatogenesis**

- Mitosis: fetal in woman; after puberty in man
- Meiosis: halted in woman; can last many years
- Relatively few oocytes released
- Release is episodic at ovulation; not a continuous stream
- Organization is comparable to testis (stromal tissue containing primordial follicles, tubules) and glandular tissue (interstitial glands, Leydig cells)
- Mitotic proliferation is less
- Time-course of gamete production is much longer

During the first meiotic prophase, the primordial germ cells stimulate organization of the surrounding cells to form the granulosa cells (flattened cuboidal epithelial cells) which condense and encircle them forming the primordial follicles. The follicular cells secrete a basement membrane around the outside forming a cellular unit (Fig. 4.4). These granulosa cells are connected to the oocyte by gap junctions through which nutrients can be transported. The primitive oocyte therefore has two layers and is about 18 μm in diameter. A few follicles may resume development spontaneously and incompletely throughout fetal and neonatal life. However, regular recruitment of the primordial follicles into the pool of growing follicles begins at puberty when levels of FSH increase, so the primordial follicles containing oocytes may stay arrested in meiosis for decades.

Preantral (primary) follicles

From puberty, a few primordial follicles spontaneously restart their development each day, forming a continuous stream of growing preantral or primary follicles. Most of these early follicles fail to develop fully and undergo atresia (fail to develop any further); less than 0.1% of follicles will ovulate and develop into a corpus luteum. The granulosa cells of follicles undergoing atresia accumulate lipid droplets and reduce protein synthesis. Both the granulosa cells and the oocyte become apoptotic (undergo 'programmed cell death'). White blood cells invade the dying follicular cell mass and scar tissue forms.

As the majority of the follicles regress rather than progress through development, the ovary has a dense population of atretic follicles resulting in an irregular corrugated outer surface of the ovary. The development of primordial follicles into primary or preantral follicles takes about 85 days; the preantral phase is the longest phase of development of the oocyte. Initiation and progress through this early follicular development is independent of pituitary hormones but there may be paracrine regulation by cytokines (see Chapter 3), such as epidermal growth factor

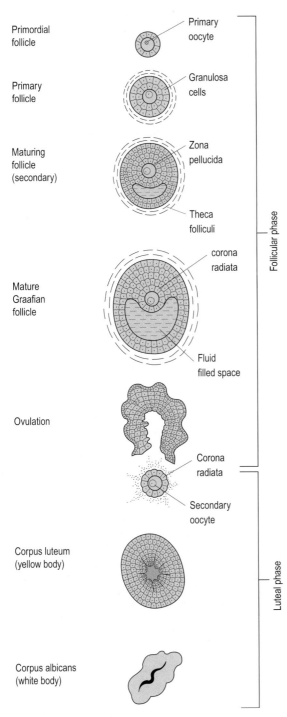

Primordial follicle
Primary oocyte

Primary follicle
Granulosa cells

Maturing follicle (secondary)
Zona pellucida
Theca folliculi

Mature Graafian follicle
corona radiata
Fluid filled space

Ovulation
Corona radiata
Secondary oocyte

Corpus luteum (yellow body)

Corpus albicans (white body)

Follicular phase

Luteal phase

Fig. 4.4 Follicular development. (Reproduced with permission from Brooker, 1998.)

(EGF; Box 4.4). These developing follicles do not secrete significant amounts of steroid hormones. Further follicular development requires pituitary support (secretion of FSH and LH).

Early in the cycle, the concentration of FSH is sufficient to support the further development of some preantral follicles. The preantral follicles that are optimal for further development are of the appropriate size and maturity to respond and have adequate FSH receptors. Recruitment of the follicles is related to the interaction between the FSH concentration and the number of FSH receptors on the developing follicles. Therefore, the number of follicles surviving is related to the amount of FSH present. The antral development phase, ovulation and luteal phase comprise one cycle in the humans. In other mammalian species, antral expansion occurs in the luteal phase of the previous cycle, thus shortening non-fertile cycles.

Antral (secondary) follicles

Usually about 15–20 preantral follicles are rescued from atresia each month and undergo initial stages of development and marked enlargement in response to the increasing FSH concentration at the beginning of each cycle. Several components contribute to the growth of the follicle: the oocyte enlarges, the follicular cells divide and further stromal cells are recruited to form the expanded outer layers of the follicle. The oocyte itself increases in diameter to 60–120 μm. It synthesizes large amounts of ribosomal RNA (rRNA) and messenger RNA (mRNA) to increase its protein stores ready for the maturation of the oocyte and fertilization, but does not resume meiosis. The follicular cells divide into several layers of granulosa cells, which secrete an amorphous and acellular translucent jelly, the zona pellucida. The zona pellucida is formed from condensation of glycoprotein and accumulates between the granulosa cells and the oocyte, acting as an extracellular coat of the oocyte. It has an important role in sperm binding and penetration during fertilization (see Chapter 6). Although the zona pellucida acts to separate the oocyte from the avascular granulosa cells, cytoplasmic processes penetrate the zona pellucida forming gap junctions at the oocyte surface. These allow delivery of low molecular weight substrates, such as nucleotides and amino acids, and cellular signalling molecules into the oocyte. Gap junctions also exist between granulosa cells.

The third component of follicular growth is condensation of ovarian stromal cells on the basement membrane (membrana propria) of the follicle. These recruited cells form a loose matrix of spindle-shaped cells around the follicle, known as the thecal layer. The cells differentiate into two layers: the theca interna, an inner layer of highly vascular glandular cells, and the theca externa, a poorly vascularized fibrous capsule.

Box 4.4 Cytokines and growth factors

Inhibin and activin

The gonadotrophins (FSH and LH) stimulate the production of the cytokines, activin and inhibin. The cytokines modulate actions of steroid hormones and gonadotrophins. Inhibin appears to affect only reproduction (see Fig. 4.7), whereas the closely related activin affects cell growth and differentiation in other tissues. Inhibin is produced by the granulosa cells of small antral follicles in response to FSH (Roberts et al., 1993) and suppresses FSH secretion. It is also produced by the Sertoli cells of the testis. Levels peak mid-cycle but remain high in the luteal phase, because the corpus luteum produces inhibin in response to LH. Inhibin production in the pituitary has a local inhibitory effect on FSH release (Hillier, 1991). Inhibin stimulates androgen output by the thecal cells and moderates aromatizing activity of the granulosa cells (Hillier, 1991). Activin is produced by granulosa cells, which also secrete follistatin, which may modulate the effects of activin. The thecal cells of the dominant follicle also produce activin (Roberts et al., 1993). The anterior pituitary gland also produces activin, which is co-secreted with the gonadotrophins and enhances FSH production. It inhibits pituitary production of growth hormone GH, ACTH and PRL. It may also have a role in embryogenesis (Hamilton-Fairley and Johnson, 1998). Activin is present in follicular fluid but is inhibited by follistatin. Activin suppresses the androgen output by thecal cells but stimulates aromatizing capacity of granulosa cells. It therefore inhibits progesterone production. Activin is present early in the cycle, and inhibin later in the cycle, thereby producing a balance between androgen output and conversion.

Follistatin

Follistatin was identified in 1987 as an inhibitor of FSH secretion (Roberts et al., 1993). It is synthesized in the ovary and inhibits activin activity by acting as an activin-binding protein.

Interleukins

Interleukins are a group of cytokines, small protein molecules, that communicate between the immune system cells and between immune and other cells. They are usually secreted by immune cells and usually have a local action. Interleukins include histamine, prostaglandin, tumour necrosis factor (TNF), IL-1 and IL-6. IL-1 is a polypeptide cytokine, usually produced by activated macrophages, which induces an acute phase reaction in the liver in response to inflammation. However, it is also produced by granulosa cells in a hormone-dependent manner with a peak production mid-cycle. IL-1 affects follicular maturation and a number of aspects of ovulation, including increasing production of prostaglandins, collagenase, nitric acid and hyaluronic acid (Hurwitz et al., 1992) and steroidogenesis. It is not known whether other members of the interleukin family are involved in follicular development.

Epidermal growth factor (EGF)

EGF is produced by many tissues including granulosa cells. It appears to inhibit FSH-stimulated oestrogen and inhibin production and proliferation and differentiation of granulosa cells. EGF may be involved in the selection of the dominant follicle (Hamilton-Fairley and Johnson, 1998).

Transforming growth factors (TGF)

Transforming growth factors, TGF-α and TGF-β, have been identified in thecal cells (Adashi et al., 1989). TGF-α has similar properties to EGF and suppresses granulosa cell differentiation. It also regulates differentiation of other cell types including fetal ovaries and ovarian carcinoma cells. Members of the TGF-β family are structurally similar to inhibin and increase FSH receptor expression, positively modulating granulosa cell proliferation and differentiation.

Insulin-like growth factors (IGFs)

Insulin-like growth factors stimulate mitotic division and cell differentiation. Their effects are mediated by insulin-like growth factor binding proteins (IGF-BP). In follicular development, they appear to coordinate the production of steroid hormones from the granulosa and thecal layers of the follicle (Giudice, 1994). IGF-I enhances follicular development and hormone production. IGF-II enhances the response to insulin. IGF-BP bind to the IGFs decreasing the concentration of free growth factor. Decreased levels of binding proteins are associated with follicular growth and increased concentrations of binding proteins are found in atretic follicles (Mason et al., 1993). The large follicles from women with polycystic ovaries have lower concentrations of growth factors and higher concentrations of binding proteins (Mason et al., 1994). IGFs seem therefore to have an important role in follicular growth, maturation and ovulation. In pregnancy, IGFs and their binding proteins play essential roles in modulating fetal growth and development (see Chapter 9).

Tumour necrosis factor (TNF)

TNF was initially identified as having a role in inflammation and in inhibiting tumour growth. It is produced by follicular cells and stimulates steroidogenesis, and may have a role in ovulation.

There is critical bidirectional paracrine and juxtacrine communication between the oocyte and the surrounding somatic or follicular cells of the ovary, the granulosa and thecal cells. FSH is required both for granulosa cell differentiation and division (Richards and Pangas, 2010).

The granulosa cells acquire receptors for FSH and oestrogen and the theca interna cells acquire receptors for LH. Synthesis of steroid hormones by the follicle requires cell cooperation (Fig. 4.5; Hillier et al., 1994). Interstitial glands lie within the stroma and between the developing

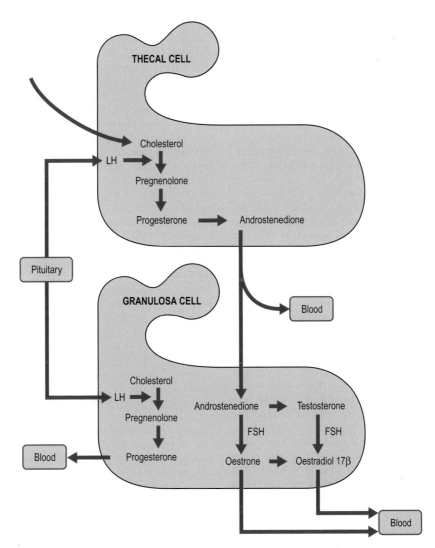

Fig. 4.5 'Two-cell model' of steroid synthesis.

follicles. They are formed of steroidogenic cells and produce androgens for secretion and aromatization to oestrogen in follicles. LH stimulates the theca interna cells to synthesize androgens (testosterone and androstenedione) from acetate and cholesterol but these cells initially have limited capacity to synthesize oestrogens. Androgens from the theca interna cells diffuse to the avascular granulosa cells. The granulosa cells are unable to synthesize androgens but can aromatize androgens to oestrogens (oestradiol-17β and oestrone). The enzyme aromatase (CYP19) is involved in the steroid biosynthesis pathway leading to increased oestrogen production. FSH stimulates production of insulin-like growth factor I (IGF-I), which stimulates aromatase activity and hence oestrogen production. Activins and oestradiol enhance the actions of

FSH (Richards and Pangas, 2010). Small amounts of LH are required to amplify follicular oestrogen production. The steroids are secreted into the bloodstream, where they have a systemic effect, and into the follicular fluid, where they may have a paracrine role. Androgens also stimulate aromatase. Oestrogens stimulate granulosa cells to proliferate and express further oestrogen receptors. Therefore, oestrogen further stimulates oestrogen output, an example of positive feedback. This increases the amount of circulating oestrogen from the most advanced or 'dominant' follicle (therefore, monitoring oestrogen output is a guide to the maturity of the most mature follicles). The dominant follicle, which undergoes the most growth, will enlarge from 20 to 200–400 μm diameter. The dominant follicle produces oestradiol, which inhibits FSH secretion.

However, the dominant follicle develops exquisite sensitivity to FSH and can continue to respond to the decreasing concentration of FSH. The smaller follicles, destined to become atretic, lose their responsiveness to FSH and do not develop LH receptors (Scheele and Schoemaker, 1996).

Early in the antral phase under the influence of FSH, the granulosa cells produce inhibin B and activin which suppresses androgen output and increases the aromatizing capability of the granulosa cells, thus promoting oestrogen synthesis. Later in the antral phase under the influence of both FSH and LH, the granulosa cells switch to producing inhibin A which stimulates androgen output and attenuates the aromatizing activity. Thus, androgen output is regulated by activin and inhibins and the ratio of inhibin A:inhibin B acts as a marker of follicular growth

The dominant antral follicle

The single follicle emerging as dominant undergoes preovulatory growth. This dominant follicle produces more oestrogen, which inhibits production of FSH from the pituitary gland. This is an example of negative feedback where a product limits its own production. The effect of oestrogen inhibiting production of FSH is that further development of the other follicles is limited. These follicles with fewer FSH receptors exposed to a diminishing supply of FSH are least able to respond to FSH and therefore undergo a downward spiral and become atretic. The dominant follicle continues to produce inhibin A which stimulates androgen production by the thecal cells and aromatization by the granulosa cells, thus leading to the surge of oestrogen. The dominant follicle also has a high ratio of insulin-like growth factor 2 (IGF-2) to IGF-BP which mediates LH-stimulated androgen output and FSH-dependent aromatization.

Angiotensin II (A-II), the product of the renin–angiotensin system (RAS, see Chapter 2), may be involved in oocyte maturation and ovulation. There is a RAS that is specific to the ovary and A-II occurs in high concentrations in preovulatory follicles. This ovarian RAS is implicated in the pathogenesis of ovarian tumours, ovarian hyperstimulation syndrome, ectopic pregnancy and hypertension (Hassan et al., 2000). Symptoms of ovarian hyperstimulation syndrome include serious metabolic and fluid disturbances which are associated with abnormal control of the RAS (note that ovarian hyperstimulation syndrome is a recognized complication of IVF treatment – see Chapter 6). It has also been suggested that A-II may have a role in the formation and maintenance of the corpus luteum, regulation of progesterone production and angiogenesis (Hamilton-Fairley and Johnson, 1998). The biggest or dominant follicle, which is best able to respond to FSH, further develops on the pathway to expansion and ovulation. Oestrogen and FSH stimulate the mid-cycle expression of LH receptors on the outer layers of granulosa cells of the dominant follicle, which means that it will be able to respond to the mid-cycle surge of LH secretion. Entry into the preovulatory phase depends on both the expression of these receptors and a surge of LH from the anterior pituitary gland.

The granulosa cells continue to divide and increase in size. However, most of the increase in follicular size is due to accumulation of follicular fluid formed from mucopolysaccharides, secreted from granulosa cells, and serum transudate. The fluid coalesces forming an antrum (or cleft) filled with follicular fluid. The antrum separates the granulosa cells into two regions: the corona radiata (a rim of granulosa cells) around the oocyte and the outer membrana granulosa. The oocyte becomes isolated and suspended in the fluid connected to the rest of the granulosa cells by a thin strand of cells, the cumulus oophorus (egg stalk). The oocyte does not increase in size but continues to synthesize RNA and protein.

Follicular development is dependent on pituitary support. Removal of the pituitary gland (hypophysectomy) results in the cessation of follicular growth and the death of the oocyte. This can be halted by adding back LH and FSH, which stimulate further growth. It takes 8–12 days for the primary follicle to grow into the antral follicle. Failure of follicular growth for any reason results in a restarting of the cycle of follicular development, and hence both a longer first phase of the cycle and a longer cycle. It seems likely that women who regularly have a longer than normal menstrual cycle have either a slow rate of follicular development and increasing oestrogen secretion or the dominant follicle starts developing but fails, so the next most appropriate follicle takes over the role as the dominant follicle.

Although the increasing concentration of oestrogen (predominantly oestradiol, E_2) initially has a negative feedback on the hypothalamus and pituitary, there is a critical concentration of oestrogen that is stimulatory provided it lasts for a critical duration. When the diameter of the follicle is 18–22 μm and the oestradiol concentration reaches 600–1200 pmol/L, there is positive feedback on the anterior pituitary gland leading to a sudden increase or 'surge' of LH release (Hamilton-Fairley and Johnson, 1998; Fig. 4.6).

The LH surge

The effect of the LH surge is twofold. First, it stimulates the terminal growth phase of the preovulatory follicle and the meiotic and cytoplasmic maturation of the oocyte, culminating in expulsion of the oocyte from the ovary. These effects include re-initiation of oocyte meiosis and expansion of the cumulus cell–oocyte complex (Richards and Pangas, 2010). Second, it causes luteinization, a series of endocrine changes within the follicular cells that result in a different hormone secretory profile in the second half of the cycle.

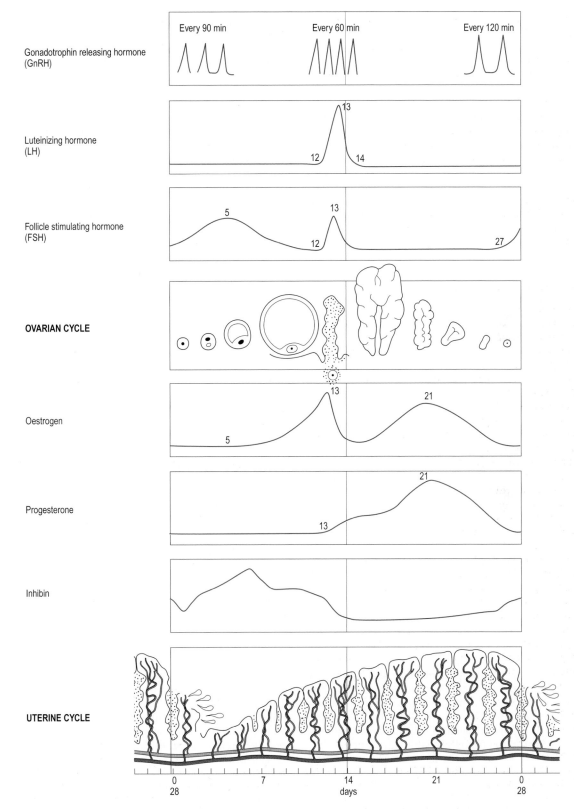

Fig. 4.6 The reproductive cycle and hormone levels.

Within a few hours of the LH surge, there are dramatic changes in the oocyte, which resumes meiotic division. There may also be a positive signal from the granulosa cells or a reduction of gap junction communication, which decreases the flow of meiosis-arresting substances to the oocyte. Progression through the remainder of the first meiotic division results in half the chromosomes (as paired chromatids) and almost all the cytoplasm being enclosed in the secondary oocyte, which is destined to become the ovum. The remaining chromosomes and very little cytoplasm are enclosed in a membrane forming a very small cell, known as the first polar body (see Fig. 4.3). Thus, the secondary oocyte keeps the bulk of the materials that were synthesized earlier in follicular development; these are conserved for the zygote. The chromosomes of the secondary oocyte enter the second meiotic division and go on to the next stage of division, called metaphase (see Fig. 7.11), where they align on the spindle. However, meiosis is then immediately arrested for a second time; this is regulated by CSFs. Meiosis resulting in the production of a mature female pronucleus will not resume until successful fertilization following ovulation. By this time, the oocyte will already contain the sperm nucleus. Thus, there is actually no time when the oocyte is a true gamete in the sense of being a cell with only 23 chromosomes, as is the case of a spermatozoon.

Concurrently, the LH surge promotes maturation of the cytoplasmic compartment of the oocyte. The cytoplasmic processes between the oocyte and the granulosa cells withdraw and contact is lost. The Golgi apparatus (see Table 1.1) synthesizes lysosome-like cortical granules, which align under the surface of the oocyte. Protein synthesis continues but the profile of the proteins synthesized changes as the oocyte prepares for fertilization. The gonadotrophin surge stimulates the cumulus cells surrounding the oocyte (see Fig. 4.4) to secrete hyaluronic acid, which disperses the cumulus cells embedding them in a mucus-like matrix.

Ovulation

Ovulation is triggered by the mid-cycle surge of LH, which occurs in response to sustained high levels of oestrogen released from the developing dominant follicle. The single mature preovulatory follicle has a diameter of 2–2.5 cm in an ovary that is approximately 3 cm long. It was this structure that de Graaf identified and named in 1672. The increased size and changed position of the follicle mean that it protrudes from the surface of the ovary (see Fig. 4.2). This results in the thinning of the layer of epithelial cells between the wall of the follicle and the peritoneal cavity. As expansion continues, the wall becomes thinner and avascular, and the cells appear to dissociate.

About 36 h after the LH surge, ovulation occurs and the oocyte is expelled from the ovary (see Fig. 4.2). The LH surge stimulates the production of a cascade of proteolytic enzymes, including renin and other trypsin-like enzymes from thecal cells, which digest the follicle wall. The biochemical changes, including generation of oxygen free radicals, that precede ovulation are similar to those seen in inflammation. Plasminogen activator, which converts procollagenase to collagenase, is produced by granulosa cells resulting in the breakdown of the connective tissue. Progesterone production rises immediately after the LH surge and the preovulatory increase in progesterone may be important in follicular rupture as it decreases formation of collagen. Prostaglandins increase vascular permeability, which maintains the intrafollicular pressure as fluid begins to leak through the eroded follicular wall. Small contractile waves also ripple across the ovary increasing the intrafollicular pressure. The force is cushioned by the follicular fluid, so the pressure generated is targeted at the weakened ovarian surface, causing it to rupture. Some women experience abdominal pain around the time of ovulation on the same side of the ovary producing the ovum. This is referred to as Mittelschmerz pain (derived from German 'middle pain'). As the follicle ruptures and the ovarian surface is breached, the fluid washes out the oocyte, which is surrounded by the granulosa (cumulus) cells, from the ovary to the exterior. The oocyte is swept into the uterine tube by the fimbria. It is then propelled towards the uterus by peristaltic muscular activity and cilia movements of the epithelial cells lining the tube. After taking years (12–50 years) to complete maturation, the oocyte is then viable and fertilizable for only about a day.

THE LUTEAL PHASE

Within 2 h of the LH surge, there is a transient rise in the oestrogen and androgens secreted by the follicle as the thecal layers become stimulated and hyperaemic. The outer granulosa cells with their newly expressed receptors for LH no longer convert androgens to oestrogen but synthesize progesterone instead. The cells no longer bind oestrogen or FSH. The result is a marked increase in progesterone secretion, which begins several hours before ovulation.

The corpus luteum

After ovulation, the residual parts of the follicle remaining in the ovary collapse into the space and form the corpus luteum ('yellow body'; see Fig. 4.4). There is some bleeding and fibrotic activity in the cavity, which allows formation of a fibrin core around which the remaining granulosa cells congregate. The structure is enclosed by a capsule of fibrous thecal cells. The basement membrane between the granulosa cells and thecal cells breaks down allowing vascularization of the interior. This allows increased transport of cholesterol precursor to the luteinizing granulosa cells to maintain a high rate of progesterone secretion. A few of the thecal cells disperse to the stroma tissue. The granulosa cells first luteinize, then stop dividing and hypertrophy into large luteal cells. The luteal cells are rich in mitochondria, endoplasmic reticulum and Golgi bodies and have numerous lipid droplets and lutein, a yellow carotenoid pigment.

Hormonal changes

Luteinization is associated with a progressive increment in progesterone secretion from the corpus luteum. The outer thecal cells form a stem cell population of smaller luteal cells which have numerous LH receptors and produce progesterone and androgens. Levels of progesterone rise until the middle of the luteal phase (see Fig. 4.6). The corpus luteum produces oestrogen and inhibin as well as progesterone. All three hormones inhibit secretion of FSH from the anterior pituitary gland and therefore prevent further development of follicles.

It has been suggested that a cause of fertility problems may be inadequate production of progesterone at the time of ovulation and during the subsequent luteal phase. However, exogenous administration of progesterone or human gonadotrophin (hCG) has had limited success in clinical practice. It appears that most women have a proportion of their cycles with a low progesterone output without their overall fertility being affected (Hamilton-Fairley and Johnson, 1998). A shortened luteal phase can lead to intermenstrual bleeding, premenstrual 'spotting' and short cycles.

The corpus luteum also synthesizes relaxin, secretion of which peaks in the middle of the luteal cycle (Johnson et al., 1993), probably regulated by LH. Relaxin may be involved in promoting the growth of the myometrium and cervix and growth and secretory activity of the endometrium (Huang et al., 1991).

Effectively, the corpus luteum is an endocrine gland producing oestrogen and progesterone. The LH surge stimulates its growth and activity. Unless fertilization occurs, the life of the corpus luteum is very short, and it undergoes spontaneous luteolysis (degeneration and regression) after about 6 days. The corpus luteum appears to have an age-related decrease in responsiveness to LH (Zeleznik and Hillier, 1996) and so requires progressively more LH for survival. Following the LH surge, LH concentration in the luteal phase is low, so luteolysis will occur. Blood flow to the corpus luteum falls and the follicular tissue becomes ischaemic. The concentrations of oestrogen and progesterone begin to fall as the degenerating corpus luteum stops hormone production. Thus, luteolysis terminates a non-fertile cycle. As the level of oestrogen falls, the inhibition on the hypothalamus will be abrogated and FSH secretion will resume, ready for the next

cycle. The atrophying corpus luteum loses its yellow pigment, so it becomes known as a corpus albicans ('white body'). It gradually contracts over a period of months, leaving a white scar tissue which is absorbed into the stromal tissue of the ovary.

Changes on fertilization

If fertilization occurs, then hCG, which has structural similarities to LH, rescues the corpus luteum from luteolysis, stimulating its further growth and production of steroid hormone up to the 10th week when placental endocrine function becomes established. Human chorionic gonadotrophin has a longer half-life than LH, so it provides a sustained and more intense stimulus. If fertilization occurs, then the concentration of relaxin also continues to rise until the end of the first trimester.

REGULATION OF GONADOTROPHIN SECRETION

The brain controls and regulates the ovarian cycle. The gonadotrophs in the anterior pituitary secrete the glycoprotein hormones LH and FSH (which together are known as gonadotrophins). There appear to be two distinct populations of cells in the anterior pituitary, each producing one particular type of hormone; however, fluorescent labelling shows that some cells contain both hormones. Synthesis and secretion of LH and FSH are dependent on gonadotrophin-releasing hormone (GnRH) from the hypothalamus, which acts as the common mediator of influences via the CNS. (GnRH is also known as luteinizing hormone releasing hormone, or LHRH.) The hypothalamus releases GnRH into the hypophysial portal circulation that runs to the pituitary gland.

This pathway means that control of the reproduction can be modulated and affected by other inputs from the higher brain centres. The GnRH neurons convert neural signals into endocrine signals. Stress, nutritional status and environmental influences, for instance, affect the timing and success of the reproduction. Ovulation appears to be seasonally regulated in populations experiencing seasonal variation in food availability; suspending reproductive function when nutrition is poor favours maternal health and outcome of pregnancy.

There are two levels of regulation. First, the GnRH neurons of the hypothalamus have an inherent pulsatile activity. The steroid hormones, the gonadotrophins (LH and FSH) and GnRH feedback on the hypothalamic–pituitary axis exert a second level of endocrine control. Prolactin (PRL) also has an effect on the control of reproduction.

GnRH and gonadotrophins are released in a pulsatile manner (see Box 4.5). The cells releasing GnRH appear to be widely and diffusely distributed (Rance et al., 1991)

Box 4.5 Biological rhythms

The study of biological rhythms is termed 'chronobiology'. All living cells, organs, organisms and groups of individuals demonstrate rhythmical changes within their internal (endogenous) physiology that can also result in external changes in behaviour. The rhythms can be categorized according to the length of the cycle or period of oscillation.

- *Ultradian:* the rhythm is less than 1 day, for example, rapid eye movement in sleep.
- *Circahordal:* the period of oscillation is around 1 h.
- *Circadian:* the period of oscillation is about 1 day; levels of many hormones such as cortisol fluctuate on a daily basis.
- *Infradian:* the rhythm is repeated in a cycle greater than 1 day, for example, menstrual and oestrus cycles.
- *Circaseptram:* the period of oscillation is about 1 week.
- *Circatidal:* the rhythm relates to tidal movement of water.
- *Circalunar (synodic):* the rhythm relates to the cycle of the moon.
- *Circannual:* the rhythm has a cycle of about 1 year.

These fluctuations are often affected by the external environment and appear to enable the individual to respond to forthcoming changes within the environment. Factors that influence or reset the cycle are described as entraining the cycle. In the human brain, the suprachiasmatic nuclei of the hypothalamus may influence daily fluctuations. The pineal gland, which produces the hormone melatonin at night, appears to affect the suprachiasmatic nuclei, acting as an entrainer. The circadian pattern of melatonin secretion is achieved through inhibition via a neural pathway (outside the optic nerve) that is activated by light stimulation upon the retina. Therefore, within temperate zones, light acts as an entrainer on a daily basis and, because of the fluctuation of the photoperiod (length of daylight exposure), entrainment of annual cycles can also be achieved.

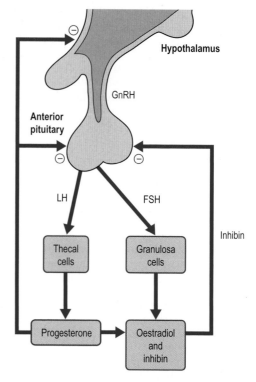

Fig. 4.7 Hormonal regulation of the menstrual cycle. (Reproduced with permission from Johnson and Everitt, 1995.)

but are remarkably synchronized to produce pulses of GnRH. During the follicular phase, the pulses are of low amplitude and high frequency, occurring every 60 min (Clarke, 1996). In the luteal phase, they are more irregular and have high amplitude and occur with a low frequency of about every 2 h. The output of the gonadotrophins, LH and FSH, is changed by increasing or decreasing the amplitude or frequency of the pulses or by modulating the response of the gonadotrophs to the pulses. Prior to the LH surge, gonadotroph GnRH receptor density increases and the cells become more sensitive to GnRH. Inhibin and activin affect secretion of FSH without affecting secretion of GnRH. Two phenomena are observed: first, a depressant effect on output of gonadotrophins by increased oestrogen, progesterone and inhibin; and second, an increased surge of LH and FSH secretion induced primarily by oestradiol

(Fig. 4.7). The pattern of pulsatile secretion of GnRH is regulated by a complex mechanism that allows multiple signals, such as neurotransmitters and sex steroids, to determine ovulation.

In the early part of the follicular phase, rising levels of FSH stimulate oestrogen production from the developing follicles. Rising concentrations of oestradiol have a negative feedback effect on gonadotrophin production from the anterior pituitary, so FSH secretion falls. Activin and inhibin also affect FSH secretion. Inhibin is involved in the negative feedback of FSH secretion. However, the dominant follicle is exquisitely sensitive to even a diminishing concentration of FSH and continues to produce oestrogen, which markedly increases by two- to fourfold. These concentrations are maintained for 48 h, which produces a positive feedback effect resulting in the dramatic surge of LH and FSH release seen in mid-cycle prior to ovulation. The effect of oestradiol is very sensitive: a low concentration has a marked and rapid effect that is evident within 1 h and maximal within 4–6 h. During the luteal phase, increased progesterone concentrations reinforce the negative feedback effects of oestradiol. The production of both LH and FSH secretion is very low; therefore, the positive effect of oestradiol is blocked.

CYCLICAL EFFECTS OF OESTROGENS AND PROGESTERONE

Effects on the uterus

Organs that respond to hormonal changes have receptors for the hormones. Responses can change because hormone levels fluctuate or because receptor density on the target organs alters. The principal actions of oestrogen and progesterone during the monthly cycle are on the endometrium which is one of the tissues most sensitive to ovarian steroid hormones. The endometrium undergoes cyclical changes: the growth of the uterine wall in expectation of an embryo, and its degeneration if fertilization does not take place. In the first half of the cycle, the uterus goes through a proliferative phase. Oestrogen stimulates the epithelial cells of the basal layer of the endometrium to divide and proliferate, forming a thick mucosal wall with numerous endometrial glands (Fig. 4.8). Oestrogen also stimulates proliferation of the stoma and glands and angiogenesis (growth of new blood vessels): extensive vascular tissue, spiral arteries and veins develop within the endometrium. Within the space of a few days, the effect of oestrogen is to increase the height of the wall from 0.5 to 5 mm, a remarkable 10-fold increase. The thickness of the endometrium is monitored by ultrasound in assisted conception (see Chapter 6) to assess whether it is optimal for implantation; the insertion of embryos into a uterine cavity with an endometrium less than 5 mm thick is unlikely to be successful. The myometrium does not grow extensively during the menstrual cycle. During the proliferative phase, oestrogen primes the endometrial cells by inducing the synthesis of progesterone receptors.

After ovulation, the cells of the enlarging corpus luteum begin to secrete progesterone, which has a dramatic effect on the secretory activity of the endometrial glands. In this secretory phase, the effects of progesterone are dominant, although oestrogen is still secreted from the corpus luteum. The spiral arteries continue growing and thus become more prominent and coiled as the height of the endometrium remains unchanged. The endometrial glands become dilated and convoluted with secretions rich in glycogen, mucus, proteins, sugars, amino acids and enzymes. The secretory products are important for the survival and nutrition of the zygote and blastocyst prior to implantation. Failure of conception results in diminishment of the corpus luteum and decreased steroid hormone production. By the 7th postovulatory day, the secretory process ceases and the glands become exhausted and regress.

Cyclical effects are particularly evident within the female reproductive tract. Activity of the myometrium is inversely related to progesterone secretion. During menstruation, when progesterone levels are low, the uterine contractions, mediated by prostaglandins, have a higher frequency and strength than in labour (Lyons et al., 1991). These uterine contractions are responsible for dysmenorrhoea (period pains). Non-steroidal anti-inflammatory drugs (NSAIDs) such as aspirin inhibit prostaglandin synthesis, and are therefore effective in reducing pain. After menstruation, there is a slow decline in myometrial activity during the follicular phase; it reaches negligible activity mid-cycle. Thus, the uterus is at its most quiescent (still) at the time of implantation. Uterine quiescence is maintained until the late luteal phase when levels of progesterone fall. If pregnancy intervenes, levels of progesterone remain high and the myometrium remains inactive. Uterine blood flow, on the other hand, correlates positively with the pattern of oestrogen secretion. Because of low levels of oestrogen, blood supply to the endometrium during menses and early follicular phase is reduced. A marked increase occurs just prior to ovulation followed by a slight nadir. A secondary peak occurs in the luteal phase which mirrors the rise in oestrogen production. This means that endometrial blood flow is relatively high at the time of implantation but lower at menstruation, which helps to limit the blood loss at the latter time.

Uterine contractile activity varies with the stage of the menstrual cycle (Kunz and Leyendecker, 2001). These periovulatory waves of muscle contraction are directional, moving inwards from the cervix to the fundus, encouraging the semen to travel towards the egg (Bulletti and de Ziegler, 2005). In the preovulatory period, uterine peristaltic activity within the uterine tube also directs sperm transport preferentially to the uterine tube lateral to the ovary containing the dominant follicle. The uterine activity is relatively quiescent in the late luteal phase which favours implantation. However, there are still some gentle peristaltic waves which may promote high fundal implantation. Uterine peristalsis causes some retrograde menstruation. It is thought that this may be of evolutionary benefit and help preserve body iron (Kunz and Leyendecker, 2001). Dysfunction of uterine activity may be involved in the development of endometriosis, uterine adenomyosis and infertility.

Effects on the uterine tubes, cervix and vagina

Uterine tubes

Oestrogen stimulates epithelial cell activity, increasing cilia movement and secretion. This facilitates the movement of the ovum along the uterine tubes following ovulation. These effects are reversed by progesterone, which inhibits the peristaltic activity of the uterine tube smooth muscle.

Cervix

Oestrogen relaxes the myometrial fibres supplying the cervix and increases stromal vascularization and oedema. Collagenase is activated, which causes some dispersal of

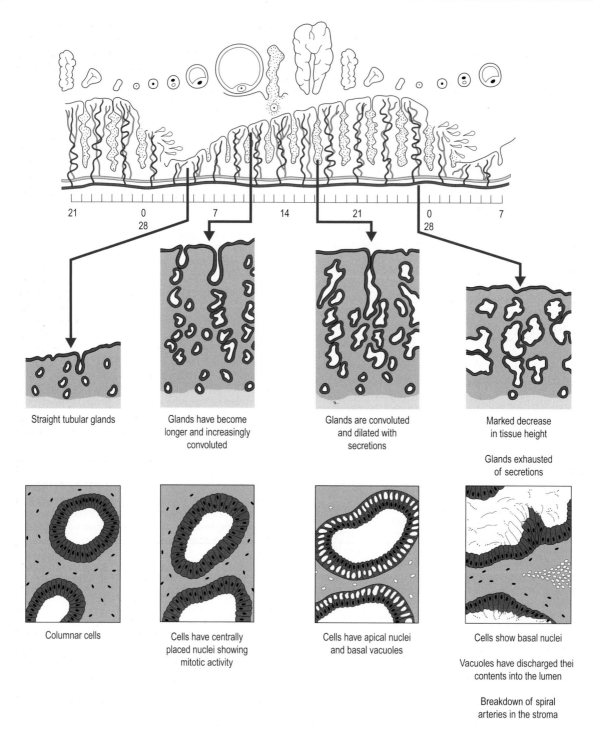

Fig. 4.8 Cyclical effects on the endometrium.

Straight tubular glands

Glands have become longer and increasingly convoluted

Glands are convoluted and dilated with secretions

Marked decrease in tissue height

Glands exhausted of secretions

Columnar cells

Cells have centrally placed nuclei showing mitotic activity

Cells have apical nuclei and basal vacuoles

Cells show basal nuclei

Vacuoles have discharged thei contents into the lumen

Breakdown of spiral arteries in the stroma

the tightly bound collagen bundles into a looser matrix. The result is that the cervix becomes softer to touch. The external os everts prior to ovulation. Progesterone causes the cervical muscle to retract and the stroma to become more compact as the collagen matrix reforms. The external os becomes tighter. The change in texture of the cervix is used as part of natural family planning (see Box 4.6). The cervix is softer at ovulation and a few days before, coinciding with the fertile period. At this stage, it has the consistency of lips compared with the harder 'nose-like' cartilaginous consistency of the cervix later in the cycle when the effects of progesterone are dominant.

The cyclical changes in blood flow are reflected by the composition of cervical mucus, which is copious and receptive to sperm penetration in mid-cycle (Table 4.1). When progesterone levels are high, small volumes of thick cervical mucus are secreted that are hostile and impenetrable to sperm. The increased viscosity of the mucus in the latter half of the menstrual cycle reduces the risk of ascending infection at the time of implantation.

Both oestrogen and progesterone are secreted from the corpus luteum in the second half of the cycle. The concentrations of oestrogen and progesterone will continue to rise if successful fertilization results in secretion of hCG and consequent survival of the corpus luteum. Therefore, the effects of the hormones in the second half of the cycle on the female body portend the changes that would take place in pregnancy.

Box 4.6 Concepts of natural family planning

- On the basis of periodic abstinence
- Also known as 'rhythm method' or 'safe period'
- Assumes that the interval between ovulation and menstruation is constant
- On the basis of recognition of signs of ovulation and fertile phases of menstrual cycle
  - temperature rise after ovulation
  - increased cervical mucus and watery vaginal secretions
  - softer consistency of cervix
- Probably most effective for birth spacing

Vagina

Oestrogen increases mitotic activity and secretion in the vaginal epithelial cells. Stimulation by progesterone results in an increased size of the nucleus of vaginal epithelial cells. It is important when examining cervical cells, obtained from a smear, to relate the morphological differences to the stage of a woman's menstrual cycle. Earlier in the cycle, cells appear flatter, whereas under the influence of progesterone they tend to become clumped and folded. There are also cyclical changes in the pH of the vagina as oestrogen stimulates the growth of commensal lactobacilli (Döderlein's bacilli). These lactobacilli metabolize glycogen from the cervical secretions producing lactic acid as a metabolic by-product, which decreases pH to a level that

Table 4.1 Changes in cervical mucus	
PROLIFERATIVE PHASE (FOLLICULAR)	**SECRETORY PHASE (LUTEAL)**
'E' MUCUS	**'G' MUCUS**
Oestrogen	Progesterone
Network of long parallel	Meshwork of polypeptide polypeptide chains strands
Carbohydrate side chains	Increased carbohydrate side chains
Forms channels 5 μm	Smaller space between wide molecules
High water content (98%)	Lower water content
Copious volume	Scanty volume
Clear	Cloudy
Acellular	Cells present
Spinnbarkeit = 10–20 cm	Spinnbarkeit ~ 3 cm (stretching between glass plates)
Dehydration: ferning	No ferning
Assists transport of sperm	Forms mucus plug to protect against infection

protects the reproductive tract from opportunistic pathogenic microorganisms.

The resident flora of the vagina also produces volatile aliphatic acids, which have distinctive odours. The profile of acids changes throughout the cycle under the influence of the changing hormones, and may result in changed sexual behaviour. It is suggested that male responses to their partners are affected by the cyclical fluctuations in olfactory stimuli stimulating sexual responsiveness and interaction. These olfactory signals do not seem to be consciously perceived in humans. Another example is women who live together are often observed to demonstrate menstrual synchrony: they ovulate and menstruate at the same time. Recently, it has been demonstrated that humans have the potential to communicate by pheromones. Odourless body secretions from women in different phases of the menstrual cycle can advance or delay the phases of other women (Stern and McClintock, 1998). Sexual desire, sexual activities and sexual satisfaction are all reported to increase around ovulation (see Chapter 5).

Other effects

There are additional effects and benefits of oestrogen on women's health. Oestrogens appear to protect the cardiovascular system; thus, women of reproductive age and normal endocrine function have a lower incidence of hypertension and a reduced risk of cardiovascular disease owing to higher levels of high-density lipoproteins (HDL), which lower circulating levels of cholesterol. Oestrogens stimulate osteoblasts, the cells involved in bone formation, thereby maintaining bone mass. Oestrogens may depress appetite and are mildly anabolic. There is a preovulatory drop in food intake; this decrease in female 'foraging' behaviour is hypothesized to allow the woman more time for activity, including 'shopping' for alternative mates (Fessler, 2003). This hypothesis is also supported by the suggestion that because ovulation is concealed in humans, the woman is able to select her mate at ovulation as opposed to other female mammals that become sexually attractive to males around ovulation (Ridley, 1994). Increased consumption of food is observed in the late luteal phase.

Postovulatory levels of progesterone are high, causing a slight increase in the basal metabolic rate. The basal body temperature rises owing to the influence of progesterone on the thermoregulatory centre of the hypothalamus. A temperature rise of 0.2–0.6°C confirms ovulation has taken place but does not predict it. In the second half of the cycle, the skin may appear more pigmented and acne may worsen as progesterone increases constriction of sebaceous glands. Progesterone also increases appetite during the luteal phase (Buffenstein et al., 1995). Women with premenstrual syndrome (PMS) may report cravings for carbohydrate, which are often associated with feelings of depression (Dye and Blundell, 1997; see Box 4.7). It is

Box 4.7 Premenstrual syndrome (PMS)

PMS is very common, with physical and psychological symptoms occurring in about 50% of women of reproductive age during their lifetime. Premenstrual dysphoric disorder (PMDD) is a more severe form of PMS that is associated with the luteal phase of the menstrual cycle. PMDD is classified as a depressive disorder by the American Psychiatric Association and affects about 3–5% of women. It is characterized by anxiety, anger and severe irritability. It is more severe than PMS and usually requires treatment to allow an affected woman to function in her environment. Both PMS and PMDD are characterized by mood swings including depression, but clinical depression occurs in PMDD. Some women have been acquitted of crimes conducted when they were affected by PMS and PMDD.

The cause of PMS is not clear. It may be due to a hormonal imbalance and low progesterone secretion in the luteal phase, abnormal neurotransmitters response, disorganized aldosterone function leading to water retention, deficient adrenal hormone secretion due to abnormal hypothalamic–pituitary–adrenal function, carbohydrate intolerance, a nutrient deficiency, stress or a combination of these factors (Girman et al., 2003). Women may be prescribed antidepressants such as serotonin reuptake inhibitors. Many women select lifestyle modification and complementary or alternative medicine approaches rather than conventional medicine. Women with PMS tend to consume more dairy products, refined sugar and high-sodium foods, so many clinicians recommend reducing intake of these. As fat contributes to oestrogen levels and fibre helps to reduce the effects of oestrogen on gut flora, high-fibre low-fat diets may be recommended. Reducing caffeine intake, from coffee, tea and caffeinated soft-drinks, can also be helpful. Vitamin B_6 can affect neurotransmitter release but the evidence that it improves PMS symptoms is inconclusive. As excess vitamin B_6 can cause nerve damage before symptoms of toxicity are evidenced, the daily dose should be limited. There is some evidence that calcium supplements can be beneficial. Of the herbal preparations more commonly used to relieve symptoms, the evidence is stronger for chasteberry (vitex) and ginkgo than for black cohosh, kava and St John's wort; the effects of evening primrose oil are thought to be a placebo effect. Exercise, such as yoga, helps reduce depression and anxiety symptoms. Many women find that keeping a symptom diary helps to identify exacerbating and relieving strategies.

frequently reported that common medical and mental health disorders are exacerbated at specific phases of the menstrual cycle (Pinkerton et al., 2010). Patterns of fluctuations in energy intake, appetite and depression may be associated with low serotonin or dopamine activity or other hormonally induced alterations in the brain which influence responses to pleasure and desire and thus affect food ingestion (Van Vugt, 2010). Changes in appetite and cravings can influence energy intake and expenditure (Davidsen et al., 2007). Changes in metabolic responses due to ovarian hormones can influence exercise performance (Oosthuyse and Bosch, 2010). Metabolism of drugs and alcohol may also cyclically alter during the menstrual cycle (Terner and de Wit, 2006).

Oestrogen and progesterone affect connective tissue oedema and hyperaemia and can cause increased breast size and tenderness. Progesterone binds to renal aldosterone receptors, causing natriuresis (sodium excretion) and blocking aldosterone occupation. Aldosterone increases to restore sodium retention, so there is a net effect of sodium retention. Oestrogen stimulates angiotensinogen production, which also tends to enhance sodium retention. Thus, in the luteal phase of the cycle, salt and water retention may be increased causing generalized weight gain and premenstrual feelings of bloatedness. The fluctuations in oestrogen and progesterone throughout the menstrual cycle affect the skin including skin structure (thickness, collagen production and breakdown and fluid retention), hydration, pigmentation, elasticity, wound healing and vasodilation (Farage et al., 2009). Thermoregulation, immune function and sleep patterns also exhibit a cyclical pattern in parallel with hormonal changes. In addition, reproductive hormones impact on psychoneurological processes affecting cognitive, emotional and sensory functions even at the level of hormone fluctuations that occur during the menstrual cycle (Farage et al., 2008).

MENSTRUATION

Menstruation is the loss of most of the decidual (superficial) layers of the endometrium accompanied by some blood loss that occurs after withdrawal of steroid hormones at the end of each menstrual cycle. During the menstrual cycle, the spiral arteries supply the endometrial stroma in preparation for implantation of the blastocyst; they have a remarkable ability to vasoconstrict during menstruation in order to limit blood loss. In humans, menstrual loss usually lasts about 5–7 days. Humans and other primates, together with elephant-shrews and some types of bats, are the only animals that menstruate. In these species there is marked progesterone-related proliferation of the endometrium and implantation is invasive. It was suggested that menstruation evolved as a protective mechanism (cleansing process) against sperm-borne pathogens by shedding any infected endometrial tissue and delivering immune cells to the uterine cavity. However, an alternative hypothesis is that cyclical regression and proliferation of the endometrium is energetically more economical in term, of reproductive costs than constantly maintaining a receptive endometrium (Strassmann,

1996). In many species, regression of the endometrium is accompanied by reabsorption of tissue debris. It is suggested that the copious menstrual bleeding in humans relates to the relatively large size of the uterus and the organization of the microvasculature (Strassmann, 1996). It has also been suggested that cyclical menstruation protects the uterine tissue from hyperinflammation and oxidative stress associated with deep placentation (Brosens et al., 2009).

Menstruation is an inflammatory process which results in tissue remodelling. The endometrial wall is described as being in a state of 'secretory exhaustion' (Clancy, 2009) and begins to breakdown because there is no embryonic signal. The mechanism of menstruation is thought to be either tissue destruction following necrosis and/or an inflammatory response (Salamonsen, 2003). In the destructive model, anoxia causes necrosis of the endometrium. The degeneration of the corpus luteum results in a fall in oestrogen and progesterone levels, which causes a modest but significant decrease in endometrial tissue height so the spiral arteries are coiled tighter and compressed. This results in a reduced blood flow, ischaemia and denudement of the endometrial tissue and interstitial haemorrhage. The withdrawal of progesterone stimulates the production of prostaglandins which are released by the spiral arteries stimulating vasoconstriction and vasodilatation resulting in rhythmic waves of contraction and relaxation in the latter. (The effect is like breaking a wire by rhythmically bending it backwards and forwards.) The waves become longer and more profound causing the decidual endometrium to break away along the natural plane of cleavage. The straight arteries in the basal layer maintain the blood supply. It is from these that new spiral arteries will regenerate. Alternatively, menstruation can be regarded as an inflammatory response. There is a marked increase in the number of leukocytes, particularly mast cells, immediately before menstruation as progesterone levels fall. These are probably attracted by chemokines produced by the endometrial cells. Mast cell degranulation may trigger the extracellular activation of matrix metalloproteinases, proteases that have the capacity to degrade components of the tissue. Prostaglandins are also involved in stimulating uterine contractions, which aid the removal of endometrial debris and blood.

Within 12 h, the height of the endometrium falls from 4 to 1 mm. At the end of the secretory phase, there is an ischaemic phase followed by the menstrual phase leading to the next proliferative phase. Endometrial repair is very rapid and occurs without scarring.

Menstrual flow is usually between 35 and 95 mL and consists of endometrial debris and blood. Blood loss is limited by vasoconstriction of the spiral arteries and formation of thrombin–platelet plugs in the terminal portions of the straight arteries. When oestrogen secretion resumes at the beginning of the next cycle, it stimulates healing and new tissue growth. Menstrual blood does

Case study 4.1

Njuka is in England with her husband who is a diplomatic representative of a central African country. When they first meet, the midwife asks Njuka when her baby is due and is informed that four full moons are left to pass before the baby will come. The midwife, intrigued by this answer, asks Njuka how she knows this. Njuka explains that six full moons have passed since her last period and that is how she knows.

- How accurate is Njuka's calculation of her gestation?
- Why is it important for a midwife to be able to estimate the length of gestation?
- What other information can help in this estimation?

not coagulate in the pattern seen normally. The damaged endometrial cells secrete proteolytic and fibrinolytic enzymes, which inhibit the formation of fibrin and therefore clot formation. The average volume of blood lost is 50 mL, which accounts for 0.7 mg of iron, a loss that is just matched by dietary iron absorption.

Case study 4.1 looks at the problem of calculating the length of gestation from the date of the last menstrual period.

HORMONAL CAUSES OF INFERTILITY

Hormonal causes of infertility account for about a third of the known causes (Box 4.8).

Hypogonadotrophic hypogonadism

Hypogonadotrophic hypogonadism is due to malfunction of the hypothalamic–pituitary axis and is characterized by low levels of oestrogen. Women with normal pituitary functions can be successfully treated with pulsatile exogenous GnRH from a small infusion pump. The hypothalamus is frequently entrained by the pump so normal rhythms of pulsatile secretion continue after the pump is removed. Alternatively, women can be treated with exogenous gonadotrophins. Human menopausal

---

Box 4.8 **Hormonal causes of infertility**

- Hypogonadotrophic hypogonadism
- Anorexic states
- Weight fluctuations
- Obesity
- Hyperprolactinaemia
- Polycystic ovary syndrome (PCOS)

---

gonadotrophin (hMG) extracted from the urine of post-menopausal women (the effects of ovariectomy or the menopause are to decrease oestradiol concentration, which results in raised circulating levels of FSH and LH) is used because it contains both FSH and enough LH to stimulate synthesis of androgenic precursors for oestrogen production. Ultrasound monitoring of follicular development is important to assess the development of excess follicles and the risk of multiple pregnancy. Ovarian stimulation can cause ovarian hyperstimulation syndrome which has serious implications because vascular permeability can suddenly increase, resulting in a movement of fluid out of the vascular system (McClure et al., 1994). In many respects, hypogonadotrophic hypogonadism resembles menopause (see below).

Anorexic states and weight fluctuations

Weight loss can also disrupt the hypothalamic–pituitary axis. Anorexic patients often have disrupted menstrual cycles, but acute weight loss or disruptions in energy intake (such as those associated with 'crash' dieting) even within a normal body weight range may disrupt hormone secretion. A body mass index (BMI) greater than 19 kg/m^2 and at least 22% fat as a proportion of body weight seem to be necessary for the maintenance of normal ovulatory cycles. It has been suggested that the critical fat mass for fertility is equivalent to the energy requirements of pregnancy (Frisch, 1990). Low body fat delays puberty and the menarche. Weight loss particularly affects LH secretion and can result in an abbreviated luteal phase.

Appetite is stimulated by the orexigenic neuropeptide Y (NPY) from the hypothalamus. NPY is involved in the regulation of food intake and energy balance. It has both stimulatory and inhibitory effects at the pituitary gland. In the well-nourished state, NPY release is acute and intermittent, a mode of secretion that potentiates GnRH-induced LH release. However, fasting decreases plasma glucose concentrations and extremes of exercise result in chronic secretion of NPY and continuous NPY receptor activation, which is inhibitory to LH release and thus fertility.

Eating causes storage of triacylglycerides in adipose cells, which stimulates the cells to release leptin. Leptin seems to be the satiety signal, which modulates the release of NPY. In starvation, leptin levels are low and NPY levels are high, which inhibits GnRH. The nutritional control of reproduction probably had an important evolutionary role in suppressing fertility at times of poor food supply. Suspending reproductive function at times of food shortage is protective.

Case study 4.2 looks at the problem of underweight in the calculation of gestation.

Case study 4.2

Lisa, a 17-year-old primipara, presents herself at the midwives' clinic, giving a vague history and saying that she thinks she might be pregnant. On palpation and abdominal examination, Lisa seems to be 26 weeks' pregnant and this is supported by a fundal height of 26 cm. The presence of fetal heart sounds confirms that Lisa is indeed pregnant. On questioning Lisa, the midwife discovers that Lisa has had only two scanty periods in the last 2 years and does not know the date of her last menstrual period. Lisa smokes 60 cigarettes a day, and has the appearance of being very underweight.

- Can you identify any possible reasons why Lisa might have irregular periods?
- Why must the midwife not assume that Lisa is 26 weeks' pregnant?
- Are there any clues that the midwife may investigate in order to estimate more precisely the actual gestation of Lisa's pregnancy?

Obesity

Paradoxically, obesity also affects fertility; obese women are over-represented in fertility clinics and have increased incidence of menstrual abnormality and a higher risk of miscarriage. The effects of obesity may persist even after weight loss has occurred. One of the reasons is that the adipose tissue is metabolically active, producing altered ratios of oestrogens and androgens. Obesity also affects insulin secretion (obese people are more likely to demonstrate insulin resistance) and affects production of leptin.

Hyperprolactinaemia

Hyperprolactinaemia can result from PRL-secreting tumours, which are usually benign. However, other factors including stress, breast stimulation or examination, hypothyroidism, polycystic ovary syndrome (PCOS) and dopaminergic antagonists can also raise circulating PRL levels. Hyperprolactinaemia can cause oestrogen deficiency, amenorrhoea and galactorrhoea (milk production). The management of hyperprolactinaemia is usually by administration of bromocriptine, a dopamine agonist, although tumours may be surgically removed.

Polycystic ovary syndrome

Polycystic ovary syndrome (PCOS) affects 5–10% of women; it is the most common endocrine disorder in women of reproductive age and is one of the leading causes of infertility. It is usually suspected from clinical signs and symptoms, and confirmed by ultrasound examination that shows enlarged ovaries containing more than 10 large cysts. Some women exhibit symptoms of disrupted cycles, central obesity and hyperandrogenism, which can cause acne, alopecia and hirsutism. The endocrine causes are hypersecretion of LH, glucose intolerance and increased levels of testosterone, insulin and PRL. Oestrogen levels are high but not cyclical and ovulation frequently does not occur. The follicles retain the oocyte, forming ovarian cysts which may take on a string-of-pearls appearance. Weight loss often improves the hormonal profile and alleviates the symptoms. Women with PCOS are at greater risk of developing impaired glucose tolerance and type II diabetes (Legro et al., 1999). Pregnant women with PCOS are at greater risk of developing gestational diabetes and therefore should be screened (Radon et al., 1999, Vollenhoven et al., 2000).

Clomifene citrate (Clomid) is an anti-oestrogenic drug that can be used to re-establish a normal pattern of ovulation in women with PCOS; however, its use is associated with an increased risk of multiple pregnancies. In cases where women fail to respond to clomifene citrate, especially if the BMI is above 25 kg/m^2, combined treatment with metformin and clomifene citrate improves ovulation and pregnancy rates (National Collaborating Centre for Women's and Children's Health, 2004).

ARTIFICIAL CONTROL OF FERTILITY

Oral contraceptives

The first oral contraceptives were extracts from yam. Although yams are rich in progesterone-like compounds, the active ingredient was actually mestranol, an oestrogenic agent. The combination of progestogen and mestranol was essential for good cycle control. Natural progesterone and most other steroid hormones are digested in the gastrointestinal tract and are usually effective only if injected. Chemically modified hormones are resistant to proteolytic digestion in the gut but retain their biological activity. Many synthetic steroid hormones have been developed that have similar biological activity as the naturally occurring hormones and are metabolized very slowly by the liver, increasing their half-life. The term progestogens is used to describe the family of natural and synthetic progesterone-like compounds.

The first contraceptive pills, used in Britain since 1961, were combined oral contraceptive pills (COC), combinations of an oestrogen and a progestogen. Currently, the most common progestogen and oestrogen combinations used are norethisterone and ethinyloestradiol, respectively (Fig. 4.9). A course of COC pills is taken for 21 days followed by 7 pill-free (or placebo) days when hormone levels fall, mimicking natural hormonal cycles and allowing a withdrawal bleed. Monophasic pills have a constant concentration of the active agents whereas biphasic and triphasic preparations attempt to mimic the characteristic

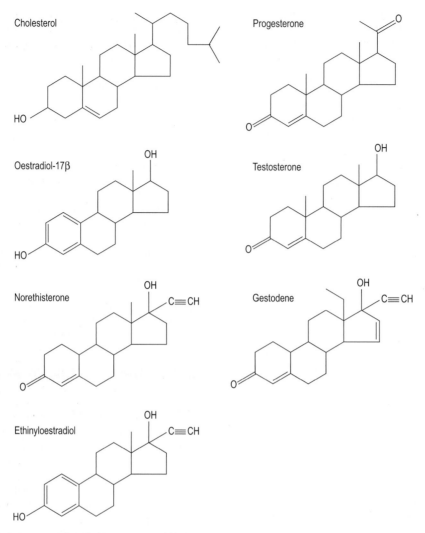

Fig. 4.9 Chemical structures of synthetic contraceptive hormones.

fluctuations in oestrogen and progesterone throughout the cycle. Alternatively, progesterone-only preparations, known as 'minipills', containing small doses of only progesterone are taken on a continuous basis. Progesterone can also be administered as a depot injection or as a slow-releasing preparation from a subcutaneous or uterine source.

It takes at least one complete menstrual cycle for the pill to become effective. Some drugs reduce the effect of the pill and can cause breakthrough bleeding, or even permit pregnancy. These include barbiturates, antibiotics and some anti-epileptic drugs.

Emergency contraception ('the morning-after pill') usually consists of two or four high-dose pills which can be combinations of oestrogen and progesterone or only progesterone. The morning-after pill has strong side-effects and relatively low reliability so it is not recommended as the main method of birth control (Halpern et al., 2010); it also does not protect against sexually transmitted diseases (STDs). Use of the morning-after pill is controversial. For those who believe that pregnancy begins at implantation, the morning-after pill prevents pregnancy, but for those who believe that pregnancy begins at conception, prevention of implantation is classified as abortion because fertilization has already occurred. The morning-after pill should not be confused with mifepristone, which is a synthetic steroid used as an abortifacient for the chemical termination of early pregnancy.

Effects on reproductive cycle

Synthetic oestrogens feedback on the hypothalamus during the antral phase of the menstrual cycle, reducing the levels and the rate of pulsatile secretion of GnRH. Therefore, the release of FSH is inhibited and follicular maturation and expression of LH receptors do not occur. The oestrogens also prevent the LH surge and subsequent ovulation. Production of endogenous oestrogen is reduced.

Synthetic progestogens interfere with the pulsatile secretion of GnRH and decrease the production of LH. Small doses of progesterone may not suppress ovulation but large doses do inhibit maturation of follicles and ovulation. Norethisterone also slows down the breakdown of natural progesterone by the liver. It can be used in low doses because it specifically binds to the progesterone receptors, rather than to androgen receptors as well. Progestogens also reduce secretory activity of the endometrium, so it is not favourable to implantation. Under the influence of progestogens, the cervical mucus is thick and tenacious and so is unreceptive to sperm. The peristaltic muscle activity and cilia movement of the uterine tube become uncoordinated, so transport of the ovum and sperm are affected; this may directly affect successful fertilization. This effect on tubal motility is the reason why there is a slight increase in risk of ectopic pregnancy (implantation in the uterine tube) associated with progesterone preparations.

COCs have their effect by inhibiting ovulation (interrupting feedback on the hypothalamic–pituitary–ovarian axis and reducing FSH and LH), preventing follicular maturation, reducing sperm penetrability of the mucous and affecting endometrial growth and receptivity (Biswas et al., 2008). The progestogen-only pill works by reducing sperm penetrability of the mucous, reducing endometrial receptivity and reducing ovulation. It is well-tolerated but has a higher pregnancy rate as timing of pill taking is more important.

Side-effects

Reported side-effects of oral contraceptives include weight gain, headaches and nausea, depression, vaginal infection or discharge, urinary tract infection, breast changes, skin problems and gum inflammation. Oestrogens affect coagulation factors and promote intravascular coagulation. They also tend to increase plasma lipid levels. Therefore, they can be used safely in young, healthy, motivated women who have no history of circulatory disease. However, smoking and obesity significantly increase the risk of side-effects, particularly thromboembolic complications. Although chemical contraceptive agents have been linked to an increased risk of breast cancer, the doses of synthetic hormone used in current contraceptive preparations are now extremely low, so it is difficult to assess their risk. Contraindications to COC use include arterial disease, smoking, hypertension, migraine, stroke, venous thromboembolism and some cancers (Biswas et al., 2008). Although hormonal treatment has known thromboembolic health concerns, the morbidity complications from pregnancy and labour far outweigh the risks of using oral contraceptives.

Non-oral contraception

The popularity of non-oral hormonal contraception is increasing because it is convenient and efficient and safer for women at risk. Methods include the vaginal ring and contraceptive patches which contain sustained release oestrogen preparations (Black and Kubba, 2008). Progestogen-only methods include contraceptive implants and injectable depo-preparations. Intrauterine methods such as the copper intrauterine device and long-lasting plastic devices such as the T-shaped levopnorgestrel intrauterine system are also effective. Barrier methods of contraception include male and female condoms, diaphragms and caps and spermacides. Sterilization for both men and women is used in many countries as a permanent method of contraception (Melville and Bigrigg, 2008) and worldwide is the most common method of contraception. Female sterilization is more common, although male sterilization is safer, more effective and cheaper. Regret following sterilization is reported to be rare, particularly when individuals are at an older age at sterilization, but requests for reversal following vasectomy are fairly commonplace and usually related to new partnerships or death of children.

Puberty

Puberty describes the morphological, physiological and behavioural changes that occur as the gonads change from infantile to adult condition. The most obvious sign of sexual maturation in women is menarche (the first menstrual cycle), which indicates that the levels of oestrogen and progesterone are adequate to induce development of the uterus. The equivalent step in men is the first ejaculation, which is often nocturnal. However, menarche or the first ejaculation does not necessarily mean that the adolescent body is able to reproduce; early menstrual cycles are frequently anovulatory and the ejaculate of pubertal boys may be mostly seminal plasma, lacking sperm. The underlying hormonal changes are initiated 2–4 years before menarche and the first ejaculation. The sequence of pubertal changes is constant in that the changes occur in the same order (described as the harmony or 'consonance' of puberty) but the starting age and the time for the changes to take place vary. The hormonal changes at puberty lead to a growth spurt and attainment of adult height. In girls, the pubertal growth spurt occurs early in puberty, whereas in boys the growth spurt occurs late in puberty (Fig. 4.10).

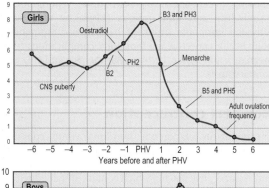

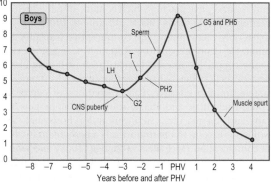

Fig. 4.10 Order of sexual maturation events for girls and boys during the adolescent growth spurt. CNS puberty represents the changed activity of the hypothalamus and nervous system controlling the pubertal changes; stages prefixed B, G and PH represent the development of the breasts, male genitalia and pubic hair, respectively on a 5-point scale. Note that sexual maturation in girls (marked by menarche) follows the peak height velocity (PHV), but in boys (marked by sperm production) occurs before the peak height velocity. (Reproduced with permission from Bogin, 1999b.)

There is thought to be an evolutionary advantage to the differential timing of adult appearance (attainment of adult height) and sexual development (fertility). Bigger girls may be treated as equals by other females in society and taught 'female life-skills', whereas smaller males will not be construed as competitive by other males in society while they undergo development; indeed, becoming fertile while not appearing to be an adult may allow an adolescent male to sneakily mate (Bogin, 1999a).

Physical changes

Physical changes include the development of secondary sex characteristics, the adolescent growth spurt and marked changes in height, psychological states and fertility. All muscle and skeletal dimensions change and the body composition also alters. The earliest changes are measurable in young girls from the age of 6 years. Secondary sex characteristics become evident as secretion of

oestrogen (from ovaries) and androgens (from ovaries and adrenal glands) increases. Changes are seen in the breasts, genitalia, pubic hair and voice.

Hormonal changes

The hypothalamic–pituitary–gonadal axis, which has been developing since fetal life, is activated in early infancy but inhibited in childhood before being reactivated ('re-awoken') at puberty. Immediately after birth, levels of hCG and placental steroid hormones fall. LH and FSH levels increase; they are released in a pulsatile pattern, with nocturnal dominance, throughout infancy and childhood. FSH levels are higher in females and LH levels are higher in males. In the prepubertal period, FSH levels are relatively high compared with LH levels.

At puberty, the pulse amplitude of GnRH increases, resulting in dramatically increased magnitude and frequency of LH secretion, particularly during sleep. In late puberty, day-time secretion of LH also increases until the adult pattern of higher basal LH levels is reached. The 'on' switch for puberty is unknown but may be related to body mass, energy metabolism, leptin secretion or other nutritional factors. There is a progressive change in pituitary responsiveness to GnRH, and a lifting of the restraint on the hypothalamus, which may be related to maturation of the central nervous system and hypothalamus. One of the important signals appears to be activation of the kisspeptin system (Tena-Sempere, 2010). Kisspeptins are a family of peptides which bind to the kisspeptin receptors in the hypothalamus which are closely associated with the GnRH neurons. They have recently been identified as essential neuropeptide regulators of reproductive maturation which influence the onset of puberty, ovulation and the metabolic regulation of fertility. Adrenal function matures independently before gonadal function. Adrenal secretion of sex steroids increases. Adrenal androgens stimulate pubic and axillary hair growth and have a small effect on growth and bone development. The timing of gonadal maturity and the onset of puberty correlate more closely with bone development than with chronological age. The central nervous system can restrain the onset by affecting the hypothalamic GnRH pattern.

Delayed puberty may result from Kallman's syndrome, hypogonadotropic hypogonadism, which is due to a genetic abnormality that results in a deficiency of GnRH from the hypothalamus. Precocious puberty, when puberty is initiated at a very early age, is usually unexplained and probably due to natural variation but it can also be a result of brain injury or a tumour such as a hypothalamic or pituitary tumour and unusually high production of GnRH or gonadotrophins. Whatever the cause, precocious puberty has serious consequences for social and psychological development and can influence adult height (as the pubertal hormone surges cause the early closure of the bone epiphyses and the cessation of subsequent growth). The increasing incidence of childhood obesity has tended to result in girls entering puberty earlier and boys entering puberty later (Ahmed et al., 2009). It has been suggested that the earlier timing of puberty over the last few decades has resulted in a dissociation between biological maturity which occurs at an earlier age and psychosocial maturity which lags behind and that this mismatch of modern puberty is instrumental in some of the social issues faced by adolescents today (Gluckman and Hanson, 2006).

Age of menarche

Over half of early menstrual cycles are anovulatory and do not result in the release of an ovum. Ovulation usually occurs about 10 months after menarche. After a period of 5 years, the incidence of anovulatory cycles has decreased to about 20%. There are secular trends in the age of menarche which got progressively earlier, particularly in the early to mid 20th century. The average age of menarche in Europe is currently 12–13 years compared with 14–15 years a century ago. However, with the marked increase in childhood obesity over the last 20 years, one might expect the age of menarche to have fallen in parallel with increased body size; this has not happened.

Various influences on the age of menarche have been investigated, such as photoperiod and body mass. One suggestion was that the earlier age of menarche has coincided with the introduction of electricity, increasing the photoperiod and the individual's exposure to light (Bullough, 1981). However, a more plausible theory is that it is related to better nutrition. Women seem to have a critical body mass for successful reproduction; if their body mass falls much below, the menstrual cycle becomes erratic and stops. Body fat levels seem to play a role. Anorexic women have lower levels of FSH and LH (see p. 86). Moderate obesity is associated with earlier menarche but severe obesity

delays it. The combination of heavy exercise and undernutrition is synergistic, as can be observed in ballet dancers and athletes (see Chapter 12). Chronic illness can also delay menarche; the exact mechanisms are unknown. An alternative view is that there are genetic factors influencing the rate of development and that body fatness and age at menarche are both driven by the 'blue-print' or genetic plan rather than age at menarche being a consequence of fat deposition. Children who are taller tend to have earlier pubertal development and the age at menarche correlates better with height than with weight (Cole, 2003). The age at menarche is clearly affected by body mass, exercise, stress, nutrition and altitude (Frisch, 1990).

Sequence of changes at puberty

The normal sequence in females is breast budding (at 8–13 years), growth of pubic hair, peak growth velocity (9.5–14.5 years) and then menarche (10–16.5 years). The pattern in boys is testicular growth, pubic hair growth, penile growth and growth spurt. These characteristic changes in pubic hair distribution and breast development in girls and external genitalia in boys have been classified as Tanner stages and are used to assess pubertal development (Table 4.2).

From about 6 months of age, childhood growth depends on adequate growth hormone (GH) secretion. Growth declines progressively and reaches its slowest velocity just before the onset of the pubertal growth spurt. In boys, the growth spurt starts slightly later, and is faster (9.4 cm/year compared with 8.3 cm/year in girls) with delayed fusion of the epiphyseal plates, so men attain a higher adult height. The pubertal growth spurt depends on sex hormones secreted from the gonads. Optimal growth depends on both sex steroids and GH; GH levels are highest in the pubertal period.

Table 4.2 Tanner stages of pubertal development

STAGE	PUBIC HAIR	BREAST DEVELOPMENT IN FEMALES	EXTERNAL GENITALIA IN MALES
1	None	Prepubertal; no breast tissue and papilla elevated	Pre-adolescent stage
2	Sparse growth of long downy hair along labia	Areolar enlargement with breast bud	Scrotum and testes enlarged (>4 mL); changes texture/colour of scrotal skin
3	Coarser and curly pigmented hairs	Enlargement of breast and areolar as a single mound	Further growth of testes (6–10 mL) and scrotum; increase in penis size
4	Small adult configuration	Projection of areolar above breast as a double mound	Further enlargement of testes (10–15 mL), scrotum and penis; glans penis development
5	Adult pubic hair distribution	Mature adult breast as a single mound	Adult stage

MENOPAUSE

Women continue to have menstrual cycles until the finite population of oocytes in the ovary is exhausted. The term 'menopause' is literally the cessation of menstrual cycles. It is defined as permanent cessation of menstruation because of the loss of ovarian follicular activity after 12 consecutive months of amenorrhoea without another cause and, hence, can only be determined retrospectively 12 months after the final menstrual period. However, the term 'menopause' is frequently applied to the climacteric (perimenopausal phase), which is the transitional decline of reproductive activity over a period of 2–3 years leading up to the final menstrual period, usually occurring between the ages of 45 and 55 years (median 51 years). The climacteric begins when fertility is already rapidly declining and continues until the ovaries cease secreting oestrogen. Ovarian senescence is actually a gradual process beginning from around 35 years of age; it is marked by a progressive decline in fertility and increased rate of menstrual irregularity and miscarriage. The hormonal changes affect particularly the tissues which have a high density of oestrogen receptors such as skin, epithelium of the vagina and bladder, neuronal tissue (changes in neurotransmitter release affect libido, irritability, mood, sleep, concentration and memory) and factors which influence cardiovascular and bone health. Thermoregulation is also affected.

The decline in oestrogen production is related to the number of remaining primordial follicles, the number of recruitable follicles in each cycle and the proportion of follicles that reach maturity before ovulation (Al Azzawi and Palacios, 2009). As the pool of oocytes gets smaller, hormonal changes occur; these precede the final depletion of follicles. Defective follicular phases result in fewer granulose cells in the follicle and therefore reduced oestrogen production. As oestrogen exerts a negative feedback effect at the hypothalamic–pituitary axis, the drop in oestrogen level causes FSH level to rise from about 35 years onwards. The first notable hormonal change preceding the climacteric is a drop in inhibin secretion, which results in a lowering of the negative feedback on the hypothalamic–pituitary gonadal axis. Therefore FSH secretion increases, which means more follicles are recruited at this early stage of the climacteric. The increased level of follicular development results in enhanced oestrogen production from the greater number of follicles; twin ovulations (and pregnancies) are more common. This, paradoxically, means that fertility towards the end of reproductive life is increased (reflected in an increased rate in twinning in older women) but it also increases the rate at which the dwindling pool of oocytes are recruited. So the hormonal changes move from being compensated to decompensated as there follicles are rapidly depleted below a critical number.

The compromised hormonal status then results in a decreased follicular phase of the cycle and a shorter cycle length. Functioning of the ovary becomes more erratic with a variable cycle length and an increased number of anovulatory cycles. Luteinization does not occur; there is no increase in progesterone secretion but oestrogen drives endometrial proliferation which can be excessive, as can be menstrual loss when there is a cycle with successful luteinization. Eventually, as the follicles are depleted, oestrogen and progesterone levels fall and menstrual cycles cease. The loss of steroid hormone negative feedback results in a gradual rise in FSH secretion which tends to fluctuate from cycle to cycle.

The loss of follicles means that there is no oestrogen production from granulose cells and no recruitment of thecal cells which produced androgens. Although the postmenopausal ovary no longer synthesizes oestradiol, there is some peripheral conversion of androstenedione by adipose tissue providing a source of oestrone. So body fat essentially acts like inbuilt hormone replacement therapy (HRT). The adrenal gland produces a small amount of progesterone and some testosterone. DHEA production by the ovaries falls which means ovarian androstenedione production falls (although some amount is still produced by the adrenal gland), so testosterone levels fall. The secretion of sex hormone binding protein (SHBP) from the liver diminishes because its production is stimulated by oestrogen and inhibited by androgens (and obesity). So postmenopausally levels of SHBP fall and bioavailability of free testosterone is enhanced. However, overall the net effect is one of androgen deficiency, which can affect sense of well-being, muscle mass and strength, sexual desire and sexual receptivity, sexual arousal and orgasm, memory and cognition, and cause depression, adding to the effect of oestrogen deficiency.

Premature menopause is defined as menopause before 40 years of age; it is usually a result of autoimmune disorders, genetics, or problems with ovarian development or chromosomal abnormalities. Menopause can also be induced, for instance by surgery (removal of ovaries usually with a hysterectomy) or by treatment for cancer. With recent increases in longevity, an average woman may spend about 35–40% of her lifespan in the postmenopausal period. Menopause is a complex and natural process of ageing. It is unique to humans (and a few other species such as the short-finned pilot whale and the Asian elephant) and is thought to have an evolutionary advantage. There are advantages to the species in preventing late childbearing and ensuring that the dependent human offspring are more likely to have the care and protection of their mother (and she to have the support of her mother; Shanley and Kirkwood, 2001). The Grandmother Hypothesis (Kuhle, 2007) suggests that the presence of postmenopausal women is beneficial for the species; compared to other species, human infants are altricial (very helpless and dependent), maturation is delayed (because childhood is an important learning time for a species with a big brain), infant mortality rates are high and inter-birth intervals are short. Grandmothers are socially established, reliable and skilled, possess specialized knowledge and have a vested interest in the survival of their grandchildren. Indeed, there are examples of grandmothers (who have their own infants), able to take over breastfeeding of their grandchildren (Scelza, 2009).

A number of factors affect the age of menopause. These include leanness and nutritional status, ethnicity and genetics. Smokers, women who have not had children and women of lower socio-economic status tend to have an earlier menopause as do women who have shorter menstrual cycle length. There is no relationship between age at menarche and age at menopause.

Effects on the reproductive system

Morphologically, the ovaries at menopause appear smaller and relatively devoid of follicles (Santoro and Chervenak, 2004). There is a finite number of ova; however, hormonal changes precede the depletion of follicles. There are about 25 000 follicles remaining at the time of menopause. One of the earliest changes is a decrease in inhibin production by the granulosa cells. This results in decreased negative feedback at the hypothalamic–pituitary axis and an increase in GnRH level, which promotes secretion of FSH and follicular development. This is the reason for the paradoxical increase in twinning rate that is observed in women conceiving late in reproductive life. After this brief increase in follicular development, the menstrual cycles tend to become shorter, particularly in the follicular phase. This results in oestrogen secretion diminishing, so the production of androgens increases. Menstrual cycles become increasingly erratic with variable cycle lengths and an increase in anovulatory cycles. Anovulation is associated with progesterone deficiency, which is associated with prolonged or irregular vaginal bleeding. As the cycles become less frequent, there is increased time for endometrial proliferation, which can lead to excessive menstrual blood loss. Ultimately, oestrogen and progesterone levels decrease and cycling ceases.

From menopause onwards, levels of FSH and LH are high and levels of oestrogen and inhibin are decreased. FSH increases because of the lack of a negative feedback from oestrogen influencing the anterior pituitary gland. The postmenopausal ovary continues to produce considerable amounts of androgens and some progesterone; thus, natural menopause is not equivalent to the effects of a surgically induced menopause following oophorectomy (removal of ovaries). There is some oestrogen production by the adipose tissue; this (and the protective cushioning provided by fat) is the reason why fatter women are protected, at least partially, from osteoporosis.

Effects on other physiological systems

In addition to the reproduction tract itself, there are many other target organs bearing oestrogen receptors, which respond to the fall in circulating oestrogen levels. The resulting vasomotor instability produces symptoms of hot flushes (or 'hot flashes'), sweats and palpitations. The thermoregulatory centre in the hypothalamus falsely signals that body temperature is too high. It is thought that the decreased oestrogen level abrogates the catechol–oestrogen inhibition of tyrosine hydroxylase so noradrenaline levels are increased. This results in physiological processes such as increased peripheral vasodilation that attempt to reduce core body temperature. Hot flushes are not always visible but may be extreme; skin temperature may increase by as much as 7–8 °C for a few minutes accompanied by a rapid increase in heart rate. Emotional and psychological problems such as anxiety, depression, loss of libido and mood swings may occur. Insomnia is also a frequently cited problem.

All the tissues of the female reproductive tract have a high density of oestrogen receptors and are profoundly affected by oestrogen withdrawal. The uterus shrinks. The vaginal epithelium diminishes and becomes less elastic. The vaginal cells decrease production of glycogen, affecting lactobacillus colonization, so the pH increases, resulting in increased susceptibility to vaginal infections. Vaginal atrophy causes vaginal secretions to diminish, which may result in painful intercourse. Menopausal women have an increased frequency of urinary problems, which is probably related to oestrogen withdrawal as there are many oestrogen receptors in the urinary tract (which shares the same embryonic origin as the lower reproductive tract). The walls of the lower bladder and urethra become thinner and the urethral muscles weaken, which increases the risk of stress incontinence.

Oestrogen protects the cardiovascular system; the risk of cardiovascular disease doubles in postmenopausal women. The incidence of coronary heart disease in premenopausal women and postmenopausal women treated with HRT is much lower than in men. Oestrogen inhibits the uptake and degradation of low-density lipoprotein (LDL) by the coronary blood vessel endothelium. It may also inhibit coronary vasospasm. Oestrogen has been shown to decrease vascular resistance (and therefore blood pressure), increase cardiac output and increase synthesis of nitric oxide (NO, a potent locally acting vasodilator). Postmenopausal women have significantly higher levels of serum cholesterol and triacylglycerides. Oestrogen inhibits endothelial hyperplasia, smooth muscle cells growth and platelet activation. Oestrogen withdrawal is associated with raised levels of certain blood-clotting factors and an increased tendency for thrombosis, and thus with increased risk of myocardial infarction and cerebrovascular accident (stroke). Insulin resistance is more common in postmenopausal women.

Skeletal changes occur as the decrease in oestrogen results in increased bone resorption, increasing the tendency to stoop and the likelihood of fractures. Osteoblasts (bone-producing cells) have oestrogen receptors. Osteoclast activity increases postmenopause and osteoblast activity decreases. Oestrogen deficiency uncouples bone formation and bone resorption. This effect is increased by changes in the hormones controlling calcium balance. Levels of calcitonin fall in parallel with oestrogen levels. Calcitonin inhibits the activity of osteoclasts (bone-absorbing cells). The progressive loss of calcium from the bones and the long postmenopausal lifetime mean that a woman can lose about half of her trabecular bone density and about a third of her cortical bone and is therefore predisposed to osteoporosis. Collagen is lost from the skin, tendons and bones.

There are also changes in metabolism and body composition postmenopause. Women tend to gain fat, especially visceral fat, and to lose muscle mass.

Hormone replacement therapy

Hormone replacement therapy (HRT) aims to reduce the diverse symptoms and adverse effects of menopause (Box 4.9). HRT provides low doses of various combinations of hormones. It is effective during its use but not in the long-term. Oestrogen on its own is mitogenic and promotes endometrial hyperplasia (which is associated with increased risk of cancer). Oestrogen with progesterone is safer as progesterone abrogates cell division and increases endometrial secretory activity. The Women's Health Initiative (WHI) studies in the United States looked at long-term health outcomes of women taking HRT using randomized controlled primary-prevention trials. The WHI studies found that HRT increased the risk of heart disease, stroke, deep vein thrombosis, pulmonary embolism and some types of cancer. This was at odds with previous studies which tended to select healthy women as subjects and omitted women who smoked or might be at increased risk of vascular disease. However, the figures need to be considered in context; although the risk of disease was increased significantly, the actual numbers of women affected were very low. Rather than being a panacea for all menopausal problems, there are benefits and risks to HRT which need to be assessed, as for all medications. Some women have extreme symptoms of menopause which have a very negative influence on the quality of life.

Key points

- The ovary produces the female gametes (ova) and steroid hormones, oestrogen and progesterone.
- Relatively few female gametes are produced during a woman's reproductive life, between puberty and the menopause.
- The meiotic division of the ovum begins in the female fetus and is suspended until ovulation, halts again, and is completed at fertilization.
- Follicular development begins about 3 months prior to ovulation but key stages in development of the follicles are stimulated by FSH in the first half of the menstrual cycle in which the ovum is released. The developing follicles produce oestrogen; usually a single dominant follicle matures and ovulates.
- The first half of the menstrual cycle (follicular phase) is dominated by oestrogen and prepares the reproductive system for ovulation, for instance by stimulating growth of the endometrial lining.
- Ovulation is triggered by the surge of LH. The ovum surrounded by a rim of cumulus cells is released and swept into the uterine tube.
- Follicular cells remaining in the ovary become the corpus luteum, which produces progesterone and oestrogen.
- The second half of the cycle (luteal phase) is dominated by the effects of progesterone, which prepare the body for pregnancy.
- LH promotes secretion from the corpus luteum. However, the effect is short-lived, so the corpus luteum regresses, unless rescued by hCG from the dividing cells of the embryo, and menstruation ensues.
- Pituitary secretion of FSH and LH is under the control of pulsatile GnRH release from the hypothalamus. Oestrogen and progesterone exert negative feedback effects on the hypothalamic–pituitary axis except at mid-cycle, when oestrogen exerts positive feedback leading to the LH surge and ovulation.
- The hypothalamus integrates other signals regulating reproductive function. Fertility can be disrupted by abnormal endocrine activity such as abnormal production of GnRH and hyperprolactinaemia, abnormal follicular development and extremes of weight loss or gain.
- Understanding the hormonal regulation of reproduction has allowed manipulation of fertility using chemical analogues of the steroid hormones in contraceptives.

Box 4.9 **Hormone replacement therapy (HRT)**

- Exogenous oestrogen replaces ovarian oestrogen
- Prevents long-term consequences
- Oral route or directly to genital tract or systemically (transdermal patch or subcutaneous implant)
- Abrogates flushing and sweating
- Stimulates replication of, and secretion from, vaginal epithelial cells
- Progesterone given to induce menstruation (and prevent endometrial hyperplasia)
- Progesterone-withdrawal bleeding is major reason for non-compliance
- Protects against coronary heart disease and osteoporosis

Application to practice

There are many environmental influences, both internal and external, that may affect the regulation of reproductive cycles. There is increasing evidence that many pollutants and chemicals in the environment can have negative effects upon human reproduction; knowledge of this is important in understanding some possible causes of subfertility and congenital abnormalities of the genitalia.

It is important to realize that the menstrual cycle prepares women for pregnancy. The physiological changes, in preparation for and support of pregnancy, are initiated prior to ovulation and conception.

An understanding of the variance in the menstrual cycle is important when considering the estimated due date. Knowledge of the reproductive cycles is essential in understanding the various methods of birth control.

ANNOTATED FURTHER READING

Balen AH, editor: *Infertility in practice*, ed 3, UK, 2008, Informa.

A practical guide, based on the author's clinical practice, which provides an overview of human infertility problems, aetiology and evidence-based possible interventions.

Guillebaud J: *Contraception today*, ed 6, UK, 2007, Informa.

This book provides an evidenced based guide to all forms of contraception available. This latest edition includes information for contraceptive use in the older women.

Gougeon A: Human ovarian follicular development: from activation of resting follicles to preovulatory maturation. *Ann Endocrinol (Paris)* 71:132–143, 2010.

An in-depth but clearly explained review of follicular growth in the human ovary which describes the interactions of hormones and local growth factors in controlling oocyte maturation and follicular growth.

Hirschberg AL: Polycystic ovary syndrome, obesity and reproductive implications, *Womens Health (Lond Engl)* 5:529–540, 2009.

A recent review about polycystic ovary syndrome (PCOS) and its biological basis which covers effects on fertility, pregnancy and metabolic syndrome and discusses effective lifestyle programmes.

Glasier A: *Handbook of family planning and reproductive healthcare*, ed 5,

New York, 2007, Churchill Livingstone.

A practical handbook covering all forms of contraception, pill prescribing, possible complications, advantages and disadvantages of each method and the clinical management of women with psychosexual disorders, sexually transmitted infections, menopausal symptoms and gynaecological problems.

Johnson MH: *Essential reproduction*, ed 6, Oxford, 2007, Blackwell Science.

An integrated and well-organized research-based textbook that explores comparative reproductive physiology of mammals, including anatomy, physiology, endocrinology, genetics and behavioural studies.

Kreitzman L, Russell FG: Rhythms of life: the biological clocks that control the daily lives of every living thing, 2004, Profile Books.

A very readable text covering fascinating details about the rhythms of the natural world and how time influences life.

Nappi RE, Lachowsky M: Menopause and sexuality: prevalence of symptoms and impact on quality of life. *Maturitas* 63:138–141, 2009.

A review of sexual and urogenital symptoms at menopause and their impact on quality of life.

Leung PCK, Adashi EY: *The ovary*, ed 2, London, 2004, Academic Press.

A detailed description of ovarian structure and function at the cellular and molecular level, including normal development and pathophysiology.

Mistlberger RE, Skene DJ: Social influences on mammalian circadian rhythms: animal and human studies, *Biol Rev Camb Philos Soc* 79 (3):533–556, 2004.

A readable review, which describes how light and social stimuli ('zeitgebers' or time-cues) entrain mammalian circadian rhythms.

Ridley M: *The red queen: sex and the evolution of human nature*, London, 1994, Penguin.

A new and exciting approach to understanding reproductive behaviour and physiology from an evolutionary perspective.

Shuttle P, Redgrove P: *The wise wound: menstruation and every woman*, ed 3, London, 1999, Victor Gollancz.

This text provides an exploration of the sociological and anthropological perspectives of human reproduction including the facts, fantasies, taboos and cultural aspects surrounding menstruation.

Szarewski A: Choice of contraception, *Curr Obstet Gyn* 16:361–365, 2009.

A short discussion of the factors affecting choice of contraception which illustrates the issues with three case studies.

REFERENCES

Adashi EY, Resnick CE, Hernandez ER, et al: Ovarian transforming growth factor-beta (TGF beta): cellular site(s), and mechanism(s) of action, *Mol Cell Endocrinol* 61(2):247–256, 1989.

Ahmed ML, Ong KK, Dunger DB: Childhood obesity and the timing of puberty, *Trends Endocrinol Metab* 20:237–242, 2009.

Al Azzawi F, Palacios S: Hormonal changes during menopause, *Maturitas* 63:135–137, 2009.

Biswas J, Mann M, Webberley H: Oral contraception, *Obstet Gyn Reproduct Med* 18:317–323, 2008.

Black KI, Kubba A: Non-oral contraception, *Obstet Gyn Reproduct Med* 18:324–329, 2008.

Bogin B: Evolutionary perspective on human growth, *Ann Rev Anthropol* 28:109–153, 1999a.

Bogin B: *Patterns of Human Growth*, ed 2, Cambridge, 1999b, Cambridge University Press.

Brooker CG: *Human structure and function*, ed 2, St Louis, 1998, Mosby 480, 488, 489.

Brosens JJ, Parker MG, McIndoe A, et al: A role for menstruation in preconditioning the uterus for successful pregnancy, *Am J Obstet Gynecol* 200:615–616, 2009.

Buffenstein R, Poppitt SD, McDevitt RM, et al: Food intake and the menstrual cycle: a retrospective analysis with implications for appetite research, *Physiol Behav* 58:1067–1077, 1995.

Bulletti C, de Ziegler D: Uterine contractility and embryo implantation, *Curr Opin Obstet Gynecol* 17:265–276, 2005.

Bullough VL: Age at menarche: a misunderstanding, *Science* 213:365–366, 1981.

Clancy KB: Reproductive ecology and the endometrium: physiology, variation, and new directions, *Am J Phys Anthropol* 140(Suppl. 49):137–154, 2009.

Clarke IJ: The hypothalamic–pituitary axis. In Hillier SG, Kitchener HC, Neilson JP, editors: *Scientific essentials of reproductive medicine*, Philadelphia, 1996, WB Saunders, pp 120–132.

Cole TJ: The secular trend in human physical growth: a biological view, *Econ Hum Biol* 1(2):161–168, 2003.

Dale B, Marino M, Wilding M: The ins and outs of meiosis, *J Exper Zool* 285 (3):226–236, 1999.

Davidsen L, Vistisen B, Astrup A: Impact of the menstrual cycle on determinants of energy balance: a putative role in weight loss attempts, *Int J Obes Lond* 31:1777–1785, 2007.

Dye L, Blundell JE: Menstrual cycle and appetite control: implications for weight regulation, *Hum Reprod* 12:1142–1151, 1997.

Farage MA, Osborn TW, MacLean AB: Cognitive, sensory, and emotional changes associated with the menstrual cycle: a review, *Arch Gynecol Obstet* 278:299–307, 2008.

Farage MA, Neill S, MacLean AB: Physiological changes associated with the menstrual cycle: a review, *Obstet Gynecol Surv* 64:58–72, 2009.

Fessler DMT: No time to eat: an adaptionist account of periovulatory behavioural changes, *Q Rev Biol* 78:3–21, 2003.

Frisch RE: The right weight, body fat, menarche and ovulation, *Baillière's Clin Obstet Gynaecol* 4:419–439, 1990.

Girman A, Lee R, Kligler B: An integrative medicine approach to premenstrual syndrome, *Am J Obstet Gynecol* 188: S56–S65, 2003.

Giudice LC: Growth factors and growth modulators in human uterine endometrium: their potential relevance to reproductive medicine, *Fertil Steril* 61:1–17, 1994.

Gluckman PD, Hanson MA: Evolution, development and timing of puberty, *Trends Endocrinol Metab* 17:7–12, 2006.

Halpern V, Raymond EG, Lopez LM: Repeated use of pre- and postcoital hormonal contraception for prevention of pregnancy, *Cochrane Database Syst Rev* CD007595, 2010.

Hamilton-Fairley D, Johnson MR: The ovary. In Chamberlain G, Broughton Pipkin F, editors: *Clinical physiology in obstetrics*, ed 3, Oxford, 1998, Blackwell, pp 396–417.

Hassan E, Creatsas G, Mastorakos G, et al: Clinical implications of the ovarian/endometrial renin–angiotensin–aldosterone system, *Ann N Y Acad Sci* 900:107–118, 2000.

Hillier SG: Regulatory functions for inhibin and activin in human ovaries, *J Endocrinol* 131:171–175, 1991.

Hillier SG, Whitelaw PF, Smyth CD: Follicular oestrogen synthesis: the 'two-cell, two-gonadotrophin' model revisited, *Mol Cell Endocrinol* 100:51–54, 1994.

Huang CJ, Stromer MH, Anderson LL: Abrupt shifts in relaxin and progesterone secretion by aging luteal cells: luteotrophic response in hysterectomized and pregnant rats, *Endocrinology* 128:165–173, 1991.

Hurwitz A, Loukides J, Ricciarelli E, et al: Human intraovarian interleukin-1 (IL-1) system: highly compartmentalized and hormonally dependent regulation of the genes encoding IL-1, its receptor, and its receptor antagonist, *J Clin Invest* 89 (6):1746–1754, 1992.

Johnson MH, Everitt BJ: *Essential reproduction*, ed 4, Oxford, 1995, Blackwell Science, pp 64, 65, 108, 109.

Johnson MR, Carter G, Grint C, et al: Relationship between ovarian steroids, gonadotrophins and relaxin during the menstrual cycle, *Acta Endocrinol (Copenh)* 129:121–125, 1993.

Johnson J, et al: Germline stem cells and follicular renewal in the postnatal mammalian ovary, *Nature* 428:145–150, 2004.

Kuhle BX: An evolutionary perspective on the origin and ontogeny of menopause, *Maturitas* 57:329–337, 2007.

Kunz G, Leyendecker G: Uterine peristaltic activity during the menstrual cycle: characterization, regulation, function and dysfunction, *Reprod Biomed Online* 4:5–9, 2001.

Legro RS, Kunselman AR, Dodson WC, et al: Prevalence and predictors of risk for type 2 diabetes mellitus and impaired glucose tolerance in polycystic ovary syndrome: a prospective, controlled study in 254 affected women, *J Clin Endocrinol Metab* 84:165–169, 1999.

Lyons EA, Taylor PJ, Zheng XH, et al: Characterization of subendometrial contractions throughout the menstrual cycle in normal fertile women, *Fertil Steril* 55:771–774, 1991.

Mason HD, Margara R, Winston RML, et al: Insulin-like growth factor-I (IGF-I) inhibits production of IGF-binding protein-I while stimulating estradiol secretion in granulosa cells from normal and polycystic human ovaries, *J Clin Endocrinol Metab* 76:1275–1279, 1993.

Mason HD, Willis DS, Holly JMP, et al: Insulin preincubation enhances insulin-like growth factor-II (IGF-II) action on steroidogenesis in human granulosa cells, *J Clin Endocrinol Metab* 78:1265–1267, 1994.

McClure N, Healy DL, Rogers PAW, et al: Vascular endothelial growth factor as capillary permeability agent in ovarian hyperstimulation syndrome, *Lancet* 34:235–236, 1994.

Melville C, Bigrigg A: Male and female sterilization, *Obstet Gyn Reproduct Med* 18:330–334, 2008.

National Collaborating Centre for Women's and Children's Health: *Clinical guideline 11. Fertility:*

assessment and treatment for people with fertility problems, 2004, National Institute for Clinical Excellence.

Oosthuyse T, Bosch AN: The effect of the menstrual cycle on exercise metabolism: implications for exercise performance in eumenorrhoeic women, *Sports Med* 40:207–227, 2010.

Pinkerton JV, Guico-Pabia CJ, Taylor HS: Menstrual cycle-related exacerbation of disease, *Am J Obstet Gynecol* 202:221–231, 2010.

Radon PA, McMahon MJ, Meyer WR: Impaired glucose tolerance in pregnant women with polycystic ovary syndrome, *Obstet Gynecol* 94:194–197, 1999.

Rance NE, Young WS, McMullen NT: Topography of neurons expressing luteinizing hormone releasing hormone gene transcripts in the human hypothalamus and basal forebrain, *J Comp Neurol* 339:573–586, 1991.

Richards JS, Pangas SA: The ovary: basic biology and clinical implications, *J Clin Invest* 120:963–972, 2010.

Ridley, M: *The red queen: sex and the evolution of human nature*, 1994, Penguin Science.

Roberts VJ, Barth S, El-Roeiy A, et al: Expression of inhibin/activin subunits and follistatin messenger ribonucleic acids and proteins in ovarian follicles and the corpus luteum during the human menstrual cycle, *J Clin Endocrinol Metab* 77(5):1402–1410, 1993.

Salamonsen LA: Tissue injury and repair in the female human reproductive tract, *Reproduction* 125:301–311, 2003.

Santoro N, Chervenak JL: The menopause transition, *Endocrinol Metab Clin North Am* 33(4):627–636, 2004.

Scelza BA: The grandmaternal niche: critical caretaking among Martu Aborigines, *Am J Hum Biol* 21:448–454, 2009.

Scheele F, Schoemaker J: The role of follicle stimulating hormones in the selection of follicles in human ovaries: a survey of the literature and a proposed model, *Gynecol Endocrinol* 10:55–66, 1996.

Shanley DP, Kirkwood TB: Evolution of the human menopause, *Bioessays* 23 (3):282–287, 2001.

Stem K, McClintock MK: Regulation of ovulation by human pheromones, *Nature* 392:177–179, 1998.

Strassmann BI: The evolution of endometrial cycles and menstruation, *Q Rev Biol* 71:181–220, 1996.

Tena-Sempere M: Kisspeptin signaling in the brain: recent developments and future challenges, *Mol Cell Endocrinol* 314:164–169, 2010.

Terner JM, de Wit H: Menstrual cycle phase and responses to drugs of abuse in humans, *Drug Alcohol Depend* 84:1–13, 2006.

Van Vugt DA: Brain imaging studies of appetite in the context of obesity and the menstrual cycle, *Hum Reprod Update* 16:276–292, 2010.

Vollenhoven B, Clark S, Kovacs G, et al: Prevalence of gestational diabetes mellitus in polycystic ovarian syndrome (PCOS) patients pregnant after ovulation induction with gonadotrophins, *Aust N Z J Obstet Gynaecol* 40:54–58, 2000.

Zeleznik AJ, Hillier SG: The ovary: endocrine function. In Hillier SG, Kitchener HC, Neilson JP, editors: *Scientific essentials of reproductive medicine*, Philadelphia, 1996, WB Saunders, pp 133–146.

Chapter | 5 |

Sexual differentiation and behaviour

LEARNING OBJECTIVES

- To discuss the advantages of sexual dimorphism.
- To describe how sexual differentiation is achieved during embryological development.
- To describe possible causes of indeterminate sex.
- To outline the phases of gonadal development.
- To identify the main differences in gonadal function between the male and female.
- To discuss factors affecting sexual behaviour.

INTRODUCTION

Evolutionary biologists have long questioned why evolution has led to sexual dimorphism: the differentiation of the sexes into male and female forms. Hermaphroditism remains limited to lower life forms, such as the annelids (worms) and molluscs (slugs and snails), although it is widespread throughout the plant kingdom. It is widely accepted that the development of sexual reproduction increased the speed of evolution resulting in the wide diversity of life forms upon the planet. The essential characteristic of sexual reproduction is that the new individual is generated from two distinct packages of genes: half from the male gamete (spermatozoon) and half from the female gamete (oocyte). The meiotic division that produces the gametes not only halves the normal (diploid) number of chromosomes but also increases genetic variability within each chromosome by exchange of bits of homologous chromosomes (see Chapter 7). Fertilization results in the gametes combining to form a genetically unique zygote (see Chapter 6).

Sexual reproduction results in a wide diversity of genetic material within a species, enabling the species to adapt to long-term environmental changes. The advantage of this diversity is that the population is likely to be more resilient to environmental challenges. Asexual reproduction, however, allows genetic adaptation only by mutation. The question as to why higher life forms evolved a reproductive strategy involving dimorphism remains unanswered. However, mammalian gametes are morphologically different, which lessens the potential for same-sex fertilization, which is not far removed from self-sex fertilization, thus ensuring optimal mixing of genes. So the gametes have distinct male or female forms and are made in morphologically different male and female gonads which produce a distinct pattern of sex hormones.

Chapter case study

Zara and her husband, James, would very much like to know the sex of their babies and had been informed by one of their friends, who happens to be a doctor and who they met while in Africa, that they would be able to find out the sex when they have the 12-week ultrasound scan.

- When Zara informs you, her midwife, that they wish to be told the sex of the babies when the scan is performed, what do you think would be important to discuss with Zara and her husband regarding the identification of the sex of the babies?
- Are there any situations where it can be justified to identify the sex of the baby at the 12-week scan?
- What should the midwife do if a woman requests a termination of pregnancy solely because she knows the sex of her baby?

These control both the development of the distinct male and female phenotype and affect behaviour and physiology thus ensuring that the gametes have an optimal chance of delivery and that mating occurs at the optimal time for fertilization. The sex hormones also prepare the female to carry the developing embryo throughout pregnancy and to nurture it through the period of lactation and dependency.

Sexual dimorphism is genetically controlled in many animals. However, in some species, such as crocodiles and tortoises, sexual dimorphism is principally determined by environment. The temperature of incubation of the egg promotes the development of either male or female offspring. Intermediate temperatures of egg incubation result in the ratios of the sexes altering in relation to the differing temperature gradients. In birds, the female carries the ZW chromosomes and the male the ZZ chromosomes, whereas some species of fish are able to change sex during a single lifetime. Differentiation of the sexes in mammals also involves sexual dimorphism of the urinary system because the two systems are closely linked in their development.

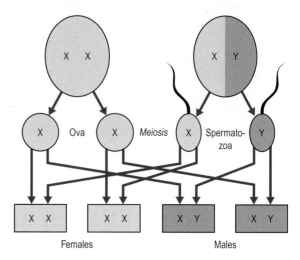

Fig. 5.1 Paternal genetic determination of sex in humans. Sex determination is genetically influenced by the SRY gene normally located on the Y chromosome; therefore it is fertilization by either a gynosperm or an androsperm that influences sexual dimorphism.

DIFFERENTIATION INTO MALE AND FEMALE

In humans, differentiation into either a male or female fetus is almost always under genetic control, depending on whether the ovum is fertilized by a sperm carrying an X chromosome (gynosperm; female) or a Y chromosome (androsperm; male). However, events such as maternal pyrexia in the first trimester of pregnancy can result in abnormal cell division and development, in some cases contributing to indeterminate (ambiguous) sexual characteristics as well as other physical malformations. As in all mammals, the human female is the homogametic sex and usually carries the XX chromosome arrangement whereas the male is the heterogametic sex and carries the XY arrangement for reproductive function to be successful. Therefore, it is the sperm that determines the sex of the fetus (Fig. 5.1). Rarely, mosaic individuals (carrying a patchwork of XX and XY cells) or those individuals with mutations in genes important for sex determination may express a phenotype opposite to their karyotype leading to XX males or XY females. If a Y chromosome is present, the individual develops testes (male gonads) regardless of the number of X chromosomes. The Y chromosome is much smaller than the X chromosome. The DNA of the Y chromosome is very condensed and so incapable of synthesizing RNA (see Chapter 7). Essentially, the Y chromosome switches on or controls the other genes required for testes formation; these genes are on the other autosomal chromosomes and the X chromosome.

The indifferent embryo

The development of the fetus, both male and female, is initially the same. The gonads are formed from the mesenchymal tissue of the genital ridge primordia which develop each side of the descending aorta. Until approximately the 4th week of gestation, the fetus is in a sexually undifferentiated state. After this phase, the differentiation process is initiated by the activation of the SRY (sex-determining region of the Y) gene, usually found only upon the Y chromosome (Sinclair et al., 1990). The SRY gene triggers a complex cascade of events leading to testicular development (Vilain, 2000) either by activating genes leading to male development or inhibiting a repressor of male development. SRY is also expressed in a number of brain structures and may be involved in sexual behaviour. If the SRY gene is not activated (even though the genotype is XY), the female morphological form will develop. Occasionally, the SRY gene may be translocated on to an X gene, so if it is activated a male morphological state may develop from an XX genotype. Other genes are involved in SRY gene activity; it seems that the ratio of these genes to SRY is more important than the absolute amount of the genes (Johnson, 2007).

Abnormal numbers of sex chromosomes are often compatible with fetal development, and therefore occur with a relatively high birth frequency (Table 5.1). The major consequence of an aberrant number of X chromosomes is infertility. If there is an additional one or more X chromosome, as in Klinefelter's syndrome (47 chromosomes, XXY), the fetus will differentiate along the male pathway, as the Y chromosome is present. The absence of a Y

Table 5.1 Normal and abnormal sex chromosome complements

STATE	KARYOTYPE	PHENOTYPE (EXPRESSED SEX)	INCIDENCE PER LIVE BIRTHS	NOTES AND EFFECTS
Normal female	46, XX	Female		
Turner's syndrome	45, X0	Female	0.1 per 1000 females	Females are usually short in stature, possibly with a broad chest, webbed neck, cubitus valgus (extreme outward displacement of the extended forearm) and autism. They are infertile (primary amenorrhoea) and sexually immature. Associated with younger mothers
'Super female'	47, XXX	Female	1.0 per 1000	Normal in females appearance and fertility, may be mentally retarded
Normal male	46, XY	Male		
Klinefelter's syndrome	47, XXY (up to four X chromosomes have been found)	Male	1.3 per 1000 males	Affected males are tall and thin with long limbs and small tests. May be infertile (azoospermia) and have gynaecomastia (breast development). May be mentally retarded. More common in sons of older mothers
'Super male'	47, XYY	Male	1.0 per 1000 males	Affected males tend to be tall, have reduced IQ and show 'antisocial' behaviour. Some studies show increased incidence (2–3%) in institutes for the criminally insane
Sex reversed	46, XXsxr	Male	1.0 per 20 000	Small piece of Y chromosome containing SRY gene is translocated on to an X chromosome

chromosome, as in normal female development (XX) or Turner's syndrome (45 chromosomes, X0, where 0 indicates an absent sex chromosome), will result in the fetus developing as a female.

The factors that activate the SRY gene remain unknown; however, its effects are orchestrated through its influence on the production of androgens. The effects of these hormones upon tissue differentiation and development result in sexual dimorphism of the male during the embryonic phase. During the embryonic phase, female form develops in the absence of endocrine activity although oestrogen is required for puberty and fertility. Therefore, a genetic male may develop female characteristics if the SRY gene is either absent or not activated (Fig. 5.2).

The undifferentiated gonad

The early human embryo is bipotential at all levels of sexual differentiation. The gonads are derived from three embryonic tissue sources: the coelomic epithelium, the underlying mesenchyme and the primordial germ cells (PGCs; Fig. 5.3). The coelomic epithelium develops into the genital ridge, which is found on the medial side of the mesonephros (which develops from the mesenchyme). The primitive germ cells, which are ultimately responsible for the production of the gametes (spermatozoa and ova), originate from the yolk sac. Here, they undergo rapid mitosis before migrating from the yolk sac wall towards the genital ridge, about 4 weeks after fertilization. The genital ridges appear to produce chemotactic substances that attract the primitive germ cells, stimulating them to develop pseudopodia and undergo amoeboid movement. Colonization of the primitive gonad by the PGCs is completed during the 6th week of embryonic development. The primitive sex cords develop from the gonadal ridges into the underlying mesenchyme forming the medulla and cortex of the gonad. In the testes, the medulla develops and will go on to form Sertoli cells and the cortex regresses; this is reversed in the development of the ovary where the cells of the sex cords condense into clusters around the PGCs (oogonia) and go on to form the primordial ovarian follicles. Two sets of primitive internal genitalia begin development. Further development will follow either the male or the female route depending on the hormonal influences.

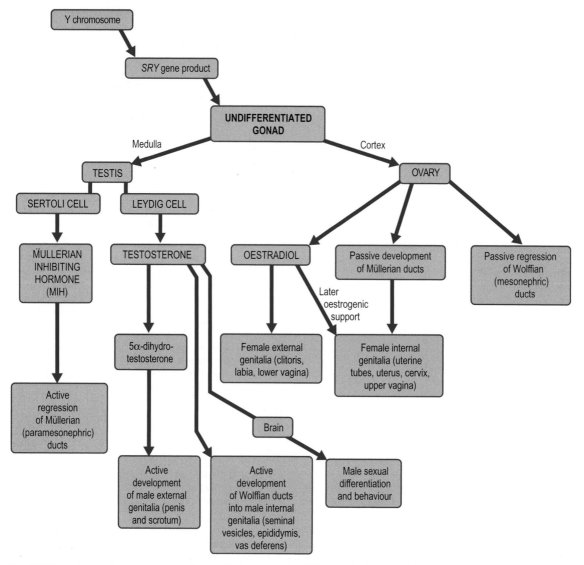

Fig. 5.2 Sex determination factors: activation and influence of the SRY gene. Activation of this gene instigates a number of endocrine influences that determine the male morphology. In the absence of SRY gene activation, female morphology develops under a genetic influence.

THE DEVELOPMENT OF THE MALE MORPHOLOGY

Embryological development

The embryo has two sets of primitive unipotential internal genitalia, each of which has the potential to develop depending on the hormonal environment. The SRY gene and the male gonad are essential for the development of male morphology. The SRY gene stimulates the medulla of the undifferentiated gonad to develop into the testes and produce two hormones, testosterone and anti-Müllerian hormone (AMH; also known as Müllerian-inhibiting substance, MIS or Müllerian-inhibiting hormone, MIH), which promote male genital duct development. In the absence of AMH and testosterone secretion, female sexual differentiation occurs. AMH, from Sertoli cells, drives the regression of the Müllerian structures (paramesonephric 'female' ducts) and testosterone, from Leydig cells, stimulates development of the Wolffian (mesonephric 'male') ducts into the male internal genitalia, the epididymis,

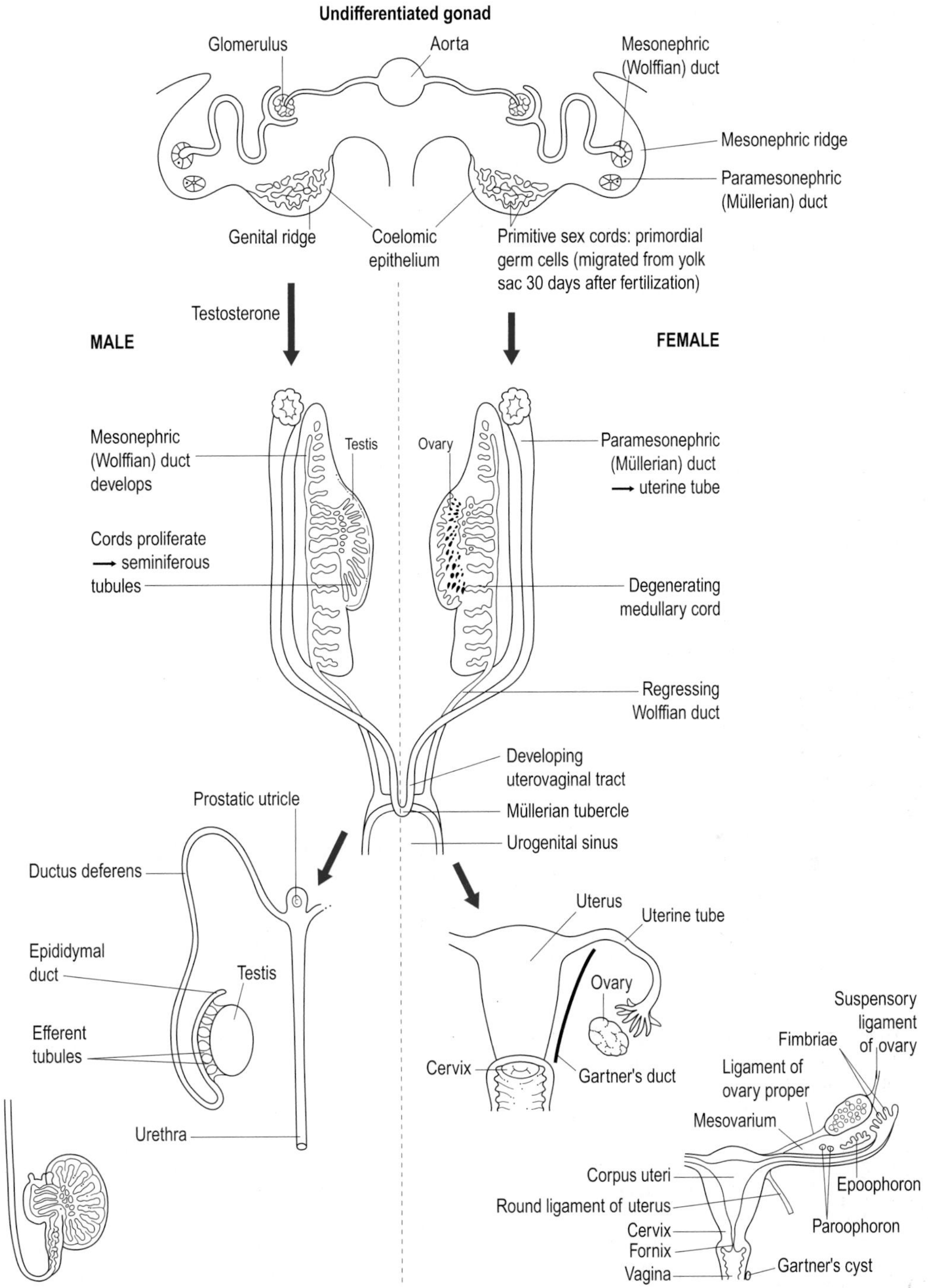

Fig. 5.3 Development of the internal genitalia. Once differentiation of the gonads has occurred, the resulting endocrine production coordinates the development of the internal genitalia. In the male, the reproductive tract is an evolutionary adaptation of a vestigial urological system.

vas deferens and seminiferous tubules. In the absence of testosterone, the Wolffian structures regress and the Müllerian ducts continue to develop into the uterus, uterine tubes and the upper part of the vagina. Sexual differentiation along the male pathway requires active diversion, whereas differentiation into a female embryo follows an inherent pattern or 'default pathway'. However, some genes have been recognized as important in ovarian development (Goodfellow and Camerino, 1999).

The Wolffian, or mesonephric, ducts initially develop as part of the embryological renal system. The adaptation of the mesonephric ducts to form the male morphology is a significant development in sexual dimorphism, in evolutionary terms. Sexual differentiation at this stage is very efficient; it is extremely rare for individuals to have both testicular and ovarian tissues. These true hermaphrodites often have an internal testis on one side and an ovary on the other side (or a mixed structure known as ovatestis) which may be a result of chimerism (the fusion of a male and female embryo; Strain et al., 1998).

The phenotypic sex is determined by the sexual characteristics of the individual. The external genitalia are bipotential (can become either male or female) and initially exist as a urogenital slit flanked by urethral folds, a genital swelling and a genital tubercle or bud. Steroid hormones directly influence the development of male external genitalia (unlike the female). Testosterone from the testes is converted into 5α-dihydrotestosterone (5α-DHT) within the target cells. Under the influence of this biologically more potent androgen, the tissues of the external genitalia form the penis and scrotum (Fig. 5.4). The urethral folds fuse enclosing the urethral tube to form the shaft of the penis and genital swellings fuse to form the scrotum. The genital tubercle expands to form the glans penis. The testes, like the ovaries, initially develop within the abdominal cavity but do not remain there. They descend to their normal position within the scrotal sac, suspended outside the abdominal cavity, just before or soon after birth. However, it is quite common (in ~1 in 50 live-born males) for either one or both testes to fail to descend at this time (the condition is described as cryptorchidism). Spontaneous descent usually occurs within the first year of life. Testicular damage, potentially resulting in later failure of spermatogenesis and a higher incidence of malignant tumours, occurs if the testes remain within the abdominal cavity, so the testes are surgically lowered (orchiopexy or orchidopexy) if spontaneous resolution has not occurred (Thorup and Cortes, 2009).

Testosterone is also converted into oestrogens within the brain. The presence of oestrogen is believed to be responsible for differentiation of certain brain structures along a male or female pathway. This resulting difference in morphology underpins the biological explanations for behavioural patterns differing between the sexes. Male sexual activity appears to depend on the presence of testosterone above a critical threshold. Female sexual activity in the human may be cyclical in response to changes in male behaviour. There are cyclical changes in the organic acid content of vaginal secretions (derived from normal bacterial flora), which may be a mechanism of olfactory communication to the woman's sexual partner (see Chapter 4).

Puberty

The male embryo produces testosterone with a peak of about 2 ng/mL at about weeks 13–15 (Johnston, 2007). Levels fall from then but peak to about the same level about 3 months after birth. Thereafter levels fall but slowly increase from about 12 months. As in the female, puberty commences when the secretory pattern of follicle-stimulating hormone (FSH) and luteinizing hormone (LH), under the influence of gonadotrophin-releasing hormone (GnRH), becomes mature. Initially, secretion of LH increases nocturnally which explains the pattern of nocturnal sperm emission in pubertal boys. FSH and LH orchestrate spermatogenesis within the male (see Chapter 2). At puberty, the testes increase in size as the seminiferous tubules canalize, the Sertoli cells increase in size and the germ cells resume mitotic activity. Unlike the ovarian cycle, spermatogenesis is a continuous process resulting in the production of many gametes. The testes produce testosterone from the Leydig cells, which influences the development of the male secondary sex characteristics (Box 5.1). Unlike the female, the male retains the capability of spermatogenesis indefinitely but failure to achieve copulation becomes more common with the progression of age (Corona et al., 2010) and overall production of testosterone gradually falls from the 4th decade onwards (Schill, 2001).

THE DEVELOPMENT OF THE FEMALE MORPHOLOGY

Embryological development

As the X chromosome does not contain the SRY gene, the Müllerian ducts differentiate into the female internal genitalia, the uterine tubes and fimbriae, the uterus, cervix and upper two-thirds of the vagina. The undifferentiated gonad develops into the ovary; the cortex develops and the medulla regresses. This is the route of differentiation in the absence of testosterone and MIH. Female external genitalia form independently of any hormonal influences; therefore, the ovary has little endocrine activity until puberty. The genital tubercle becomes the clitoris and the urethral folds and genital swellings remain unfused, forming the labia minora and majora, respectively.

Common abnormalities

During development, the body of the uterus, cervix and upper vagina are formed by the fusion of the two Müllerian (paramesonephric) ducts. Abnormalities may range

Fig. 5.4 Development of the external genitalia: formation of the external genitalia is hormonally influenced; absence of testosterone or functioning testosterone receptors will result in the female morphology developing regardless of genotype. (Adapted with permission from Johnson and Everitt, 1995.)

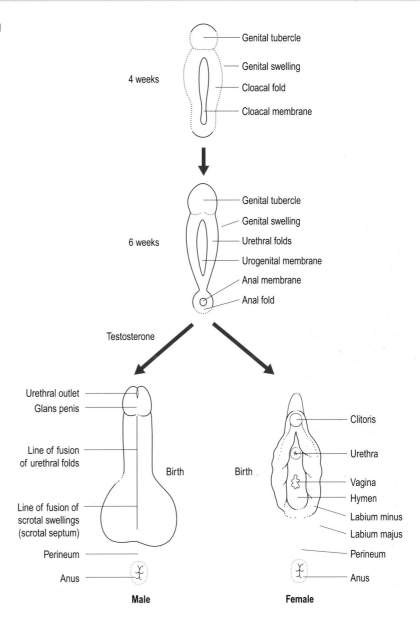

Box 5.1 **Male secondary sex characteristics**

- Enlargement of the penis
- Pubic and axillary hair growth
- Deepening of voice (due to growth of larynx)
- Masculine pattern of fat distribution
- Development of the skeletal muscle (protein anabolism)
- Secretion of skin oil glands (predisposes to acne)
- Bone growth and adolescent growth spurt (via growth hormone secretion)
- Male sexual behaviour and aggression

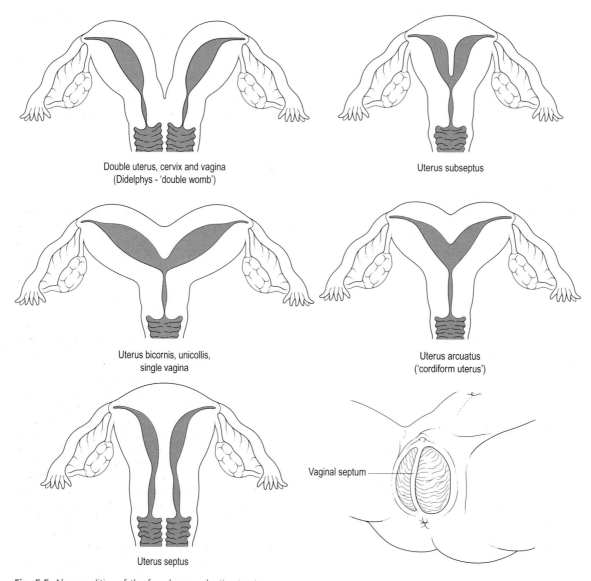

Double uterus, cervix and vagina
(Didelphys - 'double womb')

Uterus subseptus

Uterus bicornis, unicollis,
single vagina

Uterus arcuatus
('cordiform uterus')

Uterus septus

Vaginal septum

Fig. 5.5 Abnormalities of the female reproductive tract.

from a simple uterine septum to the complete duplication of the reproductive system (Fig. 5.5). The failure of one of the paramesonephric ducts to develop will result in a unilateral rudimentary horn.

Puberty: the initiation of fertility cycles

In the female, the germ cells or oogonia cease mitotic division and enter their first meiotic division (becoming primary oocytes) and most of them die before birth so the number of oocytes a woman has is finite and determined before her birth. Meiotic division is then arrested until the oocyte is triggered to resume development. Recruitment of primordial follicles into the pool of developing follicles begins at puberty. Puberty commences with the activation of the hypothalamus to produce GnRH in a mature pattern of secretion. It is suggested that the menarche is initiated when a critical mass of body fat, which may be genetically defined, is accumulated (Frisch, 1990). GnRH stimulates the anterior pituitary to produce FSH and LH, which orchestrate the reproductive cycles in the female (see Chapter 4). The ovaries begin to produce oestrogens, which influence the development of the female secondary sex characteristics. The breasts develop, the deposition of adipose tissue is responsible for the distinct female body curvature, and the growth of hair in the axilla and genital region commences.

The menopause

The menopause (see Chapter 4) marks the end of the ability of the female to reproduce. The menstrual cycle ceases and the ovarian cycle is lost, resulting in atrophy of the ovaries. Therefore, there is a marked decrease in the amount of systemic oestrogen present in the postmenopausal woman. Modern fertility treatments can reverse the menopause to restore the menstrual cycle but not ovarian function. Hence, postmenopausal fertility treatment requires the donation of an ovum from a fertile, premenopausal woman.

INDETERMINATE SEX

Indeterminate, or ambiguous, sexual features at birth are usually attributable to genetic abnormality, endocrine dysfunction (see Fig. 5.6) or developmental failure. In cases of ambiguous genitalia, the karyotype of the individual is assessed to determine the chromosomal sex (i.e. the presence of a Y chromosome for a male or the absence of a Y chromosome for a female regardless of the number of X chromosomes present within the karyotype).

Genetic abnormalities

The aetiology of genetic disease is discussed in Chapter 7. There are genetic conditions that result in a range of variable sexual development, such as Klinefelter's syndrome and Turner's syndrome. These disorders have been useful in understanding the control of normal sexual development. In Klinefelter's syndrome (47, XXY; normal number of autosomes but two X and one Y), the testes form normally but the germ cells die as they enter meiosis so following puberty testicular structure become fibrosed and hyalinized affecting spermatogenesis (Wilstrom and Dunkel, 2008). Studies have shown that surgical sperm retrieval is possible from around 44% of men with non-mosaic Klinefelter's syndrome and when used with ICSI has resulted in the birth of infants (Fullerton et al., 2010). It is common in men with Klinefelter's syndrome to develop breast tissue (gynaecomastia) at the onset of puberty.

In Turner's syndrome (45, X0), the single X chromosome initiates development of the ovary normally. However, the oocytes die before birth and the follicular cells become atretic, causing ovarian dysgenesis. The ovary becomes extremely regressed during fetal development, forming a highly regressed streak ovary similar to a postmenopausal ovarian structure. Although there are reports of spontaneous pregnancies in Turner's syndrome (Mortensen et al., 2010), this is rare and women with

Turner's syndrome usually require hormone replacement, ovum donation and IVF to become pregnant (Abir et al., 2001). Recent research suggests that a proportion of women with Turner's syndrome (who are probably genetic mosaics of 46,XX and 45,X0) may have ovarian follicles present at adolescence which could be frozen and then theoretically be utilized with assisted conception techniques at a later date to successfully conceive (Borgstrom et al., 2009).

Endocrine dysfunction

Fetal endocrine dysfunction

It is thought that about 1% of live births exhibit some degree of sexual ambiguity (Fausto-Sterling, 2002). The dissociation of gonadal and genital sex is usually due to failure of appropriate endocrine communication (Johnson, 2007). The embryonic stage of male sexual differentiation is under endocrine influence. This may be disrupted by the failure, total or partial, of production of, or response to, the necessary hormones (Fig. 5.6). Therefore, the genetic male may fail to develop male genitalia, and appear female at birth. As described previously, the gene that codes for the androgen receptor is situated on the Y chromosome and the activation of the SRY gene results in the formation of the testes, which produce testosterone. However, if the receptor is defective, the response to testosterone will be ineffectual so the Wolffian ducts will fail to develop into the male reproductive tract. The defective receptor may also be present on other tissues so the external genitalia will also be unable to respond to testosterone and the infant will appear female. AMH will continue to inhibit the growth of the female internal reproductive tract. Thus, the child will be born with the external appearance of a female but lack both male and female internal structures. The testes remain within the abdominal cavity and as a result become dysfunctional.

Sufficient amounts of testosterone may be produced, but if the target cells lack the functional androgen receptors, or if the enzyme (5α-reductase) required to convert the testosterone into 5α-DHT is lacking, then virilization will not occur. This condition is described as testicular feminization or androgen-insensitivity syndrome (AIS). The genotype is XY and the gonads develop as testes producing androgens but the external genetalia are insensitive to the androgens and so appear female. The lack of normal endocrine communication between the gonads and genitalia causes secondary or pseudo-hermaphroditism, a disparity between the gonadal sex (having testes or ovaries) and the phenotypic sex (appearing male and female).

Müllerian duct syndrome can occur if the AMH receptor is defective (persistent Müllerian duct syndrome) or if production of AMH is inadequate. Both the Wolffian and Müllerian ducts develop simultaneously, which results in the development of both the male and female

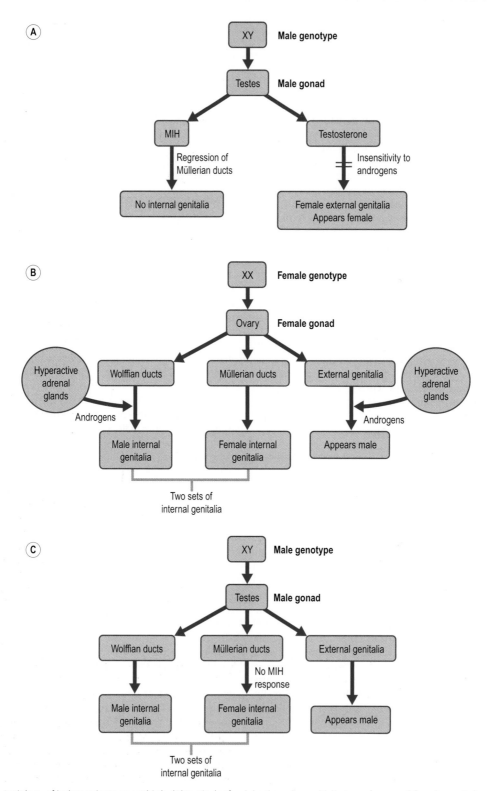

Fig. 5.6 Aetiology of indeterminate sex at birth. (A) testicular feminization – insensitivity to androgens; (B) androgenital syndrome – excess androgens; (C) Müllerian duct syndrome – insensitivity to AMH (MIH or MIS).

internal genitalia. The baby is genetically and gonadally male but retains the female internal structures, which developed from the Müllerian ducts. Men undergoing surgery for unrelated problems are sometimes found to have an unusual development of female internal genitalia without it causing any problem.

If a female embryo is exposed to androgens during development, the internal and external genitalia may develop on the male pathway. Congenital adrenal hyperplasia (CAH) is an autosomal recessive disease usually caused by a defect in the enzyme 21-hydroxylase, resulting in underproduction of corticosteroid synthesis and overproduction of steroid hormones, including androgens. CAH can cause early masculinization of males and causes the majority of cases of female virilization (androgenital syndrome), accounting for most cases of ambiguous genitalia at birth. In the female fetus with CAH, androgens stimulate the development of the Wolffian ducts and stimulate the external genitalia to resemble the male form. The Müllerian system remains because there is no AMH. Although the baby is genetically and gonadally female (XX with ovaries), it has the internal genitalia of both sexes and male external genitalia. With high androgen concentrations, the sex of the baby may not initially be questioned and thus the problem may be evident only because there are no testes to descend. In the 1950s and 1960s, high levels of progestogenic drugs were given to mothers who had previously had a mid-term spontaneous abortion. It was thought that the pregnancies failed because of inadequate production of progesterone. However, progestogens are androgenic and can stimulate testosterone receptors causing pharmacological virilization of the fetus ('progestogen-induced hermaphrodites').

In response to rulings from the European Court of Human Rights, the UK passed the Gender Recognition Act in 2004. This allows a transsexual individual to have a gender recognition certificate which means that their 'acquired' gender can be legally reassigned to be different to the one on their original birth certificate which was assigned at birth.

Case study 5.1 is an example of possible endocrine dysfunction.

Developmental failure

The physiological processes resulting in the development of the reproductive tracts are complex, arising from the induction and differentiation of embryonic tissue. If the tissues, such as the pronephros upon which the gonads develop, are missing, then the gonads fail to develop because essential induction factors produced by the pronephros are lacking.

Induction, differentiation and growth of tissues are also affected by several other factors. Optimal development occurs at body core temperature. Maternal pyrexia at critical stages of embryonic development may severely disrupt

---

Case study 5.1

Milly, who is 43, has had an uncomplicated third pregnancy. Following a chorionic villus sample, she was informed that her baby appeared to have a normal female karyotype. As Milly's other children are boys, she was thrilled to be expecting a daughter because she had decided that this was to be her last pregnancy, regardless of the outcome. Milly spontaneously went into labour at 39 weeks' gestation and, following a rapid and uncomplicated delivery, a 4.2-kg male infant, of normal appearance, was presented to her.

- What are the possible reasons to explain this?
- Do you think there is a need for any further investigations and, if so, what should they be?

Box 5.2 **Teratogens and endocrine disrupters**

- Teratogens are chemical substances that are known to interfere with embryological development and so result in the manifestation of fetal abnormalities
- Teratogens may be produced by pathogens, ingested by the mother either intentionally or unintentionally, or may be present within the external environment
- Many drugs such as Thalidomide (used in the late 1950s as an antiemetic agent in early pregnancy) are now known to produce physical deformities

---

the process. Many pathogens produce chemicals or toxins that can also severely affect embryological development (Box 5.2). There is growing concern among environmentalists over the increasing amounts of manmade chemical pollutants within the environment (see Box 3.5, p. 66). Many of these chemicals may disrupt endocrine function in a variety of ways, not only by inhibition but also by mimicking the effects of endogenous hormones. Case study 5.2 describes an example of ambiguous genitalia.

SEXUAL BEHAVIOUR

Hormonal control of sexual dimorphism results not only in physical differences between the male and female, but also in behavioural differences. There are many brain structures that are sexually dimorphic (different in males and females). Males have slightly larger brains and tend to perform better in visuospatial skills; they tend to show more physical aggression and display more sensation-seeking and risk-taking behaviour (Craig et al., 2004).

Case study 5.2

The midwife examines a newborn baby and is concerned over the appearance of the genitalia. Initially, the parents had been congratulated upon the birth of a daughter but on closer examination the labia appear fused and the clitoris seems unusually large and so a referral to a paediatrician is made.

- What are the possible causes for this ambiguity?
- What investigations will be performed to establish the true sex of the baby?
- Why is it important to confirm the sex of the baby before registering the birth?
- What are the implications of assigning the wrong sex at birth?

Case study 5.3

Lisa is a 20-year-old primigravida who has conceived by donor insemination. The biological father of the baby is Lisa's brother's partner and Lisa has agreed to act as a surrogate mother for the two men.

Would Lisa's care by the midwife be any different than to a women who had conceived normally?

How could the midwife include Lisa's brother and his partner in her care and facilitate the couple's preparation for parenthood?

Are there any legal considerations that Lisa needs to consider over the parenting of the child and if so how can the midwife facilitate this?

Females, however, perform better in verbal skills, memory tasks, language and emotional processing and seem to have greater communication between the two halves of the brain. The differentiation of certain brain structures, together with biochemical differences, is thought to explain the differences in sexual behaviour between the sexes. However, it is important to acknowledge that social construction also influences the development of sexual behaviour in humans (Carlson, 1998). It is generally accepted that gonadal steroids induce brain sexual dimorphism but there may also be a direct genetic influence. Testosterone acts either directly or via local conversion into oestradiol and appears to stimulate formation of neural circuits involved in masculine behaviour.

The correct assignment of sex at birth is thought to be important in gender development, sexual orientation and attitudes later in life. Young children appear to demonstrate gender-related patterns of energy expenditure, parental rehearsal, explicit sexual behaviour and attentiveness to personal appearance. It is suggested that children recognize their own gender identity by the time they are about 2.5-years old and ambiguity may have long-term developmental consequences. It is not clear whether there is any link between transsexualism and biological or social gender ambiguity.

Human sexuality is complex; sex appears to serve a social, as well as a reproductive, function. There is a wide diversity of sexual behaviour patterns within humans, ranging from complete homosexuality, to bisexuality, to complete heterosexual behaviour (see Case studies 5.3 and 5.4). Traditionally, in Western cultures, heterosexual behaviour has always been regarded as normal and any other variation as being abnormal. This assumption was based upon many animal observations where copulation appeared to be involved only in reproduction. Justification of such behavioural patterns has been strongly argued from a sociological perspective. Recently, however, there has been an increasing amount of evidence arising

from biological perspectives that attempts to explain the existence of diverse sexual behaviour (Crew, 1994).

Anatomical studies have shown that there may be biological differences within certain brain structures associated with the expression of homosexual behaviour in both males and females (LeVay and Hamer, 1993). These studies can be criticized for many reasons; for instance, they are small and the differences have been demonstrated only upon post-mortem inspection. It has been questioned whether these changes might be caused by death and whether the samples studied were representative of the entire population. Many of the males studied died from AIDS-related conditions; the possibility of physical changes in the brain being affected by these conditions needs to be excluded. There does, however, seem to be a genetic predisposition to homosexuality (Hamer et al., 1993), although sexual orientation is also affected by social, familial, environmental and endocrine factors. Finding genetic differences between homosexual and heterosexual brains may increase social acceptance of homosexuals; alternatively, it could provide a pseudoscientific rationale for discrimination and homophobia.

The emergence of genetic fingerprinting has enabled the identification of parents. Many biologists formerly accepted that many animals pair bonded, reproduced and then cooperated to bring up their young, sometimes on a seasonal basis or for life. However, recent genetic studies have revealed that the offspring of many animals

Case study 5.4

Joan and Pippa are both pregnant and present themselves to the midwives' clinic where they inform the midwife that the babies have the same biological father who is an anonymous sperm donor. Joan and Pippa are in a stable relationship and are excited over the prospect of becoming parents. How should the midwife manage this situation and how would she plan the care of both these women?

were conceived outside the pair-bonding arrangement. Promiscuity appears to be widespread throughout the animal kingdom. Society often portrays the human male as sexually promiscuous but studies have shown that females are six times more likely to commit adultery at the time of ovulation than during any other time of the menstrual cycle (Ridley, 1993). This has a clinical significance in relation to family history-taking because as many as one in six children may be fathered outside of a relationship. Animal studies have also revealed that some animals use sex as a means of providing social stability. Studies of the Bonobo (pygmy chimpanzee) show that sex is used as a form of greeting, bonding and submission and that a full range of sexual behaviour from homosexuality to heterosexuality is present (De Waal, 1995).

The programming of sexual behaviour may occur by endocrine organizational influences during the embryological period. However, reproductive behaviour may also be influenced by the endocrine system on a cyclical basis. Human females copulate throughout the menstrual cycle, but sexual motivation appears to increase during the ovulatory period and to decrease during the luteal phase.

Some animal studies have shown that the presence of sex steroids is required for positive sexual behaviour to be initiated. An example of this is the female rat that is receptive to the male only at certain times. During the fertile period, the female will adopt a specific position for mating called lordosis, which is induced by the presence of oestrogens and progesterone. The sex steroids also appear to make the female chemically attractive to the male by the production of pheromonal substances. Therefore, sexual behaviour in the female rat can be described in three ways:

1. Receptive: develops an ability to copulate
2. Proceptive: increase in sexual motivation
3. Attractive: physiological changes that arouse sexual interest in the male.

Some animals have a visual signal to the attractiveness component, such as the female baboon who advertises her sexual receptiveness by developing swollen genitalia. These components of female sexual behaviour are most clearly evident in animals that have an oestrus cycle, where ovulation is stimulated by copulation to maximize the chance of fertilization. In the human female, it appears that all three components are present throughout the cycle, which suggests that sexual activity in humans has evolved to have a social role. In many animals, it appears that various forms of stimuli produced by the female influence male reproductive behaviour that promotes successful reproduction. Human male sexual behaviour, however, may have developed to be more responsive to the social aspects of sex.

Key points

- Females have two X chromosomes, whereas the presence of the *SRY* region on the Y chromosome causes maleness. If there is an abnormal number of sex chromosomes, the presence of a Y chromosome leads to the phenotypic expression of maleness.
- If the embryo has a Y chromosome, the indifferent gonads differentiate into testes, which produce testosterone and Müllerian-inhibiting hormone. Testosterone promotes male differentiation of the internal and external genitalia. Müllerian-inhibiting hormone causes the structures that would have formed the female internal genitalia to regress.
- The endocrine changes at puberty cause development of secondary sex characteristics and the start of reproductive maturity.
- Indeterminate or ambiguous sex at birth can be due to genetic, endocrine or development problems.
- An abnormality of sex chromosome number is frequently associated with effects on fertility and mental ability.
- Sexual behaviour has been associated with endocrinology, brain development and cultural factors.

Application to practice

- Knowledge of sexual differentiation is essential in the examination of the newborn.
- Abnormalities of the sex organs and genitalia have their aetiology in the failure or dysfunctioning of the endocrine system. This may have a genetic origin or may be influenced by external factors such as pollutants.

An increasing number of individuals with restricted fertility due to genetic conditions are being offered assisted conception techniques to achieve pregnancy. The midwife must be able to support and understand the anxieties and stress related to these situations.

ANNOTATED FURTHER READING

De Waal F: *The ape and the sushi master: cultural reflections of a primatologist,* London, 2001, Allen Lane.
This book proposes an interesting theory that suggests primates learn behaviour from observing the behaviour of other older individuals. This theory may explain social and sexual behaviour that cannot be fully explained by innate or genetically influenced behaviour patterns.

Domoney C: Psychosexual problems, *Obstet Gynaecol Reprod Med* 19:291–295, 2009.
A short review of the more common psychosexual problems seen in gynaecology clinics and approaches to their management.

Gooren LJ, Kruijver FP: Androgens and male behavior, *Mol Cell Endocrinol* 198:31–40, 2002.

This article reviews sexual dimorphism and the differentiation of the male brain in response to androgens, which affects gender identity and sexual orientation, sexual functioning and spatial ability and verbal fluency.

Imperato-McGinley J, Zhu YS: Androgens and male physiology the syndrome of 5alpha-reductase-2 deficiency, *Mol Cell Endocrinol* 198:51–59, 2002.

This review examines the effects of mutations in the 5α-reductase isozymes which convert testosterone to the more potent androgen dihydrotestosterone (DHT). Affected individuals have ambiguous external genitalia at birth so they are believed to be girls and are often raised as such; however, virilization occurs at puberty, frequently with a gender role change.

Johnson MH: *Essential reproduction*, ed 6, Oxford, 2007, Blackwell Science.

An integrated and well-organized research-based textbook that explores comparative reproductive physiology of mammals, including anatomy, physiology, endocrinology, genetics and behavioural studies.

Jorge JC: Statistical management of ambiguity: bodies that defy the algorithm of sex classification, *Int J Crit Stat* 1:19–37, 2007.

This article challenges the current management of ambiguous genetalia cases and presents an algorithm to aid diagnosis based on management of intersexuality proposed by the American Academy of

Pediatrics. It also presents an analysis of case reports of individuals who underwent gender assignment in relation to specific clinical diagnoses.

Martin CL, Ruble DN: Patterns of gender development, *Annu Rev Psychol* 61:353–381, 2010.

A comprehensive theory of gender development which discusses how children recognize gender distinctions and understand stereotypes, and the emergence of prejudice and sexism and other topics related to gender using interesting examples.

Migeon CJ, Wisniewski AB: Human sex differentiation and its abnormalities, *Best Pract Res Clin Obstet Gynaecol* 17:1–18, 2003.

This article reviews the presentation and management of patients affected by conditions of abnormal sex differentiation; it includes descriptions of the medical, surgical and psychological treatment options for people affected by various intersex conditions, practice points and information about relevant Internet websites and patient support groups.

Mobler M, Frazer L: Donor insemination guide: written by and for lesbian women, 2002, Harrington Parker Press.

This guide provides an insight into same-sex parents and the use of donor insemination.

Sinha A, Palep-Singh M: Taking a sexual history, *Obstet, Gynaecol Reproduct Med* 18:49–50, 2007.

A succinct guide about the importance of, and approaches to, taking a sexual history

which focuses on sensitive topics and aspects of sexual concern.

Studd J, Schwenkhagen A: The historical response to female sexuality, *Maturitas* 63:107–111, 2009.

A fascinating history of medical attitudes to normal female sexual development and female sexuality.

Sykes B: *Adam's curse: a future without men*, London, 2003, Bantam Press.

Written by Brian Sykes, Professor of Human Genetics at the University of Oxford, this book explores the biological and behavioural mysteries of the male sex and discusses the cannibalization of the Y chromosome by the X chromosome drawing the conclusion that men are headed for extinction.

Wilhelm D, Palmer S, Koopman P: Sex determination and gonadal development in mammals, *Physiol Rev* 87:1–28, 2007.

A comprehensive review of the biological consequences of fertilization with either an X or a Y chromosome from the sperm and the different journeys of male and female fetal development which describes the molecular and cellular events (differentiation, migration, proliferation, and communication) that distinguish testis and ovary and the changes in gene regulation underlying these two pathways.

Wylie K, Mimoun S: Sexual response models in women, *Maturitas* 63:112–115, 2009.

A short and useful description of a number of models which have been developed to understand the female sexual response.

REFERENCES

Abir R, Fisch B, Nahum R, et al: Turner's syndrome and fertility: current status and possible putative prospects, *Hum Reprod Update* 7:603–610, 2001.

Borgstrom B, Hreinsson J, Rasmussen C, et al: Fertility preservation in girls with turner syndrome: prognostic signs of the presence of ovarian follicles, *J Clin Endocrinol Metab* 94:74–80, 2009.

Carlson NR: *The physiology of behaviour*, Boston, 1998, Allyn & Bacon, pp 290–323.

Corona G, Lee DM, Forti G, et al: Age-related changes in general and sexual health in middle-aged and older men: results from the European Male

Ageing Study (EMAS), *J Sex Med* 7:1362–1380, 2010.

Craig IW, Harper E, Loat CS: The genetic basis for sex differences in human behaviour: role of the sex chromosomes, *Ann Hum Genet* 68:269–282, 2004.

Crew D: Animal sexuality, *Sci Am* 271(1):96–102, 1994.

De Waal FBM: Bonobo sex and society, *Sci Am* 272(3):82–88, 1995.

Fausto-Sterling A: Gender identification and assignment in intersex children, *Dialog Pediatr Urol* 25(6):4–5, 2002.

Fullerton G, Hamilton M, Maheshwari A: Should non-mosaic Klinefelter syndrome men be labelled as

infertile in 2009? *Hum Reprod* 25:588–597, 2010.

Frisch RE: The right weight, body fat, menarche and ovulation, *Baillières Clin Obstet Gynaecol* 4:419–439, 1990.

Goodfellow PN, Camerino G: DAX-1, an 'antitestis' gene, *Cell Mol Life Sci* 55:857–863, 1999.

Hamer DH, Hu S, Magnuson VL, et al: A linkage between DNA markers on the X chromosome and male sexual orientation, *Science* 261:321–327, 1993.

Johnson MH, Everitt BJ: *Essential reproduction*, ed 4, Oxford, 1995, Blackwell Science, p 10.

Johnson MH: *Essential reproduction*, Oxford, 2007, Blackwell.

LeVay S, Hamer DH: Evidence for a biological influence in male homosexuality, *Sci Am* 270(5):44–49, 1993.

Mortensen KH, Rohde MD, Uldbjerg N, et al: Repeated spontaneous pregnancies in 45,X Turner syndrome, *Obstet Gynecol* 115:446–449, 2010.

Ridley M: *The red queen: sex and the evolution of human nature*, London, 1993, Penguin.

Schill WB: Fertility and sexual life of men after their forties and in older age, *Asian J Androl* 3:1–7, 2001.

Sinclair AH, Berta P, Palmer MS, et al: A gene from the human sex-determining region encodes a protein with homology to a conserved DNA-binding motif, *Nature* 346:240–244, 1990.

Strain L, Dean JCS, Hamilton MPR, et al: A true hermaphrodite chimera resulting from embryo amalgamation after in vitro fertilization, *N Engl J Med* 338:166–169, 1998.

Thorup J, Cortes D: Surgical treatment and follow up on undescended testis, *Pediatr Endocrinol Rev* 7:38–43, 2009.

Vilain E: Genetics of sexual development, *Annu Rev Sex Res* 11:1–25, 2000.

Wikstrom AM, Dunkel L: Testicular function in Klinefelter syndrome, *Horm Res* 69:317–326, 2008.

Chapter | 6 |

Fertilization

LEARNING OBJECTIVES

- To describe the physiological processes involved in coitus.
- To describe the morphology and characteristics of the male and female gametes and how they are adapted to their specific function.
- To discuss factors thought to be involved in the conception of either a male or a female baby.
- To describe capacitance, the acrosome reaction and the cortical reaction in the stages of fertilization.
- To describe events in the first week after fertilization: the first mitotic divisions, cell cleavage, compaction, hatching, implantation and maternal recognition of pregnancy.
- To outline the relevance and implications of parental imprinting.
- To outline common causes of infertility.
- To discuss the approaches used in assisted reproduction technologies.

INTRODUCTION

Fertilization is a series of processes that culminate with the union of the male gamete (the sperm) and the female gamete (the oocyte) to form a diploid zygote. Following fertilization, one cell progressively divides into six trillion cells (6×10^{12}), forming a unique individual in about 38 weeks. Understanding fertilization is important for the following events during pregnancy and understanding some of the causes of infertility and failed pregnancy. Knowledge about fertilization had led to the development of sophisticated methods of *in vitro* fertilization (IVF) and, conversely, strategies for preventing fertilization (the basis for contraception).

Chapter case study

Zara and James have attended the local hospital for the 12-week scan and have been informed that there is now only one baby present in the uterus. It would appear that one of the sacs, observed at Zara's earlier scans, had failed to develop further and the ultrasound scan could no longer detect any evidence of the sac's remnants. Zara and James are understandably upset over the loss of one of their babies but are reassured that the other baby has an extremely low risk of having Down's syndrome, is growing well and appears normal.

- How would you explain to Zara and James what were the possible reasons for one of the embryos failing to develop and is it more likely to occur in heterozygous or homozygous twins?
- How common is the loss of a twin in early pregnancy and what reasons could explain why this happens?

Mammalian fertilization occurs within the female reproductive tract. Less than one in a million sperm, or spermatozoa, reach the oocyte. The sperm are deposited in the vagina during intercourse (coitus) and then make the long journey through the female reproductive tract (equal to about 10 000 times their own length). The hazards and challenges imposed on the successful fertilization are thought to help ensure that the individual sperm that actually fertilizes the oocyte is strong and healthy. There is extensive and intricate crosstalk between the oocyte and the fertilizing sperm, which leads to activation of the egg and sperm head decondensation. Following fertilization, the female and male pronuclei form, syngamy occurs and the zygote undergoes the first cleavage divisions while travelling through the uterine tube to the uterus where it implants in the uterine wall.

COITUS

Coitus in humans lasts on average 4 min, which is quite long compared to our closest animal cousin, the chimpanzee, which averages 8 s (De Waal, 1995). Masters and Johnson (described in Levin, 1998) described a four-phase model for sexual responses in humans. This is known as the EPOR model:

- E: excitement phase, when stimuli increase sexual arousal or tension.
- P: plateau phase, when arousal becomes intense; if the level of stimulation is inadequate, arousal subsides and there is no further progression to the next phase.
- O: orgasmic phase, which is a few seconds of involuntary climax during which sexual tension is relieved, usually accompanied by a wave of profound pleasure.
- R: resolution phase, when sexual arousal is dispersed; in males, it is believed that there is an absolute refractory period in which further sexual arousal and orgasm are impossible.

In the male

The principal event necessary for male sexual activity is acquisition and maintenance of penile erection. This is primarily a vascular phenomenon, initiated by neurological controls and facilitated by appropriate psychological and hormonal components. Initial stimulation of the penis can be both psychogenic (from erotic stimuli and sexual fantasy) and tactile (via touch receptors in the penis and perineum) and necessitates autonomic nervous system activity to coordinate increased blood flow into the vascular tissues. Centrally perceived sensual stimuli are relayed via the spinal thoracolumbar erection centre (T11 through L2), and reflex erections, initiated by tactile stimuli to the genital area, activate a reflex arc involving the sacral erection centre (S2 through S4; Dey Shepherd, 2002). Involuntary non-sexual nocturnal erections occur during rapid eye movement sleep. There are three components of erection: increased arterial flow, relaxation of the sinusoidal spaces and venous constriction. In the excitement phase, increased inflow of blood converts the low-volume, low-pressure vasculature to a large-volume, high-pressure system (Andersson and Wagner, 1995).

The arterioles and arteriovenous shunts dilate so there is an increase in blood flow which engorges the erectile vascular tissues (cavernous and spongiosum bodies, see Chapter 2). The corpus spongiosum does not increase in turgor as much as the two corpora cavernosa so the urethra is not compressed. Blood outflow is occluded by compression and constriction of the veins so the sinusoids (blood-filled spaces) enlarge further. This results in hardening and erection of the penis as the blood volume is increased by about 50%.

The control of an erection is by stimulation of parasympathetic nerves, and probably simultaneous inhibition of sympathetic outflow, which reduces arterial smooth muscle tone causing dilatation and increase in blood flow. Many central and peripheral neurotransmitters are involved in mediating the erectile response. Centrally, dopamine, nitric oxide (NO), oxytocin and adreno-corticotrophin (ACTH)/melanocyte-stimulating hormone (α-MSH) seem to have a facilitatory role; serotonin may be either facilitatory or inhibitory, and enkephalins are inhibitory. Peripherally, the balance between vasoconstrictive factors (such as noradrenaline, endothelin and angiotensin) and vasodilatory factors (such as NO, vasoactive intestinal peptide (VIP) and prostanoids) controls the tone of the smooth muscle of the corpora cavernosa and determines the functional state of the penis. Other neurotransmitters implicated in the erectile response are acetylcholine, endothelins and Rho-kinases. NO is considered the most important factor facilitating vasodilatation, thus maximizing blood flow and penile erection; it promotes the generation of cyclic guanosine monophosphate (cGMP) which increases smooth muscle relaxation and inflow of blood. Detumescence (loss of erection) occurs because NO-induced vasodilation abates as cGMP is broken down predominantly by the intracavernosal cGMPphosphodiesterase (cGMP–PDE5). Sildenafil citrate (Viagra) and related oral therapies for erectile dysfunction (ED), such as vardenafil (Levitra) and tadalafil (Cialis), selectively inhibit the breakdown of cGMP by PDE5. Side effects of these drugs may include headache, flushing, rhinitis, urinary tract infections, visual disturbances, diarrhoea and dyspepsia, and they may be contraindicated for men with heart and various other medical conditions.

Descending pathways can be either excitatory (such as those initiated by the perceived attractiveness of the partner) or inhibitory (such as anxiety or guilt). Testosterone, mediated by oestradiol, is required to maintain intrapenile NO synthase levels, which mediate local vasodilatation by increasing NO production. In hypogonadal men, testosterone therapy can restore libido and erectile function. Other hormones, such as prolactin, adrenal steroids and thyroid hormone, contribute to male sexual functioning.

ED ('impotence'), defined as the inability to achieve and/or to maintain an erection for long enough to permit satisfactory sexual intercourse, can be caused by abnormalities of circulation or of neural inputs affecting the nervous control of erection. ED can result from psychogenic, organic (neurogenic such as spinal trauma, hormonal, vascular, cavernosal or drug induced) or mixed causes. Most cases of ED have an organic origin, mostly vascular disease. Atherosclerosis results in endothelial damage, cellular migration and smooth muscle proliferation influenced by cytokines, thrombosis, growth factors, reactive-oxygen species (ROS) and metabolic changes. Ageing affects NO production by the endothelium. Smoking is a risk factor for ED because it affects the vascular endothelium and nicotine, both increases sympathetic tone leading to smooth muscle contraction in the cavernosal body and decreases activity of the enzyme nitric oxide synthase. Failure of erection can be caused by damage to the spongy bodies, impaired flow in the vessels supplying the penis, drugs that interfere with neurotransmitter action or psychogenic factors. Local atherosclerosis can affect blood flow as can nicotine, which has vasoconstrictive properties.

ED is usually treated with vacuum devices, intraurethral suppositories, intracavernosal injections of vasoactive drugs (such as prostaglandin E_1 (PGE_1, alprostadil) and papaverine, which increase cAMP levels) and, more recently, with oral antagonists of cGMP–PDE (see above). (However, note that many men do not like or cannot tolerate PDE inhibitors.) Neurogenic ED can also arise from lesions in the nervous system, such as peripheral nerve damage. At the cellular level, alterations in potassium efflux may lead to a state of hypercontraction and lack of erectile response. ED is a common age-related problem so the incidence of ED will increase as longevity increases; ageing is associated with a decline in testosterone which may compromise the oestrogen–androgen crosstalk involved in the control of erection. Diabetes, particularly if coexisting with obesity, is a risk factor for ED and is related to accelerated atherosclerosis, alterations in erectile tissue, neuropathy and changes in hormone levels (Tamler, 2009). Diabetes-associated changes include smooth muscle degeneration, endothelial cell dysfunction, abnormal collagen deposition and high levels of glycosylated end products which reduce NO levels; these result in impaired relaxation of the corpus cavernosum smooth muscle (Sullivan et al., 2002). Medications for hypertension can contribute to ED; β-blockers can cause 'dry' ejaculation which is probably due to retrograde ejaculation because the β-blockers are causing bladder neck relaxation.

ED can also be a manifestation of cardiovascular disease; hyperlipidaemia and hypercholesterolaemia affect the production of NO by the vascular endothelium. ED is a symptom not a disease; it may act as a barometer of cardiovascular health and be the first presenting sign of previously undiagnosed hypertension, atherosclerosis and diabetes. Although the incidence of ED is common and increasing, it is underreported, underdiagnosed and undertreated as many men are reluctant to seek help. The condition can have considerable psychological and social impact on the affected man and his partner and their quality of life, causing depression, anxiety and loss of self-esteem.

As the penis becomes erect, the testes increase their blood volume and are drawn up towards the perineum. The dartos muscle contracts so the scrotal skin thickens and contracts. As stimulation proceeds, the plateau phase of emission occurs, where the muscles of the prostate, vas deferens and seminal vesicle undergo coordinated responses that propel spermatozoa and seminal fluid into the urethra. Ejaculation, the orgasmic phase, is the process of ejecting sperm from the urethra following contraction of the urethra smooth muscle. This is accompanied by contraction of the pelvic floor muscles and the accessory muscles including the vesicular urethral sphincter, which prevents retrograde ejaculation into the bladder. Orgasm, or contraction of the muscles, can occur without ejaculation. Oxytocin has a key role in the regulation of erection and, together with endothelin-1, in coordinated contraction of the epididymis and tubules at orgasm (Filippi et al., 2003); oxytocin responsiveness seems to be mediated by oestrogen. The composition of ejaculate changes because the contractions are sequential and there is relatively little mixing of the components (Table 6.1).

Premature or rapid ejaculation is the most common ejaculatory dysfunction and is usually caused by anxiety or emotional stress (Master and Turek, 2001); it is treated with behavioural therapy, pelvic floor muscle exercises, α-adrenoceptor antagonists ('sympathetic α-blockers'), topical anaesthetics, tricyclic antidepressants and selective serotonin reuptake inhibitors such as fluoxetine and sertraline. There have also been some clinical trials investigating the use of PDE5 inhibitors in the treatment of rapid ejaculation. Neurological lesions, such as spinal cord damage or damage following injury or surgery to the colon or abdomen, can also cause ejaculatory dysfunction; the sympathetic nerves associated with control of sexual functioning can easily be damaged. Other problems, such as diabetes and multiple sclerosis, can cause ejaculatory problems. Drugs, such as medication for hypertension and the common cold, may cause a lack of emission (deposition of the seminal fluid into the posterior or back part of the urethra), resulting in failure of ejaculation. Bladder neck damage in men who have undergone prostate surgery (particularly, transurethral resection of the prostate) can result in retrograde ejaculation. Bloody ejaculation is usually due to haematospermia, a benign, self-limited

Table 6.1 Composition of ejaculate during orgasm		
FRACTION	**DOMINANT GLAND**	**PARTICULARLY RICH IN**
Initial	Prostate	Acid phosphatase
Mid	Vas deferens	Sperm
Late	Seminal vesicles	Fructose

condition resulting from inflammation of the seminal vesicles, colon or prostate, which is treatable by antibiotics.

In the female

Women have similar responses in coitus to those of men. Tactile stimulation of the perineal region and the glans clitoris as well as psychogenic stimuli elicit the response. The corpora of the clitoris and the labia undergo vascular engorgement. Increased blood flow to the vagina increases transudation and vaginal lubrication. The vagina increases in width and length and the uterus is elevated upwards, which lifts the cervical os to produce a 'tenting effect'. At orgasm, vaginal and uterine contractions increase in intensity. During orgasm, women may expel fluid from the urethra; the Skene's glands produce this fluid. Sexual responses in the female tend to be more prolonged. Detumescence of the female organs is similar to detumescence of the penis. Orgasm in women seems to be learnt, whereas in men, it is a reflex action; female orgasm is not essential for pregnancy.

Systemic effects occur in both males and females: heart rate and blood pressure increase, accompanied by peripheral vasodilatation. This is followed by the resolution phase.

THE GAMETES

Male gametes

The sperm (Fig. 6.1) develop in the seminiferous tubules of the testes (see Chapter 2). At about 40–50 μm long, of which only approximately 5 μm is the head, the sperm cell is one of the smallest human cells. It retains fertilizing ability for about 2–5 days once deposited in the female reproductive tract. The genetic material of the male gamete is carried in the head of the sperm at the tip of which is located the acrosome, a vesicle containing digestive enzymes. The mid-piece is located between the head and the tail and is packed with mitochondria which generate the ATP required for movement. The tail of the mature sperm has a whip-like action which generates the propulsion for the sperm to swim about 30 cm/h. Abnormalities in human sperm morphology (such as having no tail, two tails or a coiled tail, or no head, two heads or a small head) are very common. Table 6.2 summarizes these and their possible causes. Abnormal motility or morphology of sperm is associated with infertility, causing problems with both fertilization and implantation. As well as the paternal haploid genome (23 paternal chromosomes), the sperm contributes the signal which initiates metabolic activation of the oocyte and also the centriole which causes the microtubules to form the mitotic spindle.

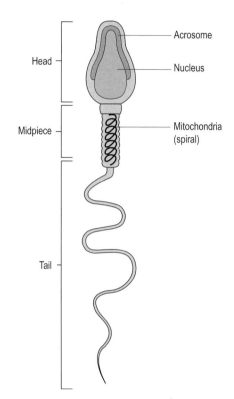

Fig. 6.1 The male gamete: the spermatozoon or sperm. (Reproduced with permission from Brooker, 1998.)

Sperm competition

Female choice and male-to-male competition prior to copulation are examples of sexual selection (Lewis et al., 2008). However, it seems that in many species, females typically mate with more than one male at a time when they could conceive. Sperm competition is the competition between sperm from two or more males to fertilize an ovum. There are various mechanisms involved such as sperm number and sperm length, removal of rival sperm, switching off female receptivity to subsequent males and plugging the female reproductive tract. It was proposed that morphologically abnormal human sperm, rather than being due to errors in production, have a role to play in fertilization (Baker and Bellis, 1988). This highly controversial theory suggested that there are two types of sperm: 'egg-getters' and 'blockers'. The morphologically abnormal sperm may be adapted to non-fertilizing roles, particularly preventing passage and successful fertilization by a competitor's sperm. However, the theory has been contested because the metabolic cost of producing non-fertilizing sperm is high and sperm competition is probably better achieved by better swimming and fertilizing ability rather than by producing sperm to compete in other ways (Lewis et al., 2008). Comparative

Table 6.2 Abnormalities of sperm

TYPE OF ABNORMALITY	DESCRIPTION	POSSIBLE CAUSES
Azoospermia (aspermia)	No sperm present within the ejaculate	Primary testicular failure; blockage to the vas deferens, that is, infection or trauma
Oligozoospermia (oligospermia)	Reduced numbers of sperm in the ejaculate (low sperm count)	Gonadotrophin insufficiency; drugs (social and medical, alcohol, toxins, etc.)
Idiopathic oligospermia	Low sperm count but physiological parameters normal	Unexplained
Teratozoospermia (teratospermia)	Abnormal morphology, for example, giant heads, double tails	Genetic, toxins, viral infection
Asthenospermia	Reduced (or lack of) mobility	Toxins, infection
Sperm agglutination	Sperm clump together in groups	Infection, Production of antigens against sperm (autoimmune response)

physiology predicts that mammalian species that have a large testis:body weight ratio are more likely to benefit from a promiscuous mating system in which sperm competition operates (because larger testes produce more sperm); by these criteria, men were not designed to be promiscuous (Short, 1997).

Female gametes

The ovum (i.e. the oocyte surrounded by the corona radiata) is expelled from the mature follicle of the ovary (see Chapter 4) and picked up by the fimbria of the uterine tube. The oocyte is the largest human cell, approximately 120–150 μm in diameter, and is therefore just visible to the naked eye. In comparison, follicular cells are typical-sized human cells of about 10 μm diameter. A rim of these follicular cells known as cumulus cells or the corona radiata surrounds the released oocyte. During follicular growth, the oocyte accumulates RNA and protein and numerous large mitochondria, which provide the needs of the dividing zygote. At birth, meiotic division has been suspended (see Chapter 7).

The fertile window

The lifespan of the human oocyte is thought to be about 6–24 h. Sperm have a viability of up to about 5 days in oestrogenized cervical mucus, so sperm in the reproductive tract up to 5 days before ovulation have a chance of fertilizing an oocyte. This means that the 'fertile window', when conception is possible, is about 4–5 days before ovulation. Conception on the day after ovulation has never been reported (Stanford et al., 2002). Sperm concentrations fall with increasing frequency of intercourse

but not to an extent that daily intercourse reduces benefit. Sperm counts are maximal after about 5 days of abstinence. Thus, daily intercourse during the fertile window optimizes conception because each day of intercourse increases the probability of pregnancy. The best outcome might be achieved by couples abstaining from intercourse for about 5 days prior to the fertile window and then aiming for daily intercourse.

Sex of the zygote

In meiotic division, the cells have their genetic complement reduced from 46 to 23 chromosomes. Each normal sperm will have 22 autosomes and either an X or a Y sex chromosome. If the oocyte is fertilized by a sperm bearing an X chromosome (a gynosperm), the zygote will be female, and if it has a Y chromosome (an androsperm), the offspring will be male (see Chapter 5). Theoretically, there will be equal numbers of gynosperm and androsperm. However, the sex ratio is not constant. The number of male babies born exceeds the number of female babies all over the world and, since the actual number of male conceptions is proportionately higher, male embryos have a higher failure rate (Bromwich, 1991).

It was observed that the incidence of male babies was markedly higher in cultures where menstruating women were considered unclean and had a ritual cleansing period (niddah) before resuming sexual relations (Harlap, 1979). It was therefore suggested that sperm bearing X and Y chromosomes swim at different rates. If there is a longer period between menstruation and the first intercourse, sperm deposition is less likely to occur much before ovulation, so a recently ejaculated sperm will achieve fertilization. It is hypothesized that androsperm, which are slightly smaller than gynosperm and have rounder heads, can swim faster.

There are a number of methods that are proposed to alter the sex chromosome ratio in sperm and allow sex selection. The difference in mass of gynosperm and androsperm in some species is much more marked than it is in humans. Bulls' sperm, for instance, can be effectively separated by differential centrifugation. The bottom fraction in the tube will be enriched with the heavier gynosperm, which can be used to impregnate cows to increase the female dairy proportion of the herd. Separation of human androsperm and gynosperm seems more difficult but is practised albeit with questionable success rates. Some environmental factors may influence the ratio of X- and Y-bearing sperm (James, 2008). Although a number of practices may have no scientific foundation, an increased number of female babies are born as the father ages, infants with blood group O are more likely to be male and environmental pollution seems to increase the number of female babies born. Sex selection is practised but usually not at the time of fertilization. In some parts of the world, selective abortion or infanticide is reported. In the West, sex selection is evident in that couples who have both a male and a female child are less likely to have further children.

Case study 6.1 looks at the question of sex determination.

In the days leading up to ovulation, the epithelial cells lining the uterine tubes become more ciliated and smooth muscle activity of the tubes increases. At ovulation, the fimbriae of the uterine tube move closer to the ovary and rhythmically stroke its surface. These sweeping movements, together with the currents generated by the moving cilia, facilitate the capture of the ovum released at ovulation. Ovum capture is remarkably efficient. Some women have only one functional ovary and one functional uterine tube; even if the ovary and uterine tube are from opposite sides, pregnancy can still occur. The oocyte is transported towards the uterus by movements generated

by peristaltic contractions of the uterine tube aided by the beating movement of the cilia. The oocyte has no inherent motility but is washed along by tubal fluid secreted by the epithelial cells and serum transudate. It takes about 3 or 4 days to reach the uterus. Initially, the movement through the ampulla, where fertilization is most likely to occur, is slow, but the zygote travels faster through the isthmus into the uterus. The junction between the uterine tube and the uterus relaxes under the influence of progesterone and allows the oocyte through. If the oocyte has not been fertilized, it degenerates and is phagocytosed.

STAGES OF FERTILIZATION

Gamete motility and sperm deposition

Spermiogenesis (see Chapter 2) occurs in the seminiferous tubules but, although the sperm are morphologically mature, they are not fully motile. The sperm develop swimming ability during a maturation phase of 4–12 days in the epididymis. At intercourse, about 200–300 million sperm are released in about 3 mL of seminal fluid (Box 6.1), which is deposited in the vagina. Repeated ejaculation normally results in a fall in sperm concentration, but the proportion of motile sperm decreases in men who are infertile, suggesting that impaired transport through the male genital tract affects motility (Matilsky et al., 1993). The sperm coagulate in the vagina, which appears to facilitate their retention and to buffer them against the normally unfavourable acidic environment (pH $\approx$ 4–5) of the vagina. The pH of the vagina is increased by the buffers in the seminal fluid favouring sperm motility and access to the cervix. The coagulum dissolves in about 20–60 min.

Between days 9 and 16 of the menstrual cycle, during the fertile period of the few days preceding and including ovulation, the watery composition of cervical mucus facilitates passage of sperm (see Table 4.1, p. 83). The cervical mucus interacts with the sperm and provides protection and nourishment. It also acts as a reservoir and may filter out sperm with abnormal morphology and motility

---

 Case study 6.1

Molly, who has four healthy daughters, is expecting her fifth child. She jokes with the midwife that she knows that this will be a girl as well. The midwife asks her why and Molly informs her that her husband works on an oil rig and is always home for 10 days and then away for 10 days. She laughingly states that every time she has conceived she has always started her period on the day her husband returns home.

- What factors in Molly and her husband's life may influence the sex of their children?
- How unusual is it to have five children all of the same sex?

Box 6.1 **Composition of ejaculate**

- 40–250 million sperm
- Prostatic fluid (30%): citric acid, acid phosphatase, magnesium and zinc ions
- Seminal fluid (60%): fructose (energy source for sperm), alkaline
- pH 7.0–8.3
- Volume: 2–6 mL

(Suarez and Pacey, 2006). Most sperm (99%) do not enter the uterus. A few hundred sperm reach the uterine tubes within a few hours of coitus; this first wave of rapid transport probably depends on rhythmic muscular contractions of the female reproductive tract. Some sperm appear to be stored in a reservoir (or at least remain in a functional and fertile state associated with the isthmic epithelium) within the uterine tubes for up to 24 h; they are activated by ovulation. Muscular activity of the female genital tract does not seem to be essential for fertilization; some sperm will be stored in cervical crypts and then travel in a relatively slow second wave through the cervical mucus, reaching the uterine tube a few days after ejaculation. Chemoattractants, released from the ovum and the surrounding cumulus cells and temperature changes, guide the sperm to the cumulus cell oocyte complex (Sun et al., 2005).

Capacitation

Ejaculated sperm are unable to fertilize an oocyte immediately; in order to fertilize the oocyte, ejaculated sperm undergo capacitation, interact with the zona pellucida and undergo the acrosome reaction. *In vitro*, there may be a delay of several hours before unprepared sperm can fertilize an oocyte. However, *in vivo* (and in sperm reclaimed from the uterus), the action of female enzymes and the oestrogen-stimulated high salt concentration of the uterine secretions speed up the preparation of the sperm. These biochemical and functional changes undergone by the sperm in the uterus and uterine tubes are known as capacitation. The changes include removal of adherent seminal plasma proteins from the sperm, remodelling of the sperm plasma membrane, including changes in cholesterol and phospholipid content, influx of extracellular calcium, increase in cAMP, phosphorylation of proteins and a decrease in intracellular pH (Wassarman, 2009). The modifications alter ion channels in the membrane allowing a transmembrane flux of ions, which direct protein phosphorylation, thereby initiating hyperactivation of the sperm. Sperm metabolism changes from oxidative to glycolytic. The hyperactivated sperm tail movements change to become whiplash-like so the sperm thrusts vigorously forward, moving from the sperm storage reserve in the isthmus of the uterine tube to the ampulla (Suarez, 2008). The accentuated lateral head movements generate a boring action, which aids access through the cumulus cells and ZP to the oocyte. The tail is also involved in sperm movement within the oocyte (Van Blerkom et al., 1995).

Access to the oocyte

The ovulated oocyte is surrounded by two layers which need to be penetrated by the sperm in order for it to reach the oocyte membrane and to acquire fusibility. The first barrier preventing access of the sperm to the oocyte is the outer layer of cumulus cells, the corona radiata, embedded in an intercellular matrix of carbohydrates, protein and hyaluronic acid. Hyaluronidase, released from the sperm acrosome, breaks down the hyaluronic acid matrix between the follicular cells so sperm can pass through to the zona pellucida. The hyperactive swimming movements of the sperm aid penetration of the corona radiata. The gradual release of sperm from the reservoir of cervical mucus and their activation close to the oocyte means that the time limit of fertility is extended.

Binding to the zona pellucida

The oocyte is surrounded by the zona pellucida, which is about 14–15 μm thick. It is an extracellular matrix composed of sulphated glycoproteins that were produced by the growing oocyte. It is permeable to some viruses, immunoglobulins and enzymes. Before ovulation, cytoplasmic processes from the corona radiata cells penetrate the zona pellucida, allowing communication to, and nourishment of, the oocyte via gap junctions. When these are withdrawn in response to the luteinizing hormone (LH) surge, they may leave gaps in the zona pellucida that offer easier access for sperm penetration, thus facilitating fertilization (Familiari et al., 1992). The zona pellucida acts as a barrier that allows only species-specific sperm–egg interaction.

The human zona pellucida is composed of four glycoproteins ZP1, ZP2, ZP3 and ZP4 (Gupta et al., 2009). ZP2 and ZP3 are implicated as sperm receptors; ZP3 and ZP4 are involved in the binding of sperm to the oocyte and induction of the acrosome reaction. Penetration through the zona pellucida gives the sperm access to the perivitelline space where interaction with the oocyte membrane can take place. The zona pellucida confers a high degree of species specificity; if it is removed, sperm from a different species are able to fertilize an oocyte, though development will rapidly arrest. This is the basis of the hamster zona-free ovum (HZFO) test or sperm penetration assay (SPA) in which hamster oocytes, with their zona chemically removed, are used to test the ability of human sperm to penetrate an oocyte.

The zona pellucida is antigenic: anti-zona pellucida antibodies may be the cause of some cases of infertility. The composition of the zona pellucida changes with the cortical reaction after fertilization so it prevents polyspermy but allows secretions of the uterine tube to reach the oocyte during the early stages of cell division. The zona pellucida also has a role in preventing the blastocyst from prematurely implanting into the wall of the uterine tube before it reaches the uterus. It is possible that an excessively thick zona pellucida could cause problems with blastocyst hatching and subsequent implantation.

Interaction of sperm with the zona pellucida seems to occur in several stages (Ikawa et al., 2010). At first, the capacitated sperm loosely and reversibly adhere to the surface of the zona pellucida. Then, the sperm become strongly and irreversibly bound to the zona pellucida.

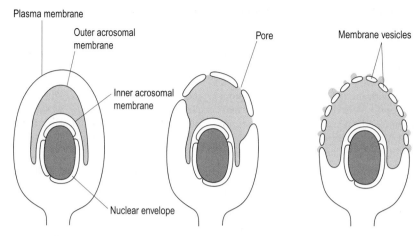

Fig. 6.2 The acrosome reaction.

Many sperm bind to the oocyte zona pellucida but usually only a few sperm penetrate into the perivitelline space and only one will fuse with the oocyte plasma membrane.

The acrosome reaction

After binding to the zona pellucida, the sperm undergo the acrosome reaction (Fig. 6.2). The sperm binding to the ZP receptor is a carbohydrate-mediated event which initiates a signal transduction cascade and raised intracellular calcium concentration. Carbohydrate-binding proteins on the sperm surface recognize glycoproteins on the ZP. This molecular interaction is associated with inhibition of both the innate and adaptive immune responses (Barroso et al., 2009) which may help to protect the gametes and developing embryo ('fetoembryonic defence system hypothesis;' Clark et al., 2001). The acrosome reaction can also be triggered by follicular fluid and progesterone (Brucker and Lipford, 1995). The outer acrosome membrane fuses with the covering plasma membrane of the sperm. Small vesicles containing acrosomal enzymes are pinched off and their contents are released. The inner acrosomal membrane is then exposed. A tunnel is digested through the zona pellucida by acrosin, a serine protease that remains bound to the inner acrosomal membrane, and the acrosomal enzymes released from the vesicles. The lurching movements of the sperm propel it forward through the zona pellucida and the perivitelline space so that its head is in contact with the oocyte vitelline (surface) membrane. Penetration through the zona pellucida requires both hyperactivated sperm and lysis of the zona pellucida.

Gamete fusion

The acrosome reaction triggers changes in the sperm membrane that allow sperm–oocyte binding and then fusion to occur. The acrosome reaction reveals antigens such as Izumo on the sperm which can interact with receptors on the surface of the oocyte (Ikawa et al., 2010). Similar egg cell surface proteins on the oocyte membrane are recognized by the sperm. The surface of the oocyte is covered with microvilli, except in the region overlying the meiotic spindle. Oocyte microvilli surround the head of the sperm preceding fusion and then the sperm plasma membrane is incorporated into the oocyte membrane. Various docking and recognition molecules on both the sperm head and the oocyte are implicated in sperm–oocyte binding and fusion; these include sperm ADAMs (a family of proteins with a disintegrin and metalloprotease domain) and CD9 and other proteins on oocytes (Kaji and Kudo, 2004). In human fertilization, the sperm tail remains motile and is incorporated into the oocyte (Payne et al., 1997). Paternal mitochondria entering the oocyte are selectively degraded (Kaneda et al., 1995). The zygote and resulting embryo have only maternal mitochondria (Gyllensten et al., 1991); the oocyte seems to lose mitochondrial DNA (mtDNA) with increasing maternal age, a factor that may be important in fertility. One technique to deal with this is transfer of the cytoplasm from a younger woman's oocytes to 'rescue' oocytes from older women (Barroso et al., 2009). As well as the male nuclear component, the fertilizing sperm also contribute to the centriole and microtubule-organizing centre, from which the first mitotic spindle will develop (Van Blerkom et al., 1995). Fertilization takes about 10–20 min.

The cortical reaction and block to polyspermy

Polyploidy is usually fatal and is often detected in spontaneously aborted fetuses (Gardner and Evans, 2006). Most human triploidy is due to polyspermic fertilization where two sperm fertilize an ovum. The number of sperm reaching the newly ovulated egg is partly regulated by sperm transit from reservoirs in the female reproductive tract. Oocytes from most mammals develop mechanisms during growth and development to block polyspermy, the entry of more than one sperm. Following fertilization by one sperm, polyspermy is prevented by a sequence of events which modifies the structure of the plasma membrane and/or the zona pellucida. The relative importance to the plasma membrane versus the zona pellucida block to polyspermy varies with species. In most mammalian oocytes, the zona pellucida is thought to provide the most important block to polyspermy. The number of supernumerary sperm found in the perivitelline space between the ZP and the plasma membrane is usually 1–10 in humans, suggesting that the membrane block occurs almost simultaneously with the ZP block. Two events are involved: the cortical reaction and modification of the zona pellucida by enzymes released from the cortical granules (the 'zona reaction'). Failure of either of these steps results in polyspermy. Polyspermy results in non-diploid zygotes which are usually not viable but, in some cases, can develop into gestational trophoblastic neoplasias and tumours such as the benign hydatidiform mole or the malignant choriocarcinoma (Hauzman and Papp, 2008). The incidence of non-diploid zygotes increases with alcohol, drug use, anaesthesia and fertilization of 'aged' oocytes (i.e. aged in terms of hours after ovulation). Intracytoplasmic sperm injection (ICSI) does not trigger the membrane block to polyspermy; this is not important in the clinical scenario, as ICSI-fertilized eggs are not going to be exposed to additional sperm, but it does indicate that ICSI is not fully equivalent to IVF or *in vivo* fertilization.

The secretion of cortical granules into the perivitelline space is triggered by a rise in intracellular calcium ion (Ca^{2+}) concentration. In experimental species used to study fertilization, such as sea urchin eggs, two mechanisms have evolved to reduce the occurrence of polyspermy. Prior to the ubiquitous zona reaction, sperm binding rapidly triggers an influx of sodium ions, leading to depolarization of the oocyte membrane which transiently blocks binding of additional sperm. This is known as the 'fast block' to polyspermy. There is no evidence for membrane depolarization being involved in the fast block to polyspermy in mammals.

The initial calcium increase triggers calcium release from the intracellular stores, which promotes fusion of the cortical granules with the oocyte membrane (Hoodbhoy and Talbot, 1994). The calcium signal starts from the site of fusion and moves as an oscillating wave through the oocyte, sequentially activating about 4000 cortical granules (Fig. 6.3). The trigger for this calcium-induced calcium rise seems to be a soluble cytosolic factor released from the fertilizing sperm. This sperm factor is probably a novel phospholipase C, PLC-ζ (PLC-zeta) which diffuses into the oocyte cytoplasm following fusion of the sperm and oocyte plasma membranes, initiating the calcium release that leads to the oscillations of calcium (Swann et al., 2004).

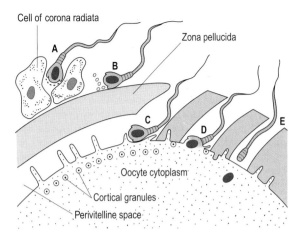

Fig. 6.3 Fertilization: (A) acrosome reaction; (B) binding to zona pellucida; (C) penetration of zona pellucida; (D) fusion of oocyte and sperm, and cortisol reaction; (E) fertilization.

These calcium oscillations may last for several hours (Palermo et al., 1997) and act as the signal for the oocyte to activate and begin development. During the ICSI procedure used in IVF (see below), it is common practice to immobilize the sperm by mechanical damage to the sperm tail just before injecting it into the egg (Yanagida et al., 2001). The extensive disruption of the sperm membrane wrought by this damage may help the sperm factor to be released, as there is a more rapid onset of calcium oscillations after ICSI.

Egg activation is triggered by the rise in intracellular calcium concentration; the earliest indicators are the resumption of meiosis and secretion of cortical granules. The rise in calcium subsequently initiates the first division of the embryo (Jones, 2007).

The zona reaction

The contents of the cortical granules (enzymes, such as proteases and peroxidase, and polysaccharides) are released into the perivitelline space and diffuse through the zona pellucida to digest the ZP3 sperm receptors. The zona pellucida loses its ability to bind to sperm and to induce the acrosome reaction. The changed texture of the zona pellucida is described as 'zona hardening'. This reaction is known as the zona reaction. The composition of the oocyte plasma membrane is also altered.

Events leading to the first mitotic division

Possible benefits of arrested meiosis

Prior to fertilization, the chromosomes of the oocyte had been arrested in metaphase of the second nuclear division (see Fig. 7.11, p 151). It has been suggested that growth of the oocyte requires a diploid number of chromosomes. Meiotic arrest in the diplotene stage of metaphase means that both maternal and paternal alleles can be expressed during oocyte maturation. Observation of IVF has shown that the human meiotic spindle is unstable and very sensitive to external influences.

As a species, humans have a high frequency of aneuploidy in products of fertilization. This results in zygotes and embryos with the wrong number of chromosomes, for example, Down's syndrome with 47 chromosomes (see Table 7.1, p. 152). Down's syndrome is an example of trisomy, a chromosome complement that is compatible with fetal survival; other examples are thought to be just as likely but may result in failed implantation or failed *in utero* development. Although chromosome 21 and 22 are both small chromosomes, chromosome 21 has only 225 active genes, whereas chromosome 22 has 545 active genes. Therefore, trisomy 21 results in a relatively small number of genes in triplicate form, which may explain why trisomy 21 is compatible with life. Genes on chromosome 21 are of particular interest because of their role in Down's syndrome, a type of Alzheimer's disease and several types of cancer. These diseases and the small number of genes on chromosome 21 led to it being the second fully sequenced human genes in the Human Genome Project (Hattori et al., 2000).

Aneuploidy is mostly due to non-disjunction of bivalent chromosomes in the first meiotic division (see Fig. 7.11) and is associated with pregnancy loss. Aneuploidy is the most common cause of mental retardation where the fetus survives (Hassold and Hunt, 2001). The frequency of aneuploidy increases with increased maternal age; ageing oocytes seem more prone to errors in meiosis and abnormal segregation of chromosomes. Studies have shown that the risk of Down's syndrome where the extra chromosomal material is maternally derived increases with age. A lower incidence of Down's syndrome results from extra paternal chromosomal material; however, this is less likely to be linked to increasing age of the male partner.

Other factors such as alcohol abuse, chemotherapy and smoking (Zenzes et al., 1995) have been found to disrupt meiosis. Arrest in the second meiotic division may help to prevent aneuploidy and the inclusion of an extra or absent chromosome in the oocyte.

Completion of the second meiotic division

The calcium rise that triggers the cortical reaction is also the stimulus for the oocyte to increase its metabolism. Calcium regulates the cell cycle (Whittaker, 1995); it promotes resumption of meiosis, probably via activation of the M-phase-promoting factor, and completion of second meiotic division (Fig. 6.4). The increase in oxidative metabolism is preceded by a rise in intracellular pH.

The 23 paired chromatids then separate, half being expelled as the second polar body into the perivitelline space. A pronuclear membrane appears around the remaining 23 chromosomes forming the female pronucleus, thus completing the meiotic division.

Decondensation of the sperm nucleus

The chromatin or genetic material of the mature sperm is transcriptionally inert and compacted tightly in the head. After the head of the sperm enters the cytoplasm of the oocyte, it is affected by cytoplasmic factors that cause the chromatin threads of the DNA to decondense and become transcriptionally competent. The decondensation takes place while the sperm pronucleus is moving towards the pronucleus of the oocyte. The centrioles radiate microtubules in a formation known as a sperm aster, which aids the movement of the two pronuclei (Schatten, 1994). Then, oocyte histones begin to associate with the male chromosomal material (see Chapter 7). As the developing pronuclei near each other in the centre of the cell, they synthesize DNA in preparation for the first mitotic division and the chromosomes replicate into chromatids.

First mitotic division

In the first mitotic division, the membranes of both pronuclei break down and the male and female chromosomes become organized around a mitotic spindle ready for the first cell division. The combination of the male and female chromosomes is called syngamy. It is at this point that conception has occurred. Fertilization is complete about 18–24 h after fusion, and the fertilized oocyte is known as a zygote (the steps of fertilization are summarized in Box 6.2). A cleavage furrow then appears and the zygote becomes two identical cells.

The random assortment of nuclear material in meiosis and the random exchange of nuclear material create new combinations of genes so the gametes are both haploid and genetically unique. Fertilization of one gamete with another results in a unique combination of genetic material in the zygote, which is important in variation of the species (see Chapter 7). Whether the sperm carries an X or Y chromosome will determine the primary sex of the zygote so it will differentiate into either a female or male embryo (see Chapter 5). Fertilization restores the diploid number of chromosomes and initiates the cleavage of the zygote.

The mitochondria contained in the mid-piece of the sperm enter the egg at fertilization but seldom survive beyond 2 or 3 days after fertilization. The number of mitochondria present in somatic cells ranges from a few hundreds to a few thousands depending on the energy requirements of the specific cell type. Each mitochondrion contains 5–10 identical, circular molecules of

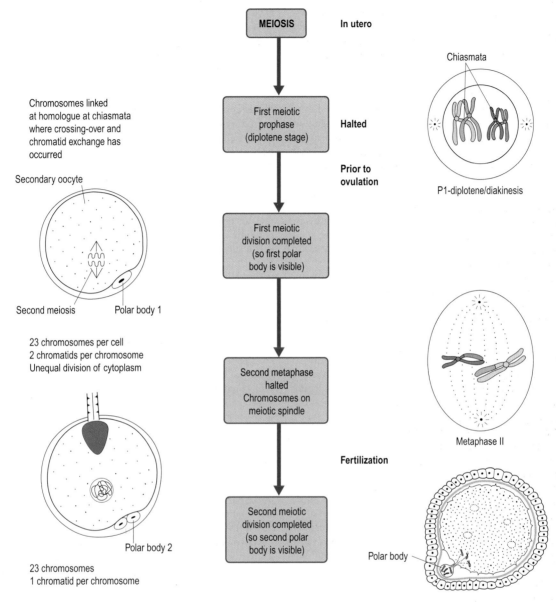

Fig. 6.4 Fertilization and the generation of the second polar body.

Box 6.2 **Sequence of steps in fertilization**

- Deposition of sperm
- Sperm capacitation in the female reproductive tract
- Penetration of the corona radiata
- Binding of capacitated sperm to the zona pellucida
- Acrosome reaction
- Penetration of zona pellucida
- Fusion of sperm with oocyte plasma membrane

- Cortical reaction and prevention of polyspermy
- Increased respiration and metabolism by the oocyte
- Completion of the second meiotic division of the oocyte
- Extrusion of the second polar body
- Decondensation of the sperm nucleus
- Development and fusion of the male and female pronuclei

mtDNA which codes for 13 proteins involved in the mito-chondrial respiratory chain as well as ribosomal RNA (rRNA) and transfer RNA (tRNA) molecules. Mature oocytes are very large cells with high energy requirements and contain approximately 1 million mitochondria. The fertilizing sperm introduces up to 100 mitochondria into the oocyte cytoplasm at fertilization. The sperm mtDNA are highly vulnerable to ROS and mutagenesis during the lengthy process of spermiogenesis, storage, migration through the male and female reproductive tracts and fer-tilization, particularly as the sperm has little antioxidant capability. So, destruction of potentially defective sperm mitochondria is important to ensure that the developing embryo has a healthy stock of mtDNA. The mechanism by which sperm mitochondria, but not the mitochondria derived from the oocyte, are selectively destroyed relies on the tagging of spermatozoa with ubiquitin during sper-matogenesis. Ubiquitin is a small polypeptide universally used by cells to tag protein molecules which are destined for degradation. After initial tagging, sperm mitochondria are subsequently masked by disulphide bond formation during maturation and storage in the epididymis but fol-lowing fertilization, the glutathione-rich environment of the early embryo exposes the ubiquitin-tagged sperm mid-piece which is then recognized by the oocyte's ubiquitin-proteasome-dependent proteolytic pathway so the sperm mid-piece is lyzed and its component mito-chondria and their mtDNA are destroyed. The outcome of this efficient destruction of male-derived mitochondria and their mtDNA is that all mtDNA in human offspring are maternally derived (matrilinear). There is no change in the base pair sequence (of about 16 500 base pairs) when the mtDNA is passed on from mother to child so it is a useful tracking tool for tracing ancestry through the female line (Sykes, 2004). The relatively simple analy-sis of, for example, buccal smears can therefore establish maternal ancestry (see Chapter 7). In forensic investiga-tions, mtDNA rather than nuclear DNA is used to identify human remains such as the remains of the Russian royal family. However, mtDNA has a high mutation rate and aberrant mtDNA are thought to be involved in cancers and disease of ageing such as sporadic Alzheimer's disease (Wallace, 2010).

DEVELOPMENT BEFORE IMPLANTATION

The zygote spends about 4–6 days travelling to the uterus. It is moved through the uterine tube by the peristaltic action of the smooth muscle and the sweeping move-ments of the cilia and the fluid produced by the ciliated epithelium. The embryo at first divides approximately every 15 h; the division time becomes progressively shorter. During the initial cleavage steps, the embryo is enclosed within the restraining zona pellucida and its total mass remains approximately constant. Cytoplasmic factors regulate cleavage, which occurs without net growth (Fig. 6.5) so cell number increases but the cells become progressively smaller.

Initially, the cleavage divisions are synchronous and each cell (blastomere) is identical, but then the cells divide at an independent rate. Later synchrony is lost, so the pattern of doubling of cell number is also lost. In human and mouse embryos, at the eight-cell stage, each of the cells is totipotent (i.e. is able to generate all cell lineages in the embryo/fetus and extraembryonic tissues) and its fate is not irreversible (Hardy et al., 1990). Experi-ments on mouse embryos have demonstrated that each of the cells has the capability of independently developing into an embryo. Cells from different origins can also be combined to form a mosaic or a chimera. In human IVF, a single blastomere can be removed from the blasto-cyst at this stage for genetic testing using the technique of preimplantation genetic diagnosis (PGD) without preju-dicing the outcome for the embryo if it is transferred to the uterus (see Chapter 7).

After the eight-cell stage, the cells change morphologi-cally so some of the cells at the outer edge of the embryo become flatter. About day 4, as it reaches the uterus, the embryo is a mass of cells known as the morula (derived from the Latin word for mulberry). The dividing ball of cells enters a phase called compaction. The inner cells are sealed off by outer cells, which adhere tightly in a sphere, developing a polarity and communicating via gap junc-tions. A fluid-filled cavity, or blastocoele, forms between the inner and outer cell layers; the embryo is now known as a blastocyst. By the 64-cell stage, the cells of the concep-tus are irreversibly differentiated on the pathway to becom-ing embryonic or extraembryonic tissue. Differentiation into a particular cell type seems to be related to positional information of the cells, which induces particular genes to be expressed. Cells of the blastocyst initially differentiate into two distinct cell lines. Most of the outer layer of cells forms the trophoblast, which will develop into the pla-centa, chorion and extraembryonic tissue. Most of the cells of the inner cell mass will develop into the embryo, umbil-ical cord and the amnion (Fig. 6.6).

PARENTAL IMPRINTING

Chromosomes from the oocyte and sperm express differ-ent alleles depending on their origin. Both maternal and paternal chromosomes are required for normal zygote for-mation and development but genes from both chromo-somes are not always expressed. This is described as imprinting and is due to gamete-specific patterns of DNA modification such as methylation. This means that, although the pairs of chromosomes carry the same genetic

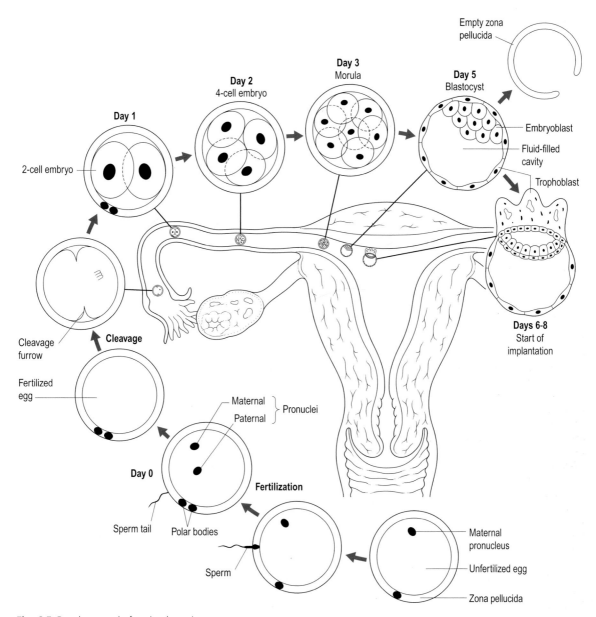

Fig. 6.5 Development before implantation.

information, this information is expressed differently depending on whether it originates from the oocyte or the sperm (see Chapter 8). Paternal imprinting favours development of the placenta and inhibits development of the embryo. Maternal imprinting seems to switch off some of the genes involved in placental development. Normally, the paternal copy of the X chromosome is preferentially activated in cells derived from the trophoblast. Conversely, in the inner cell mass, the paternal and maternal chromosomes are randomly inactivated (see Chapter 7).

X chromosome inactivation is irreversible, except in oogonia. Parental genetic imprinting is lost (reordered) on formation of the new gametes, which have new parental imprinting on the formation of new chromosome sets. Most imprinted genes are associated with placental tissue and so affect growth and development (Miozzo and Simoni, 2002).

In mouse embryo cells, removal and replacement of one of the pronuclei with another of opposite sex (so both pronuclei are of the same sex) results in abnormal

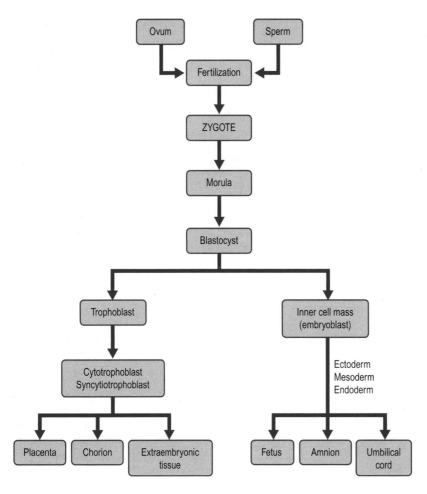

Fig. 6.6 The pathway of cell division.

development. If both the pronuclei are female, early embryo development appears normal but placental development is impaired. If both pronuclei are male, placental development appears normal but embryonic development is extremely stunted. Hydatidiform mole development in humans occurs as a result of diandric diploids, that is, when two sperm fertilize an oocyte and the maternal chromosome complement does not participate in development (Jacobs et al., 1980). The result is extreme overdevelopment of the placental tissues and extreme underdevelopment of the embryonic tissues. This situation could also arise from the fertilization of an oocyte with a diploid sperm. Digynic triploids (i.e. two maternal and one paternal chromosome sets) can occur if the polar body is retained.

Human oocytes can be induced to undergo spontaneous cleavage in the absence of fertilization by a sperm and develop into parthenotes. Early stages of cleavage, therefore, seem to be maternally imprinted. However, mouse parthenogenic oocytes arrest after the first cleavage divisions, at the time the embryonic genes would be expressed. Some maternal genes are expressed in the blastocyst but overall, embryonic genes are required for blastocyst formation. Imprinting causes difficulties in cloning such as premature ageing and increased risk of cancer; the clones may not have DNA which is methylated in the correct places. It is also thought that there is an increased risk of low birthweight in otherwise healthy infants born after assisted reproduction technologies (see p. 132), which may be partially related to different conditions very early in life affecting the imprinting of genes involved in fetal growth (Miozzo and Simoni, 2002). Kaguya, a parthenogenic mouse that survived to adulthood (a 'virgin birth'), has been developed (Kono et al., 2004) by engineering eggs to produce the normally paternally imprinted growth factor, IGF-2. The method was very problematic and only 2 of 457 reconstructed eggs developed; there is a consensus that cloning of humans would be of little merit and be likely to have major risks for maternal health and offspring development (Mollard et al., 2002).

TWINS

Throughout history, twinning has fascinated civilizations. The incidence of twins in the United Kingdom was about 15 in 1000 livebirths in 2002 (Siddiqui and McEwan, 2007), a increase over previous years because of the increased use of ART, though this figure may drop a little because of the HFEA guidelines to limit the number of embryos transferred during IVF cycles (Milingos and Bhattacharya, 2009). Approximately two-thirds of the twins are dizygotic (fraternal or non-identical) and one-third is monozygotic (identical). The rate of monozygotic twins is fairly constant worldwide but the ratio of monozygotic to dizygotic twins varies markedly from country to country and is affected by season, ethnic origin, parity and maternal age. Dizygotic twins arise from multiple ovulation and two fertilized oocytes implanting and developing; they have separate placentas and membranes (though sometimes these are fused). Monozygotic or identical twins are derived from one fertilized oocyte; the single embryo divides and then splits. Although it is possible that a two-celled embryo could split and result in twins, most twins in practice result from the subdivision of the inner cell mass at the blastocyst stage (Fig. 6.7). About 75% of monozygotic twins share one placenta; the remainder have separate placentas and membranes. Twin pregnancies have a higher rate of obstetric complications, including fetal death, miscarriage and preterm labour, compared to singleton pregnancies.

IMPLANTATION

The blastocyst may remain free-floating in the uterine cavity until implantation at day 7. The blastocyst accumulates fluid and expands. This, together with the digestion and thinning of the zona pellucida by uterine enzymes, results in shedding of the zona pellucida, described as 'hatching', at about 6–7 days post-fertilization. The disappearance of the zona pellucida allows the cells of the blastocyst to come into contact with the epithelium of the uterus. The blastocyst consists of at least 100 cells, but some programmed cell death (apoptosis) has already occurred even at this very early stage of the life cycle (Hardy et al., 1989). In most blastocysts, there is a degree of degeneration of some trophoblast cells and some of the inner cell mass. After hatching, growth is no longer physically restricted and the blastocyst grows in mass as well as cell number. Embedding or nidation of the blastocyst normally occurs in the upper part of the body of the uterus (the fundal region). The blastocyst implants at the embryonic pole,

where the inner cell mass lies. The inner cell mass forms the embryonic disc (see Chapter 9).

The outer cells of the blastocyst secrete proteolytic enzymes and collagenase, which break down and destroy some of the cells of the endometrial surface, forming a depression in which the blastocyst lies. Implantation in humans is a very invasive mechanism. Uterine muscle activity is low at this time because secretion of progesterone is high. Once implantation has occurred, the lining of the uterus closes over the blastocyst and the pregnancy is established. The trophoblast cells absorb nourishment from the decidua and secrete human chorionic gonadotrophin (hCG) which stimulates growth and secretory activity of the corpus luteum to produce steroid hormones, which support continued growth of the decidua. Critical amounts of hCG are required for blastocyst survival.

MATERNAL RECOGNITION OF THE PREGNANCY

Successful implantation requires crosstalk (reciprocated two-way communication between mother and embryo; Hill, 2001). The menstrual cycle, under the control of ovarian steroids, induces the biochemical, physiological and morphological changes which prepare the uterus for blastocyst implantation. Many signals are involved in the crucial role of maintaining the corpus luteum, regulating uterine vascular permeability and maternal immunosuppression. Not all of the signals have been identified. hCG is involved in maintaining the corpus luteum and its essential endocrine role. hCG is luteotrophic, binding to the LH receptors and stimulating a progressive rise in progesterone and oestrogen secretion. Levels of hCG are abnormally low if implantation is inadequate, if trophoblast cell division is insufficient, if implantation is ectopic or if growth of the corpus luteum is deficient (Check et al., 1992). Secretion of hCG from the trophoblast is regulated by trophoblastic gonadotrophin-releasing hormone (GnRH). hCG also binds to the embryonic trophoblast cells and affects the differentiation of cytotrophoblast into syncytiotrophoblast (see Chapter 8). Before it becomes receptive, the uterus contains high levels of the endogenous cannabinoid, anandamine. The concentrations of anandamine fall as receptivity increases, leading to the suggestion that lower birthweight associated with maternal marijuana use occurs because the cannabinoid level is not optimal (Piomelli, 2004).

Implantation and the three stages of apposition, adhesion (attachment) and penetration (invasion) require the endometrium to change and to become responsive. The endometrial stroma is modified (see Chapter 8); vascular permeability increases, and the endometrial cells become hypertrophied and produce prolactin. The processes

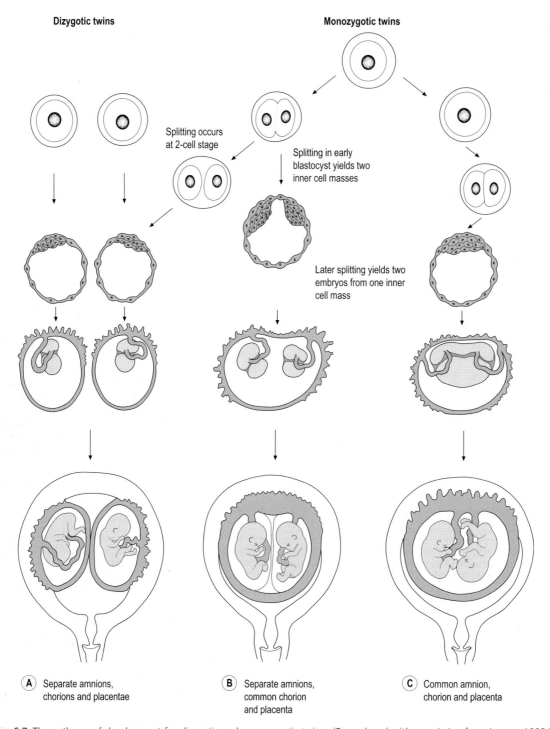

Dizygotic twins

Monozygotic twins

Splitting occurs at 2-cell stage

Splitting in early blastocyst yields two inner cell masses

Later splitting yields two embryos from one inner cell mass

(A) Separate amnions, chorions and placentae

(B) Separate amnions, common chorion and placenta

(C) Common amnion, chorion and placenta

Fig. 6.7 The pathway of development for dizygotic and monozygotic twins. (Reproduced with permission from Larsen, 1993.)

inducing the changes are known as decidualization; the changed uterine lining is called the decidua. The initial changes begin in the luteal phase of the menstrual cycle. The uterine glands become more tortuous, the spiral arteries develop and the endometrium becomes thicker and oedematous. Uterine secretions increase and intercellular spaces develop. The decidua forms a physical barrier to invasive trophoblast cell migration and generates a cytokine environment that promotes trophoblast attachment rather than invasion (Fazleabas et al., 2004). The decidualized endometrial cells produce IGFBP-1 which modulates interactions at the maternal–fetal interface and is involved in regulating growth.

Effectively, a nidation or implantation window, related to changes in the endometrial epithelium, occurs at about day 20–23 of the cycle (6–8 days after ovulation). The timing of the endometrial changes is mediated by preovulatory increase in 17β-oestriol and subsequent luteal progesterone secretion and has to synchronize with the time the fertilized ovum enters the uterus (Csemiczky et al., 1998). Problems with coincident timing can cause infertility or impaired fertility. During this receptive period, tiny hair-like microvilli protruding from the endometrial cells transiently fuse into single smooth flower-like apical membrane protrusions called pinopodes or uterodomes (Nikas and Aghajanova, 2003). The pinopodes form a week after ovulation and are present for only 2 days before regressing. They absorb fluid and molecules from the uterine lumen which tends to decrease the size of the uterine cavity and to increase the chance of apposition between the embryo and the endometrium. The transient absence of cilia may also prevent the blastocyst being swept away from the site of implantation. Progesterone stimulates pinopode formation, as well as increased uterine secretions, increased blood flow and oedema.

The microenvironment of the reproductive tract is influenced by the secretion of maternal proteins which may then be further modified by proteins secreted by the developing embryo. Embryo-derived platelet-activating factor (ED-PAF) influences vasodilatation and oedema of the decidua. It increases vascular permeability, induces thrombocytopenia, regulates prostaglandin synthesis and activates platelets. Prostaglandins are also involved in regulating decidual factors. Other substances thought to be involved in maternal–conceptus crosstalk include chemokines and cytokines (such as interleukins, interferons and tumour necrosis factor), inhibin and other growth factors (see Box 4.4, p. 74), adhesion molecules (such as integrins), angiogenic and apoptotic factors, leptin and vitamin D (Vigano et al., 2003). The expression of these proteins and peptides can act as a marker of uterine receptivity. The uterine immune system plays an important role in implantation and trophoblastic growth and development; more than 40% of decidua cells are immune cells, predominantly uterine natural killer (NK) cells.

CAUSES OF INFERTILITY

Strictly speaking, infertility is a failure to produce gametes capable of fertilization and thus, conception never happens. But in practice, the term infertility is used for failure to continue a pregnancy to term (resulting in a 'take home' baby). Some female infertility is due to primary ovarian failure (independent of hypothalamic and pituitary defects) or premature ovarian failure; these probably have genetic components but these have not been clearly identified (Matzuk and Lamb, 2008).

Women who undergo prolonged shock resulting from major haemorrhage (sometimes associated with surgery or a previous pregnancy) can develop anterior pituitary necrosis which can result in Sheehan's syndrome; the pituitary necrosis means that FSH and LH cannot be produced so menopause abruptly begins and fertility is lost.

About a third of female fertility is related to tubal and peritoneal factors (Coughlan and Li, 2009). This includes damage or obstruction to the uterine tubes, often related to pelvic inflammatory disease (PID) or sometimes pelvic or tubal surgery. PID is associated with irreversible damage and loss of the ciliated cells lining the uterine tubes, and thus the loss of transport of the fertilized embryo to the uterus. Persistent tubal damage increases with each episode of infection. Previous ectopic pregnancy, prior abdominal surgery especially if it caused peritubal adhesions, endometriosis, hydrosalpinx (where the uterine tube is blocked and filled with fluid), sepsis following abortion, appendicitis associated with rupture, uterine fibroids and tubal sterilization can also affect tube patency and function. Female fertility can also be curtailed by failure to ovulate or to produce or respond to hormones during the menstrual cycle. Polycystic ovarian syndrome is a relatively common cause of impaired fertility. Ageing affects the success of the menstrual cycle, and it is thought that many women overestimate the length of their reproductive life. Menopause, particularly early or premature menopause, can lead to unexpected early infertility.

In a third to half of infertile couples, the male has poor semen quality which can include low sperm count and/or sperm with abnormal morphology or poor motility (Pacey, 2008). Although male reproductive functions do not cease abruptly in a way equivalent to female menopause, paternal age has marked effects on semen quality, hormone levels, libido and erectile function (Fisch, 2009). Damage to the cells and tissues involved in spermatogenesis such as that caused by trauma or infection (like mumps or malaria) can affect sperm production. Defects of the genital tract (usually obstruction), antibodies or problems with ejaculation usually due to retrograde ejaculation or impotence are the more common causes of male infertility.

There are some factors which can affect fertility in both men and women. These include genetic factors such as Robertsonian translocation (see Chapter 7) where one of the parents has chromosomal rearrangement which means that their own genetic constitution is fine but they have an increased risk that their gametes are unbalanced and could potentially produce a non-viable embryo. Chromosomal abnormalities, especially where the number of sex chromosomes is abnormal, are associated with infertility. Endocrine abnormalities, particularly if they affect the hypothalamic pituitary axis such as pituitary tumours (like prolactinaemia), Kallman's syndrome and hypopituitarism, can affect fertility. Some metabolic/endocrine disorders such as diabetes, liver, kidney, thyroid and adrenal diseases have effects on reproduction. Generally, untreated endocrine disorders are associated with infertility and treatment restores fertility. Sexually transmitted diseases, extremes of body weight in either partner and age can affect fertility. Environmental factors such as virus infections, toxins, pesticides, solvents, pollutants (including cigarette smoke), alcohol and recreational drugs are all associated with reduced fertility (measured as a longer time to conception and/or increased risk of miscarriage). Some medications, particularly those used to treat cancer, such as the chemotherapy regimens, can permanently affect fertility. There is also a significant probability that either both partners have fertility problems or that there is no explanation for failure of conception.

ASSISTED REPRODUCTIVE TECHNOLOGY (ARTIFICIAL FERTILIZATION)

Infertility is medically defined at the point when it is appropriate to offer intervention which is when conception has not occurred after 12 months of unprotected intercourse in couples wishing to start a family or after 6 months if the woman is over 35 years old. Subfertility is thought to affect about 15–20% of couples. However, this figure depends on how subfertility is defined as couples may also experience delays in achieving second and subsequent pregnancies. In practice, infertility cannot be cured but subfertility may be treated; medical intervention attempts to optimize conditions that will aid conception. The study of infertility is a relatively new field, open to new research. It involves not just biological aspects of fertility but also social and psychological aspects. Many couples seeking fertility treatment will not succeed. In the United Kingdom, fertility treatment is regulated by the Human Fertilisation and Embryology Act 1990 and monitored by the Human Fertilisation & Embryology Authority (HFEA).

If gametes are available, either from the couple themselves or from a donor, assisted conception techniques

---

Box 6.3 **Commonly used assisted reproduction procedures**

- *In vitro* fertilization and embryo transfer (IVF+ET)
- Gamete intrafallopian transfer (GIFT)
- Zygote intrafallopian transfer (ZIFT)
- Intracytoplasmic sperm injection (ICSI)
- Donor insemination (DI)
- Intrauterine insemination (IUI)

---

can be used. Laboratory techniques can be used to prepare the gametes and bring them closer together to enhance fertility (Box 6.3). Such techniques can be utilized in situations where there is damage to the uterine tubes (the site of normal fertilization), endometriosis, which may alter the uterine environment, male infertility (reduced number, motility or fertilizing ability of sperm) or coital dysfunction. They are also used to treat unexplained fertility where they will test the fertilizing ability of the sperm or where preimplantation diagnosis of genetic disorders is advisable.

Methods of selecting the gametes used for IVF are extremely important especially when legal, ethical or religious reasons mean that destruction of supernumerary embryos has to be avoided. There may be an association between a lower level of ovarian stimulation and better oocyte and embryo quality (Ubaldi and Rienzi, 2008). An oocyte is considered normal when, after the removal of the cumulus cells which are also examined, it has a round clear zona pellucida, a small perivitelline space enclosing a single whole first polar body and cytoplasm which appears pale, moderately granular and without inclusions. However, oocytes with morphological abnormalities can still be fertilized by ICSI, although abnormally shaped oocytes and giant oocytes are not associated with good outcomes. A large perivitelline space may be due to oocyte overmaturity. Likewise, sperm morphology can also be assessed; when strict selection criteria are applied, the success rate is improved and the ICSI technique is known as intracytoplasmic morphologically selected sperm injection (IMSI; Bartoov et al., 2003). The criteria are based on the morphology of the sperm acrosome, neck, mitochondria, tail and nucleus but IMSI is expensive and time-consuming and so is not used routinely.

In vitro fertilization

IVF is now a routine procedure for certain types of infertility. Although IVF has given amazing opportunities to otherwise infertile couples to conceive, there are concerns that the technologies used traverse natural barriers which normally prevent the transmission of genetic defects. There are a number of stages in a cycle of IVF treatment (Box 6.4; Van Steirteghem et al., 1996). The couple may have more than one cause of infertility. IVF can also be

Box 6.4 Stages in an IVF cycle

- Patient selection
- Ovarian stimulation
- Oocyte retrieval
- Semen preparation
- Possible cryopreservation of gametes (variable success rates)
- Insemination
- Assessment of fertilization
- Embryo cleavage
- Embryo replacement
- Cryopreservation of excess embryos
- Detection of pregnancy

Box 6.5 Naegele's rule

This rule was devised by Dr. Franz Karl Naegele who was a German obstetrician in the nineteenth century.

The rule estimates the expected date of delivery (EDD) from the first day of the woman's last menstrual period (LMP) by adding a year, subtracting three months and adding seven days to that date. This approximates to the average normal human pregnancy which lasts 40 weeks (280 days) from the LMP, or 38 weeks (266 days) from the date of fertilization.

Example:
LMP = 8 May 2011
+1 year = 8 May 2012
−3 months = 8 February 2012
+7 days = 15 February 2012

Based on a menstrual cycle of 28 days, add 9 months + 7 days to the first day of the last period to calculate the EDD. Many women have a longer and some have shorter menstrual cycle. If this is the case, ovulation nearly always happens 14 days before period is due – so it is the first part of the menstrual cycle that varies. Therefore, short cycles of 26 days, for instance, need to have another 2 days added on and long cycles, for instance 32 days, need to have four additional days taken off.

It is estimated that only around 5% of babies actually arrive on their due day. Normal term is considered from the completion of the 37th week of pregnancy up until the completion of the 42nd week of pregnancy (often written as T + 14) so under Naegele's rule working from the first day of the last menstrual period, the pregnancy would normally last between 266 and 294 days. After the 41st week, the term 'post-mature' is used; current practice is to recommend induction of labour once 42 weeks have been completed. Some babies (around 15%) will be born premature (before the completion of the 37th week).

used with oocyte donation, for instance, where the woman has ovarian dysfunction (such as premature menopause or Turner's syndrome) or has a high risk of transmitting a serious chromosomal abnormality. Ovarian stimulation is used to increase the number of mature oocytes that will be harvested as some are likely to fail to be fertilized. The method is based on suppressing the natural menstrual cycle by inhibiting the LH surge with a GnRH agonist and then stimulating follicular development with hMG (human menopausal gonadotrophin, which contains FSH and LH), a technique called superovulation. Ultrasound techniques can be used for both follicular assessment and the retrieval of oocytes. When several follicles have grown to a particular size (17–18 mm), ovulation is induced with human gonadotrophin. The oocytes are collected at a preovulatory stage so they are not truly mature. Ovarian hyperstimulation syndrome (OHSS) is a significant complication of fertility treatment involving ovarian stimulation (Nastri et al., 2010); it can cause ovarian enlargement which may result in abdominal distension, increased vascular permeability, intravascular dehydration and the consequences of raised cytokine production such as thrombosis. Progesterone or hCG is necessary to support the luteal phase. The collected oocytes are then cultured. The semen is prepared by separating the motile sperm from the seminal fluid and allowing them to capacitate in an artificial 'capacitating medium'. The capacitated sperm are introduced to the oocyte within a few hours of oocyte retrieval. The oocyte is enclosed by the corona radiata. The presence of the first polar body shows that the oocyte is at the metaphase II stage (see Fig. 7.11, p. 151) and ready to be fertilized.

At about 18 h after insemination, the oocytes are denuded by mechanical removal of the cumulus cells. If fertilization has occurred, two distinct pronuclei, and usually two polar bodies, will be observable under a microscope. Twenty-four hours later, embryonic cleavage is evident and the quality of the embryo can be assessed morphologically for its potential to continue developing by the number of anucleate fragments and the evenness of the cells. Embryos with fragmented or uneven cells rarely continue developing. At the four-cell stage, a blastomere can be removed for preimplantation diagnosis (Handyside et al., 1992). Two or three embryos are then selected for transfer to the uterus about 48 h after the two-cell stage; morphological scoring systems are used to assess embryo quality and potential viability. The zona pellucida tends to harden in culture and has to be eroded mechanically or by acid digestion to aid hatching prior to the transfer. Multiple births are common with IVF, although nowadays only three oocytes are implanted into older women, as the success rate is higher in younger women and the protocols try to avoid multiple gestation to increase well-being of the infants. Successful implantation relies on both embryo quality and endometrial receptivity. Excess embryos can be cryopreserved (carefully frozen using protectant fluid and specific rates of freezing and thawing). Increased hCG levels 10–12 days after fertilization confirm a successful pregnancy; levels of hCG usually double every 1.3 days.

In IVF treatment, injections of hCG can be given to prepare the follicles for ovulation following ovarian stimulation as it mimics the action of LH closely. Once the follicles have matured, the oocytes can be harvested. The administration of GnRH agonists administered in the luteal stage of the menstrual cycle has been shown to increase the implantation success of IVF and ICSI treatments (Razieh et al., 2009).

Intracytoplasmic sperm injection

ICSI now accounts for about half of all IVF treatment in the United Kingdom (HFEA, 2009); the other half is conventional IVF. Where there is severe male factor infertility, the sperm are unable to fertilize the oocyte. In ICSI, a single sperm is injected directly into the oocyte cytoplasm (Palermo et al., 1997). The advantage of this method is that it is successful even with very severe sperm dysfunction. Sperm do not need to be motile and can even be harvested from the epididymis by microepididymal sperm aspiration (MESA) or percutaneous epididymal sperm aspiration (PESA). The success rates of ICSI are usually high because the oocyte and endometrium are healthy and apparently not damaged by the procedures (although the cytoplasm of the egg is disrupted during injection and because the hydrolytic enzymes from the sperm acrosome are released into the cytoplasm of the oocyte so there is a small risk of mechanical injury to the meiotic spindle that could potentially lead to aneuploidy). ICSI bypasses almost all of the natural selection mechanisms that challenge the sperm in a normal conception.

It will be important to monitor the health of children born following assisted conception procedures. For instance, the fertility of male offspring resulting from fertilization with a sperm incapable of normal fertilization may be affected. Also, male offspring born following ICSI from fathers with Y chromosome deletions may inherit the same deletion (Chandley, 1998). There are also increased incidences of *de novo* sex chromosomal aberrations, inheritance of cystic fibrosis mutations and Y microdeletions (Bowdin et al., 2007). Over 1% of births in the United Kingdom and the United States are now due to ART which also accounts for more than 30% of twin births. There is an increased complication rate in infants conceived by IVF, though some of this is probably due to the increased frequency of multiple births. However, singleton IVF infants are more likely to be of lower birthweight and have birth defects. There is an increased risk of the rare growth disorders, such as Beckwith–Weidemann Syndrome and Angelman Syndrome, which are due to defects in gene imprinting (see p. 164). This may be related to the embryo culture conditions used in IVF or the genetic instability

underlying the infertility, but the absolute number of children with these disorders is very small.

Cryopreservation techniques have resulted in increased fertility rates; cryopreserved embryos that are surplus to requirement may be offered to other couples who are either infertile or carry a genetic disease but find antenatal diagnosis and termination of an abnormal pregnancy unacceptable. Embryo donation has many ethical, legal and psychosocial implications. There is an increasing trend for patients facing intensive chemotherapy and other procedures to request gamete retrieval and cryopreservation; a more ethically complex area is requests for gamete retrieval from men who are terminally ill, dead, near-dead (for instance, in a persistent vegetative state) or brain-dead.

Case study 6.2 is an example of artificial fertilization.

Case study 6.2

Elizabeth is a 42-year-old primipara who has been married for 20 years to Thomas. They had never used contraception. After initial investigations at a subfertility clinic, they were told that Thomas had a very low sperm count and that the sperm present were morphologically abnormal and displayed little motility. After eight attempts of IVF, Elizabeth and Thomas were offered ICSI and as a result, a pregnancy occurred.

- Should the advice that the midwife gives to Elizabeth and Thomas be any different to that given to a fertile couple?
- What kinds of anxieties and concerns would Elizabeth and Thomas have and how might these be addressed?
- Are there any more serious risks and complications for a developing fetus conceived by ICSI?

Key points

- The male gamete (sperm) is one of the smallest human cells and is motile, whereas the female gamete (oocyte) is one of the largest human cells and is immotile.
- Fertilization is the union of the sperm and the oocyte, resulting in a diploid zygote.
- Coitus requires circulatory and neuronal activity resulting in erection of the penis by increasing blood volume. Sexual arousal causes analogous physiological changes in the female.
- Although sex selection is practised in the husbandry of domesticated animals, there is little evidence to suggest that it can be successfully manipulated in humans.
- In order to fertilize the oocyte, sperm undergo a series of changes: (a) development in the testes, (b) maturation in the epididymis and (c) capacitation in the female reproductive tract which alters their tail movements and metabolism and enables them to fertilize the oocyte.

- The acrosome reaction, and release of enzymes, results in digestion of a pathway through the follicular cells and zona pellucida. Interaction between the sperm and the oocyte is mediated by species-specific receptors.
- Fusion of the gametes results in the cortical reaction (which prevents polyspermy), metabolic changes, completion of the oocyte meiotic division, extrusion of the second polar body, DNA replication and initiation of the first mitotic division.
- The embryo or zygote undergoes cell cleavage as it is moved towards the uterus.
- As the number of cells increases, the embryo is described as a morula. The inner and outer cells undergo compaction and differentiate.
- The accumulation of fluid causes the embryo to 'hatch' out of the zona pellucida and it is then described as a blastocyst. The blastocyst has an outer layer of trophoblast cells (the future placenta) and an inner cell mass (the future embryo).
- The trophoblast cells secrete hCG, which promotes the survival and further growth of the corpus luteum.

- Maternal recognition of the pregnancy allows embryonic development and uterine receptiveness to be coordinated.
- Implantation occurs about 7 days after fertilization.
- Assisted fertility techniques have been developed for couples who have subfertility.

Application to practice

Primarily, the midwife is not involved with the treatment of infertility. However, with the advance of technology, there are an increasing number of conceptions and successful pregnancies as a result of fertility treatment.

An understanding of the complexities and interventions required to achieve conception is essential in order for the midwife to support women and partners. A knowledge of fertilization is also required in the understanding of contraceptive techniques.

ANNOTATED FURTHER READING

Balen AH, editor: *Infertility in practice*, ed 3, London, 2008, Informa Healthcare.

A practical guide, based on the authors' clinical practice, which provides an overview of human infertility problems, aetiology and evidence-based possible interventions.

Bancroft JHJ: *Human sexuality and its problems*, ed 3, New York, 2008, Churchill Livingstone.

A comprehensive text of factors determining human sexuality which covers sexual development, anatomy and physiology, biochemistry and endocrinology in addition to sociological and psychological aspects of sexuality. Topics include development of sexual preferences, investigation of sexual dysfunction, marriage, marital therapy, prostitution, AIDS, ageing, sexual abuse and sexual abuse survivors.

Carlson BM: *Human embryology and developmental biology*, ed 4, 2008, Mosby.

An illustrated textbook detailing the development of the human embryo from conception to birth, including the molecular and mechanistic basis of normal and abnormal development; provides a particularly good description of control of development at the cellular and molecular level.

Coughlan C, Ledger WL: In-vitro fertilisation, *Obstet Gynaecol Reprod Med* 18:300–306, 2008.

A review which succinctly and clearly summarizes the steps involved in in-vitro fertilization.

Devroey P, Fauser BC, Diedrich K: Approaches to improve the diagnosis and management of infertility, *Hum Reprod Update* 15:391–408, 2009.

A summary of the current best practice relating to patient pretreatment assessment, ovarian stimulation, embryo assessment and laboratory standards and procedures during ART, together with some brief comments on the future of ART.

Fleming S, King R: *Micromanipulation in assisted conception*, Cambridge, 2003, Cambridge University Press.

This is a practical handbook which provides comprehensive and well-illustrated descriptions of the micromanipulation techniques used in IVF laboratories, clearly explaining the procedures and potential difficulties.

Furse A: *Your essential infertility companion: a user's guide to tests, technology and therapies*, London, 2009, Thorsons.

A useful and sensitively written reference on all aspects of human infertility, including practical information on the

medical help available, the procedures involved, potential side effects of fertility drugs, self-help, complementary therapies and emotional aspects of fertility treatment.

Hammarberg K, Fisher JR, Wynter KH: Psychological and social aspects of pregnancy, childbirth and early parenting after assisted conception: a systematic review, *Hum Reprod Update* 14:395–414, 2008.

A review on the interesting and emerging topic of how ART affects parenting and the development of a confident parental identity.

Johnson MH: *Essential reproduction*, ed 6, Oxford, 2007, Blackwell Science.

An excellent, well-organized research-based textbook which explores comparative reproductive physiology of mammals, including anatomy, physiology, endocrinology, genetics and behavioural studies.

Matzuk MM, Lamb DJ: The biology of infertility: research advances and clinical challenges, *Nat Med* 14:1197–1213, 2008.

A detailed review presenting a summary of the current state of knowledge about infertility, including the mechanisms and gene mutations involved.

Sauer MV, Kavic SM: Oocyte and embryo donation 2006: reviewing two

decades of innovation and controversy, *Reprod Biomed Online* 12:153–162, 2006.
An overview of the use of oocyte and embryo donation which discusses reasons for their use, screening of donors and recipients, legal and

psychosocial issues and some of the wider implications.
Siddiqui F, McEwan A: Twins, *Obstet Gynaecol Reprod Med* 17:289–295, 2007.
A brief description of the causes and management of obstetric complications

in twin pregnancies, including in utero death of one twin, discordant growth and anomalies, twin reversed arterial perfusion and twin-to-twin transfusion syndrome.

REFERENCES

Andersson KE, Wagner G: Physiology of penile erection, *Physiol Rev* 75:191–236, 1995.

Baker RR, Bellis MA: Kamikaze sperm in mammals, *Anim Behav* 36:936–939, 1988.

Barroso G, Valdespin C, Vega E, et al: Developmental sperm contributions: fertilization and beyond, *Fertil Steril* 92:835–848, 2009.

Bartoov B, Berkovitz A, Eltes F, et al: Pregnancy rates are higher with intracytoplasmic morphologically selected sperm injection than with conventional intracytoplasmic injection, *Fertil Steril* 80:1413–1419, 2003.

Bowdin S, Allen C, Kirby G, et al: A survey of assisted reproductive technology births and imprinting disorders, *Hum Reprod* 22:3237–3240, 2007.

Bromwich P: The sex ratio, and ways of manipulating it, *Prog Obstet Gynaecol* 7:217–231, 1991.

Brooker CG: *Human structure and function*, ed 2, St Louis, 1998, Mosby, p 477.

Brucker C, Lipford GB: The human sperm acrosome reaction: physiology and regulatory mechanisms, *Hum Reprod Update* 1:51–62, 1995.

Chandley AC: Chromosome anomalies and Y chromosome microdeletions as causal factors in male infertility, *Human Reprod* 13(Suppl 1):45–50, 1998.

Check JH, Weiss RM, Lurie D: Analysis of serum human chorionic-gonadotropin levels in normal singleton, multiple and abnormal pregnancies, *Human Reprod* 7:1176–1180, 1992.

Clark GF, Dell A, Morris HR, et al: The species recognition system: a new corollary for the human fetoembryonic defense system hypothesis, *Cells Tissues Organs* 168:113–121, 2001.

Coughlan C, Li TC: Surgical management of tubal disease and infertility, *Obstet Gynaecol Reprod Med* 19:98–105, 2009.

Csemiczky G, Wramsby H, Johannisson E, et al: Importance of endometrial quality in women with tubal infertility during a natural menstrual cycle for the outcome of IVF treatment, *J Assist Reprod Genet* 15:55–61, 1998.

De Waal FBM: Bonobo sex and society, *Sci Am* 272(3):82–88, 1995.

Dey J, Shepherd MD: Evaluation and treatment of erectile dysfunction in men with diabetes mellitus, *Mayo Clin Proc* 77:276–282, 2002.

Familiari G, Notola SA, Macchiarell G, et al: Human zona pellucida during in vitro fertilization: an ultrastructural study using saponin, ruthenium red and osmium thiocarbohydrazide, *Mol Reprod Dev* 32:51–61, 1992.

Fazleabas AT, Kim JJ, Strakova Z: Implantation: embryonic signals and the modulation of the uterine environment – a review, *Placenta* 25: S26–S31, 2004.

Filippi S, Vignozzi L, Vannelli GB, et al: Role of oxytocin in the ejaculatory process, *J Endocrinol Invest* 26(Suppl 3):82–86, 2003.

Fisch H: Older men are having children, but the reality of a male biological clock makes this trend worrisome, *Geriatrics* 64:14–17, 2009.

Gardner AJ, Evans JP: Mammalian membrane block to polyspermy: new insights into how mammalian eggs prevent fertilisation by multiple sperm, *Reprod Fertil Dev* 18:53–61, 2006.

Gupta SK, Bansal P, Ganguly A, et al: Human zona pellucida glycoproteins: functional relevance during fertilization, *J Reprod Immunol* 83:50–55, 2009.

Gyllensten U, Wharton D, Josefsson A, et al: Paternal inheritance of mitochondrial DNA in mice, *Nature* 352:255–257, 1991.

Handyside AH, Lesko JG, Tarin JJ, et al: Birth of a normal girl after in vitro fertilisation and preimplantation diagnostic testing for cystic fibrosis, *N Engl J Med* 327:905–909, 1992.

Hardy K, Handyside AH, Winston RML: The human blastocyst-cell number, death and allocation during late preimplantation development in vitro, *Development* 107:597, 1989.

Hardy K, Martin KL, Leese HJ, et al: Human preimplantation development in vitro is not adversely affected by biopsy at the 8-cell stage, *Hum Reprod* 5:708–714, 1990.

Harlap S: Gender of infants conceived on different days of the menstrual cycle, *N Engl J Med* 291:1445–1448, 1979.

Hattori M, et al: The DNA sequence of human chromosome 21, *Nature* 405:311–319, 2000.

Hassold T, Hunt P: To err meiotically is human: the genesis of human aneuploidy, *Nat Rev Genet* 2:280–291, 2001.

Hauzman EE, Papp Z: Conception without the development of a human being, *J Perinat Med* 36:175–177, 2008.

Hill JA: Maternal–embryonic cross-talk, *Ann N Y Acad Sci* 943:17–25, 2001.

Hoodbhoy T, Talbot R: Mammalian cortical granules: contents, fate and function, *Mol Reprod Dev* 39:439–448, 1994.

Human Fertilisation Embryology Authority, *Fertility facts and figures 2007*, London, 2009, HFEA.

Ikawa M, Inoue N, Benham AM, et al: Fertilization: a sperm's journey to and interaction with the oocyte, *J Clin Invest* 120:984–994, 2010.

Jacobs PA, Wilson CM, Sprenkle JA, et al: Mechanism of origin of complete hydatidiform mole, *Nature* 286:714–717, 1980.

James WH: Evidence that mammalian sex ratios at birth are partially controlled by parental hormone levels around the time of conception, *J Endocrinol* 198:3–15, 2008.

Jones KT: Intracellular calcium in the fertilization and development of mammalian eggs, *Clin Exp Pharmacol Physiol* 34:1084–1089, 2007.

Kaji K, Kudo A: The mechanism of sperm–oocyte fusion in mammals, *Reproduction* 127:423–429, 2004.

Kaneda H, Hayashi JL, Takahama S, et al: Elimination of paternal mitochondrial DNA in intraspecific crosses during early mouse embryogenesis, *Proc Natl Acad Sci USA* 92:4542–4546, 1995.

Kono T, Obata Y, Wu Q, et al: Birth of parthenogenetic mice that can develop to adulthood, *Nature* 428:860–864, 2004.

Larsen WJ: *Human embryology*, ed 2, New York, 1993, Churchill Livingstone, p 481.

Levin RJ: Sex and the human female reproductive tract: what really happens during and after coitus, *Int J Impot Res* 10(Suppl 1):514–521, 1998.

Lewis Z, Price TA, Wedell N: Sperm competition, immunity, selfish genes and cancer, *Cell Mol Life Sci* 65:3241–3254, 2008.

Matilsky M, Battino S, Ben-Ami M, et al: The effect of ejaculatory frequency on semen characteristics of normozoospermic and oligozoospermic men from an infertile population, *Hum Reprod* 8:71–73, 1993.

Master VA, Turek PJ: Ejaculatory physiology and dysfunction, *Urol Clin North Am* 28:363–375, 2001.

Matzuk MM, Lamb DJ: The biology of infertility: research advances and clinical challenges, *Nat Med* 14:1197–1213, 2008.

Miozzo M, Simoni G: The role of imprinted genes in fetal growth, *Biol Neonate* 81:217–228, 2002.

Mollard R, Denham M, Trounson A: Technical advances and pitfalls on the way to human cloning, *Differentiation* 70:1–9, 2002.

Nastri CO, Ferriani RA, Rocha IA, et al: Ovarian hyperstimulation syndrome: pathophysiology and prevention, *J Assist Reprod Genet* 27:121–128, 2010.

Nikas G, Aghajanova L: Endometrial pinopods: some more understanding on human implantation? *Reprod Biomed Online* 4:18–23, 2003.

Pacey AA: Male fertility and infertility, *Obstet Gynaecol Reprod Med* 19:42–47, 2008.

Palermo GP, Avrech OM, Colombero LT, et al: Human sperm cytosolic factor triggers Ca^{2+} oscillations and overcomes activation failure of mammalian oocytes, *Mol Hum Reprod* 3:367–374, 1997.

Payne D, Flaherty SP, Barry MF, et al: Preliminary observations on polar body extrusion and pronuclear formation in human oocytes using time-lapse video cinematography, *Hum Reprod* 12:532–541, 1997.

Piomelli D: THC: moderation during implantation, *Nat Med* 10:19–20, 2004.

Razieh DF, Maryam AR, Nasim T: Beneficial effect of luteal-phase gonadotropin-releasing hormone agonist administration on implantation rate after intracytoplasmic sperm injection, *Taiwan J Obstet Gynecol* 48 (3):245–248, 2009.

Schatten G: The centrosome and its mode of inheritance; the reduction of the centrosome during gametogenesis and its restoration during fertility, *Dev Biol* 165:299–335, 1994.

Short RV: The testis: the witness of the mating system, the site of mutation and the engine of desire, *Acta Paediatr Suppl* 422:3–7, 1997.

Stanford JB, White GL, Hatasaka H: Timing intercourse to achieve pregnancy: current evidence, *Obstet Gynecol* 100:1333–1341, 2002.

Sullivan ME, Keoghane SR, Miller MA: Vascular risk factors and erectile dysfunction, *Br J Urol Int* 87:838–845, 2002.

Suarez SS: Control of hyperactivation in sperm, *Hum Reprod Update* 14:647–657, 2008.

Suarez SS, Pacey AA: Sperm transport in the female reproductive tract, *Hum Reprod Update* 12:23–37, 2006.

Sun F, Bahat A, Gakamsky A, et al: Human sperm chemotaxis: both the oocyte and its surrounding cumulus cells secrete sperm chemoattractants, *Human Reproduction* 20:761–767, 2005.

Swann K, Larman MG, Saunders CM, et al: The cytosolic sperm factor that triggers $Ca2^{+}$ oscillations and egg activation in mammals is a novel phospholipase C: PLCzeta, *Reproduction* 127:431–439, 2004.

Sykes B: *The seven daughters of Eve*, London, 2004, Corgi Books.

Tamler R: Diabetes, obesity, and erectile dysfunction, *Gend Med* 6(Suppl 1):4–16, 2009.

Ubaldi F, Rienzi L: Morphological selection of gametes, *Placenta* 29 (Suppl B):115–212, 2008.

Van Blerkom J, Davis P, Merriam J, et al: Nuclear and cytoplasmic dynamics of sperm penetration, pronuclear formation and microtubule organization during fertilization and early preimplantation in the human, *Hum Reprod Update* 1:429–461, 1995.

Van Steirteghem A, Liebaers I, Devroey P: Assisted reproduction. In Hillier SG, Kitchener HC, Neilson JP, editors: *Scientific essentials of reproductive medicine*, Philadelphia, 1996, WB Saunders, pp 230–241.

Vigano P, Mangioni S, Pompei F, et al: Maternal–conceptus cross talk: a review, *Placenta* 24:S56–S61, 2003.

Wallace DC: Mitochondrial DNA mutations in disease and aging, *Environ Mol Mutagen* 51:440–450, 2010.

Wassarman PM: Mammalian fertilization: the strange case of sperm protein 56, *Bioessays* 31:153–158, 2009.

Whittaker M: Regulation of the cell division cycle by inositol phosphate and the calcium signalling pathway, *Adv Second Messenger Phosphoprotein Res* 30:299–310, 1995.

Yanagida K, Katayose H, Hirata S, et al: Influence of sperm immobilization on onset of Ca(2() oscillations after ICSI, *Hum Reprod* 16(1):148–152, 2001.

Zenzes MT, Wang P, Casper RF: Cigarette smoking may affect meiotic maturation of human oocytes, *Hum Reprod* 10:3213–3217, 1995.

Chapter | 7 |

Overview of human genetics and genetic disorders

LEARNING OBJECTIVES

- To describe the packaging of genes in the chromosome and how they are expressed.
- To describe the general characteristics of dominant, recessive and X-linked genetic traits.
- To interpret a pedigree chart and make simple genetic predictions.
- To discuss the principles of genetic screening.
- To relate current genetic research to midwifery practice.
- To discuss evolutionary influences upon human reproduction.

INTRODUCTION

Genetics is the science of genes, heredity and the variation of organisms. Although genetics is a component of virtually all areas of biology, it tends to be reductionist in nature. Life is the result of the genetic codes that all living things carry in almost all of their cells. The mechanisms that govern the manner in which genetic information is duplicated, altered, transferred and expressed provide a wealth of information about the biochemical processes of all living organisms. The advent of molecular biology has meant that many problems considered formidable until very recently may now be understood and resolved. Molecular biology has added new dimensions to understanding the origin of the human species, to creating new drugs, and to sequencing of entire genomes of a variety of species, including disease-causing microorganisms, plants, insects and animals including humans.

Chapter case study

As part of the routine antenatal care, which Zara is receiving from her midwife at her local maternity unit, Zara is offered a 20-week anomaly ultrasound as part of the screening policy of the local maternity services. This scan examines the physical structures of the baby and enables a skilled ultrasonographer to identify major structural abnormalities of the internal organs and other signs of structural problems such as polyhydramnios, oligohydramnios, placental abnormalities and so on. Often the presence of a number of abnormalities (frequently referred to as a syndrome) could indicate the presence of many possible genetic disorders.

Zara is quite upset because one of her friends has just undergone amniocentesis as her ultrasound scan had revealed cardiac, brain and limb abnormalities. Zara's scan appears to be normal and the baby appears to be growing well but Zara is still concerned that all may not be well and wishes to discuss what further tests are available that would reassure her all is well.

- How would you, as Zara's midwife, reassure and counsel her and James through this difficult period?

Within living organisms, the genetic information is usually carried in chromosomes where organization of the DNA provides a gene or 'blueprint' (genotype) directing protein synthesis and thus the expression of the genes into physical characteristics (phenotype). Characteristics are passed from one generation to the next in the form of genes. In sexually reproducing species, the genes are shuffled and repackaged into the gametes. Variations between genes affect survival so the individuals with the best-adapted characteristics to cope with environmental conditions have an advantage. This is described as natural selection. Although DNA codes for the genes, not all the genes are expressed in any one cell or any one time. The phenotype is determined by which genes are expressed (turned on) and which are not. Epigenetics is the term used to describe the modifications to DNA which controls which genes are expressed. As well as the functions of the genes being identified as part of the determination of the DNA sequence (human genome), thousands of small non-coding RNAs have roles in mRNA stability, protein translation, protein modification and changes in the germline. All eukaryotic organisms (animals) have both nuclear DNA and mitochondrial DNA (mtDNA) (outside the nucleus) which is probably due to a serendipitous event in evolution whereby ancestral bacterial forebears of mitochondria were incorporated into eukaryotic cells (see Chapter 1).

The study of genetics focuses on inherited characteristics, particularly those that are considered abnormal, how these arise and their effects on the individual. Genetics is a predictive science and its rules are based upon the application of mathematical statistics and probability. Evolutionary effects on genetics may determine the penetration of recessive genetic disorders such as cystic fibrosis into gene pools. The impact of genetics upon antenatal screening to predict the probability of fetal abnormalities is of particular relevance for midwives.

A BRIEF HISTORY OF GENETICS

Historically, humans unknowingly but successfully applied genetics to the breeding and domestication of animals and plants. However, the first systematic study of genetic interactions is associated with the breeding experiments of Gregor Mendel, an Austrian monk, in the 1860s. Mendel established inheritance patterns of certain traits in pea plants and demonstrated that application of statistics to inheritance could be very useful. Subsequently, more complex forms of inheritance have been identified.

Mendel correctly identified the concept of genes long before the structures of DNA and chromosomes were understood. He proposed that 'particles of inheritance' were transmitted from one generation to the next and defined a concept that he described as an allele. The term 'allele' is now used to describe a specific variant or alternative form of a particular gene occupying a given locus (position) on a chromosome.

The term 'eugenics' was coined by Francis Galton (a cousin of Charles Darwin) who advocated that application of Darwinian theories and selective breeding could improve the quality of entire populations, particularly with respect to talent and intelligence. In the late nineteenth century, eugenics societies formed in various parts of the world sought to promote such practices as marriage restriction, sterilization and custodial commitment of those thought to have unwanted characteristics and positively encouraging reproduction in those individuals perceived as the best and brightest. The popularity of the eugenics movement was already waning when infamous eugenics programmes of Nazi Germany were revealed at the end of World War II.

Darwin's 'survival of the fittest' theory promoted the concept of natural selection and how environmental conditions determine survival and reproduction of organisms with particular traits. If environmental conditions do not vary much, these traits continue to be adaptive and become more common within the population.

Neo-Darwinism (or 'modern evolutionary synthesis') extends the scope of Darwin's ideas of natural selection by including modern genetic knowledge about DNA and concepts such as speciation, kin selection and altruism. It advocates that survival of a species is not necessarily by the fittest but by those that are most likely to reproduce successfully. This is reflected in the work of William Hamilton, popularized by Richard Dawkins, who asserted that the gene, rather than the organism or species, is the true unit of reproduction and the primary driver and beneficiary of evolution. The genes are provocatively described as 'selfish' because in order to replicate and be successful they use organisms that contain them solely as vehicles to ensure survival (1989). Obviously, reproduction is vital to ensure that the genes survive.

This controversial view portrays organisms solely as mechanical methods of survival to pass genes on to as many offspring as possible. However, there are a number of arguments against this view. Organisms are not perfectly adapted; for instance, humans seem to have some non-advantageous genes such as those coding for the vermiform appendix. It could be argued that these genes have not been obliterated because other linked genes are advantageous and effectively protect them. The other important point is that species not only interact with their environment but also positively alter their environment to optimize survival. The selfish gene hypothesis also accounts for how genes that seem to be harmful can evolve by natural selection (Badcock and Crespi, 2008).

The environment interacts with genes (the nature/nurture debate) and has a tremendous influence on how they are expressed, affecting susceptibility and resistance to disease. Genes may act in competition with each other, which may explain certain pathophysiological conditions and their aetiology. Some organisms may use their genes to alter the phenotype of another animal to increase their chances of survival. For example, infection with the trematode parasite causes its snail host's shell to become thicker (Dawkins, 1999). Co-evolution explains how the change of one organism can be linked to the change in a related organism. Each organism exerts selective pressure on the adaptation and evolution of the other. Examples include how angiosperm (flowering trees) and primates evolved, the existence of mitochondria in eukaryotic cells (see Chapter 1) and co-evolution of parasites with the acquired immunity of their hosts. Epigenetics and genetic imprinting (see p. 164) explain how gene expression can be affected by the environment.

Box 7.1 **Areas of genetic research**

- Screening for fetal abnormality
- Genetic counselling for parents with a family history of genetic disorders
- Identification of fetal sex in the early (indifferent) embryological phase
- Cloning of whole organisms
- Gene manipulation not only to eradicate disease but also to improve existing disease states
- Treatment by gene manipulation in animals to produce human proteins, hormones and so on
- Genetic modification
- Identification of individuals by genetic 'fingerprinting'

Box 7.2 **Genetics as a language**

Genetics can be considered as a language based on the DNA molecule. Linguistic development and evolution have a number of similarities. Studies looking at the origins of a particular word and how it has evolved to be slightly different in different languages are similar to the changes in genes (Jones, 1994). Genetic mutations are analogous to new words being introduced into the language (such as 'email').

- Language = genetics
- Vocabulary = genes
- Grammar = rules about the arrangement of information
- Literature = the instructions to make a human
- Alphabet = four bases of DNA
- Word = codon (three 'letter' code for an amino acid)

Within the modern medical world there now exist ethical dilemmas surrounding the screening for, detection of and termination of abnormal fetuses. Current research in genetics is not solely medical (Box 7.1) as it can be applied to population studies, such as tracing the origins of human migration movements, and to genealogy, such as tracing the real families of children of the Argentinean 'Disappeared' (Jones, 1994) and the route the early Polynesians took to reach New Zealand (Sykes, 2001).

GENES AND CHROMOSOMES

Genes are the units of inheritance. Each gene is a length of DNA on a chromosome that contains the coded information to direct the synthesis of a specific protein chain. The differences between organisms are related to different proteins being synthesized that have different structures and functions. Effectively the genes act as a blueprint, or instruction manual, for the total development of the organism and how it will function and change during its lifetime (Box 7.2). Chromosomes are packages of DNA in the nucleus, on which the genes are linearly arranged. Chromosomes have two arms: a shorter p arm and a longer q arm, with a centromere between them. Chromosomes are important in cell replication and the passing of the genetic message from one generation to the next. Usually the DNA, about 180 cm per nucleus, exists as an unstructured mass of threads in the nucleus. However, when the cell is undergoing division the DNA becomes organized and compacted into chromosomes, which can be visualized by microscopy (see Chapter 1). This chromosomal organization allows biologists to identify genes and localize them to a particular chromosome to follow their pattern of inheritance. Each cell has the same genetic information in its nucleus as the original zygote (fertilized ovum) and all of the cells derived from it. Different cells behave in different ways because they express different subsets of information from the DNA.

THE STRUCTURE OF DNA AND RNA

Watson, Crick, Franklin and Wilkins elucidated the biochemical structure of DNA in 1953. Their description of the helical structure revealed how the molecule was able to replicate itself and thus explained the cellular mechanism of reproduction. DNA is composed of two strands of sugar phosphate molecules that are joined together to form long chains (Fig. 7.1). The strands of DNA are made up of repeating units called nucleotides. The DNA nucleotide has three components: a deoxyribose sugar, a phosphate group and a base. There are four types of bases: thymine and cytosine, which have single-ring structures, and adenine and guanine, which have double-ring structures. DNA exists as a double-stranded molecule wound into a helix. The strands are kept together by hydrogen bonding between the bases. The bases are of different sizes and have a different potential number of hydrogen bonds so they always pair in the same ways. Adenine (A) and thymine (T) pair with two hydrogen bonds: cytosine (C) and guanine (G) pair with three. This means that the sequence of the bases is complementary; the sequence of bases on one strand can be deduced from the sequence on the other strand.

DNA REPLICATION AND CELL DIVISION

The arrangement of base pairs of the two strands is like the rungs of a ladder or teeth of a zip. When DNA replicates, the strands unwind and the hydrogen bonds holding the

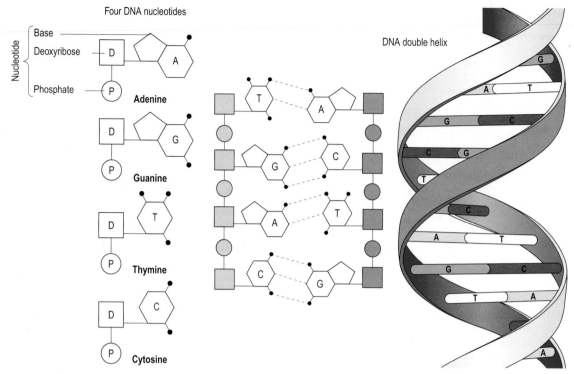

Fig. 7.1 The structure of DNA.

base pairs together separate (unzip). Each strand acts as a template for the synthesis of another new strand of complementary DNA bases to form from nucleotides that enter the nucleus through the nuclear pores (Fig. 7.2). So two new DNA double helices are formed, each with one strand of 'old' DNA and a newly synthesized strand. Thus the replication is described as semiconservative. Replication occurs as part of mitosis or cell division. Replication of DNA means that the chromosomes have double their nuclear material in preparation for dividing into two separate cells. Therefore, the chromosome is formed of two identical chromatids.

Mitosis

The replication of the entire human genome is achieved through the process of mitosis, which is part of the cell cycle (Fig. 7.3). Cellular replication results in growth of tissues through hyperplasia (an increase in the number of cells); each cell has the identical genetic message (DNA content) to its parent cell. Mitotic rates are different for different types of cells. Cells that divide rapidly (have a high mitotic index) include skin and gut epithelial cells, spermatogonia and tumour cells. With increased age the mitotic rate slows down so skin renewal, for instance, takes longer and the appearance of the skin is more aged. Drugs used to treat cancers also inhibit mitosis so their

side effects are mostly clearly manifested in normal cells with high mitotic rates, causing problems with nutrient absorption and decreasing male fertility. Many cells, such as brain, heart and liver cells, have an extremely slow rate of mitosis and do not regenerate or heal well after injury. Mitosis is a continuous process but for ease of description is traditionally described in distinct phases: prophase, metaphase, anaphase and telophase (Fig. 7.4). Interphase is the name given to the gap between mitotic divisions.

THE GENETIC MESSAGE

The structure of DNA allows both ease of replication and duplication of the genetic message prior to cell division, and also a method of directing protein synthesis and ultimate cell function. The DNA message is interpreted as a specific protein product. The genes in the DNA strand contain exons, regions that will be translated to proteins, interspersed with introns, regions which are not transcribed into proteins. Proteins are synthesized at the ribosomes of the cell, whereas the encoded information, in the form of DNA, remains within the nucleus. The information is carried from DNA to the site of protein synthesis by the second type of nucleic acid, RNA. Whereas DNA is a double strand, RNA exists as a single strand of sugar

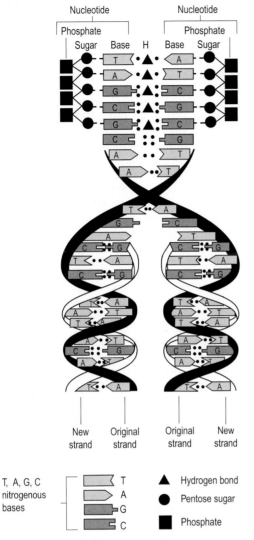

Fig. 7.2 DNA replication. (Reproduced with permission from Brooker, 1998).

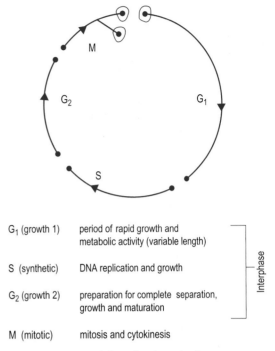

G_1 (growth 1)	period of rapid growth and metabolic activity (variable length)
S (synthetic)	DNA replication and growth
G_2 (growth 2)	preparation for complete separation, growth and maturation
M (mitotic)	mitosis and cytokinesis

Fig. 7.3 The phases of the cell cycle and cell content. (Reproduced with permission from Brooker, 1998.)

the protein. Splicing allows genes to form different proteins because the exons can be spliced in different patterns with each pattern generating a specific protein. The process of splicing is carried out by small nuclear RNAs (smRNA) called spliceosomes. The process where one gene can code for multiple proteins ('splice variants') means that there are about three times as many possible proteins as there are genes which is why the human genome project identified far fewer genes than was originally anticipated.

The DNA contains genes but only specific genes will be expressed in any particular cell at any particular time. Gene expression describes the means by which information from a gene drives the synthesis of a functional gene product which is usually a protein. Molecular biology techniques have allowed in-depth investigation of the function of single genes. There are several ways in which gene expression can be regulated. These include controlling which particular genes are transcribed, selective processing of the transcribed DNA to control which RNA become cytoplasmic mRNA, selective translation of mRNA and post-translational modification of the proteins produced from mRNA (Sadler, 2010).

Transcription

The process starts with the DNA strands separating like a zip pulling open in the middle. This is the reverse process to the way it coils when condensing into chromosomes

phosphate units, and has ribose sugar units (instead of deoxyribose) and similar complementary base molecules to those found in DNA, except that uracil instead of thymine pairs with adenine. RNA also exists as different forms with different functions. Initially a gene is transcribed as nuclear (or 'premessenger') RNA (nRNA). nRNA is modified to form mRNA. It is messenger RNA (mRNA) that carries the message from the nucleus to the ribosome, as a complementary strand of mRNA is formed using a stretch of unwound DNA as a template. mRNA is shorter than nRNA because nRNA contains the introns that are spliced out (removed) as the nRNA moves from the nucleus where it is formed to the cytoplasm where it is translated to form an amino acid chain that will form

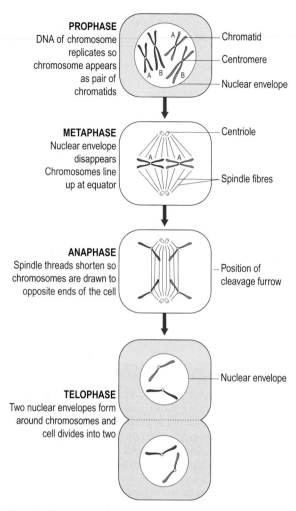

PROPHASE
DNA of chromosome
replicates so
chromosome appears
as pair of
chromatids

— Chromatid
— Centromere
— Nuclear envelope

METAPHASE
Nuclear envelope
disappears
Chromosomes line
up at equator

— Centriole
— Spindle fibres

ANAPHASE
Spindle threads shorten so
chromosomes are drawn to
opposite ends of the cell

— Position of
cleavage furrow

TELOPHASE
Two nuclear envelopes form
around chromosomes and
cell divides into two

— Nuclear envelope

Fig. 7.4 The stages of mitosis.

(Fig. 7.5). Only one strand of DNA, the coding or 'sense' strand, is used as the template; the other is described as non-coding or 'non-sense'. The mRNA chain is built by RNA polymerase enzymes as the bases pair with the DNA template. This is called transcription (Fig. 7.6).

The whole gene is transcribed but not all of it is used so the primary transcription product mRNA is modified (cut and spliced) into functional mRNA (Fig. 7.7). The parts of the mRNA that are removed have been copied from parts of the gene called introns and those that are retained come from the parts of the DNA known as exons. It is estimated that only about 2–5% of the total genome (genetic code or DNA) is composed of exons and actually codes for protein synthesis. Some of the DNA modulates genetic expression, switching the process of protein synthesis on and off; these control genes are referred to as operator, regulator and inducer genes. Introns form the majority of the

DNA sequence and do not appear to be involved in coding for protein synthesis, although they may allow different proteins to be formed from the same length of DNA. Much of the genome (about 98%) may be composed of redundant genes that are no longer activated and involved in the synthesis of proteins. These unused stretches of DNA are used to compare tissue samples for DNA fingerprinting.

Single nucleotide polymorphisms or SNPs (pronounced snips) are DNA sequence variations that occur when a single nucleotide in the genome is altered, often with the substitution of cytosine with thymine. Variations that occur in at least 1% of the population are considered to be SNPs. There are more than 1.4 million SNPs in the human genome, occurring approximately every 100–300 bases and accounting for up to 90% of all human genetic variation. These variations in the human genome alter how individuals respond to disease, infection, drugs and so on. SNPs are valuable because they do not change much from generation to generation and can be targeted for biomedical research and developing drugs.

The term 'genome' refers to a complete DNA sequence of one set of chromosomes of an organism. As such, it does not describe the genetic polymorphism (diversity) of a species. To understand how variations in DNA cause particular traits or diseases will require comparison between individual genomes. The Human Genome Project (HGP) was established as a multinational cooperative research project in 1990 to map the common human nucleotide sequence of more than 3 billion DNA bases in some reference human genomes (the DNA of a few anonymous donors). It was hoped that identification of the 20 000–25 000 genes in the human genome would accelerate progress to diagnosing, treating and ultimately preventing diseases as well as answer questions about evolution. As individuals (except for identical twins) have unique genomes, the project involved determining the sequence of many versions of each gene. In April 2003, it was announced that 99% of the genome had been sequenced and in May 2006 the sequence of the final chromosome was published. There are still a few DNA sequences to be resolved including the repetitive central regions close to the centromeres and the telomeres, the repetitive terminals of the chromosomes which become progressively shorter with age. The mapping of the genome allows a framework for looking at differences in DNA sequences in individuals so variations in DNA sequence associated with diseases could be identified. The HGP has been supported by remarkable technological progress in bioinformatics, statistics and biotechnology. The HGP raises some complex ethical, legal and social implications such as gene patenting

Protein synthesis

When transcription and post-transcription modification are complete, the finished functional mRNA strand detaches from the DNA and leaves the nucleus, via a

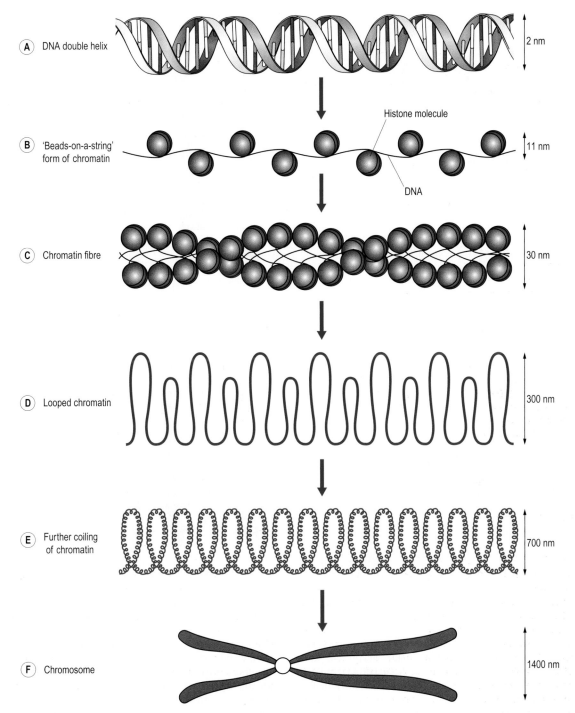

A DNA double helix — 2 nm

B 'Beads-on-a-string' form of chromatin — Histone molecule — DNA — 11 nm

C Chromatin fibre — 30 nm

D Looped chromatin — 300 nm

E Further coiling of chromatin — 700 nm

F Chromosome — 1400 nm

Fig. 7.5 (A–F) The stages of DNA packaging; in order for transcription to take place, the chromosomes must be uncoiled and 'unzipped' in the reverse process to that shown. (Adapted with permission from Goodwin, 1997.)

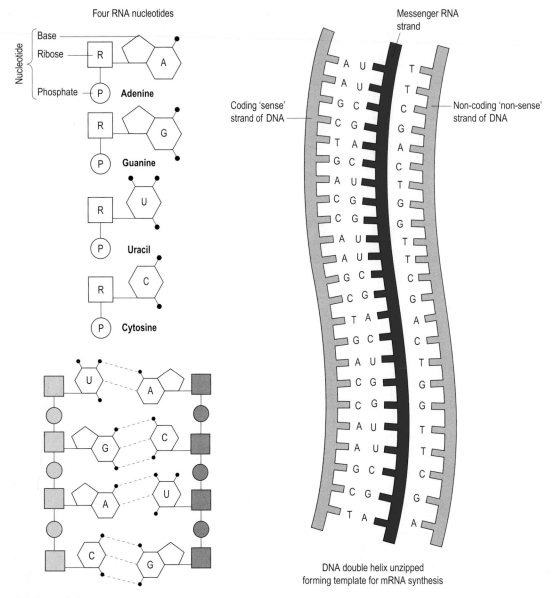

Four RNA nucleotides

Base

Ribose

Nucleotide

Phosphate

Adenine

Guanine

Uracil

Cytosine

Messenger RNA strand

Coding 'sense' strand of DNA

Non-coding 'non-sense' strand of DNA

DNA double helix unzipped forming template for mRNA synthesis

Fig. 7.6 Transcription.

nuclear pore, to go to the ribosomes. Ribosomes are structures formed of two subunits made of protein and another type of RNA, ribosomal RNA (rRNA). mRNA attaches to ribosomes and the sequence of bases of the mRNA is decoded to direct the synthesis of a protein. This step is called translation (Fig. 7.8). The mRNA sequence is 'read' three bases at a time. A particular sequence of three bases is called a codon; each codon prescribes that a specific amino acid is incorporated into the final amino acid chain of the overall protein structure. There are 20 amino acids; however, as a three-base genetic code allows the

potential of $4 \times 4 \times 4 = 64$ permutations, most amino acids are coded for by more than one codon (Fig. 7.9).

Another form of RNA in the cytoplasm, called transfer RNA (tRNA), carries amino acids to the ribosome to be incorporated into the protein chain. There are different types of tRNA, each one with a specific binding site for a particular amino acid at one end and an 'anticodon', which recognizes the codon on the mRNA at the other end. The first amino acid of a new protein is methionine. The next amino acid joins to the carboxyl group of methionine with a peptide bond. Successive amino acids join,

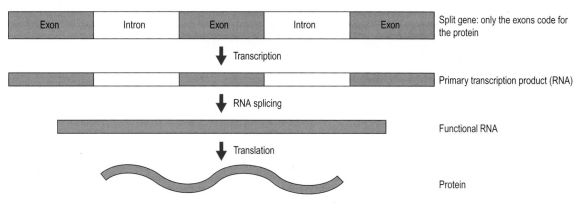

Fig. 7.7 Splicing. (Reproduced with permission from Goodwin, 1997.)

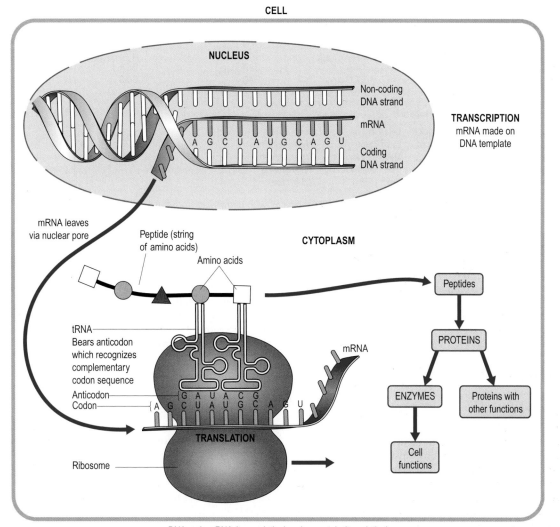

DNA makes RNA (transcription) makes protein (translation)

Fig. 7.8 The stages of protein synthesis translation.

Second letter

First letter	U	C	A	G	Third letter
U	UUU ⎤ Phe UUC ⎦ UUA ⎤ Leu UUG ⎦	UCU ⎤ UCC ⎦ Ser UCA ⎤ UCG ⎦	UAU ⎤ Tyr UAC ⎦ UAA stop UAG stop	UGU ⎤ Cys UGC ⎦ UGA stop UGG Trp	U C A G
C	CUU ⎤ CUC ⎦ Leu CUA ⎤ CUG ⎦	CCU ⎤ CCC ⎦ Pro CCA ⎤ CCG ⎦	CAU ⎤ His CAC ⎦ CAA ⎤ Gln CAG ⎦	CGU ⎤ CGC ⎦ Arg CGA ⎤ CGG ⎦	U C A G
A	AUU ⎤ Ileu AUC ⎦ AUA ⎤ Met AUG ⎦	ACU ⎤ ACC ⎦ Thr ACA ⎤ ACG ⎦	AAU ⎤ Asn AAC ⎦ AAA ⎤ Lys AAG ⎦	AGU ⎤ Ser AGC ⎦ AGA ⎤ Arg AGG ⎦	U C A G
G	GUU ⎤ GUC ⎦ Val GUA ⎤ GUG ⎦	GCU ⎤ GCC ⎦ Ala GCA ⎤ GCG ⎦	GAU ⎤ Asp GAC ⎦ GAA ⎤ Glu GAG ⎦	GGU ⎤ GGC ⎦ Gly GGA ⎤ GGG ⎦	U C A G

The abbreviated names of amino acids are:

Ala = alanine	**Gln** = glutamine	**Leu** = leucine	**Ser** = serine
Arg = arginine	**Glu** = glutamic	**Lys** = lysine	**Thr** = threonine
Asn = aspargine	**Gly** = glycine	**Met** = methionine	**Trp** = tryptophan
Asp = aspartic acid	**His** = histidine	**Phe** = phenylalanine	**Tyr** = tyrosine
Cys = cysteine	**Ileu** = isoleucine	**Pro** = proline	**Val** = valine

Fig. 7.9 Codons and the amino acids they code for. (Reproduced with permission from the Open University, 1988.)

forming a chain of amino acids until a 'stop' codon on mRNA signals the end of the chain. The sequence of amino acids determines the primary structure of the protein. The further configuration of the protein is determined by the interactions between different amino acids on the chain, which change the protein shape into a 'folded' structure, the final shape determining its function. Hence the sequence of bases of the gene, or region of DNA, determines the sequence of amino acids, which in turn prescribes the structure and function of the protein.

MUTATION

The copying of DNA has to be accurate. If mistakes are introduced into a region of DNA that is expressed as a protein (i.e. into an exon), the altered sequence of amino acids can change the structure of the protein. This permanent and transmissible change in base sequence of DNA is described as a mutation. Mutations can lead to death of a cell or cause cancer. They are considered to be the driving force of evolution; favourable mutations tend to accumulate and less favourable ones tend to be removed by natural selection. It is estimated that mutations occur every half an hour in each person but a mutation in a functional gene only occurs once in five generations. A mutation can be described as 'descent with modification'. DNA has regions of 'hotspots' where the mutation rate can be up to 100 times more frequent than normal. New gene mutations are associated with increasing paternal age (above 35 years); it is suggested that new gene mutations are exclusively inherited from the father and occur during spermatogenesis. All dominant mutations seem to arise in the male germline and may be caused by fragmentation induced by free radical damage (Aitken and Graves 2002). In mitosis, there are accumulated errors in copying the genetic message. Each chromosome has a specialized length of DNA at its end, which gets shorter with each successive division. About four bases seem to be lost with each successive cell division.

A base pair may be spontaneously replaced by a different base pair (a 'point mutation') thus altering the codon and ultimately the amino acid sequence. Age, environmental pressure, radiation and chemicals increase mutation rate. One notable example is haemophilia, the sex-linked genetic condition that afflicted male members of the European Royal Family for several generations. The spontaneous mutation for changed haemoglobin structure

Box 7.3 Sickle cell anaemia

Most haemoglobin (Hb) in adults is HbA, which has two α-peptide chains and two β-peptide chains forming the haemoglobin molecule. Sickle cell anaemia is an example of a single point mutation where the substitution of one base changes the codon and results in the substitution of one amino acid (Fig. 7.10). Uracil replaces adenine so, instead of glutamic acid, valine is inserted in the protein chain at position 6. Valine has a different charge to glutamic acid so the protein folds differently. The result is that the protein structure of the β-chain of haemoglobin is changed, which affects the molecular shape and oxygen-binding properties. The red blood cells distort into a characteristic sickle shape, particularly at low oxygen tension. Sickle cell anaemia is inherited as an autosomal recessive condition; affected patients have two mutant haemoglobin S genes, one from each parent. The parents are heterozygotes (HbA/HbS) and are thus clinically normal but carry the sickle cell gene. Homozygotes (HbS/HbS) have chronic haemolytic anaemia and are prone to infarction; lifespan is shortened.

may have occurred in one of the gametes forming the zygote that became Queen Victoria. This type of mutation is referred to as a substitution. Mutations may arise as an insertion or deletion of a nucleotide into or from the DNA strand; these mutations could cause a shift in the 'reading frame' of the codons or alter splicing of mRNA thus altering the gene product. Mutations may also occur by the complete insertion of new codons or by the deletion of a complete codon, thus altering protein structure by introducing or deleting amino acids in the protein. This can be complicated if codons are duplicated and repeated one after the other, for example in fragile X syndrome.

Many mutations occur in the non-coding areas of DNA, so protein structure and function are not affected by the change; these mutations are described as 'silent' as they have no effect. If the mutation results in a different codon that codes for the same amino acid as the original, there will also be no effect. However, a different base, or a missing base, will cause a change in the final sequence of amino acids of the protein, which may have serious effects on protein structure and function. An example is sickle cell anaemia (Box 7.3 and Fig. 7.10).

MEIOSIS

The basic characteristics of meiosis – two cell divisions without intervening DNA replication, halving the chromosome complement of the resulting cells – are conserved in evolution. Each species has a characteristic number of chromosomes; humans have 46 chromosomes, arranged as 23 pairs. One chromosome of each pair is maternally derived (from the ovum); the other is paternally derived (from the sperm). (The members of each pair are called homologous; see below.) Human gametes contain only 23 chromosomes, that is half the normal number of chromosomes in other human cells. This reduction from the diploid number of chromosomes (46) to the haploid number (23) is accomplished by meiosis. Meiosis is the process whereby a diploid parent cell produces four haploid daughter cells, resulting in gametes, or sex cells, that are not identical to their parent cells. These gametes are haploid and during meiosis the genetic instructions are randomly assorted, thus generating unique combinations. Meiosis is also described as 'reduction division' because the number of chromosomes is reduced from 46 (i.e. 23 pairs) to 23. It occurs in two successive divisions (meiosis I and II), each of which can be divided into steps (Fig. 7.11). Meiosis II is very similar to mitosis.

In anaphase I, there is random segregation of each member of the chromosome pairs with a maternal and a paternal chromosome randomly going to a particular end of the cell. This would theoretically generate 2^{23} (i.e. 8,388,608) different possibilities of gamete combination. However, the crossing over of genetic material between the chromosomes adds far more variation. Meiosis allows the genomes of the parents to be combined to form an individual whose genome is related to their parents and siblings but is unique.

Mammalian oogenesis begins meiotic development during fetal development but arrests in meiosis I and does not complete meiosis I until ovulation; the second division is only completed if the egg is fertilized. Oogenesis, therefore, requires several stop and start signals and, in humans, may last for several decades. The longer an oocyte is immobilized at prophase I, the greater is the chance of failure of separation of the homologous chromosomes (non-disjunction). Often genetic abnormalities arise as extra genetic material is incorporated into the genome. If an extra chromosome is inserted, the condition is referred to as trisomic (Table 7.1). Most combinations of trisomy are not seen, but there is no reason to believe that certain chromosomes are more susceptible to failed disjunction. Those seen are probably those that are compatible with fetal survival, although they may cause congenital abnormalities or affect neonatal survival. Sometimes extra chromosomal material may become attached to a chromosome, making it abnormally long. Rarely, a condition called triploidy occurs where the chromosomes of the zygote are in triplicate rather than the normal duplicate complement. This condition is not compatible with embryo survival but is sometimes found in products of a failed conception (early miscarriage) and is associated with a high incidence of hydatidiform mole (see Chapter 6). Imperfect disjunction also causes conditions where the genome is lacking part or a whole chromosome. For example, there is only one X chromosome present in Turner's syndrome (see Chapter 5) and Wolf–Hirschhorn syndrome is caused by loss of chromosomal tissue from chromosomes 4 and 5.

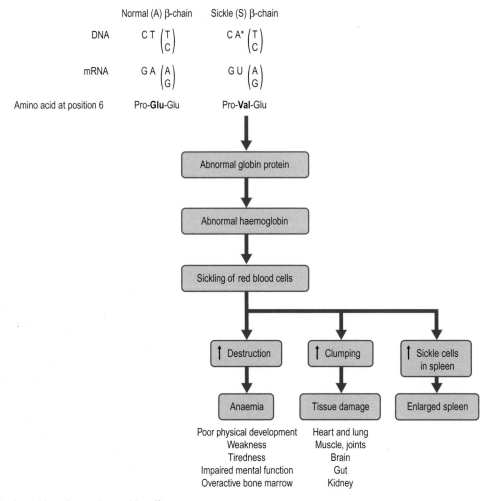

Fig. 7.10 The sickle cell mutation and its effects.

AUTOSOMES AND SEX CHROMOSOMES

Each gene has a specific location on a specific chromosome, which is referred to as a locus (plural: loci). Each chromosome may have 1000–2000 different genes, each with its own location and function. The visualization of the chromosomes from a cell is described as a karyotype (Box 7.4) (Case study 7.1). Of the 23 pairs of chromosomes that constitute the human genome, 22 pairs of chromosomes can be seen in both sexes; these are referred to as the autosomes and contain the autosomal genes. The 23rd pair of chromosomes comprises the sex chromosomes; these are homologous within the female (i.e. XX) but in the male the XY arrangement consists of a pair of non-homologous chromosomes.

Sex chromosomes

The sex chromosomes provide the mechanism for the determination of sex and the differentiation into male morphology, which is usually dependent on the inheritance of a Y chromosome (see Chapter 5). As well as sex determination and identity, other genetic traits can be inherited on the sex chromosomes (see below).

It is thought that the sex chromosomes originated from a pair of autosomes (see Chapter 7) during the evolution of sex determination (Graves, 2002). The X and Y chromosomes are very different in size and sequence compared to the other 22 pairs of autosomes. The Y chromosome is very small in comparison to the X chromosome and is completely different from the X chromosomes except at its tips. These identical regions at the tips, known as the pseudoautosomal regions, contain most of the Y chromosome genes involved in control of growth and allow the

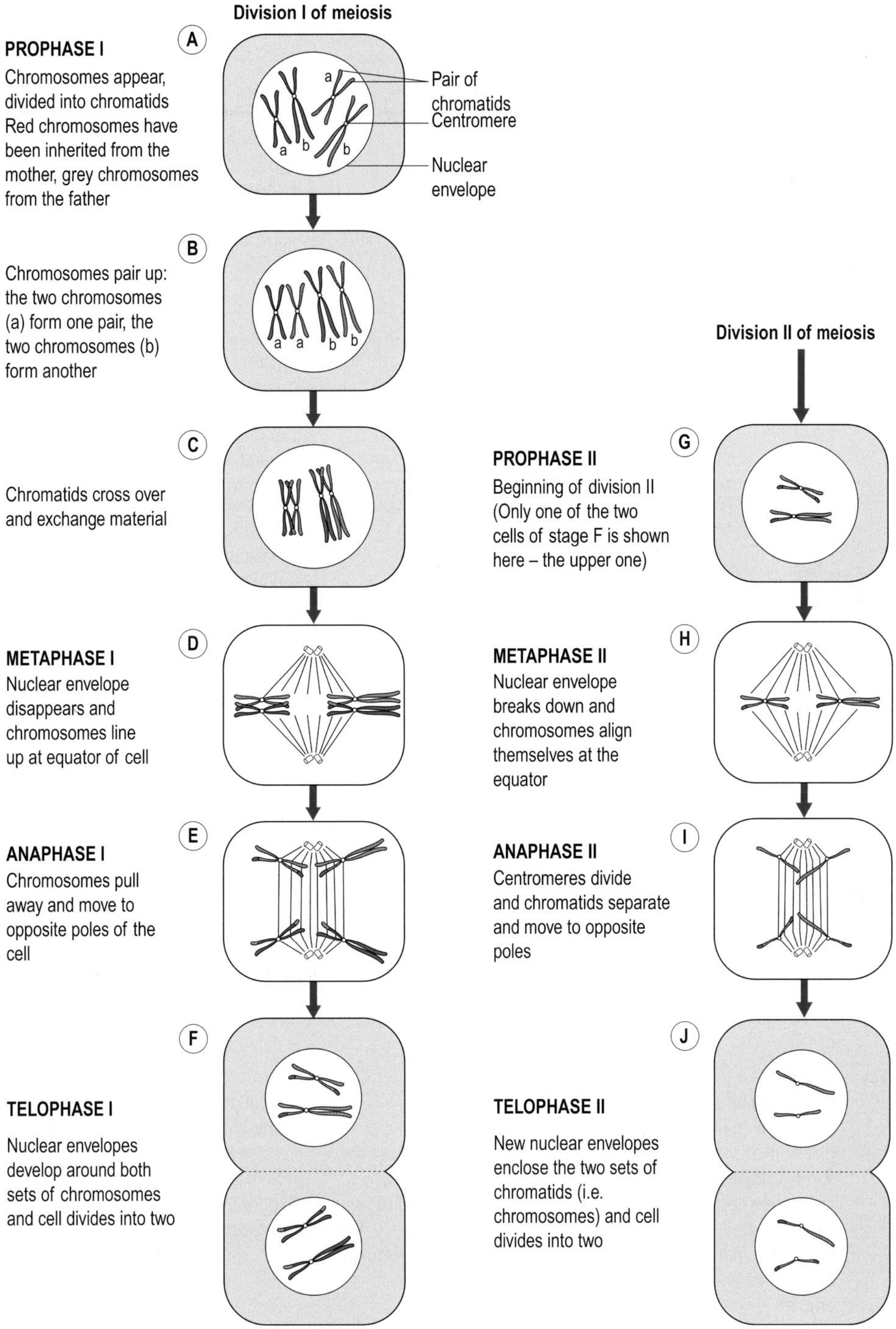

Division I of meiosis

PROPHASE I (A)
Chromosomes appear, divided into chromatids Red chromosomes have been inherited from the mother, grey chromosomes from the father

Pair of chromatids
Centromere
Nuclear envelope

(B)
Chromosomes pair up: the two chromosomes (a) form one pair, the two chromosomes (b) form another

Division II of meiosis

(C)
Chromatids cross over and exchange material

PROPHASE II (G)
Beginning of division II (Only one of the two cells of stage F is shown here – the upper one)

METAPHASE I (D)
Nuclear envelope disappears and chromosomes line up at equator of cell

METAPHASE II (H)
Nuclear envelope breaks down and chromosomes align themselves at the equator

ANAPHASE I (E)
Chromosomes pull away and move to opposite poles of the cell

ANAPHASE II (I)
Centromeres divide and chromatids separate and move to opposite poles

TELOPHASE I (F)
Nuclear envelopes develop around both sets of chromosomes and cell divides into two

TELOPHASE II (J)
New nuclear envelopes enclose the two sets of chromatids (i.e. chromosomes) and cell divides into two

Fig. 7.11 The stages of meiosis A–J. (Reproduced with permission from Goodwin, 1997.)

Table 7.1 Examples of chromosome disorders

DISORDER	EXAMPLE	INCIDENCE	OUTCOME	NOTES
Polyploidy	Triploidy 69 chromosomes (69, XXX, 69,XXY, 69, XYY)	Occurs in 2% of conceptions but early spontaneous abortion is normal	Lethal	Usually arises from fertilization of oocyte by two sperm or from a diploid gamete. 69,XXY is most common. Polyploid cells occur normally in the bone marrow and liver as a stage of cell division
Trisomy	Trisomy 13	1/5000 live births	Patau's syndrome	Usually due to non-disjunction of chromosomes or chromatids at anaphase. Trisomy increases with increased maternal age and is sometimes associated with radiation or viral infection. There may be a familial tendency
	Trisomy 18	1/3000 live births	Edward's syndrome	Maternal age effect. Incidence at conception much higher – most affected fetuses abort spontaneously. More female fetuses seem to survive
	Trisomy 21	1/700 live births	Down's syndrome	Incidence at conception is higher. Maternal age effect; the extra chromosome is maternal in 85% cases. The most serious complications are mental handicap and congenital heart problems
	47,XXY	1/1000 male births	Klinefelter's syndrome	Trisomies involving sex chromosomes usually result in a less serious outcome. Condition is usually diagnosed during investigations for infertility
	47,XYY	1/1000 male births		Often asymptomatic, some effects on IQ. Only XX and XY offspring observed
Monosomy	Monosomy X	1/5000 female births, much higher at conception	Turner's syndrome	Due to non-disjunction in either parent; 80% of affected females have maternal X so it is the paternal chromosome that is missing
Deletion and ring chromosome	Wolf–Hirschhorn syndrome (partial deletion of short arm of chromosome 4) Cri du chat syndrome (partial deletion of short arm of chromosome 5)	Incidence of deletions and/or duplications is 1/2000 births	Chromosome imbalance of autosomes is usually associated with mental retardation and multiple dysmorphic features	A deletion is the loss of part of chromosome. A ring chromosome is due to deletions in both arms of a chromosome and the fusion of the proximal sticky ends. Microdeletions are deletions that can just be detected by light microscopy
Duplication				Duplication is where there are two copies of a segment of chromosome. This is more common and less harmful than deletions

Continued

Table 7.1 Examples of chromosome disorders—cont'd

DISORDER	EXAMPLE	INCIDENCE	OUTCOME	NOTES
Inversion			The carriers of balanced inversions and translocations are healthy because the cells have all the genetic material but gamete formation is affected so there is a high rate of miscarriage and malformation	A segment of the chromosome is inverted through 180° between breaks Usually does not cause clinical problems but unbalanced gamete may result
Translocation	Reciprocal			Translocations involve transfer of chromosomal material between chromosomes. Two chromosomes are broken and repaired abnormally or there is recombination between non-homologous chromosomes at meiosis. Reciprocal translocations involve transfer of material between two chromosomes
	Robertsonian (centric fusion)			Robertsonian translocation involves transfer of material, which leaves a large chromosome, and a fragment of a chromosome, which is unable to replicate; most common centric fusion translocations are 13/14 and 14/21. Balanced carriers have 45 chromosomes and are healthy. Gametogenesis is affected

pairing of the X and Y chromosome and crossing over during cell division. The X chromosome is about 5% of the total length of a single set of chromosome and bears about 3000–4000 genes, many of which are conserved (identical to those of other placental mammals). The Y chromosome contains only about 45–50 genes, many of which appear to be non-functional; others are involved with male differentiation and spermatogenesis, implantation and promoting placental growth. It is suggested that the Y chromosome is particularly vulnerable to mutations and gene deletions because it cannot retrieve lost genetic information by homologous recombination and that, over the past 300 million years, it has already lost most of its original 1500 genes and continues to deteriorate; at its present rate of decay (losing about five genes per million years), it will self-destruct in about 10 million years (Aitken and Graves, 2002). This has already happened in the mole vole, which has lost the Y chromosome and all of its genes from the genome. An alternative view is that the Y chromosome, rather than being 'damaged', is an efficient carrier of male-specific genes, rationalized by evolutionary selection (Craig et al., 2004); there has not been any genes lost from the Y chromosome since the ancestral paths of humans and chimpanzees diverged (Goto et al., 2009).

Alleles

Each pair of autosomes is homologous; this means that their gene arrangements, although not necessarily the specific gene at each locus, are identical. So although the genes at a specific locus code for a specific physiological feature these features in themselves may vary. For instance, the genes at a particular locus may code for eye colour, but this could be blue eye colour on the chromosome inherited from one parent and brown eye colour on the chromosome inherited from the other parent. Genes that code for the same physical feature but produce variations in that feature are called alleles.

If the genes are identical alleles, then the structure and coding of the pair are referred to as being homozygous. If the genes are differing alleles then the pair is referred to as being heterozygous. If one copy of a gene is required for a trait to

Box 7.4 **Karyotyping**

Karyotyping is the method of visualizing the chromosomes in an ordered display of the chromosomes as they appear in the nucleus of a cell during metaphase of mitosis. For a fetal karyotype, a sample of amniotic fluid is removed. The cells are centrifuged to concentrate the fetal cells. The supernatant can also be used diagnostically for biochemical tests such as investigation of enzyme deficiencies, protein defects and gene alterations. Alternatively, cells may be taken from the chorionic villus. A karyotype of adult cells is usually derived from a sample of venous blood, where the anuclear red blood cells are lysed and the washed remaining cells are, therefore, white blood cells containing nuclei.

The fetal cells or white blood cells are grown in cell culture. The time taken for this depends on the number of cells in the original sample. Contamination of the sample can interfere with the success of the method. Colchicine, a chemical poison, is added to the culture medium to prevent spindle formation. Thus, mitosis in all cells is halted at the metaphase stage when the chromosomes are maximally contracted and well defined as paired chromatids (therefore they take on the typical X-shaped appearance). The cells, all halted at the same stage, can be separated from the culture medium. Exposure of the cells to hypotonic saline causes the nucleus to swell so the chromosomes are spread out. The cells are then fixed and stained. Visualization of the karyotype is done by computer-aided photographic techniques. The chromosomes are ordered according to size with the homologous autosomes being paired together. The chromosomes of pair number 1 are the longest and those of pair number 22 are the shortest. The position of the centromere is also used to sort the chromosomes into order. Stains that bind preferentially to some areas of the chromosome, producing a distinct pattern of bands, can be used to identify the chromosomes. Karyotypes can be used to identify gross abnormalities such as additional or missing chromosomes and missing or duplicated parts of chromosomes. However, a normal karyotype does not reveal the presence of abnormal genes at specific loci. In order to identify such genes, the chromosomes are stained, which produce a pattern or banding enabling an abnormal gene or a marker gene to be identified. A marker gene is a gene that is often found in close proximity to an abnormal gene; the closer the marker gene to the abnormal gene, the higher is the association.

Occasionally, results from karyotyping may be complicated by mosaicism. Mosaicism, a different number of chromosomes in different populations of cells may occur for instance where the chorionic tissue has a different number of chromosomes to the fetus.

 Case study 7.1

Surya presents herself to a midwife at 8 weeks' gestation demanding that she needs to know the sex of her baby because if it was a female infant she would rather have a termination than proceed with the pregnancy. What should the midwife do in this situation? Are there any circumstances when fetal sex determination is justified?

be expressed (i.e. for the feature to be 'visible' in the resultant individual), the gene is described as being dominant. If two copies are required, the gene is described as being recessive. Autosomal traits (genetic instructions carried on the autosomes) can be expressed as either dominant or recessive traits. Simple inheritance of these traits can be predicted diagrammatically (see Figs. 7.12 and 7.16).

PREDICTION OF GENETIC OUTCOMES

Genetic predictions forecast the chance of an ovum carrying a specific combination of genes being fertilized by a sperm carrying a specific combination of genes. The convention is to show the dominant gene as a capital letter. The genetic potential is described as the genotype; how it is expressed is called the phenotype. Combination diagrams and Punnett squares give the same results, predicting the chance of a particular outcome (Figs. 7.12 and 7.13).

The genetic rules that dictate eye colour follow the traditional form of dominant and recessive interaction (see Box 7.5). However, it is important to realize that, like so many other physiological states, expressed characteristics may be the outcome of multifactorial genes where more than one gene is involved. The environment may also influence the expression of genes. For instance, inheriting genes for tall stature does not necessarily mean the child will be tall. In the absence of appropriate nutrition at critical times of growth, the genetic potential may not be realized.

CHARACTERISTICS OF DIFFERENT TYPES OF INHERITANCE

Autosomal dominant inheritance

The trait is expressed by a gene on an autosome and is expressed provided that at least one chromosome has the dominant gene. Each person expressing the trait usually has a parent with the trait (Fig. 7.14 shows a pedigree chart for a pattern of autosomal dominant inheritance; the symbols used in these charts are shown in Box 7.6).

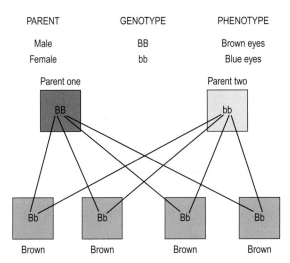

PARENT	GENOTYPE	PHENOTYPE
Male	BB	Brown eyes
Female	bb	Blue eyes

Fig. 7.12 Combination diagram to illustrate the genetic outcomes of crossing a homozygous male with brown eyes (carrying two dominant genes for brown eye colour, BB) and a homozygous female with blue eyes (carrying two recessive genes for blue eye colour, bb). All the offspring will be heterozygous, carrying one recessive gene and one dominant gene. All the children will have the phenotype of brown eye coloration.

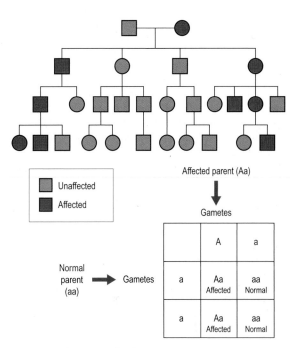

Fig. 7.14 Inheritance of a dominant trait.

	Parent one Gametes	
	B	**B**
Parent two Gametes b	Bb	Bb
b	Bb	Bb

Fig. 7.13 Punnett square.

Box 7.5 **Selected examples of recessive and dominant traits**

Autosomal trait	Recessive trait
Brown eye colour	Blue or grey eye colour
Curly hair	Straight hair
Dark brown hair	All other colours
Near or far sight	Normal vision
Normal skin pigment	Albinism
Normal hearing	Deafness
Migraine headaches	Normal
A or B antigen (A, B or AB blood group)	No A or B antigen (O blood group)
Rhesus antigen (Rh+ blood group)	No Rhesus antigen (Rh− blood group)

Box 7.6 **Symbols used in pedigree charts**

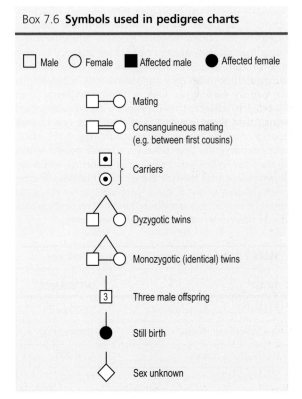

This means that a particular characteristic or disorder can be traced through several generations if it has little effect on survival. However, a trait occurring in a new generation may be the result of polygamic behaviour (illegitimacy) or a fresh mutation. Autosomal dominant traits also tend to be extremely variable in expression so they may be undetectable and appear to 'skip' a generation. For instance, polydactyly (an extra digit) may be manifest as a tiny pedicle, rather than an extra finger. Autosomal dominant disorders are often caused by defects in structural proteins.

If an affected person mates with an unaffected person, the chances of any child being affected are one in two (i.e. 50%). Some autosomal diseases or traits do not affect the predicted 50% of offspring. These are described as having incomplete penetrance. Conversely, a highly penetrant gene is expressed regardless of environmental and other factors.

In the UK, the most common dominantly inherited traits are Huntington's disease and achondroplasia (Table 7.2). Huntington's disease, a degenerative neuropsychiatric disorder initially characterized by spasmodic movements of the body and limbs and ultimately dementia, is usually not expressed until the third or fourth decade when the person affected is likely to have reproduced. The age at onset and progression of the disease is linked to the number of polyglutamine sequence repeats in the disease protein (coded by CAG bases in the gene).

A complication occurs in the case of inherited achondroplasia (dwarfism) (note that 80% of cases of achondroplasia are caused by new mutations in the offspring of parents of normal height). Humans exhibit selective rather than random mating, often being attracted to partners of similar height, intelligence and other physical attributes. In consequence, individuals with achondroplasia partner each other with a higher frequency than expected by chance. If two people with achondroplasia mate, there is an expected prediction of a one in four chance of a child having normal stature (Fig. 7.15). However, homozygosity (two genes for achondroplasia) results in the fetus having lethal respiratory problems, which are incompatible with survival. Hence the actual ratio of newborn children is one in three. (Arguably, achondroplasia could be viewed as a recessively inherited respiratory condition that confers dwarfism on the heterozygote.)

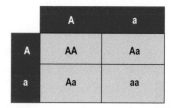

Expected outcome might be 25% chance of child with normal height, but AA is lethal lung deformity so observed outcome is 2:1 chance of achondroplasia: normal height.

Fig. 7.15 Inheritance of achondroplasia.

Autosomal recessive inheritance

As with autosomal dominant inheritance, this type of inheritance can affect both sexes equally. However, the recessive trait is expressed only if the gene is present on both alleles, which means it has been inherited from both parents. If the parents are heterozygotes, each carrying one recessive gene for the trait and one normal dominant gene, they express the dominant gene and are described as 'carriers' of the recessive gene. In some conditions, the carriers may exhibit mild signs of a disease or have an unusual level of certain biochemical markers that can be measured in genetic testing.

Most inherited enzyme disorders are recessive. Another characteristic of recessive disorders is that they show a variation in birth frequency among different populations (Table 7.3). It is suggested that the reason some recessively inherited disorders reach such a high incidence within a population is because advantages are conferred on the heterozygotes. For example, it is recognized that carriers of the gene for sickle haemoglobin (see Box 7.3), namely HbS or C, have a resistance to malaria falciparum, the most dangerous form of malaria (but not to other types). Obviously, such an advantage will selectively increase the number of people within the population who carry the gene. The incidence of malaria and the inheritance of other forms of

Table 7.2 Examples of autosomal dominant diseases

TRAIT	INCIDENCE
Familial hypercholesterolaemia	1/500 births
von Willebrand disease	1/20–30 000
Huntington's disease	1/18 000
Achondroplasia	1/26 000

Table 7.3 Examples of recessively inherited diseases

TRAIT	CARRIER FREQUENCY
β-Thalassaemia	One in six Cypriots
Cystic fibrosis	1 in 25 Northern Europeans
Phenylketonuria	1 in 10 000 Europeans
Sickle cell anaemia	Varies amongst Mediterranean, Middle Eastern and Afro-Caribbean races
Tay-Sachs disease	1 in 30 Ashkenazi Jews

altered haemoglobin, such as β-thalassaemia, can be mapped to the same parts of the world.

In the Caucasian population, the most common autosomal recessive condition is cystic fibrosis. The carrier rate within the population is about 1 in 25 people. This means that there is a 1 in 25 chance that any person might be heterozygous for (i.e. carry) the cystic fibrosis gene. The chance, therefore, of two carriers mating is 1 in 625 (25 × 25) (Fig. 7.16). If two heterozygous parents have children, there is a one in four chance that any child will be affected and a one in two chance that any child will be a carrier of the gene themselves. The live-birth rate of children with cystic fibrosis is about one in 2500 (625 × 4). Because of the relatively high incidence of the disease, parents who already have an affected child or those whose family history has a strong incidence of the disease will be offered genetic counselling. Carriers of the cystic fibrosis gene appear to have resistance to gastrointestinal conditions, tuberculosis and cholera, and to have increased fertility. Cystic fibrosis is a condition which has the potential to be treated by gene therapy (Box 7.7).

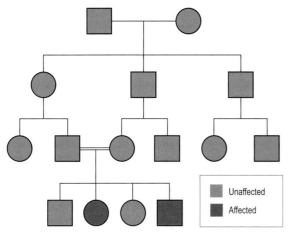

Cystic fibrosis

Carrier rate = $\frac{1}{25}$ (Cc)   Chance of two parents being carriers = $\frac{1}{25}$ x $\frac{1}{25}$ = $\frac{1}{625}$

	C	c
C	CC Normal	Cc Carrier
c	Cc Carrier	cc Affected

Live birth rate approximately $\frac{1}{25}$ x $\frac{1}{25}$ x $\frac{1}{4}$ = $\frac{1}{2500}$

Fig. 7.16 Inheritance of cystic fibrosis, a recessive trait.

Box 7.7 **Advances in gene therapy**

Recent advances in gene therapy have led to techniques to insert normal genes into human cells and tissues which express abnormal genes. Gene therapy aims to supplement a defective allele with a functional allele and focuses on single-gene defects such as cystic fibrosis, muscular dystrophy, sickle cell anaemia and haemophilia. This is achieved by using a modified virus that acts as a vehicle by which the normal gene is carried into and thus incorporated into the genome. The altered virus is unable to replicate and so causes no harm to the recipient. In treatment of cystic fibrosis, the cells of the nasal passages and lining of the lungs are exposed to the virus in the form of an inhaled spray. So far, all human gene therapy has targeted at somatic (body) cells; germline engineering (altering stem cells or gametes) remains controversial.

Sex-linked inheritance

The sex chromosomes not only determine the sex of the embryo but also have other structural genes. Female and male genetic endowments are different. Very few genes appear to be carried on the Y chromosomes so sex-linked inheritance usually relates to X-linked inheritance. Most genes carried on the X chromosome are recessive. The effects of a recessive X-linked gene are usually masked in the female by the presence of the paired normal gene upon the other X chromosome. However, should such a woman carry an abnormal gene, she may pass it on to her sons. Males inherit only one of the paired X chromosomes; therefore, if they acquire the abnormal gene on the X chromosome the disease will automatically be manifest because the Y chromosome lacks the corresponding allele of the other X chromosome that is found in the female. Also, if a female inherits two abnormal genes, one on each X chromosome, the condition is usually incompatible with life and the embryo is lost at a relatively early stage. X-linked recessive disorders therefore affect many more males than females. Very few sex-linked abnormalities are inherited as dominant traits which affect would both male and female offspring. One example is vitamin D-resistant rickets.

Most sex-linked diseases (Table 7.4) involve a female carrier partnered with a trait-free man (Fig. 7.17). There is a one in two chance that any male offspring will inherit and express the disorder and a one in two chance that any female offspring will carry the trait. An affected man cannot pass the disorder to his sons because they will receive a Y chromosome only, but all of his daughters will be carriers of the disease.

Only males have the genes from the Y chromosome which is small and contains very little active genetic coding. However, it does contain the SRY (sex-determining region of the Y chromosome) gene, which, when activated, directs male embryonic development (see Chapter 5).

Table 7.4 Examples of sex-linked recessive disorders

TRAIT	UK FREQUENCY/ 10 000 MALES
Red–green colour blindness	800
Haemophilia A (factor VIII)	2
Haemophilia B (factor IX)	0.3
Duchenne muscular dystrophy	3
Fragile X syndrome	5

The male, however, still requires the presence of an X chromosome as this contains many genes that are vital for normal development to occur.

The female inherits two X chromosomes but evidence suggests that only one of the chromosomes is activated within the cell. On examination of the cell nucleus, one chromosome is always contracted, forming a characteristic Barr body at the outskirts of the nucleus. The number of Barr bodies is one of the tests used in determining the sex of a baby born with ambiguous genitalia. The contracted

Barr body chromosome was assumed to be inert, but a small number of genes appear to remain active and expressed. Although the second X chromosome in females is inactivated this is usually incomplete so a proportion (perhaps 15%) of X-linked genes will be expressed at higher and variable levels in women. As X chromosome inactivation is random, some female cells will express the paternal X chromosome, whereas the others will express the maternal X chromosome so women are genetic mosaics with respect to X-linked gene expression.

There are examples of mosaic phenotypes where a heterozygous woman has a mix of dominant and recessive expression. For instance, in X-linked ectodermal dysplasia, affected males have smooth skin with no sweat glands. Female carriers may have patches of normal skin interspersed with patches of dysplastic skin. Similarly, females who are heterozygous for ocular albinism may have a mosaic pattern of pigmentation in their irises. There also seems to be some form of dosage compensation, as the inheritance of two X chromosomes does not result in twice the amount of proteins coded for by genes on the X chromosome. The explanation is that, early in embryonic development, a process called X-inactivation or 'Lyonization' occurs in which one of the X chromosomes is permanently inactivated (Box 7.8 and Fig. 7.18).

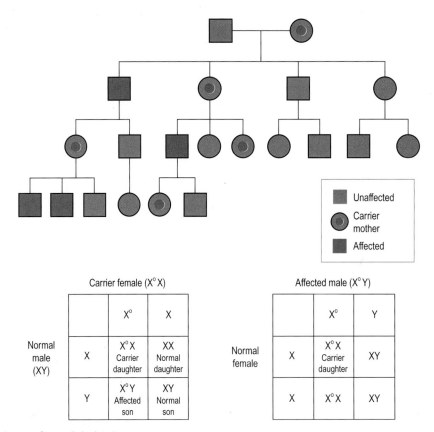

Unaffected

Carrier mother

Affected

Carrier female ($X^{o}X$)

		X^{o}	X
Normal male (XY)	X	$X^{o}X$ Carrier daughter	XX Normal daughter
	Y	$X^{o}Y$ Affected son	XY Normal son

Affected male ($X^{o}Y$)

		X^{o}	Y
Normal female	X	$X^{o}X$ Carrier daughter	XY
	X	$X^{o}X$	XY

Fig. 7.17 Inheritance of a sex-linked trait.

Box 7.8 X-inactivation or Lyonization

X chromosome inactivation or Lyonization (named after Dr. Mary Lyon who first proposed the hypothesis in 1961) occurs at approximately 15 days into the gestation (Huynh and Lee, 2005). In humans, the cell mass of the embryo at around this stage is approximately 5000 cells (Fig. 7.18). The female embryo randomly inactivates all but one X chromosome on each cell; once inactivated, all the cells descending from each parent cell retain their pattern of either paternal or maternal inactivation. In some animals, such as marsupials, it is always the paternally derived X chromosome that is deactivated but in mammals it appears that either one of the pair is inactivated. Random inactivation would predict that 50% of female cells would have an active paternal X and 50% have an active maternal X; however, skewed patterns of inactivation can arise which means that the X chromosomes from one parent may be predominantly inactivated so the X chromosomes from the other parent will then be expressed. This could lead to the dominant proportion of expressed X chromosomes carrying a disorder that can be expressed. The inactivated chromosome appears as a sex chromatin body (Barr body) and is identified as it always divides late in mitosis. However, not all the chromosomes are totally inactivated: the pseudoautosomal region of the short arm and other loci remains active to prevent the manifestation of Turner's syndrome in all normal genotypical women.

As random chromosomes are selected for inactivation, different regions of the adult body have different chromosomes inactivated.

The three main types of inheritance are summarized in Box 7.9.

Other types of inheritance

Blood groups A and B are inherited as co-dominant genes, whereas the gene for blood group O is recessive (Fig. 7.19 and Box 7.10). Some disorders are inherited via the mitochondria. The mitochondria of the zygote and subsequent cells are exclusively derived from the oocyte (see Chapter 6); therefore, no paternal mitochondria are passed on to the next generation. Disorders of mitochondrial metabolism are passed from mother to child but never from father to child. The unique matrilineal transmission of mtDNA has been particularly useful for the study of population genetics and evolutionary biology. This has been particularly useful in determining family lineage, such as the notable case of Anastasia, the Russian princess. DNA analysis showed that the mtDNA of members of the present Royal Family was different to that of the person who claimed to be Anastasia (Sykes, 2001). Determining patterns of inheritance can be complicated, however, where different inherited disorders apparently cause the same effect, such as blindness.

The presence of 23 pairs of normal chromosomes indicates a normal karyotype (see Box 7.4).

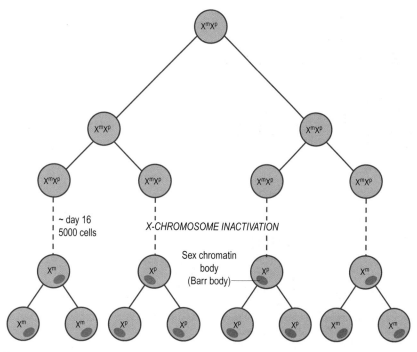

Fig. 7.18 Lyonization.

Box 7.9 **Characteristics of different types of inheritance**

Autosomal dominant inheritance

- Effects are manifest in heterozygotes
- Affected person + person: half of offspring are affected
- Unaffected persons do not transmit condition
- Fresh mutation may produce abnormal genes
- An affected person usually has an affected parent
- Traits are often variably expressed and may not be penetrant (an individual can have the mutant gene but have a normal phenotype)
- Often structural, receptor or carrier proteins are affected and clinical effects tend to be less severe than those due to recessively inherited traits

Autosomal recessive inheritance

- Effects are manifest in homozygotes
- Affected person receives genes from both parents
- Heterozygote = 'carrier'
- Heterozygote parents
  - One in four chance that offspring will be affected
  - One in two chance that offspring will be carriers
  - One in four chance that offspring will be unaffected
- Variation in birth frequency
- Recessive traits usually result in enzyme defects

Sex-linked inheritance

- Sex chromosomes carry genes and determine sex
- Sex-linked = X-linked
- Most conditions are rare
- Genes involved are usually recessive
- Female carrier
  - One in two chance that male offspring will be affected
  - One in two chance that female offspring will also be carriers
- Affected male
  - All sons will be normal
  - All daughters will be carriers

CHROMOSOMAL ABNORMALITIES

Changes within the genetic message, for instance those due to mutation, may involve large parts of the chromosome (Box 7.11). If the changes can be seen by light microscopy, they are termed gross aberrations and can be detected from an examination of the karyotype. Chromosomal abnormalities can be classified as numerical or structural, affecting

PHENOTYPES OF PARENTS	PHENOTYPES OF POSSIBLE	OFFSPRING IMPOSSIBLE
A A	A, O	B. AB
A B	A, B, AB, O	none
A AB	A, B, AB	O
A O	A, O	B, AB
B B	B, O	A, AB
B AB	A, B, AB	O
B O	B, O	A, AB
AB AB	A, B, AB	O
AB O	A, B	AB, O
O O	O	A, B, AB

Antigens A and B are inherited as dominant traits whereas O is inherited as a recessive trait

Fig. **7.19** Inheritance of ABO blood groups.

Box 7.10 **Erythrocyte surface antigens: blood group classifications**

The reason for the evolution of differing blood groups in humans remains a mystery except that at some point during evolutionary history they may have been advantageous to ensure overall survival of the population. Other animals do not have the same number or type of blood groups. The more common human blood cell antigens give rise to the blood groups A, B, AB and O (Table 7.5).

Table 7.5 ABO blood groups				
BLOOD TYPE	**A**	**B**	**AB**	**O**
Antigen on RBC (agglutinogen)	A	B	A + B	None (universal donor)
Antibody in plasma (agglutinin)	b	a	None (universal recipient)	a + b
Can donate to	A and AB	B and AB	AB	All
Can receive from	A and O	B and O	All	O
Distribution in UK (%)	42	9	3	46
Genotype	AA, AO	BB, BO	AB	OO
Phenotype	A	B	AB	O

Continued

Box 7.10 **Erythrocyte surface antigens: blood group classifications—cont'd**

Other surface antigens commonly found in practice are Duffy, Rhesus D, C, E and Kell. The presence of other antigens explains why, even with closely matched blood, recipients can react to the blood of the donor. The Rhesus antigen, which is present in approximately 85% of the population, has implications for fetal survival (see Chapter 10).

Box 7.11 **Incidence of chromosomal abnormalities**

- Incidence of major chromosomal abnormality
  - About 1 in 200 live births
  - About 1 in 20 perinatal deaths (stillbirths and early neonatal deaths)
  - About 1 in 2 early spontaneous abortions
- About 1 in 100 births: single-gene (unifactorial) disorder
- About 1 in 50 births: +major congenital abnormality

either the autosomes or the sex chromosomes. These types of abnormality are easier than a single-gene abnormality to detect.

Numerical abnormalities

The loss or gain of one or more chromosomes is described as aneuploidy (wrong number of chromosomes), whereas cells with the correct number of chromosomes are euploidic. It is estimated that 10–25% of all human fetuses are aneuploidal, predominantly due to non-disjunction in maternal meiosis (Hunt and Hassold, 2002), although trisomy 18 most often results from non-disjunction in meiosis II. Aneuploidy occurs more frequently in humans than in other species which is probably the reason for such a high rate of miscarriage in humans. Aneuploidy is usually due to non-disjunction in the formation of the gametes resulting in a zygote that does not have 46 chromosomes. Monosomy describes the loss of a complete chromosome and trisomy the addition of a single chromosome, as in Down's syndrome (trisomy 21) (see Table 7.1). Monosomy and triploidy (an extra complete set of 23 chromosomes) are usually lethal. Most autosomal trisomies are also lethal except those involving chromosomes 13, 18 or 21 but these, and the sex chromosome trisomies, are the main cause of mental retardation and developmental disability. It is interesting to note that chromosomes 13, 18 and 21 carry the fewest genes. Abnormal numbers of sex chromosomes have a less serious effect on development; for instance, a missing sex chromosome can result in a Turner's syndrome monosomy (45,X0). Although it might be possible that paternally derived aneuploidies are preferentially eliminated, it is more likely that more errors occur in maternal meiosis and/or that the mechanisms for detecting and correcting or eliminating them are less stringent. The most likely reason for non-disjunction is age-related deterioration of the meiotic spindle and the motor proteins which move chromosomes along it.

Down's syndrome

Down's syndrome is the most common chromosomal anomaly at birth affecting about one in 700 live births. The conception rate is much higher but it is associated with a high incidence of spontaneous abortion and stillbirth. Either the ovum or the sperm carries the extra chromosome 21. Although non-disjunction is associated with older maternal age, there is evidence to suggest that older men, perhaps because of a lower incidence of coitus, also have an increased rate of non-disjunction in their sperm formation. There is also a slight increase in the incidence of Down's syndrome in teenage pregnancies which may reflect a tendency to non-disjoin in early ovarian cycles (Hassold and Hunt, 2001).

Affected children have typical stigmata of Down's syndrome (Box 7.12). Their life expectancy tends to be shorter because of increased susceptibility to infection, congenital heart disease and leukaemia. It is also hypothesized that individuals with Down's syndrome have increased oxidative damage to neurons, which results in accelerated brain ageing similar to that of Alzheimer's disease.

Over half of the conceptions with trisomy 21 fail, suggesting that the extra copy of chromosome 21 interferes with intrauterine development. Although males with Down's syndrome are infertile, females with Down's syndrome can reproduce; theoretically, half the ova will have an extra copy of chromosome 21 but the effects on uterine development mean that the live-birth rate does not correlate with the conception rate. Amniocentesis

Box 7.12 **Down's syndrome: clinical features**

- Slanting palpebral fissure, almond-shaped eyes
- A roundish head and flat facial profile
- Small nose
- Low-set ears
- Simian crease (single palmar crease) in 50% of cases
- Folds of redundant skin around neck
- Clinodactyly (inwardly curved little finger) in 50% of cases
- Usually mentally retarded with IQ < 60
- Congenital heart malformations occur in 40% of cases
- Prone to presenile dementia in fifth decade

for cytogenetic screening is offered to all mothers over 35 years of age and the triple test is available to all women in the UK regardless of their age (see p. 169). Some women may also be offered ultrasonography screening.

About 4% of babies with Down's syndrome have 46, rather than 47, chromosomes. The extra chromosomal material from a chromosome 21 is attached to another chromosome (Robertsonian or balanced translocation; see Table 7.1). Usually, one of the parents is a carrier of Down's syndrome and has the translocation in a balanced form; 45 chromosomes with the extra copy of chromosome 21 attached to another chromosome (Fig. 7.20). This means that the translocation carrier is not directly affected but will produce a proportion of gametes with an unbalanced complement of chromosomes. There is frequently an associated history of recurrent spontaneous abortion due to lethal arrangements of chromosomes in the gametes.

Case study 7.2 looks at concerns related to Down's syndrome.

Structural abnormalities

Autosomal abnormalities

Structural chromosomal abnormalities include translocations, where material is exchanged between chromosomes, inversions, where a segment of the chromosome is rotated through 180°, and deletions, where segments

Case study 7.2

Josie is 48 years old and has four children between 14 and 24 years of age. She attends the midwives' clinic in a state of shock as her doctor has just informed her she is 8 weeks' pregnant.
- What advice would the midwife need to give to Josie in relation to antenatal screening?

Josie attends her local maternity unit at 12 weeks' gestation for a nuchal translucency scan and is given an estimated risk of a one in six possibility of a Down's syndrome baby.
- What further investigations could be offered to Josie and how can the midwife best support her during this period of investigation?

of chromosomes are lost (Fig. 7.21). Cri du chat syndrome is associated with deletion of the short arm of chromosome 5. Deletions leave the affected chromosomes with fragile sites that adhere to each other, forming ring chromosomes. In inversions, a parent may have the correct amount of chromosomal material and therefore no clinical problem, but the chromosomes align inappropriately in meiosis so gamete formation is affected. Many chromosomal disorders affect fertility.

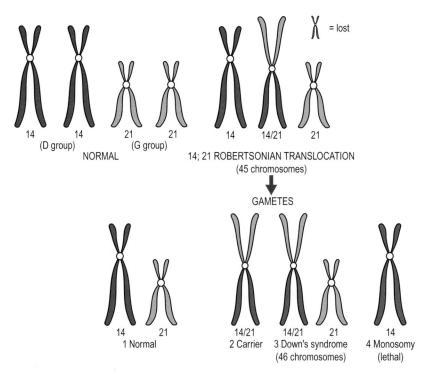

Fig. 7.20 Robertsonian translocation.

Fig. 7.21 Gross chromosome aberrations: deletions, inversion, duplication and translocation.

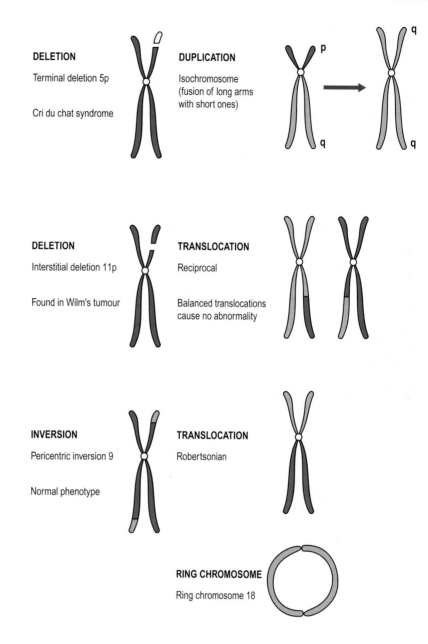

DELETION

Terminal deletion 5p

Cri du chat syndrome

DUPLICATION

Isochromosome (fusion of long arms with short ones)

DELETION

Interstitial deletion 11p

Found in Wilm's tumour

TRANSLOCATION

Reciprocal

Balanced translocations cause no abnormality

INVERSION

Pericentric inversion 9

Normal phenotype

TRANSLOCATION

Robertsonian

RING CHROMOSOME

Ring chromosome 18

Sex chromosome abnormalities

Sex chromosome anomalies are relatively common but produce fewer ill-effects than autosomal anomalies. Generally, the greater the number of extra sex chromosomes, the higher is the degree of mental retardation. Many sex chromosome anomalies also affect reproductive performance (see Chapter 5).

An example of an X chromosome abnormality is fragile X syndrome (Box 7.13).

Box 7.13 **Fragile X syndrome**

Fragile X syndrome is one of the commonest causes of mental retardation in males. It is inherited as an X-linked trait, affecting one in 1000 male babies. The fragile site on the X chromosome is on the long arm. Affected males often have a large head, prominent chin and ears and may develop large testes at puberty. A significant proportion of carrier women are mentally retarded.

EPIGENETICS AND IMPRINTING

Epigenetic modifications to the genome produce inheritable changes in gene expression which do not involve a change in sequence of bases in DNA. Thus the phenotype of the offspring is changed because bases in DNA are modified in some way without their sequence being altered. Epigenetics is the basis of genetic imprinting (see below). The expression of genes can be switched on or off by DNA methylation (the addition of a methyl group to a cytosine residue of DNA), by phosphorylation or by modification of the DNA-associated histone proteins. During embryonic development, for example, imprinting switches off the expression of key genes so that only the gene from one of the parents is expressed as the functional protein. This additional mechanism of regulation of gene expression has created challenges in animal cloning experiments and in human ovarian tissue cryopreservation.

Imprinted genes cluster in particular parts of the genome which are rich in CpG nucleotides (where a cytosine nucleotide is next to a guanine nucleotide linked by a phosphate group – CpG denotes Cytosine–phosphate–Guanine). CpG dinucleotides do not occur as often as predicted suggesting that they are vulnerable to mutation. The regions of the DNA strand which have a high prevalence of CpG nucleotides are called 'CpG islands'. CpG islands often occur at the beginning of a gene. Most of the cytosine nucleotides in CpG islands are methylated with the methyl group being attached to the cytosine. Methylation usually switches off – 'silences' – the gene. Histone modification of the DNA strand affects whether transcription factors can access the DNA to direct the transfer (transcription) of genetic material to RNA. There are about 20 000 genes in the human genome of which several hundreds are thought to be imprinted, predominantly affecting growth (including function of the placenta) and development including brain development (Keverne, 2010) (see Box 7.14).

Some genes are expressed when inherited from one parent but are not expressed when inherited from the other parent. This is genetic imprinting, the suppression or silencing of certain alleles on the chromosomes depending on their parental origin. Following fertilization, some genes are only expressed if they were inherited from the mother (the paternal gene being imprinted and therefore silenced), whereas others are expressed only if they were inherited from the father with the maternal gene being imprinted. Expression of some imprinted genes is spatially and temporally regulated and may only be active for a limited window during development.

Imprinted genes result in monoallelic gene expression and a number of diseases have been linked to defects in the normal imprinting process. The importance of genetic imprinting can be clearly seen in situations where imprinted

Box 7.14 Epigenetic control of growth

Insulin-like growth factor 2 (IGF2) is encoded by the IGF2 gene which is imprinted. A fetus inherits two copies of the IGF2 gene, one from each parent. Usually, the paternal copy is expressed and the maternal gene is silenced. If the maternal gene is expressed as well as the paternal gene, the fetus has Beckwith–Wiedemann Syndrome which results in a high birthweight and other markers of overgrowth such as macroglossia (enlarged tongue) and an increased risk of childhood cancer (Eggermann et al., 2008). If both the maternal and paternal genes are silenced, the result is Silver–Russell (or Russell–Silver) syndrome which is due to fetal undergrowth. Both conditions are rare but they occur with increased frequency in offspring derived from ICSI (see Chapter 6) suggesting the manipulation of gametes and embryos may affect imprinting.

genes are either inactivated or deleted on the normally active allele. The diseases Präder–Willi syndrome (PWS) and Angelman syndrome (AS) result, respectively, from a paternal (PWS) or a maternal (AS) deletion of the same region of chromosome 15 and since the alleles derived from the other parent are silenced by being imprinted, the genes are not expressed and their proteins are absent. In PWS, genes are deleted from the paternal chromosome 15 which are also imprinted on the maternal allele. In AS, the same region of chromosome 15 as that affected in PWS is deleted on the female allele and imprinted on the allele derived from the male.

Paternally imprinted genes tend to enhance fetal growth, whereas maternally expressed genes tend to constrict growth (see p. 220 for discussion of the 'conflict hypothesis'). Much of the research has been carried out in mice but in most genes, the imprinting status is conserved between species. Mouse genome manipulation demonstrates that androgenote mice, which have only paternal DNA, have a poor embryonic development and gynogenote mice, which have only maternal DNA, have poor placental development. In the mouse placenta, the paternal X chromosome is imprinted so that only the maternal genes are expressed and the paternal genes are silenced (Keverne, 2009). It is suggested that this may be important in avoiding a maternal immune rejection response to allogeneic fetal proteins that could be encoded by the paternal X chromosome (see Chapter 10). Gene expression in the brain is complex probably affecting behaviour, cognition and personality. In the preoptic area of the mouse brain, there is a high incidence of genes which are parentally imprinted; this area of the brain is a testosterone-dependent sexually dimorphic region which is important for male sexual behaviour and maternal care (Gregg et al., 2010).

The appropriate establishment and maintenance of the epigenetic imprints are essential for normal growth and development. Aberrant gene expressions due to imprinting problems are called 'epimutations'. These can occur during imprint erasure, when the primordial germ cells migrate to the gonadal ridges in embryonic development (see Chapter 9), during imprint establishment when gametogenesis occurs or during imprint maintenance, throughout the life of the organism. The paternal genome is actively demethylated within a few hours of fertilization, whereas the maternal genome is demethylated passively during the first few cleavages of the embryo in a species-dependent manner. This pattern of demethylation, which erases most imprinted genes from the parents in the preimplantation stage, spares some imprinted genes which are then maintained throughout development. Assisted reproductive techniques (ART) are associated with an increased risk of epigenetic disturbance which is more likely when gametes are manipulated (affecting imprint establishment) or when the preimplantation embryo is manipulated (affecting imprint maintenance). As the first ART involving invasive manipulation of gametes and embryo are fairly recent events, it is not yet clear whether there will be any long term epigenetic-medicated repercussions, the so-called 'ART ticking time bomb' (Grace and Sinclair, 2009).

GENETIC SCREENING

The detection of abnormal genetic conditions such as cystic fibrosis (e.g. Case study 7.3) has been the focus of much ongoing research. There are three particular areas in which genetic investigation can be used to assess risk factors and confirm diagnosis of genetic disorder: parental screening, preimplantation screening and antenatal assessment.

Parental screening

Individuals from families with a known prevalent genetic disorder may be tested to confirm whether they carry the abnormal gene. The findings form the basis of genetic counselling in which both the risks of passing on the abnormal gene and the possible consequences for a child are discussed. Frequently, this follows the delivery of an affected baby, especially if there is no family history. The condition may have arisen by spontaneous mutation and so the chances of it reoccurring in subsequent pregnancies may be much smaller than if the parents were actually carrying the defective gene.

Preimplantation genetic diagnosis and preimplantation genetic screening

Preimplantation genetic diagnosis (PGD) is a technique which allows diagnosis of genetic and chromosomal disorders in an embryo before pregnancy is established (Basille et al., 2009). It was developed as a test for couples carrying genetic disorders who were at risk of having a child with the disorder. However, the technique is also now used extensively for optimizing IVF outcome in couples who do not carry a genetic disorder (Spits and Sermon, 2009) because chromosomal aberrations occur at high frequency in all embryos and can be detected before implantation thus reducing the otherwise inevitable early pregnancy loss and increasing pregnancy rate in women who have poor IVF success rates. *In vitro* fertilization techniques (see Chapter 6) allow genetic analysis on polar bodies extracted from the oocyte before fertilization (first polar body) and/or after fertilization (second polar body). Genetic testing can also be carried out on a single cell from a 3-day-old embryo (at the cleavage stage) or on trophoblast cells from the blastocyst at day 5. These techniques thus allow selection of normal embryos for subsequent implantation. PGD and preimplantation genetic screening (PGS) utilize molecular techniques such as fluorescent *in situ* hybridization, DNA analysis and polymerase chain reaction (PCR; see Box 7.15) to detect single-gene disorders, such as thalassaemias or cystic fibrosis, or to screen for structural or numerical chromosome disorders. PGD offers an alternative to prenatal diagnosis and selective termination of an affected pregnancy, which may be important for couples who cannot contemplate termination of a pregnancy. The identification and selection of euploid embryos also has a positive effect on the clinical outcome of assisted reproductive technologies (see Chapter 6) as chromosomal abnormalities are one of the major causes of spontaneous abortion and implantation failure. There are, however, detrimental effects of the biopsy procedures and removal of embryonic cells (Diedrich et al., 2007).

Antenatal assessment

It is common throughout the UK for the screening for certain genetic disorders to be offered to all women. The tests predict the mathematical probability of a pregnancy being

Case study 7.3

Tania has a brother who was diagnosed as having cystic fibrosis some years ago. Tania has been identified as being a carrier. Tania presents herself at the midwives' clinic with an unplanned pregnancy at 8 weeks' gestation. Her partner, Paul, has no family history of cystic fibrosis.
- What reassurance and advice can the midwife give to Tania?
- What referrals should the midwife make and how should this be explained to Tania?

Molecular genetics studies human variations and mutations at the level of the gene and is important for understanding and identifying genetic diseases. Application of molecular genetic methods allows DNA diagnosis from very small amounts of tissue.

Fluorescent *in situ* hybridization

This involves the use of a genetic probe, which attaches to the target gene that it is designed to detect. The probe has a fluorescent label and so the abnormal gene can be visualized. Fluorescent in situ hybridization is used to identify microdeletions, aneuploidy and translocations.

Polymerase chain reaction

A small fragment of DNA is selectively amplified (at least a million times) by enzymatic procedures to produce large quantities of the relevant restriction fragments. These fragments can then be visualized by electrophoresis through an agarose gel, which is stained with a fluorescent dye. Polymerase chain reaction (PCR) is used to identify single-gene disorders such as fragile X syndrome, Huntington's disease and muscular dystrophy. PCR can be used for any condition for which gene sequencing, and therefore the information required to design primers for selective amplification, is available.

affected. If a test results in a high risk of abnormality, a diagnostic procedure such as chorionic villi sampling or amniocentesis may be offered. The aim is to detect chromosomal and anatomical abnormalities. Minor structural variants that can be detected by ultrasound are described as 'soft markers' (Loughna, 2009); these cannot be used in isolation but together with other markers can predict the probability of risk. Clinical tests include first-trimester nuchal transluceny (NT) ultrasound, second-trimester maternal serum screening and second semester ultrasound for anatomical survey. Methods of prenatal screening have to be adapted for women with multiple gestation (Cleary-Goldman et al., 2005); offspring of multiple gestation is at increased risk of abnormality but zygosity has to be first inferred from ultrasound diagnosis of chorionicity. In women, who conceive with egg donation, it is the age of the ovum donor that is important.

First-trimester NT ultrasound

At around 12 weeks' gestation, the nuchal fat pad at the back of the fetus's neck is measured using ultrasound assessment. NT increases with crown-rump length so the findings combined with maternal age and fetal size (crown-rump length) indicate a higher or lower risk of the fetus having Down's syndrome. The detection rate is about 83%. If the NT is raised, but the karyotype is normal, the fetus may be checked later for other physiological conditions such as cardiac abnormalities.

An increased NT (thicker fat pad) indicates an increased risk of a genetic or physical abnormality being present. Abnormal NT is also associated with other trisomies and fetal abnormalities (Souka et al., 1998). It is not clear why such conditions result in a thicker NT but this may be related to oedema due to cardiac conditions, or failure of the neck lymphatic structures to develop at the right time, or both. Each case has to be assessed on an individual basis taking into consideration the maternal age and fetal size, although measurements less than 1.9 mm are probably normal, whereas those greater than 3 mm are probably abnormal.

Second-trimester maternal serum screening tests

The risk of Down's syndrome can also be estimated by a combination of blood tests, such as the levels of hCG (human chorionic gonadotrophin, which is usually raised in singleton Down's syndrome pregnancies), AFP (alpha-fetoprotein, which is usually low in a Down's syndrome pregnancy), unconjugated oestriol and inhibin-A at around 16 weeks in combination with maternal age (Table 7.6). These tests have various formats and are often referred to as double, triple or Bart's, and quadruple test and so on. Trisomy becomes more common with an increase in maternal age and is linked to an increasing failure of the division of the oocyte to be completed normally. The results from the biochemical indicators are combined with the maternal age risk and compared with normal values, adjusted for gestational age, to establish the likelihood ratio (probability or risk) of the pregnancy being affected.

Combined and integrated tests

Combined testing refers to combining the results of blood tests and ultrasound scans before the completion of the 14th week of pregnancy to predict risk of Down's syndrome; this is more sensitive than using blood tests and ultrasound examination in isolation. Integrated testing involves two blood tests, one in the first trimester (ideally between 10 and 12 weeks) followed by another blood test in the second trimester (ideally between 15 and 20 weeks). The results of the tests are evaluated using sophisticated risk evaluation software.

Ultrasound

All pregnant women in the UK are currently offered an ultrasound scan at approximately 20 weeks' gestation. The scan entails the detailed examination of the gross anatomical structures, such as internal organs, head, limbs and spine, and assessment of fetal growth. Many physical

Table 7.6 Combination test screening for chromosomal abnormalities

INDICATOR	SOURCE	RATIONALE	CONSIDERATIONS
Alpha fetoprotein (AFP)	Amniotic fluid Maternal serum (MSAFP – levels about 1000 times less than amniotic fluid)	MSAFP levels are reduced in pregnancies affected by trisomy 21 and other trisomies. AFP leaks from exposed capillaries into amniotic fluid in fetuses with NTD and some other malformations	The results are interpreted using appropriate standards for ethnic background: MSAFP is lower in Asian women and higher in Black women. Levels are reduced in mothers with insulin-dependent diabetes
Human chorionic gonadotrophin (hCG)	Maternal serum	Values are higher in trisomy 21 and lower in trisomy 18	Free β-subunit may be measured
Unconjugated oestriol (E3)	Maternal serum	Values are lower in trisomy 21	
Pregnancy-associated plasma protein A (PAPP-A)	Maternal serum	Values are lower in trisomy 21	PAPP-A increases with gestation. PAPP-A measurement may be used in first-trimester screening

abnormalities, such as cardiac defects and limb length, are markers which may indicate the presence of a genetic abnormality. The more abnormal the ultrasound findings, the higher the risk of fetal aneuploidy. Abnormalities include structural malformations, increased nuchal thickness, short ear length, short femur or humerus, an extra vessel in the umbilical cord, a wide space between the toes and increased bowel echogenicity (Ott and Taysi, 2001). This has led to the development of ultrasound scoring systems to identify fetuses at risk and support to the suggestion that ultrasound alone may be an alternative method of detecting genetic abnormalities in women who are reluctant to undergo amniocentesis.

Amniocentesis and chorionic villus sampling

Diagnosis of the above disorders can be confirmed only with more invasive procedures such as chorionic villus sampling (CVS) and amniocentesis (withdrawal of amniotic fluid) (Fig. 7.22). Both of these procedures enable the karyotype of the fetus to be examined, enabling fetal sexing, the identification of a trisomy or the presence of markers indicating the presence of abnormal alleles. Other invasive techniques are fetoscopy and cordiocentesis (fetal blood sampling) and biopsy. These procedures carry a slightly increased risk of procedure-related loss; however, the spontaneous abortion rate is higher in pregnancies with chromosomal abnormalities.

The fetal cells in the amniotic fluid or villus sample are grown in culture to produce enough cells for testing. The time taken for a result depends on the number of cells in the original sample and their growth rate, which can be affected by contamination with blood or maternal cells. The cell sample is greater in CVS so results are usually quicker. Occasionally, results can be complicated by chromosomal mosaicism where an individual has two or more cell lines, each with different chromosome numbers, derived from one zygote. For example, 1% of people with Down's syndrome are mosaics with both trisomic cells and normal cells; the clinical outcome is much better in these cases but if the abnormal cells are in the gonads there may be a high risk of producing abnormal gametes.

Amniocentesis and CVS are both invasive methods of prenatal diagnosis with inherent risks for the pregnancy. Alternative less-invasive methods of obtaining fetal cells and nucleic acids (DNA and RNA) are being studied because they are not associated with the same increased risk of miscarriage. The placenta is not a totally impermeable barrier. Some fetal cells transfer to the maternal circulation (see microchimerism, p. 242); there is approximately one fetal cell per millilitre of maternal blood. These intact fetal cells can be separated from maternal cells by flow cytometry (automated cell sorting equipment) as the cells have different morphological characteristics. Developments in molecular biology mean that PCR amplification assays (see p. 169) can be used for prenatal screening and genetic diagnosis. The discovery that fetal cell-free DNA and RNA (nucleic acids probably derived from apoptosis of the trophoblast during placental development) can also be extracted from the maternal blood has potential widespread clinical applications, particularly as intact fetal cells in maternal blood are rare. Routine non-invasive prenatal diagnosis using nucleic acids extracted from maternal plasma has been used to detect blood group incompatibility, fetal sex and some single-gene disorders (Avent et al., 2009). Although DNA extraction from fetal cells isolated from cervical mucus appeared to also offer the potential

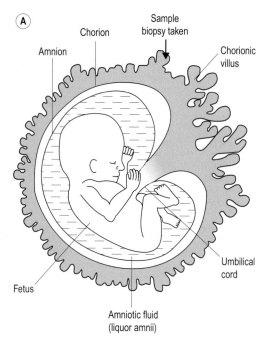

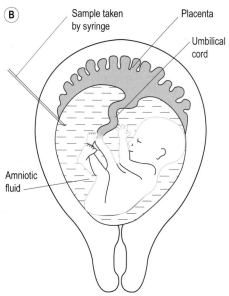

Fig. 7.22 (A) Amniocentesis; (B) transvaginal chorionic villus sampling (CVS). (Reproduced with permission from Brooker, 1998.)

Table 7.7 Prenatal diagnostic procedures

PROCEDURE	GESTATION AT WHICH TEST IS PERFORMED (WEEKS)	CONDITIONS SCREENED FOR OR DIAGNOSED
Non-invasive techniques		
NT measurement by ultrasound scan	12	Screen for trisomic conditions and other abnormalities
AFP test	16	Screen for neural tube defects
Triple/double/ Bart's test	16	Screen for Down's syndrome
Ultrasound scan	20	Diagnosis of gross physical defects
Invasive techniques		
CVS	10–12	Diagnosis of chromosomal abnormality
Amniocentesis	16	Diagnosis of chromosomal abnormality
Fetoscopy		Diagnosis of chromosomal abnormality
Cordocentesis (removal of fetal blood from the umbilical cord)		Diagnosis of metabolic disorders
		Assessment of antibody status in haemolytic disease
		Detection of fetal infection
Organ biopsy (liver, skin, etc.)		Metabolic disorders
		Hereditary disorders

for early non-invasive prenatal diagnosis, there have been some issues with cell collection and detection rate (Cioni et al., 2003).

Table 7.7 summarizes the prenatal diagnostic procedures and Box 7.15 describes the techniques for molecular detection of abnormal genes.

EVOLUTION

Evolution is the study of genetic variation within populations and how this variation allows populations to evolve in response to changes within the environment in which they live. The variation of genes within a defined population is referred to as the gene pool. Charles Darwin's famous book 'On the Origin of the Species by Means of Natural Selection, or the Preservation of Favoured Faces in the Struggle for Life' (known as 'The Origin of the Species') (1859) presented the argument that all organisms descended from a common ancestor and advocated natural selection as the mechanism of evolution. The mechanism of evolution is still contested, particularly how other mechanisms such as random genetic drift have contributed to evolution and the effects of gradual accumulation of small genetic changes rather than fewer large ones.

As described earlier in this chapter, many disease processes have their aetiology in the physical expression (phenotype) of an abnormal gene (genotype). They are normally recessive, so the effects of the abnormal gene are masked by the presence of a normal gene. The physical effects of recessive genes are only seen when there are two recessive genes present in the genome, for instance, in cystic fibrosis (see also in Case study 7.4, which looks at the Rhesus-negative blood type). Some abnormal genes may be partially expressed or modified by the presence of a normal gene. Many heterozygous, partially expressed genetic conditions may, in the right environment, impart a beneficial effect on the individual. An example is the sickle cell trait HbA/HbS or HbA/HbC (see Box 7.3). If one recessive gene is present, the anaemia condition is expressed in a minor form. Whilst this can cause problems for individuals in periods of stress and physiological change, such as pregnancy, the symptoms are usually not life-threatening; on the contrary, in the malaria zones of the world the sickle cell trait is beneficial to heterozygotes as it affords some protection from the malaria parasite. This is because entry of the parasite into

the red blood cell causes the cell to die before the parasite has time to reproduce. In the major form of the disease when the individual inherits two abnormal genes, one from each parent, the haemoglobin configuration is abnormal. The erythrocytes are sickle-shaped and fragile which leads to severe complications of blood cell lysis and coagulation. Hence, although the homozygous form has implications for the survival of the affected individual, the abnormal gene is maintained within the gene pool because its partial form confers advantage in the gene pool of the population by increasing resistance to falciparum malaria. The absence of the Duffy surface antigen, which is usually present on the erythrocyte cell membrane, also affords protection against malaria as the malarial parasite attaches itself to this particular antigen to enable it to enter the cell.

The environment is ever changing and so the process of evolution as a result continues to facilitate adaptation to such changes. The process of evolution itself may then complicate our own understanding of human physiological processes. More than one regulatory system may develop at different times within our evolutionary progression. Different prevailing environmental conditions would thus influence the evolution of changes within the regulation mechanisms to match the change within the environment. Human physiological processes can be described as being in two evolutionary states that are either progressing or declining. Our reproductive physiology may still be influenced by processes that evolved to cope with the Pleistocene environment, in which it is believed that the genus Homo first evolved, even though these may now be in a state of evolutionary decline. In contrast, it is believed that our physiological processes may be responding to 'younger' evolutionary influences and therefore be in a state of evolutionary progression. Depending on the external (exogenous) and internal (endogenous) conditions present, the response to either of these evolutionary types may still be initiated.

 Case study 7.4

Jane is a 30-year-old woman expecting her second baby. Her first baby was born 3 years ago in rural Africa. She has now returned to this country at 36 weeks' gestation. The blood group results from her first antenatal visit show that Jane's blood group type is O, Rhesus negative.

- What are the implications of this?
- If it is known that her partner has the same blood group, what are the risks of the pregnancy being affected?
- If Jane's first baby was Rhesus positive, what risk is there to the current fetus and how does it depend on its own blood group?
- If a baby is affected by haemolytic disease of the newborn, what clinical symptoms are likely to be evident and how can they be treated?
- If the first baby had been born in England, how would Jane have been treated?

Key points

- Genetics is a reductionist science that uses mathematical probability to predict the risk of inheriting certain characteristics, usually of medical relevance. Techniques such as combination diagrams and Punnett squares can be used to predict the probability of inheriting single-gene traits.
- DNA is the 'blueprint' of the organism, which is organized into chromosomes within the cell nuclei. A gene is a unit of a chromosome, or length of DNA, that codes for a particular instruction. Humans have 23 pairs of chromosomes: 22 pairs of autosomes and a pair of sex chromosomes (XX in females and XY in males).

Continued

169

Key points—cont'd

- The structure of DNA facilitates its semiconservative replication prior to cell division, thus each cell of an organism has the same DNA.
- Mitosis is normal cell division producing daughter diploid cells with 23 pairs (i.e. 46) of chromosomes. Meiosis is a specific cell division in gamete formation that results in the number of chromosomes being reduced to 23 (the haploid number).
- DNA controls protein synthesis by acting as a template for the formation of mRNA (transcription); mRNA induces protein synthesis by directing the incorporation of amino acids into the protein (translation).
- There are accumulated errors in replicating DNA, which may manifest as mutations causing proteins with abnormal structure and function to be formed.
- A trait that is dominantly inherited is expressed if the individual has at least one copy of the gene, whereas a recessively inherited trait is expressed only if the individual inherits the gene from both parents. Sex-linked traits affect males more than females, who may be carriers.
- Chromosomal abnormalities may be numerical or structural and have serious clinical implications for those affected.
- Detection of fetal abnormalities is a routine part of antenatal care, which has developed screening programmes to assess risk and tests to confirm diagnosis.

Application to practice

It is important to realize that the genetic diversity of a population drives the process of evolution and adaptation to changes in the external environment.

Many genes are labelled as abnormal but they may be essential variants that may at least contribute to the survival of the population as a whole.

The focus of antenatal screening of the fetus is based upon the detection of the abnormal using tests that are both invasive such as CVS and non-invasive such as ultrasound scanning. In many situations, the conditions being screened for have a genetic cause or dysfunction. Knowledge of this is essential for the midwife to be able to understand and explain what the tests actually involve and what the results may indicate.

Midwives have an increasing role in the care of women suffering from pregnancy loss for whatever reasons, so an in-depth knowledge of fetal abnormalities is essential in providing care for the women.

Preimplantation genetic diagnosis can be performed on early embryos following IVF before implantation. This means that some genetic conditions can be identified as part of the embryo selection procedures so that only non-affected embryos are replaced into the uterine cavity. This does not, however, guarantee a healthy infant and couples undergoing this technique may have high anxiety levels.

ANNOTATED FURTHER READING

Burley J, Harris J, editors: *Companion to genetics*, 2004, Wiley-Blackwell.

An interesting multidisciplinary and well-explained collection of essays describing the many ethical, legal, social and political issues raised by the recent developments in human genetics.

Butler MG: Genomic imprinting disorders in humans: a mini-review, *J Assist Reprod Genet* 26:477–486, 2009.

A clear explanation of genomic imprinting and the effects of aberrant expression and silencing of genes, illustrated by the examples of Prader–Willi and Angelman syndromes.

Department of Health 2008 NHS Fetal Anomaly Screening Programme – Screening for Down's syndrome: UK NSC Policy recommendations 2007–2010: Model of Best Practice UK National Screening Committee.

This booklet gives in-depth details of current methods used in the UK for antenatal screening.

Dupont C, Armant DR, Brenner CA: Epigenetics: definition, mechanisms and clinical perspective, *Semin Reprod Med* 27:351–357, 2009.

A recent review about epigenetic mechanisms which considers the epigenetic issues for assisted reproductive technology and the potential clinical implications.

Emery AEH, Mueller RF, Young ID: *Emery's elements of medical genetics*, ed 11, New York, 2001, Churchill Livingstone.

A comprehensive textbook which is divided into three parts. Section A focuses on genetic principles, risk prediction and factors influencing inheritance. Section B covers medical aspects of genetics including genetic diseases and genetic factors in diseases. Section C deals with clinical applications, including genetic counselling, ethical issues, screening and diagnosis.

Ferguson-Smith MA: Placental mRNA in maternal plasma: prospects for fetal screening, *Proc Natl Acad Sci USA* 100:4360–4362, 2003.

A short description of the tests used for fetal screening including the use of placental DNA in maternal plasma.

Genetic Interest Group: A Guide to Cord Blood Banking for Families with Genetic Conditions, London, 2009, GIG.

A concise and well-written pamphlet aimed at families who are considering storing or donating cord blood for treatment of a child (or other relatives or unknown recipients) with a genetic condition. Contains links to useful websites.

Hartl DL: *Essential genetics: a genomics perspective*, ed 5, 2011, Jones and Bartlett Publishers, Inc.

A popular and well-illustrated textbook, suitable for beginners, which clearly explains genetic concepts from the principles of hereditary and genetic analysis to molecular genetics.

Kingston HM: *ABC of clinical genetics*, ed 3 (revised), London, 2002, BMJ.

A slim, well-illustrated volume, targeted at clinicians, which describes genetic mechanisms, diseases and diagnosis.

Maynard Smith J, Szathmary E: *The origins of life: from the birth of life to the origin of language*, 2000, Oxford Paperbacks.

The authors present their hypothesis on the origin of life and alternative views of evolution focusing on seven transitions from the beginning of life on earth, the chemistry of molecular cycles and the origins of language.

Moore J, Bhide A: Ultrasound prenatal diagnosis of structural abnormalities, *Obstet Gynaecol Reprod Med* 19:333–338, 2009.

A succinct paper describing the detection of more common fetal anomalies by ultrasound.

National Collaborating Centre for Women's and Children's Health: *Antenatal care: routine care for the healthy pregnant woman*, 2008, National Institute for Clinical Excellence.

This guidance details the current recommendations and methods for routine antenatal screening in the UK.

Richards JE, Hawley RSSH: *The human genome: a user's guide*, ed 3, 2010, Academic Press.

A description of the human genome project and its implications which considers how genetic issues affect health and public policy; includes chapters on forensics, stem cell biology, bioinformatics and ethical issues.

Ridley M: *Nature via nurture: genes, experience and what makes us human*, New York, 2004, Harper Collins.

A readable discourse about the effects of environment on genetics which covers historical and social facets as well as biological aspects of various topics such as child development, schizophrenia and the experience of twins.

Russell PJ: *iGenetics: a Mendelian approach*, New York, 2005, Harper Collins.

A modern approach to genetics which covers fundamentals of genetics using an experimental enquiry-solving approach includes experimental data from research studies, critical thinking skills, problems and worked examples.

Shenfield F: Ethical aspects of pre-implantation diagnosis, *Obstet Gynaecol Reprod Med* 18:312–313, 2008.

A brief overview of some of the ethical issues raised by PGD including eugenic practices, fair access to technology, 'saviour siblings', social sex selection and late onset disorders.

Tobias ST, Connor JM, Ferguson-Smith MA: *Essential medical genetics*, ed 6, Oxford, 2011, Blackwell.

An updated and well-written text that introduces the basic principles and clinical applications of genetics with a focus on the molecular mechanisms involved in genetic disorders and diseases. Also covers the genetics of common diseases and cancer, prenatal screening and gene therapy.

Turnpenny P, Ellard S: *Emery's elements of medical genetics*, ed 13, New York, 2007, Churchill Livingstone.

A comprehensive textbook which is divided into three parts. Section A focuses on genetic principles, risk prediction and factors influencing inheritance. Section B covers medical aspects of genetics including genetic diseases and genetic factors in diseases. Section C deals with clinical applications, including genetic counselling, ethical issues, screening and diagnosis.

Wolpert CM, Singer ML, Speer MC: Speaking the language of genetics: a primer, *J Midwifery Womens Health* 50:184–188, 2005.

A brief background to genetic concepts and terminology included for healthcare professionals working in primary care settings.

Wright A, Hastie N: *Genes and common diseases: genetics in modern medicine*, 2007, Cambridge University Press.

This book explores the clinical implications of the recent advances in genetic and molecular research, and considers both the potential strengths and limitations of genetics in understanding common diseases.

http://fetalanomaly.screening.nhs.uk/tests_about.

This website details current UK antenatal policy with information produced for both public and health care professionals.

REFERENCES

Aitken RJ, Graves JAM: The future of sex, *Nature* 415:963, 2002.

Avent ND, Madgett TE, Maddocks DG, et al: Cell-free fetal DNA in the maternal serum and plasma: current and evolving applications, *Curr Opin Obstet Gynecol* 21:175–179, 2009.

Badcock C, Crespi B: Battle of the sexes may set the brain, *Nature* 454:1054–1055, 2008.

Basille C, Frydman R, El Aly A, et al: Preimplantation genetic diagnosis: state of the art, *Eur J Obstet Gynecol Reprod Biol* 145:9–13, 2009.

Brooker CG: *Human structure and function*, ed 2, St. Louis, 1998, Mosby, pp 8, 20, 514.

Cioni R, Bussani C, Scarselli B, et al: Fetal cells in cervical mucus in the first trimester of pregnancy, *Prenat Diagn* 23:168–171, 2003.

Cleary-Goldman J, D'Alton ME: Growth abnormalities and multiple gestations, *Seminars Perinatol* 32:206–212, 2008.

Craig IW, Harper E, Loat CS: The genetic basis for sex differences in human behaviour: role of the sex chromosomes, *Ann Hum Genet* 68:269–282, 2004.

Darwin C: *On the origin of the species by means of natural selection*, London, 1859, John Murray.

Dawkins R: *The selfish gene*, ed 2, Oxford, 1989, Oxford University Press.

Dawkins R: *The extended phenotype: the long reach of the gene*, revised edn, Oxford, 1999, Oxford University Press.

Diedrich K, Fauser BC, Devroey P, et al: The role of the endometrium and embryo in human implantation, *Hum Reprod Update* 13:365–377, 2007.

Eggermann T, Eggermann K, Schonherr N: Growth retardation versus overgrowth: Silver-Russell syndrome is genetically opposite to Beckwith-Wiedemann syndrome, *Trends Genet* 24:195–204, 2008.

Goodwin B: *Health and development: conception to birth*, Milton Keynes, 1997, Open University.

Goto H, Peng L, Makova KD: Evolution of X-degenerate Y chromosome genes in greater apes: conservation of gene content in human and gorilla, but not chimpanzee, *J Mol Evol* 68:134–144, 2009.

Grace KS, Sinclair KD: Assisted reproductive technology, epigenetics, and long-term health: a developmental time bomb still ticking, *Semin Reprod Med* 27:409–416, 2009.

Graves JAM: The rise and fall of SRY, *Trends Genet* 18:259–264, 2002.

Gregg C, Zhang J, Butler JE, et al: Sex-specific parent-of-origin allelic expression in the mouse brain, *Science* 329:682–685, 2010.

Hassold T, Hunt P: To err (meiotically) is human: the genesis of human aneuploidy, *Nat Rev Genet* 2:280–291, 2001.

Hunt PA, Hassold TJ: Sex matters in meiosis, *Science* 296:2181–2183, 2002.

Huynh KD, Lee JT: X-chromosome inactivation: a hypothesis linking ontogeny and phylogeny, *Nat Rev Genet* 6:410–418, 2005.

Jones S: *The language of the genes: biology, history and evolutionary future,* London, 1994, Flamingo.

Keverne B: Monoallelic gene expression and mammalian evolution, *Bioessays* 31:1318–1326, 2009.

Keverne EB: Neuroscience: a mine of imprinted genes, *Nature* 466:823–824, 2010.

Loughna P: Soft markers: where are we now?, *Obstetr Gynaecol Reprod Med* 19:127–129, 2009.

Open University: *Inheritance and cell division. Unit 20 in: Science foundation course (S102),* Milton Keynes, 1987, Open University, p 48.

Open University: *DNA: molecular aspects of genetics. Unit 24 in: Science foundation course (S102),* Milton Keynes, 1988, Open University, pp 14, 36.

Ott WJ, Taysi K: Obstetric ultrasonographic findings and fetal chromosomal abnormalities: refining the association, *Am J Obstet Gynecol* 184:1414–1421, 2001.

Sadler TW: *Langman's medical embryology,* Baltimore, Lippincott Williams & Wilkins, 2010.

Souka AP, Snijders RJM, Novakov A, et al: Defects and syndromes in chromosomally normal fetuses with increased nuchal translucency thickness at 10–14 weeks of gestation, *Ultrasound Obstet Gynecol* 11:391–400, 1998.

Spits C, Sermon K: PGD for monogenic disorders: aspects of molecular biology, *Prenat Diagn* 29:50–56, 2009.

Sykes B: *The seven daughters of Eve,* London, 2001, Transworld Publishers.

Chapter | 8 |

The placenta

LEARNING OBJECTIVES

- To describe the development of the placenta, membranes and umbilical cord.
- To describe the structure of the placenta, membranes and umbilical cord and recognize common structural variants.
- To identify the roles of the placenta.
- To discuss how abnormal placental development might affect fetal development including intrauterine growth retardation and other outcomes of the pregnancy.
- To describe methods for monitoring placental function.
- To outline the development of the placenta in twin pregnancies.

 Chapter case study

At Zara's 20-week scan, the ultrasonographer documented in her report that the placenta was situated on the anterior wall of the uterus with the majority of the placental body situated in the middle and lower pole of the uterine body with the lateral edge of the placenta approximately 2 cm from the internal cervical os.
- What are the possible complications that could arise from this situation?
- How do you think the midwife should discuss these possible complications with Zara and how they could be recognized?
- Why is it common for women with this situation to have vaginal bleeding around 34 weeks of pregnancy?
- Are there any conditions or factors related to low lying placentas and if so how can these be managed?

INTRODUCTION

The development of the placenta is critical for fetal survival because of the importance of the placenta in maternal–fetal transfer. It has a range of functional activities (Table 8.1), including complex synthetic capabilities, which are essential to the development of a normal term baby. The placenta flourishes in an immunologically foreign environment and has an important role in the immunological acceptance of the fetal allograft (see Chapter 10). Essentially, the placenta acts as a vascular parasite, depending on maternal blood for oxygen and nutrients and removal of waste products. The structure of the placenta means that, although optimal diffusion gradients are established, maternal and fetal blood never actually mixes.

The placenta and the chorion (outer membrane) are derived from the trophoblast layer of blastocyst cells (see Fig. 6.6, p. 128). Other extraembryonic tissues develop from the inner cell mass. These include the amnion (inner membrane), the yolk sac, the allantois (a largely vestigial structure in humans) and the extraembryonic mesoderm. The umbilical cord and the blood vessels of the placenta are derived from the extraembryonic mesoderm.

The human placenta is haemochorial, which means that maternal blood comes into contact with the placental trophoblast cells. The uteroplacental unit is made up of both fetal and maternal components. The placenta as seen at delivery is just the fetal component or chorionic plate. The maternal component or basal plate is the placental bed which underlies the fetal component and the uteroplacental circulation that vascularizes the placental bed. Between the

Table 8.1 Summary of placental functions

FUNCTION	PLACENTAL ROLE
Respiration	Maternal oxyhaemoglobin dissociates in the intervillous spaces. O_2 diffuses through the walls of the villi where it binds to fetal haemoglobin forming fetal oxyhaemoglobin. Transfer is increased by the higher affinity of fetal haemoglobin for O_2 (see Chapter 15). The lower CO_2 level facilitates transfer of CO_2 in the reverse direction in pregnancy (see Chapter 11)
Nutrition	Active transport of glucose, iron and some vitamins and passive transport of other nutrients. The placenta can metabolize proteins, fats and carbohydrates into simple molecules. Fats cross the placenta with less ease so the fat-soluble vitamins (A, D, E and K) cross slowly. The placenta stores glycogen, which can be converted to glucose when required
Excretion	Waste products of metabolism, CO_2 and heat cross from the fetus to the mother
Protection	The placenta acts as a barrier against most bacteria (such as cocci and bacilli). However, smaller micro-organisms (such as the syphilis bacterium) and viruses (including rubella, varicella-zoster, cytomegalovirus, coxsackie and HIV) can cross the villi. The placenta transfers IgG antibodies (see Chapter 10) and Rhesus antibodies to the fetus. Drugs including teratogens (see Chapter 9), anaesthetics and carbon monoxide (from smoking) can cross the placenta
Endocrine role	Initially, the trophoblast produces hCG, which maintains the corpus luteum and its production of steroid hormones. From the third month onwards, oestrogen and progesterone are produced in large quantities by the placenta. hPL is produced from the syncytiotrophoblast. The placenta also produces a broad range of other hormones including corticosteroids, ACTH, TSH, IGFs, prolactin, relaxin, endothelin and prostaglandins
Immunological role	The trophoblast has unique immunological properties that render it immunologically inert so a maternal antigenic response does not occur (see Chapter 10)

chorionic and basal plates is the intervillous space where the maternal–fetal exchange occurs. Conversion of the maternal spiral arteries to dilated and flaccid vessels is an essential step for successful pregnancy. Abnormal placental function is strongly associated with fetal complications, but study of the human placenta, particularly the maternal component, is not easy. Placentation in the human is unique, which means that observations from other species can be applied to humans only with caution. Placental reserve needs to exceed fetal requirements (otherwise the fetus could be compromised under conditions of hypoxia). It might be expected that placental size would increase in parallel with increased fetal size; however, the placental:fetal weight ratio actually decreases during gestation (Kingdom et al., 1993). Placental efficiency is best described as grams of fetus produced per gram of placenta developed (Wilson and Ford, 2001). Indeed, as there is a relationship between size at birth and life expectancy which is associated with the placental supply of nutrients; lighter placentas are more efficient placentas and associated with better long-term health outcome (Fowden et al., 2009). Placental efficiency is affected by the surface area for exchange, the thickness of the barriers between fetal and maternal circulations and the arrangement of the fetal and maternal blood vessels ('vascular architecture'). It is the later variable that appears to account for species differences in placental efficiency. The most efficient human placentas are those which are small in diameter and thin; it is thought that these small placentas must functionally adapt to increase nutrient transporter abundance and become more efficient.

Instead, placental efficiency is enhanced by an increase in both the number of carrier proteins involved in the transport of substances across the placenta and the placental perfusion.

UTERINE RECEPTIVITY

The first phase of the development of uterine receptivity is regulated by oestrogen and progesterone which stimulate the presence of microvilli on the columnar epithelial cells of the endometrium. Smooth muscle myosin also increases and the stromal cells proliferate. The second phase is described as the blastocyst response phase (Banerjee and Fazleabas, 2010). The signals involved in the exquisitely sensitive dialogue between the embryo and the endometrium include human chorionic gonadotrophin (hCG), interleukin-1 and insulin-like growth factor (IGF) 2 (see Chapter 3). In the third phase following attachment and implantation, signals between the newly formed embryo and primed endometrium cause endometrial changes, or decidualization, whereby the stromal cells under the endometrial epithelium accumulate lipid and glycogen and become known as decidual cells. The stroma thickens and blood flow increases. Decidualization promotes changes in the endometrium that make it receptive to implantation. Synchronous development and communication between the maternal endometrium and the embryonic tissue are required for successful establishment of pregnancy. Whereas mammalian embryos have intrinsic invasive potential and can initiate implantation-type reactions in many different tissues, the endometrium protects itself from implantation except for the limited duration of the implantation window (Bischof et al., 2000).

During the implantation or nidation window, micro-villi on the surface of the uterine endometrial cells fuse together to form single flower-like projections called pino-pods or uterodomes (Murphy, 2000). These smooth bleb-like protrusions which lack the typical microvilli form under the influence of progesterone (during the mid-luteal phase) only in the preferred sites of embryo–endometrial interac-tion and thus act as markers of uterine receptivity (Usadi et al., 2003). The pinopods are only present for 2–3 days during which implantation must occur. The interaction between the endometrium and the developing trophoblast is facilitated by a number of cytokines, metalloproteinases, surface integrins and growth factors, including IGFs and their binding proteins, which create a specific microenviron-ment which modulates trophoblast function. It is evident that implantation is a rather inefficient process in the human; the probability of conception during a menstrual cycle (defined as fecundity) is about 30% and over three quarters of failed pregnancies are thought to be due to implantation defects (Wilcox et al., 1999).

IMPLANTATION

Implantation is the consequence of a well-organized sequence of events involving synchronized crosstalk between the receptive endometrium and a functional blas-tocyst (Achache and Revel, 2006). It occurs in three stages: apposition, adhesion and invasion. The trophoblastic cells overlying the inner cell mass are known as the polar trophoblast; it is these cells that initiate the adhesion and implantation processes. The morula enters the uterus about 4 days after fertilization. It may float freely in the uterus before it hatches out of the protective zona pellu-cida (Kingdom and Sibley, 1996). About 7 days after fer-tilization, the blastocyst hatches and comes into contact with the endometrium. The blastocyst rolls freely over the endometrium until it reaches a receptive area. This process is thought to be mediated by glycoproteins called selectins which are expressed on the polar trophoblast cells of the newly hatched blastocyst (Vitiello and Patrizio, 2007). The blastocyst then orientates itself so that the embryonic pole implants first. Inappropriate implantation

of the blastocyst so there is reduced contact between the polar trophoblast and the uterine endothelium is thought to lead to abnormalities of umbilical cord insertion and even failure of pregnancy (Huppertz, 2008). The endome-trium produces MUC1, a mucin-rich glycoprotein, to pre-vent the blastocyst adhering to areas of the endometrium with poor chances of implantation. The optimally receptive areas of the endometrium secrete chemokines and growth factors to attract the blastocyst to the pinopods. The appo-sition of the blastocyst to the endometrium triggers the production of adhesion molecules such as integrins and cadherins which firmly anchor the blastocyst to the endo-metrial pinopods (Fig. 8.1). This process is enhanced because the endometrial surface expresses receptors for selectins. The tethering of the blastocyst to the endome-trium stimulates the polar trophoblastic cells to undergo rapid mitosis and proliferate as the invasion of the uterine wall commences. Implantation may be affected by mater-nal antiphospholipid syndrome hence the high incidence of pregnancy loss associated with this condition (Stone et al., 2006) (Case study 8.1).

DIFFERENTIATION INTO CYTOTROPHOBLAST AND SYNCYTIOTROPHOBLAST

There are two distinct cell layers in the blastocyst (see Chapter 6): the inner cell mass which is surrounded by an outer sphere of a single layer of mononucleated trophoblast cells. The trophoblast is the first cell type to

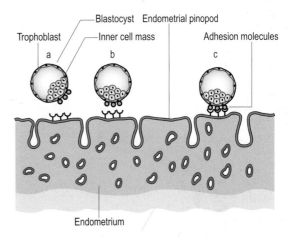

Fig. 8.1 The sequence of implantation: (a) the blastocyst comes close to the endometrial pinopods and the trophoblast overlying the embryonic pole expresses selectins. (b) the trophoblast selectins are recognised by the selectin receptors on the endometrium which (c) triggers the production of adhesion molecules. (Reproduced with permission from Achache and Revel, 2006.)

Case study 8.1

Trudy is a 36-year-old, para 1, gravida 11. She attends the midwives clinic at 6 weeks gestation, very distressed as this was not a planned pregnancy. Trudy informs the midwife that her last baby was born at 32 weeks gestation, very small for dates and that Trudy had also developed fulminating pre-eclampsia which was the main reason for the early delivery. Three days after this delivery Trudy developed severe difficulty in breathing which was diagnosed as a pulmonary embolism. Trudy then informs the midwife that all her other pregnancies had been spontaneous miscarriages at around 10 weeks gestation.

The midwife reviews Trudy's post obstetric notes and discovers that Trudy has antiphospholipid syndrome and that at her last delivery it was documented that the placenta was small and infarcted. As a result of this, the midwife immediately refers Trudy to attend a consultant clinic as an emergency.

- Why did the midwife refer Trudy to the consultant as an emergency?
- What treatment would be offered to Trudy and how will the pregnancy be managed?
- What is the significance of the placental infarcts and what was the most likely cause?

differentiate; this outer layer rapidly proliferates and develops into the placental tissue and fetal membranes.

The trophoblast differentiates into two layers: the outer syncytiotrophoblast and the inner cytotrophoblastic layer. Some of the proliferative cytotrophoblast cells lose their cell membranes and coalesce to form a multinucleated syncytium (a united mass of fused cellular material): the syncytiotrophoblast (Fig. 8.2). This outermost layer of the placenta has little proliferative and transcriptional activity; the maintenance and growth of the syncytiotrophoblast throughout gestation is dependent on the incorporation of cytotrophoblast cells into the layer. Apoptosis (programmed cell death) of trophoblast tissue increases throughout pregnancy as a normal part of trophoblast turnover and syncytiotrophoblast formation. The nuclei of the cells newly incorporated into the syncytiotrophoblast are initially similar to the nuclei of the cytotrophoblast cells but then undergo morphological changes; the chromatin condenses so the nuclei become smaller and denser eventually resembling late apoptotic nuclei. Some of these nuclei aggregate and are packaged into syncytial knots which are shred from the apical surface of the syncytiotrophoblast into the maternal circulation. In a normal pregnancy, these syncytial knots can be identified in maternal blood in the uterine veins but are destroyed in the maternal pulmonary vessels. In pre-eclampsia, syncytiotrophoblast renewal is overactive; there is an increase in apoptosis often complicated by aponecrosis. The syncytial knots are more prominent and are smaller so they can survive the maternal pulmonary vasculature and trigger a maternal systemic inflammatory response including an activated endothelium and increase in proinflammatory markers (Hawfield and Freedman, 2009).

The surface of the syncytiotrophoblast is covered in microvilli which increase the surface area. The syncytiotrophoblast expresses transporters, enzymes and receptors on its surface. It also produces hCG and hPL which are crucial to the maintenance of the pregnancy. hCG enhances differentiation of cytotrophoblasts into the syncytiotrophoblast. Electron microscopy reveals the syncytiotrophoblast to be a mass of cytoplasm containing remnants of intercellular

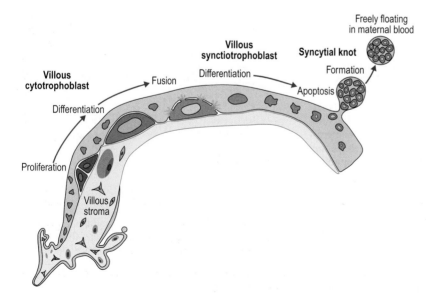

Fig. 8.2 The differentiation of villous cytotrophoblast into villous syncytiotrophoblast and the shedding of syncytial knots into maternal blood. (Reproduced from Huppertz, 2008.)

membrane, evenly dispersed nuclei and a few intermediate cells. This syncytial organization of cells is unusual; other than the trophoblast, multinucleated cells are seen only in some tumour cells and inflammatory giant cells (Chard, 1998). Interestingly, a range of tumour cells appears to secrete hCG (Iles and Chard, 1991) but at lower concentrations than those characteristic of trophoblast cells; these tumours usually affect individuals late in life.

The cytotrophoblasts, which form the inner monolayer of placental stem cells, are large clear discrete cuboidal cells each with a single nucleus, a few organelles and a well-defined cell membrane. These cells have marked mitotic activity and DNA synthesis. The syncytiotrophoblast increases in volume throughout the second week as cells detach from the proliferating layer of cytotrophoblast and fuse with the mass of syncytiotrophoblast. The syncytiotrophoblast has an invasive phenotype, secreting enzymes, which attack the endometrium, and hormones, which sustain the pregnancy. It is also involved in absorption of nutrients. The syncytiotrophoblast invasion is aggressive; between 6 and 9 days postfertilization the embryo becomes completely implanted into the endometrial stroma. The hydrolytic enzymes produced cause breakdown of the extracellular matrix between the cells of the endometrium thus eroding a pathway. The surface of the syncytiotrophoblast has tiny processes extending from it that penetrate between the endometrial cells, pulling the conceptus into the uterine wall. As implantation progresses, the expanding syncytiotrophoblast gradually envelops and encircles the blastocyst. The endometrial epithelium regenerates over the site of implantation, forming the decidua capsularis (Fig. 8.3). By 9 days, the embryo

is completely embedded within the endometrial wall with the syncytiotrophoblast forming a complete mantle around the entire conceptus so it is the only embryonic tissue in direct contact with the maternal tissue; this is important in protecting the embryo from rejection, The syncytiotrophoblast has a developmental gradient (Huppertz, 2008); it is thicker and better developed over the embryonic pole. Implantation is complete by about 10–12 days after fertilization. A plug of a cellular material called the coagulation plug or operculum seals the small hole at the point of implantation (Fig. 8.4).

In the first week of development, as the free-floating embryo or conceptus moves towards the uterine cavity propelled by the cilia movement and muscular contraction of the uterine tube, the cells can obtain nutrients from secretions of the uterine tubes and endometrium and eliminate waste products by simple diffusion. It is thought that endometrial secretions of lactate and pyruvate and possibly some amino acids may be important in the nutrition of the embryo for up to 8 weeks (Burton et al., 2001). The nutrients and oxygen are taken up by the syncytiotrophoblast; this is known as histiotrophic nutrition. By the end of the first trimester, there is a transition to haemotrophic nutrition from the uteroplacental circulation which provides a system in which the maternal and fetal circulations come

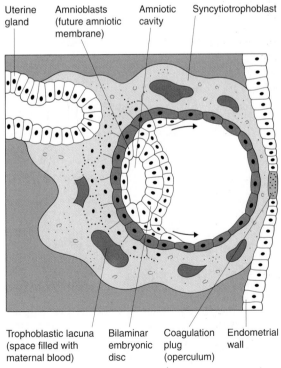

Uterine gland | Amnioblasts (future amniotic membrane) | Amniotic cavity | Syncytiotrophoblast

Trophoblastic lacuna (space filled with maternal blood) | Bilaminar embryonic disc | Coagulation plug (operculum) | Endometrial wall

Fig. 8.4 Implantation of blastocyst into the endometrial wall at 9 days postfertilization.

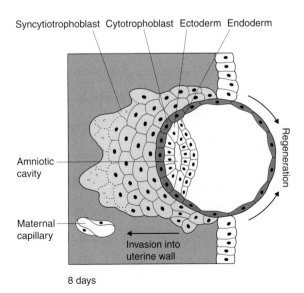

Syncytiotrophoblast Cytotrophoblast Ectoderm Endoderm

Amniotic cavity

Maternal capillary

Regeneration

Invasion into uterine wall

8 days

Fig. 8.3 Regeneration of endometrium over the site of implantation.

into close contact to facilitate transfer of substances from one system to the other.

As the syncytiotrophoblast penetrates the uterine wall, it comes into contact with the maternal endometrial capillaries and superficial veins. Fragments of these are engulfed within the syncytiotrophoblast forming fluid-filled trophoblastic lacunae (literally 'little lakes'); these coalesce to form larger lacunae which are the precursors of the intervillous spaces. As maternal blood vessels are progressively invaded, the lacunae fill with maternal blood. Maternal capillaries near the syncytio-trophoblast expand to form maternal sinusoids which rapidly anastomose with the trophoblastic lacunae. As this development continues, the lacunae become separated by columns of syncytiotrophoblast, or trabeculae, which effectively form a framework on which the villous tree of the placenta develops. The trabecular columns project radially from the blastocyst. The cytotrophoblast at the core of the columns proliferates locally to form extensions, which grow into the columns of syncytiotrophoblast. The growth of these protrusions is induced by the newly formed extraembryonic mesoderm (Fig. 8.5). The result is the primary stem villus, an outgrowth of cytotrophoblast covered by syncytiotrophoblast, which penetrates into the blood-filled lacuna (Fig. 8.6).

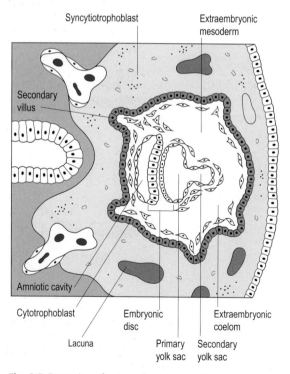

Fig. 8.5 Formation of extraembryonic mesoderm.

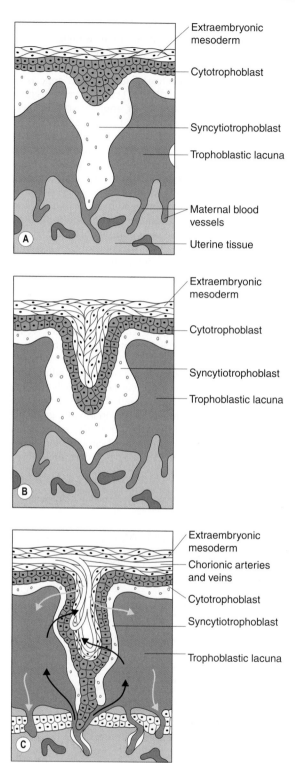

Fig. 8.6 The stem villus: (A) primary (11–13 days); (B) secondary (16 days); (C) tertiary (21 days).

EXTRAVILLOUS CYTOTROPHOBLAST AND REMODELLING OF THE UTERINE VESSELS

Cytotrophoblast migration and invasion

The cytotrophoblast layer has several distinct roles: (1) acting as proliferative progenitor or stem cell layer to generate and construct the developing syncytiotrophoblast which covers the villi; (2) forming the proliferative cell columns of the anchoring villi; (3) detaching from the cell columns and migrating into the maternal stroma to form interstitial cytotrophoblasts; and (4) migrating as non-proliferative extravillous cytotrophoblast cells to remodel the spiral arteries and replace the maternal endothelial cells (Knofler, 2010). These extravillous cytotrophoblast cells migrate from the villi beyond the leading edge of syncytiotrophoblast into the stroma. From about 12 days postfertilization, these cells invade the maternal capillaries and spiral arteries of the decidua. The extravillous cytotrophoblast cells initially plug the lumen of the maternal vessels that have been invaded and subsequently replace the maternal endothelium of these vessels. Plugging of the lumen of the invaded maternal blood vessels prevents bleeding and is achieved by day 14, which coincides with the expected date of the next menstrual period. If the maternal vessels are not plugged adequately during implantation and early development then vaginal bleeding may occur, which is associated with an increased risk of spontaneous miscarriage (sometimes haematomas can be seen on ultrasound investigation). The plugs prevent flow of maternal blood into the intervillous space in early pregnancy but allow a slow seepage of plasma (Jauniaux et al., 2003) so the lacunar spaces enclosed by the syncytiotrophoblast initially contain exudate from maternal vessels rather than blood. The developing placenta forms an effective barrier between the mother and developing embryo that persists up to 10 weeks' gestation when the trophoblastic plugs are dislodged and intervillous blood flow is established (Jauniaux et al., 1992). It is at this time that peak hCG secretion occurs (Meuris et al., 1995). The increasing oxygen level and concomitant oxidative stress also stimulate cytotrophoblast proliferation and differentiation and the increased expression of antioxidant enzymes. Doppler ultrasound shows there is no intervillous blood flow in normal pregnancies before this period and oxygen electrodes have demonstrated that an oxygen gradient exists across the placenta and decidua. This means that embryogenesis occurs in a relatively hypoxic environment. In fact, maternal–placental blood flow has been observed in the first trimester in a number of non-viable pregnancies but it is not clear whether this is a cause of the pregnancy failure or an effect (Kingdom and Sibley, 1996). The developing embryo is thought to be particularly vulnerable to damaging oxygen-free radicals during the sensitive period of organogenesis and the first-trimester placenta has limited antioxidant capacity; thus, limiting fetal exposure to oxygen may be protective. The differentiation of trophoblast cells is influenced by the local oxygen levels; hypoxia promotes trophoblast proliferation and normoxia inhibits proliferation and induces migration (Knofler, 2010). In most other mammalian species, organogenesis is complete and embryonic development is advanced before placental attachment. But in the human, implantation is highly invasive so the precocious conceptus is embedded in the uterine wall even before the primitive streak is evident (Jauniaux et al., 2006). Hence it is much more sensitive to oxidative stress. Embryonic and placental cells are particularly vulnerable because they are undergoing extensive cell division and DNA replication. The syncytiotrophoblast is exposed to the highest concentration of oxygen as it is closest to the maternal blood but it has low levels of antioxidant enzymes. Maternal metabolic disorders such as diabetes generate more oxidative free radicals and are associated with a higher incidence of miscarriage, vasculopathy and fetal structural defects which is thought to be due to oxidative stress (Jauniaux et al., 2006).

Spiral artery conversion

Between the 4th and 16th week of gestation, villus growth and considerable remodelling of the placenta occur, including remarkable changes in the maternal blood vessels underlying the fetal placenta ensuring that the spiral arteries are capable of delivering large volumes of blood to the placental intervillous spaces at an appropriate rate and pressure to protect the delicate fetal villi perfused by the low-pressure developing fetal circulation which are immersed in maternal blood which circulates at a much higher pressure and velocity. Failure of the transformation of the spiral arteries is associated with a number of common complications of pregnancy including pre-eclampsia, fetal growth restriction, recurrent first and second trimester losses, spontaneous preterm labour and premature rupture of the membranes (Burton et al., 2009a). In the early weeks, some of the cytotrophoblastic cells (described as extravillous cytotrophoblast) move from the tips of the anchoring villi to colonize the decidua and myometrium of the placental bed. It is this invasion of extravillous cytotrophoblast cells into the maternal blood vessels that promotes maternal recognition of the fetus and the subsequent production of blocking antibodies (see Chapter 10), which are important for the survival of the pregnancy. The extravillous cytotrophoblast cells are involved in physiologically remodelling the maternal spiral arteries which is completed by the end of the first trimester. After an apparent rest phase of a couple of weeks (weeks 14–16), there is a resurgence of the endovascular trophoblastic migration.

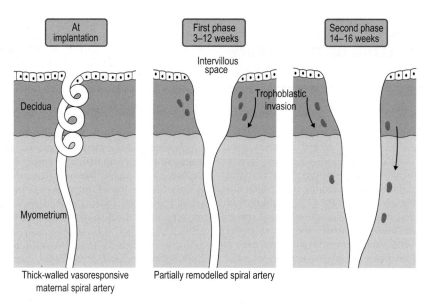

Fig. 8.7 Conversion of spiral arteries into uteroplacental arteries. The maternal spiral arteries have thick muscular walls and are responsive to vasoactive substances. They are remodelled by the trophoblastic cells in two waves, ultimately forming non-responsive dilated vessels. Where remodelling is inadequate, a proportion of the vessels retain the structure of preimplantation or partially remodelled vasoresponsive vessels.

The second wave of cytotrophoblast cells moves down the myometrial segments of the spiral arteries to their origin at the branching from the radial arteries. The cytotrophoblast cells are involved with the destruction of the maternal artery musculoelastic tissue and the replacement of the maternal endothelial wall with trophoblast resulting in a change in the vessel wall vasoresponsiveness. The result is conversion of the thick-walled muscular spiral arteries to compliant dilated sac-like uteroplacental vessels that have low impedance to blood flow (Fig. 8.7). The changes in the spiral arteries are augmented by interstitial trophoblast cells which migrate through the endometrial stroma and penetrate the spiral arteries from the outside; they continue to invade the myometrium where they transform into immotile giant cells (Burton et al., 2009a). Insufficient remodelling of the spiral arteries is associated with failure of the fetus to reach its genetic growth potential (intrauterine growth restriction (IUGR)) and pre-eclampsia (Box 8.1). Maternal spiral arteries maintaining a high vasculature resistance because of incomplete or failed remodelling are predisposed to hypoperfusion, hypoxia, reperfusion injury and oxidative stress. Although the trophoblast invasion and remodelling are limited to the spiral arteries, the radial, arcuate and uterine arteries also undergo profound dilation especially close to the site of implantation (Burton et al., 2009a,b). These vessels unusually progressively increase rather than decrease in diameter as they reach their target organ.

The remodelled vessels can passively dilate and accommodate a greatly increased blood flow (about 30% of maternal cardiac output) but they are not responsive to vasoactive agents. The effect of this interaction between the trophoblastic cells and the maternal blood vessels is that a low-pressure, high-conductance vascular system is established, which provides an adequate maternal blood flow to the placenta and thus a plentiful provision of oxygen and nutrients to the fetus. The maternal uteroplacental circulatory system is mostly complete by mid-gestation. In contrast, the fetal villous tree continues to branch and develop throughout the pregnancy, ensuring that the capacity of the placenta matches the growth of the fetus.

As the maternal cardiac output increases by about 40% (see Chapter 11), the net effect is to increase the uteroplacental blood flow by about 10-fold to over 500 mL/min (Kingdom and Sibley, 1996). Doppler ultrasound flow velocity waveforms provide diagnostic and prognostic information about maternal vessels, placental circulation and fetal vessels together with implications for both mother and fetus (Harman and Baschat, 2003). Flow in the uterine arteries gives a picture of the maternal vascular effects of the invading placenta, predicting likely pre-eclampsia and IUGR. Umbilical artery Doppler ultrasound depicts placental vascular resistance, which correlates with IUGR and effects of placental deficiency. Before pregnancy and in the first trimester, the uterine arterial waveform has a low end-diastolic flow velocity and early dichrotic notch during diastole. By 18–20 weeks' gestation, successful trophoblastic invasion alters this pattern to one showing a high diastolic flow velocity and loss of the dichrotic notch. If the dichrotic notch and low end-diastolic velocity persist, this indicates that the uterus still

Box 8.1 **Pre-eclampsia**

Pre-eclampsia is a placental condition; it can occur in the absence of a fetus in a molar pregnancy. One of the most convincing theories about the aetiology of pre-eclampsia and the associated condition of IUGR (which can occur independently or with pre-eclampsia) is that they are due to placental malperfusion secondary to deficient spiral artery conversion (Burton et al., 2009). In normal pregnancies, all spiral arteries in the placental bed are invaded by cytotrophoblast cells. In pre-eclampsia, it seems that only a proportion of the maternal vessels are invaded and that a significant number of vessels show complete absence of physiological changes. The second wave of arterial invasion may be the stage that is most compromised owing to the endovascular trophoblast failing to reach the intramyometrial portion of the vessels. This means that the spiral arteries are not completely transformed to uteroplacental vessels. Maternal uteroplacental blood flow is therefore restricted, which results in placental abnormalities and fetal complications such as IUGR. The effect is compounded by the persistence of vasoresponsiveness of the spiral arteries, which retain the ability to constrict and limit placental perfusion, like the spiral arteries of a non-pregnant uterus (see Chapter 4). Impaired placental perfusion increases the risk of ischaemia–reperfusion type insult which leads to the generation of reactive oxygen species (oxidative stress). Oxidative stress results in increased generation of oxygen-free radicals which lead to the formation of lipid peroxides which alter cell membranes. The incorporation of cholesterol, oxidized free fatty acids and LDLs into membranes is increased which leads to a biological cascade of leukocyte activation, platelet adhesion and aggregation and the release of vasoconstrictive agents (Jauniaux et al., 2006). Acute atherotic changes can lead to the development of intimal plaques which can project into the vessel lumen and restrict blood flow. In addition, endoplasmic reticulum (ER) stress is also triggered by ischaemia–perfusion and hypoxia. ER stress can lead to inhibition of protein synthesis and reduced expression of amino acid transporters (thus affecting growth) as well as activating apoptosis. There are serious maternal complications of pre-eclampsia which have been attributed to an as-yet unidentified placentally derived 'factor X' which is released into the maternal circulation; possible candidates include proinflammatory cytokines from the syncytiotrophoblast, products of placental oxidative stress, anti-angiogenic factors and trophoblastic apoptotic debris such as syncytiotrophoblast micro-fragments all of which could contribute to activation of maternal endothelial cells and cause the peripheral syndrome of pre-eclampsia (Fig. 8.8).

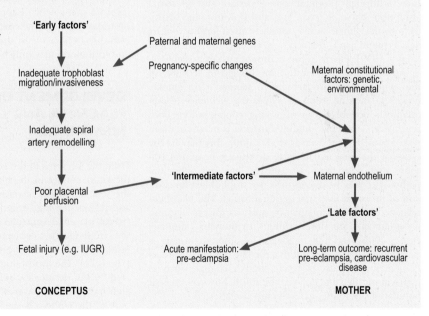

Fig. 8.8 Interactions between the conceptus and the mother in the development of pre-eclampsia. (Reproduced with permission from Lala and Chakraborty, 2003.)

has high resistance to blood flow, which is predictive of intrauterine growth retardation (IUGR) and severe pre-eclampsia (Fig. 8.9).

A number of pathologies including placental infarction or abruption, pre-eclampsia and recurrent pregnancy loss are associated with defects within the placental vascular bed. Deficiencies of vitamin B12 and folate and hyperhomocysteinaemia are risk factors for these placenta-mediated diseases (Ray and Laskin, 1999). Smoking is associated with poorer outcomes of pregnancy including

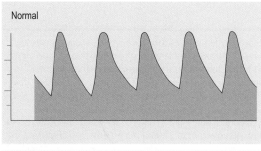

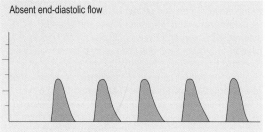

Fig. 8.9 Doppler ultrasound waveforms showing diastolic flow and dichrotic notch. (Reproduced with permission from Miller and Hanretty, 1998.)

low birthweight, spontaneous abortion and placental abruption. Nicotine, cadmium and polyaromatic hydrocarbons in cigarette smoke adversely affect fertility, oocyte development and oestrogen synthesis (Shiverick and Salafia, 1999). Effects of these compounds on trophoblastic invasion and proliferation are thought to account for the increased miscarriage rate of women who smoke; however, smoking seems to reduce the incidence of pre-eclampsia, possibly because smoking reduces endothelium sensitivity. Severe placental dysfunction is more common with a male fetus (Edwards et al., 2000); this may be the cause of the male:female ratio decreasing from 164:100 soon after conception to 106:100 at birth. Placental pathologies may be due to defective trophoblast function and/or impaired maternal decidualization. The placental-related disorders of pregnancy, such as miscarriage and pre-eclampsia, are almost unique to humans (Jauniaux et al., 2006) and the incidence in other mammals is extremely low. It is thought that the rate of these disorders is increasing because of recent lifestyle changes such as hypercaloric diets and delayed childbirth; however, current populations of hunter-gatherers are also affected.

VASCULARIZATION OF THE PLACENTAL VILLI

Fetal blood cells are derived from blood islands in the extraembryonic mesoderm surrounding the yolk sac (see Chapter 9). The blood vessels that perfuse the placenta

also develop in this tissue. In the third week of postfertilization, the extraembryonic mesoderm associated with the cytotrophoblast penetrates into the core of the primary stem villi transforming them into secondary stem villi. This mesoderm develops into the blood vessels and connective tissue of the villi. It forms at the same time as the embryonic vasculature with which it will eventually connect. Haemangioblast cells (precursors of blood cells) appear and capillaries form. The linking of the blood vessels of the villi with the vessels of the embryo results in a circulating blood system so the villi begin to be perfused by the fetal circulation at about 28 days after fertilization. The fetal red blood cells containing embryonic haemoglobin allow oxygen transfer at low partial pressures of oxygen and low pH. The villi containing differentiated blood vessels are described as tertiary stem villi. By the end of the fourth week after fertilization, these villi cover the entire blastocyst surface forming a spherical shell of villi projecting outwards into the maternal tissue (Fig. 8.10). It is possible to remove a sample of the developing placental villi for genetic testing (Box 8.2). The placental barrier now effectively limits diffusion of gases, nutrients and waste materials. There are four layers: the endothelium lining the villus capillary, the connective tissue in the villus core, a layer of cytotrophoblast cells and a maternal-facing layer of syncytiotrophoblast (Fig. 8.11). By mid-gestation, most of the cytotrophoblast layer of many villi disappears and the placental barrier becomes very thin. The syncytiotrophoblast may even come into direct contact with the fetal capillary so the maternal and fetal blood may only be about 2–4 μm apart.

DEVELOPMENT OF THE DISCOID PLACENTA AND CHORIONIC MEMBRANE

From the 4th week to the 16th week, the villus growth over the entire surface of the blastocyst is remodelled. Most of the villi orientated towards the uterine cavity degenerate and regress, leaving behind an area that develops into the typical placental structure and shape seen at delivery. As the embryo starts to enlarge, the uterine wall where it has implanted starts to protrude into the uterine cavity (Fig. 8.12). The protruding portion of the embryo is covered by the decidua capsularis, a thin layer or capsule of endometrium. The layer of decidua under the embryonic pole of the embryo is the decidua basalis. The remaining areas of the decidua are described as the decidua parietalis.

In the third month, as the fetus enlarges and grows to fill the uterus, the thin rim of decidua capsularis covering the bulge gradually thins and disappears so the chorion comes into contact with the decidua parietalis of the opposite wall of the uterus. Before the trophoblastic shell comes into contact with the uterine wall on the opposite side, cells of fetal origin can enter the uterine cavity and

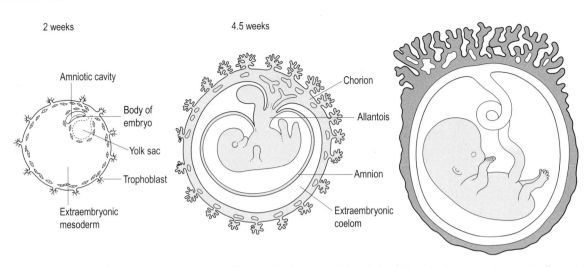

Fig. 8.10 Early villus formation occurs in a sphere-like organization around the whole of the enlarging conceptus; eventually most of the villi will degenerate leaving only the ovoid development of the fetal placenta.

Box 8.2 **Chorionic villus sampling**

In the chorionic villus sampling (CVS) procedure, 20–40 mg of placental tissue can be obtained from a villus for genetic diagnosis of trisomy 21, for instance or of a single-gene abnormality such as cystic fibrosis or β-thalassaemia. After 10 weeks' gestation, the tissue can be extracted transabdominally by needle aspiration or transcervically using curved biopsy forceps. The collected trophoblast cells, which divide very rapidly, can be cultured for 24 h and then the chromosome number can be determined (see Chapter 7). Because of the problems associated with mosaicism (see Chapter 7), a more accurate determination of chromosome number and structure is obtained by using fibroblast cells taken from the vascular core of the villus. These cells grow more slowly so they have to be cultured for 2 weeks before being stained and examined (which means the results of the test take longer). As fibroblast cells are derived from the mesoderm, they originate from the inner cell mass and are embryonic rather than the trophoblast-derived cells from the outer layers of the villus. Placental mosaicism is associated with increased fetal loss and IUGR. There is a 1–2% procedure-related loss in CVS, although it should be remembered that the procedure is being performed because there is already a concern about the pregnancy. Pregnancies associated with genetic abnormality have a much higher risk of spontaneous failure.

can be collected by flushing or aspiration from the endocervical canal (Kingdom et al., 1995). This is a route of non-invasive prenatal diagnosis, particularly for newer testing procedures that require fewer cells. The size of the chorionic, or embryonic, sac can be used to determine the gestational age of the embryo.

The uterine cavity is obliterated by 12 weeks' gestation. The enlarging blastocyst compresses the trophoblastic layer, distal to the entry pole, and limits nutrient supply and further growth by the villi in this region of the decidua capsularis. The underlying villi slowly degenerate and regress so by the fifth month this region becomes devoid of villi and smoother. This flattened surface of the decidua capsularis and atrophied chorion form the chorion laeve, the uteroplacental membrane, which is also known as the chorionic membrane or bald chorion. Effectively, the chorion is extraplacental trophoblast with similar immunological properties; it may also be an important source of hCG, particularly in early pregnancy. The portion of the trophoblastic tissue associated with the decidua basalis implants further and receives a plentiful supply of nutrients so it continues growing. This area of the chorion, therefore, retains villi that proliferate and progressively arborize forming the chorion frondosum ('frondosus' is Latin for leaf), which ultimately develops into the definitive discoid fetal placenta. The placenta is a union between the chorion frondosum derived from the fertilized ovum and the decidua basalis (basal plate) formed from the maternal uterine wall. It is anatomically complete by the end of the first trimester but continues to grow throughout the pregnancy.

DEVELOPMENT OF THE AMNION (INNER MEMBRANE)

The amniotic cavity first appears at about day 7. The primitive ectoderm cells enclosing the cavity become flattened forming amnioblasts, cells which become the fetal-facing amniotic membrane. These cells secrete amniotic fluid,

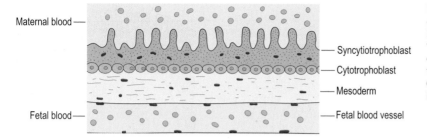

Maternal blood —

— Syncytiotrophoblast

— Cytotrophoblast

— Mesoderm

Fetal blood —

— Fetal blood vessel

Fig. 8.11 Exchange of substances across the placenta occurs across a barrier consisting of four layers of tissue: syncytiotrophoblast, cytotrophoblast, mesoderm and fetal blood vessel wall. (Reproduced with permission from Miller and Hanretty, 1998.)

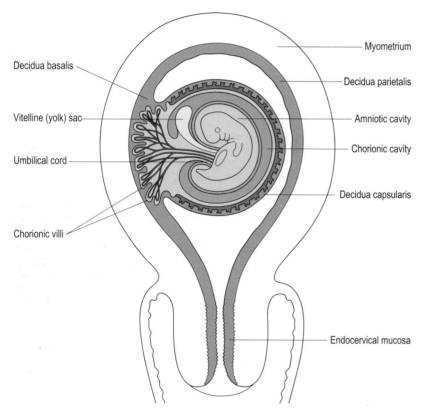

Myometrium

Decidua basalis

Decidua parietalis

Vitelline (yolk) sac

Amniotic cavity

Chorionic cavity

Umbilical cord

Decidua capsularis

Chorionic villi

Endocervical mucosa

Fig. 8.12 Protrusion of the developing conceptus into the uterine cavity and formation of the decidua capsularis.

thus the embryo is enclosed in the fluid-filled amniotic sac. The outer surface of the amnioblast cell layer becomes covered with mesoderm. As the embryo expands, the amnion comes into contact with the chorion. The chorionic cells are lined with mesoderm cells on the inner side. When the amnion and chorion meet, the two layers of mesoderm loosely fuse. The fetal membranes protect the fetus and secrete factors into the amniotic fluid which affects amniotic fluid activity and also can influence the maternal uterine physiology. An important aspect of examining the placenta and membranes is to ensure that both membranes are present following birth. The amnion and chorion should be easily separated; the chorion is attached to the edge of the placenta, whereas the amnion can be separated from the surface of the placenta with attachment around the base of the cord.

Amniotic fluid

Amniotic fluid has an important role in protecting the fetus, cushioning it from external impact and stresses preventing fetal injury. It also allows symmetrical fetal growth and movement, preventing fetal parts from adhering together or to the amnion, allows practice breathing and swallowing exercises and increases placental surface area. Amniotic fluid has bacteriostatic properties and is

184

also important in maintaining a constant body temperature; it is also involved in maintaining amnion integrity, discouraging myometrial contractions and maintaining cervical length and consistency (Harman, 2008). In the first half of gestation, before skin keratinization takes place, fluid and electrolytes can diffuse freely across the skin (Jauniaux and Gulbis, 2000). Although the amnioblasts actively secrete amniotic fluid, the composition of the fluid at this time is similar to that of fetal tissue fluid. After 20 weeks, the skin becomes keratinized and transudation from maternal and fetal blood vessels contributes less to the amniotic fluid. Fetal urine and lung secretions are also important. Fetal swallowing and exchange across the amnion mean that turnover of fluid is rapid, particularly close to term. Lung fluid may contribute abut 100 mL per day and fetal urine 7–10 mL per hour. The fetus may swallow up to 1 L of fluid per day; the extra water crosses the gut, enters the fetal circulation and can then cross the placenta. By term, the normal volume of amniotic fluid is 500–1000 mL. Polyhydramnios is an excess amount of fluid (over 2000 mL), which is usually associated with multiple pregnancies or fetal swallowing problems such as oesophageal atresia. A deficiency of amniotic fluid (<500 mL) is classified as oligohydramnios, a condition often associated with impaired fetal renal function.

Amniotic fluid provides a useful tool to monitor fetal development and well-being. A small amount of amniotic fluid can be removed in amniocentesis for measurement and testing. Amniotic fluid contains many maternal and fetal proteins and fetal cells, which can be used for genetic testing (see Chapter 7). If the fetus has a neural tube defect (see Chapter 9), concentrations of AFP (alpha-fetoprotein, derived from spinal fluid) in the amniotic fluid are very high. Levels of AFP are low in Down's syndrome (trisomy 21) and are measured as part of the triple test (see Chapter 7). It has been proposed that this could be due to the persistence of extraembryonic coelom or related to interferon receptor levels (Chard, 1998). Components of amniotic fluid may also be used to predict preterm labour, premature cervical effacement and fetal infection (Harman, 2008). Recent research has investigated the role of amniotic fluid in inhibiting bacterial growth in burns victims and in promoting healing of burns and other skin injuries. Amniotic fluid is a potential source of pluripotent (stem) cells and novel anti-inflammatory compounds (Harman, 2008).

GROWTH AND MATURATION OF THE PLACENTAL VILLI

The placental villi continue to grow for most of the pregnancy. There is a widely held belief that the placenta ages during the pregnancy and that at term it is about to decline into functional senescence. Instead, the continuous morphological changes should perhaps be viewed as an increase in functional efficiency rather than ageing. Thus in early pregnancy, the placenta is a highly invasive and proliferative tissue and in later pregnancy, although its growth rate slows down, it continues to mature and increase in efficiency. Placental efficiency is favoured by the attenuated maternal–fetal barrier and reduced diffusion distance rather than by an increase in weight. Although the rate of placental growth does decline in the later part of gestation, this decrease in growth rate is not irreversible or inevitable. If the maternal environment becomes unfavourable, for instance because of maternal anaemia or increased altitude, fresh villus growth will ensue and the placenta will expand its surface area and continue branching past term. In all placentas, total placental DNA levels continue to increase linearly beyond the 40th week of gestation.

Growth of the placenta (see Fig. 8.6, p. 178) can be divided into three stages. Earlier in pregnancy, the trabeculae develop side-branches of syncytiotrophoblast protrusions (syncytial spouts) which may be filled with a core of cytotrophoblast. These primary villi protrude into the intervillous spaces. Later on, more lateral branches develop and the layers forming the placental barrier become more refined. In the ninth week, the tertiary stem villi lengthen to form mesenchymal villi as extraembryonic mesodermal cells penetrate the cytotrophoblast; the presence of this mesenchymal core transforms the villi into secondary or mesenchymal villi. Haematopoietic stem or progenitor cells develop within the mesoderm of the secondary villi forming the first placental blood cells and endothelial cells. Maternal and embryonic vascular systems do not connect; their development is similar and coordinated but independent and separate. The formation of placental blood vessels and cells transforms the villi into tertiary villi. Placenta blood vessels are formed in two processes: vasculogenesis is the formation of the first blood vessels from cells differentiated from the mesenchymal core and angiogenesis is the development of new vessels from existing vessels (Demir et al., 2007). These processes of blood vessel development are controlled by oxygenation, and the vascular endothelial growth factor (VEGF) family of growth factors and their receptors (Arroyo and Winn, 2008).

By the 16th week, the terminal extensions of the tertiary stem villi reach their maximum length. At this stage, the villi are described as immature intermediate villi. The cells of the cytotrophoblast layer become more dispersed within the villi creating gaps in the cytotrophoblast layer of the villus wall. Near the end of the second trimester, the tertiary stem villi form numerous side-branches and are described as mature intermediate villi. The earliest mature intermediate villi finish forming by about week 32 and then begin to produce small nodule-like secondary branches characteristic of the terminal villi. This is the final structure of the placental villous tree. The terminal villi are not formed by active outgrowth of the syncytiotrophoblast but by coiled and folded villus capillaries that bulge against the villus wall and expand by unfurling. Two types of chorionic villi can be identified: deep villi anchor the placenta to the decidua basalis; shorter villi extend into the intervillous spaces and have a nutritive role.

The blood-filled intervillous space into which the villi project is formed from the trophoblastic lacunae that grow and coalesce. Therefore, the intervillous space is lined on both sides with syncytiotrophoblast. The maternal face of the placenta is the basal plate, which consists of syncytiotrophoblast lining plus a supporting layer of decidua basalis. The fetal side is formed of the layers of chorion of the chorion plate.

The functional unit within the placenta is the placentome (or placental lobe), a villous tree arising from the chorionic plate within the intervillous space, which is perfused by a spiral artery. There are about 50–100 such units within the placenta. The villous tree has rami (major branches) and smaller ramuli. The terminal villi have little impedance to flow and therefore an increased fetoplacental flow; they are probably the major sites of nutrient and gaseous exchange in late gestation. The progressive development and branching of the placental tree structure is important for fetal growth and development. For instance, in IUGR pregnancies requiring elective preterm delivery, there are fewer terminal villi, which seem to have an abnormal extravillous cytotrophoblast structure. By term, the surface area of the placental villi is estimated to be 12–14 m^2 (Jauniaux et al., 2006).

On the basal (maternal) surface, the placenta is subdivided into cotyledons by wedge-like placental septa, which appear in the third month. The placental (decidual) septa grow into the intervillous space from the maternal side of the placenta, separating the villi into 10–40 cotyledons. The placental septae do not fuse with the chorionic plate, so maternal blood can flow freely from one cotyledon to another. This means that the villi are bathed in a lake of maternal blood which is constantly exchanging; this organization of placental perfusion is described as haemochorial. Haemochorial placentation is efficient because the trophoblast is in contact with maternal blood optimizing maternal–fetal transport of gases, nutrients, water and ions. The trophoblast can also endocytose the immunoglobulin IgG. In addition, hormones produced by the fetoplacental unit can easily access the maternal circulation. There are, however, some costs to the haemochorial arrangement; bleeding may be extensive at parturition and cells can be transferred between mother and fetus, for instance, resulting in microchimerisms (see Chapter 10) or erythroblastosis fetalis (haemolytic disease of the newborn due to Rhesus incompatibility).

PLACENTAL BLOOD FLOW

The fetal blood reaches the placental blood system via the two umbilical arteries which spiral around the umbilical vein (Fig. 8.13). On reaching the chorion, the vessels usually each supply half of the placenta. The arteries (which are vessels carrying blood away from the fetal heart and therefore carry deoxygenated blood) divide repeatedly to form a branching network of smaller arteries and capillaries running through the intervillous space. The fetal blood flow through the placenta is about 500 mL/min, propelled by the fetal heart. Smooth muscle fibres contracting in the villi may help to pump blood back from the placenta to the fetus.

The maternal blood enters the intervillous space via about 50–100 of the remodelled spiral arteries. There is a pressure gradient from the maternal arteries to the intervillous space to the maternal veins. The blood leaves the intervillous space via the endometrial veins. Most organs have a progressive decrease in arterial diameter as the blood nears its target tissue. In the uteroplacental vessels, the remodelled spiral arteries increase in diameter as the vessels approach the intervillous space. Therefore, the intervillous space is a low-pressure system; the blood gently flows through and washes over the fetal placental tissue. The placenta has little resistance to maternal blood flow and a high vascular conductance so there is little fall in pressure across the intervillous space. The main determinant of the rate of maternal blood flow is the vascular resistance in the myometrial arteries. Myometrial contractions can decrease or stop afferent blood flow to the intervillous space. This effect is probably due to the compression or occlusion of the veins draining this space. During a contraction, the space distends so the fetus is not totally deprived of oxygen.

IUGR and 'placental insufficiency'

Fetal hypoxia, IUGR (see Box 8.3) or fetal death is often attributed to 'placental insufficiency'. A proportion of those babies with a low birthweight (<2.5 kg) probably failed to achieve their growth potential because placental transfer of oxygen and nutrients was inadequate. However, the fetal placenta is rarely insufficient. Like all essential organs, it has a considerable physiological reserve. It has been estimated that the placenta could lose 30–40% of its villi (and therefore surface area) without affecting its function. However, the placentas of growth-restricted fetuses may exhibit pathological changes such as reduced syncytiotrophoblast area, increased placental apoptosis or increased thickness of the exchange barrier (Arroyo and Winn., 2008).

Placental insufficiency really describes inadequate maternal uteroplacental blood flow, which is probably due to incomplete conversion of the spiral arteries during the early stages of pregnancy. Studies suggest the uteroplacental perfusion is greatly reduced because of a failure of the trophoblast invasion into the myometrium and subsequent remodelling of the spiral arteries (Brosens et al., 2002) which results in fewer terminal villi and other placental abnormalities affecting blood vessels and membranes involved in diffusion. It is possible that some small-stem arterioles may be occluded by fetal platelets

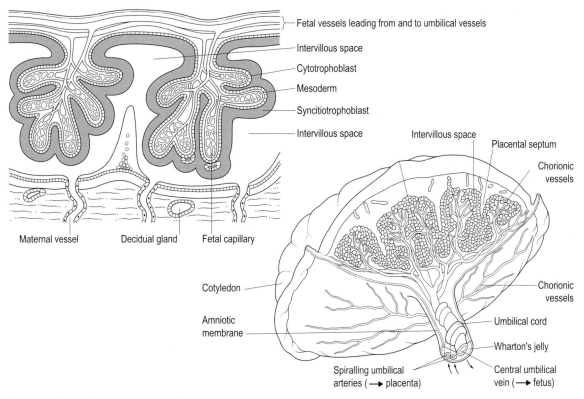

Fig. 8.13 The umbilical cord and the circulation through the placenta.

Box 8.3 **Intrauterine growth restriction**

UUGR increases the risk of disability or death for the fetus and neonate in the perinatal period and predisposes the individual born following IUGR to later adult disease (see Chapter 12). Although there is no internationally agreed definition for IUGR, it is usually defined small for gestation age (SGA) and as a birth weight below a certain percentile (10th, 5th or 3rd percentile). It may be further qualified as also including a longitudinal decrease in the growth of the abdominal circumference, increased fetal head:abdomen circumference ratio or oligohydramnios. Risk factors for IUGR include acquired blood borne infections (such as malaria, rubella and cytomegalovirus), pre-existing maternal disease (cardiovascular, endocrine, autoimmune), aneuploidies, metabolic factors and placental disorders including abnormal placental position. However, for most infants with IUGR, there is no known cause; idiopathic IUGR is often described as 'placental insufficiency'. In IUGR, there are marked reductions in the placental delivery of amino acids to the fetus (Cetin and Alvino, 2009) which is reflected in decreased deposition of tissue. This is probably due to both blood flow and arteriovenous differences in nutrient concentrations being compromised as well as reduced activity in the placental amino acid transport systems. Placental transport of glucose in IUGR seems no different to a normal placenta but the placental expression of the lipoprotein receptors and lipoprotein lipases involved in transfer of maternal fatty acids is altered. In IUGR, there also appears to be increased placental permeability and increased placental oxygen utilization. Where there is IUGR with a normal umbilical blood flow, amino acid and LCPUFA concentrations are significantly reduced and non-esterified fatty acids levels are increased. However, when umbilical blood flow is also impaired in severe IUGR, fetal blood flow to the brain, liver and heart is altered leading to the fetus becoming hypoxic and lactacidaemic with subsequent effects on the fetal growth trajectory. Associated with these changes, the fetus adapts to nutrient intake not meeting demand by increasing protein catabolism, reducing metabolic rate and making endocrine adaptations; these adaptation mechanisms are not without cost and may have lifelong health consequence (see Chapter 12). The most serious complications of IUGR occur in fetuses weighing less than 500 g. One approach to correcting IUGR might be

Continued

Box 8.3 Intrauterine growth restriction—cont'd

placental gene therapy, particularly as growth factors (such as insulin growth factors, placental growth factor and VEGF) are all implicated in failure of trophoblast remodelling of the uterine spiral arteries which appears to be the underlying abnormality in both IUGR and pre-eclampsia. Although development of such treatment is theoretical at the moment,

it does raise interesting ethical questions about whether the patient in such a scenario is the woman or her fetus and whether gene therapy could be justified if it was safe and effective, where there was reasonable certainty that the fetus would suffer irreversible and substantial harm without the intervention and where the risk to the mother was negligible.

(Wilcox and Trudinger, 1991). Measurement of abnormal oxygen and amino acid levels in the umbilical vein blood suggests a defect in placental transport mechanisms (Cetin et al., 1990). However, it is not established whether these changes are causative or adaptive. Compensatory mechanisms exist in the fetus, which result in redistribution of blood to the fetal brain at the expense of the lower body. This is supported by the finding that amniotic fluid volume is decreased presumably because blood flow to the kidneys is reduced (Kingdom and Sibley, 1996). Substances that cause vasoconstriction, such as cocaine and alcohol, are implicated in preterm labour, possibly because they cause a decrease in blood flow to the placenta affecting uterine contractility and sensitivity.

Case study 8.2 details an example of a small baby.

Fetoplacental blood flow

Blood leaving the right atrium is diverted into the ductus arteriosus, into the aorta and down to the lower body (see Chapter 15). At term, about 40–50% of the fetal cardiac output goes to the placenta via the umbilical arteries. Blood flow from the aorta to the umbilical arteries is high because the resistance to flow in these vessels is low compared with the systemic circulation of the lower body. The vessels of the fetoplacental circulation lack autonomic innervation but a variety of substances can affect the smooth muscle of the stem villous arteries. Of particular importance are paracrine agents, which have a local effect on the fetoplacental

circulation. Both prostacyclin and nitric oxide (NO), which have vasodilatory and anticoagulant effects, are produced from the vessel endothelium. It is suggested that flow-mediated release of NO may have an important role (Learmont et al., 1994). Diffusion of NO into the intervillous space affecting maternal uteroplacental vessels may also be important (Myatt et al., 1993). The heterogeneous cells of the placental vessel endothelium also produce endothelin-1 (a potent vasoconstrictor), substance P, serotonin, ATP, atrial natriuretic peptide (ANP) and neuropeptide Y (NPY) (Cai et al., 1993; Myatt et al., 1992); whether these substances have a physiological role is yet to be established.

Optimal placental exchange requires adequate vascularization of the placental bed by the maternal arteries matched by circulation of fetal blood to the placenta. The fetus does not appear to have a mechanism to increase umbilical flow in response to hypoxia or volume depletion. It has a limited ability to increase cardiac output. Therefore, the fetus adapts to hypoxia or decreased nutrient availability by decreasing oxygen consumption and growth rate. The cardiac output is redistributed to the heart, brain and adrenal glands at the expense of the flow to the body and gut. Hypoxia and acidosis cause cerebral vasodilatation and constriction of the pulmonary and femoral vessels. Blood flow to the liver is high when oxygen and nutrients are plentiful but the hepatic circulation is bypassed if placental exchange is compromised.

It is hypothesized that perfusion of the placental vessels is controlled to match the maternal perfusion of the uteroplacental vessel in a similar way to the perfusion–ventilation matching in the neonatal or adult pulmonary system (see Chapter 1). If an area of the placenta is underperfused by the maternal blood flow, hypoxia ensues. The endothelium of the placental vessels responds by vasoconstricting (by decreasing NO synthesis and increasing endothelin-1 production) so fetoplacental blood flow is diverted to a better-perfused villous tree.

PLACENTAL TRANSPORT MECHANISMS

Many substances are transported from the maternal blood in the intervillous space to the fetal blood in the capillaries of the villi and vice versa. By term, most exchange

Case study 8.2

Polly was diagnosed as carrying a small-for-dates baby. She spontaneously delivered Thomas at 39 weeks, and although he weighed only 2.4 kg, he appeared healthy and vigorous. The midwife noted that the third stage appeared complete but failed to identify that the placenta appeared relatively large.

- Do you think that there is any need to weigh placentas and to compare the placental and birth weights?
- Are there any situations where the weight and condition of the placenta may be used as a possible indicator for disease states in later life?

occurs in the terminal villi, which have a high surface area and small diffusion distance, perhaps of only a few micrometres in some areas. The surface area of the placenta is calculated to be 5 m^2 at 28 weeks, increasing to about 11 m^2 at term (Carlson, 1994). The precise mechanisms of placental transport for many substances are not clear. Transport mechanisms include simple diffusion and transporter-mediated processes; these can be active or facilitated. The effectiveness of the transport mechanism depends on the morphological characteristics of the placenta (like surface area and barrier thickness) and on the abundance and distribution of specific transporters. Simple and facilitated diffusion depends on the concentration gradient, the placental permeability and the surface area; however, passive diffusion alone is not likely to be adequate for fetal requirements for nutrients.

Lipophilic substances (soluble in lipid such as respiratory gases) are soluble in cell membranes so their transport depends on the concentration gradient and the relative rates of maternal and fetal blood flow. Because the placenta provides a large surface area, the transfer of respiratory gases depends on the maternofetal concentration difference which depends on the flow rates of the uterine and umbilical circulations (Desforges and Sibley, 2010). Diffusion of hydrophilic substances (soluble in aqueous solutions but poor solubility in lipid bilayers) is limited by the diffusion distance (placenta thickness) and the surface area of the membranes of the placental barrier. The fetal capillary endothelium probably limits transport of large proteins (such as albumin, IgG and AFP). Transport studies of the syncytiotrophoblast suggest that it is much more permeable than was previously believed and probably has channels or pores which offer a route continuous with, and containing, extracellular fluid (Kingdom and Sibley, 1996), which allows the diffusion of large proteins. The transfer of substances across the placenta occurs in both directions, to and from the fetus.

There are specific transport proteins on the placental plasma membrane involved in the efficient transfer of metabolically important substances. Some of these proteins form channels and others act as shuttles or carriers. Glucose demands are high and are estimated to be 4–8 mg/kg/min (Aldoretta and Hay, 1995). Glucose transport is predominantly carried out by the facilitative-diffusion glucose transporter GLUT1 and also by GLUT3 (Knipp et al., 1999). Glucose transport by GLUT1 is concentration-dependent, bidirectional and independent of insulin. GLUT1 expression is higher on the maternal side of the syncytiotrophoblast which favours mother-to-fetus transfer and protects glucose being transported from the fetus during maternal hypoglycaemia. GLUT1 expression is downregulated by hyperglycaemia so fetal development is partially protected if there is maternal hyperglycaemia. GLUT3 is not the major facilitator of glucose transport to the developing fetus but may be important during periods of maternal hypo- or hyperglycaemia. Fetal glucose

levels are usually slightly lower and directly related to maternal levels. The difference between fetal and maternal glucose levels increases with the severity of IUGR.

Some substances, such as certain amino acids and calcium, are transported by active (energy-dependent) transport against their electrochemical gradients. There are several amino acid transfer systems in the uterine and placental tissues. The system A amino acid transporter is sodium-dependent and transports neutral amino acids with short or linear side chains such as alanine, glutamine, methionine, serine, proline and glycine (Desforges and Sibley, 2010). System A activity is affected by substrate availability and hormones; it is also inhibited by hypoxia and oxidative stress. The sodium-independent amino acid transport systems L and γ+ transport branched chain amino acids and lysine. Placental transfer of amino acids is reduced in IUGR probably because there are fewer transporters expressed and thus a reduced maximum rate of transfer. Amino acid levels are usually higher in the fetus than in the mother as expected with active transport systems but where fetus is growth-restricted, maternal amino acid levels are not as low as in normal pregnancies.

Fatty acids, particularly the long-chain polyunsaturated fatty acids (LCPUFA), are important for synthesis of phospholipids and cell membranes, and growth and development of the brain and nervous system. The fetus is dependent on placental transfer which is mediated by specific fatty acid binding and transfer proteins and preferentially transports LCPUFA (Cetin and Alvino, 2009). The placental transfer of maternally derived fatty acids requires placental lipases which hydrolyse lipoprotein-borne triacylglycerides and phospholipids. The placenta nucleoside transporters enable the fetus to meet its high demands for nucleosides to synthesize nucleotides; transport of adenosine is decreased by ethanol. There are additional mechanisms for the transport of some very large molecules such as receptor-mediated pinocytosis for IgG (see Chapter 10). There is a net flux of water to the fetus, mostly across the placenta.

Steroid hormones cross the placenta but peptide hormones seem to be poorly transferred. Gas transfer occurs by diffusion and is probably limited by blood flow. As well as oxygen and carbon dioxide, the placenta permits diffusion of other gases such as carbon monoxide and inhalation anaesthetics. The placenta itself has a high rate of oxygen consumption; much of this oxygen is used for oxidative phosphorylation of glucose. The consequent production of ATP is used mainly for synthesis of peptide and steroid hormone and for transport of nutrients.

The placenta has a protective function and limits transfer of some xenobiotic substances to the fetus. The placenta expresses cytochrome P450 enzymes which metabolize and detoxify a number of drugs. There are also export pumps in the syncytiotrophoblast which reduce placental transfer of potentially toxic substances. However, some bacteria (such as the one that causes syphilis), some protozoa (such as the parasite that causes toxoplasmosis) and a number of viruses (including HIV, cytomegalovirus, rubella, polio and varicella) can cross the placenta and affect outcome.

The placenta acts as a nutrient sensor and regulates nutrient transfer depending on the ability of the maternal circulation to supply the nutrients. Furthermore, the placenta has its own nutrient demands; it extracts a fixed proportion of maternal nutrients (70% of the glucose and 40% of the oxygen) (Miller et al., 2008) and can also take nutrients, such as amino acids, from the fetal circulation for its own nutrient needs (Cetin and Alvino, 2009). This means the fetus is vulnerable to nutrient deprivation as it is restricted to the surplus nutrients that remain after placental demands are met. So even slight placental dysfunction can restrict nutrient transfer and blood flow to the fetus whilst maintaining the high level of placental nutrition. Likewise, placental oxygen uptake also seems to remain constant even when there are acute reductions in uterine oxygen supply, so it is the fetal level of oxygenation which is compromised in such conditions. If uterine perfusion is reduced, delivery of glucose and amino acids to the fetus can be compromised. Such a reduction in substrate availability can affect growth and metabolism of the fetus. The fetal compensatory responses include downregulation of the insulin and IGF1 axis and hepatic glucose metabolism. This results in glycogenolysis and endogenous protein breakdown which increase fetal glucose and amino acid levels but potentially compromise growth. Endocrine response includes hypothyroidism, bone demineralization and up-regulation of the adrenocortical axis. Fetal red blood cell mass increase which not only may exacerbate placental dysfunction but also results in increased risk of thrombocytopenia, increased blood viscosity, and platelet aggregation.

PLACENTAL HORMONE PRODUCTION

Placental hormones have a role in adjusting maternal physiology to provide the optimal environment for fetal development (see Chapter 11); however, roles for all of the placental products have not yet been elucidated. Concentrations of placental protein hormones are higher in the maternal blood than in the fetus because the fetal circulation limits the transfer of large molecules (Firth and Leach, 1996). Conversely, levels of steroid hormones are about 10 times higher in the fetal circulation (Chard, 1998). Although the levels of placental protein hormone fluctuate randomly, a true circadian rhythm of placental secretion has never been demonstrated (Chard, 1998). This includes secretion of hCG, which is not higher in urine specimens collected in the morning (Kent et al., 1991). Hormonal concentrations also change in response to environmental challenges such as changes in maternal blood flow,

compromised maternal diet and hypoxia. In the fetal compartment, environmental conditions that favour fetal growth increase concentrations of anabolic hormones such as thyroid hormones, insulin and IGFs and decrease concentrations of catabolic hormones such as catecholamines and cortisol (Fowden and Forhead, 2009).

The placenta has a broad endocrine capacity and diversity, producing many hormones that other endocrine organs also produce. The syncytiotrophoblast is probably the source of most placental products including hormones, growth factors and cytokines, although the cytotrophoblast may also produce hCG, human placental lactogen (hPL), inhibin, relaxin and placental releasing hormones (Chard, 1998). The major steroids produced are progesterone and oestrogens (oestriol). The production of oestrogens requires both maternal and fetal precursors, so monitoring maternal oestrogen levels during the pregnancy is a useful indicator of fetal well-being. Cholesterol from maternal low-density lipoprotein (LDL) is mostly used as the precursor for steroid hormone production. Oestriol synthesis requires 16α-hydroxydehydroandrosterone sulphate derived from the fetal liver and adrenal gland. Most of the steroid hormones produced enter the mother's circulation, affecting her physiology (see Chapter 11). The placenta also produces neuropeptides (although it has no nerves), which may regulate placental hormone production, leptin, growth factors and cytokines.

hCG and steroids

Embryo development requires progesterone to maintain uterine quiescence. Initially hCG from the trophoblast rescues the corpus luteum from atresia (see Chapters 4 and 6) thus maintaining the production of oestrogen and progesterone. Release of hCG from the trophoblast seems to begin about 7 days after fertilization (Chard, 1998). However, levels of hCG and luteal steroid hormones are not directly related in normal pregnancies (Hamilton-Fairley and Johnson, 1998). Hormone levels fall following in vitro fertilization (IVF) despite increasing levels of hCG (Johnson et al., 1993a). The relationship between hCG and steroid hormone production is stronger in anembryonic pregnancies (Johnson et al., 1993b), where embryonic development has failed, suggesting that the embryo itself takes over the control of steroid hormone production by the corpus luteum. The corpus luteum becomes redundant at about 7 weeks after fertilization when steroid hormone production is taken over by the placenta. The change in site of production is described as the luteoplacental shift; a relative progesterone and oestradiol deficiency can develop and lead to abortion (Schindler, 2004). Inadequate hormone production by the corpus luteum early in pregnancy before this shift, or insufficient placental development, is also thought to be responsible for early miscarriages.

hCG can be detected in maternal serum and urine once implantation has occurred about 9–10 days postfertilization when secretions from the trophoblast can enter the maternal vessels. hCG is composed of two subunits; the α-subunit is common to all glycoprotein hormones such as LH (luteinizing hormone), FSH (follicle-stimulating hormone) and TSH (thyroid-stimulating hormone). Dissociated α- and β-subunits of hCG, as well as the intact dimer (the complete hCG molecule formed of two subunits), are measurable in pregnancy (Kingdom and Sibley, 1996). The concentration of α-subunits progressively increases throughout the pregnancy reaching maximal levels at about 36 weeks. The concentration of free β-subunits parallels the concentration of intact dimer, reaching a peak about 10 weeks after fertilization, and then declines to a plateau. It is thought that the cytotrophoblast produces α-subunits and the more differentiated syncytiotrophoblast produces both α- and β-subunits (Kingdom and Sibley, 1996). Raised levels of β-subunits of hCG are associated with Down's syndrome, reflecting abnormal formation of the syncytiotrophoblast (Spencer et al., 1992). Levels of the hormone are also significantly higher in cases of severe pre-eclampsia (see Box 8.1, p. 181) and IUGR (Wenstrom et al., 1994). hCG promotes cytotrophoblast differentiation and migration of extravillous trophoblasts (Banerjee and Fazleabas, 2010). The role of hCG in maintaining hormone production by the corpus luteum is clearly established. However, the peak of hCG production is reached after the function of the corpus luteum has already started to decline, suggesting other roles for the hormone. hCG may have immunoregulatory roles and also be involved with fetal testosterone production and male sexual differentiation (see Chapter 5). Because of the structural similarity between hCG and LH, hCG is used in ART for controlled ovarian stimulation (see p. 133) because it reduces the risk of ovarian hyperstimulation syndrome. It has been suggested that higher levels of hCG in early pregnancy are associated with a long-term protection against breast cancer (Banerjee and Fazleabas, 2010). In the myometrium, hCG inhibits smooth muscle contraction via several mechanisms and so may be important in preventing premature delivery (Ticconi, 2007).

Human placental lactogen

hPL (also known as human chorionic somatomammotropin, hCS) is also a product of the syncytiotrophoblast; it is structurally and functionally similar to human growth hormone. Levels of hPL increase throughout gestation and correlate well with placental syncytiotrophoblast mass so it can be used clinically to evaluate placental function. By term, 1–3 g of hPL is produced per day (equivalent to 5–7 mg/mL in maternal blood). hPL affects maternal metabolism, erythropoietin activity, fetal growth, mammary gland development and ovarian function; it induces insulin resistance and carbohydrate intolerance (see p. 281) and is important in the provision of fatty acids for the fetus. Lower hPL levels are associated with pre-eclampsia, aborting molar pregnancy (hydatidiform mole), choriocarcinoma and placental insufficiency. Higher than normal hPL levels are associated with multiple pregnancies, placental tumours, intact molar pregnancy, diabetes and Rhesus incompatibility. However, there are reports of women with abnormally low or absent levels of hPL having completely normal pregnancies (Kingdom and Sibley, 1996).

Placental growth hormone

PGH is synthesized by the syncytiotrophoblast. It has high somatogenic (growth) activity and low lactogenic activity. PGH is structurally similar to hPL and pituitary growth hormone. It gradually replaces pituitary growth hormone in the maternal circulation (Evain-Brion and Malassine, 2003). It is secreted continuously only into the maternal circulation (whereas pituitary growth hormone has a pulsatile secretory pattern) and is important in facilitating maternal metabolic adaptation to pregnancy and regulating the amount of glucose and amino acids available for placental extraction from the maternal circulation. Together with hPL, PGH regulates the serum levels of insulin-IGFs; levels of PGH correlate with the birthweight of the newborns.

THE ALLANTOIS AND YOLK SAC

The allantois and yolk sac are semivestigial structures that have a more important role in other species, such as birds and reptiles, where the yolk sac is important in nutrition of the maternally isolated eggs and the allantois has a respiratory and excretory role. The allantois forms from a pocket of the hindgut embedded within the umbilical cord, which is incorporated into the developing urinary system. Blood cells develop in the wall of the allantois during weeks 3–5 and its blood vessels become the vessels of the umbilical cord which forms in the region of the body stalk and is covered by the developing amnion. The embryonic structures and the right umbilical vein disappear, leaving two arteries and one vein. The yolk sac develops on the ventral side of the embryonic disc and is important in nutrition of the embryo while the uteroplacental circulation is forming. The primordial germ cells (see Chapter 5) and the blood islands develop in the tissue of the yolk sac. The yolk sac becomes thin and elongated and is incorporated into the umbilical cord and primitive gut. Its role in haematopoiesis is taken over by the liver in the sixth week of development. The remnant of the yolk sac lies between the chorion and amnion; it is a calcified yellow nodule about 4 mm long (Kaplan, 2008).

THE PLACENTA AT TERM

The mature placenta is an oval/round disc with a diameter of about 18–22 cm and 2–3 cm thick in the middle, petering out towards the edges. At the placental margins, the basal and chorionic surfaces of the placenta unite to form the fetal chorionic membrane. On average, a placenta weighs about one-sixth of the weight of the fetus, about 470–500 g. The amniotic membrane is smooth so the fetal aspect of the placenta, the chorionic plate, appears shiny and grey. The amnion is a single layer of epithelial cells and avascular connective tissue which is weakly attached and can be easily removed from the delivered placenta. The basal plate is maternal surface of the placenta which appears grooved and lobed with a dull red coloration. This basal surface is a mixture of extravillous trophoblasts, maternal decidua cells and immune cells such as macrophages and natural killer cells, extracellular matrix, fibrinoid and blood clots. The chorionic membrane retains the ridged appearance owing to the regression of the early villi. The umbilical cord is usually inserted slightly eccentrically into the chorionic plate. The umbilical cord gets progressively longer with the duration of the pregnancy as fetal activity and traction on the cord increases its length. At term, the umbilical cord is normally between 50 and 60 cm long. If the cord is abnormally short, it can cause bleeding problems. If it is long (>70 cm), it may prolapse through the cervix or entangle with the fetus, possibly forming knots that could obstruct fetal circulation during delivery, causing potentially fetal distress and death. Abnormal cord length is used clinically as a marker of undetected intrauterine events (Calvano et al., 2000); although it is not clear whether cord length is long because of traction associated with entanglement or whether entanglements occur because the cord is long. There is thought to be a genetic component to abnormally long cords (Kaplan, 2008). For a normal vaginal delivery, a cord length of at least 32 cm is thought to be necessary to avoid fetal distress, cord tearing and possible abruption. Short cords are associated with poor fetal movement (such as in oligohydramnios) and prenatal exposure to alcohol and drugs such as cocaine; short cords have been associated with compromised neurological development (Kaplan, 2008). Most umbilical cords are twisted; usually the twists are counterclockwise 'left twists' every few centimetres. Cords without any twists are associated with single umbilical artery (SUA) and an increased risk of perinatal mortality. Excessive twisting, which can compromise blood flow, is also associated with fetal morbidity and mortality. True knots in the umbilical cord occur in about 1% of births (Moore and Persaud, 1998). The vessels of the cord, two arteries carrying blood from the fetus and one vein carrying blood to the fetus, are embedded in Wharton's jelly. This jelly is a connective tissue that protects the vessels of the cord.

EXAMINATION OF THE PLACENTA

Examination of the placenta, membranes and umbilical cord at delivery is an important responsibility of the attendant midwives. A quick visual inspection of the maternal and fetal surfaces can pick up the occasional abnormal specimen; unusual odour which could indicate a bacterial infection and substantial amounts of fresh clot could indicate premature placental separation. Cord length and diameter are assessed and the distance of insertion to the nearest placental margin. The cord is checked for vessel number, true knots, twisting, discolouration, congestion and thrombosis. There are usually two arteries and the persisting left umbilical vein. The SUA occurs in about 1% of births and is associated with an increased frequency of fetal and chromosomal abnormalities, particularly of the renal or cardiovascular systems (Benirschke, 1994); however, it is normal for the arteries to fuse together just above the fetal surface. Sometimes more vessels are present because the right umbilical vein has not regressed. Although an abnormality in the number of vessels is associated with congenital abnormalities, it is not clear whether the wrong number of vessels is a cause or a result of the abnormality. About 20% of infants with SUA will have other major congenital abnormalities; the remainder are often slightly small and have an increased risk of perinatal mortality (Kaplan, 2008). Macrosomic babies of diabetic mothers tend to have thick oedematous cords, whereas thin delicate cords are associated with IUGR. The cord can be inserted into the placental bed in different ways. Insertion of the cord is usually approximately central but may be lateral. Abnormal insertion of the cord can create problems at delivery (Table 8.2). If the cord is ruptured, it indicates that there may have been some fetal blood loss during labour. The chorionic plate opacity and colour including the amount of fibrin and thrombosis in the subchorionic region can also be assessed.

The type of membrane insertion and their completeness are assessed. The membranes are easier to examine if the placenta is held up by the cord. Usually, the two membranes hang down in a neat uniform way. The placenta is continuous with the chorion but the amnion should be able to be separated from the chorion up to the base of the cord. If the membranes are ragged and torn, some parts of the membrane may be retained in the uterus, which can impede uterine involution and staunching of blood loss. Meconium can discolour the membranes in late gestation; fresh meconium may also be present.

A healthy placenta is normally rounded and uniform but shape is quite variable. Unusual shapes may be a result of uterine cavity abnormalities. Placental weight is usually between 350 and 750 g; excessively light or heavy placentas are associated with pathological conditions. An excessively large or oedematous (soft) placenta is associated with

Table 8.2 Placental abnormalities

CONDITION	DESCRIPTION AND CAUSE
Abruptio placentae	Separation of normally situated placenta from site of implantation after 24th week of gestation but before delivery of the fetus. More common in women with high parity and history of obstetric problems. May cause uterine tenderness and tetany, and variable bleeding. Complications may include disseminated intravascular coagulation (DIC), postpartum haemorrhage (PPH) and shock. It is essential to avoid vaginal examination until placenta previa has been excluded
Placenta previa	Abnormally implanted placenta, positioned partially or totally (over the os) in the lower segment, which obstructs normal delivery. More common in multigravidae, particularly those of high parity and with multiple pregnancy. Usually causes painless vaginal bleeding. Factors that cause damage and scarring of the endometrium increase risk. Possibly due to deficient decidua in fundus at implantation. The placenta is likely to be large and may have succenturiate lobes (see below)
Abnormal insertion of cord	Vasa previa is a rare condition that may occur with velamentous insertion of cord where some of the umbilical vessels cross the internal os. Velamentous insertion occurs in 1% of singleton pregnancies. The cord is attached to the membranes outside the placental boundary and blood vessels, unprotected by Wharton's jelly, and is at risk from compression and tearing
Abnormal conformation of placenta	Placentation may be extrachorial, where the surface area of the chorionic plate is less than the basal (maternal) area. A circumarginate placenta has a flat ring at the transition from placenta to chorion. A circumvallate placenta has a raised rolled ring at the transition and is associated with increased incidence of growth retardation
Succenturiate (accessory) lobes	Variations in shape and number of lobes do not normally affect the outcome of the pregnancy. The placenta may have accessory lobes or be completely bi-lobed. This may cause problems in determining whether the placenta has been completely expelled at delivery
Hydatidiform mole and choriocarcinoma	Abnormal placental development where the embryo is absent or non-viable. Related to abnormal fertilization and survival of paternal chromosomes only (see Chapter 7). Hydatidiform mole is a non-invasive chorionic development and choriocarcinoma is a malignant tumour derived from trophoblast tissue, possibly from a hydatidiform mole. The villi are not vascularized in either case (as extraembryonic mesoderm is derived from the inner cell mass)
Abnormal adherence of chorionic villi	In placenta accreta, the villi adhere to the uterine wall, which has an abnormal decidual layer due to excessive invasion. In placenta percreta, the villi penetrate right through the myometrium to the perimetrium. The placenta fails to separate properly in the third stage of labour and maternal haemorrhage is likely

maternal diabetes, hydrops or cardiac abnormalities. Maternal diabetes tends to result in placenta with a deep red colour. The placenta is also examined for abnormal numbers of lobes (Table 8.2) or missing areas of the maternal surface, which could indicate that a lobe has been retained, potentially causing serious postpartum bleeding. Depending on whether twins are monozygotic or dizygotic, the placenta may be shared or regions fused (Box 8.4). The maternal surface is examined for completeness, adherent blood clot, lesions (such as infarcts and thrombi) and degree of calcification. Cysts are common on the surface and are associated with fibrin deposition but are usually not significant. True placental infarcts are also common,

they tend to be small (<1 cm) and located at the placental margins. Haemorrhages on the maternal surface are usually due to premature separation and are more common with hypertensive disorders, ascending infection, smoking and cocaine use (Kaplan, 2008).

Sometimes a dense raised white rim may be observed on the periphery of the fetal placental bed; this is called a circumvallate placenta. It is thought to be caused by deep implantation of the placenta into the maternal decidua and subsequent partial separation of the placental from the uterine wall. This results in the folding back of the membrane towards the chorionic surface. The rim is a double fold of fetal membranes with degenerated

Box 8.4 **The placenta in multiple pregnancies**

Dizygotic (non-identical) twins and monozygotic (identical) twins resulting from early splitting of the blastocyst prior to implantation can have separate placentas and membranes. However, if the two blastocysts implant in close proximity, the placentas and chorion may fuse. If monozygotic twins arise from division of the inner cell mass, they usually have separate amnions but share the placenta and chorion. The vascular systems within the placenta may remain separate but can fuse. If the vascular systems fuse within the placenta, twin-to-twin transfusion syndrome may occur where the twins have

an unequal blood supply. This condition, which occurs in 10–15% of monozygotic twins (thus affecting 1 in 400 pregnancies, 1 in 1600 babies) with a shared placenta, can threaten the survival of both twins because the donor twin is anaemic and the recipient twin is polycythaemic and prone to cardiac hypertrophy and heart failure. Modern treatments have increased the survival of twins but the survivors are at increased risk of brain injury and neurodevelopment consequences.

Case study 8.3

Following what appeared to be a normal delivery, the midwife inspected the placenta and membranes. She discovered a hole in the membranes that had blood vessels leading to it, radiating out from the main body of the placenta.

- What do you think the midwife concluded from these findings?
- What care and observation will the woman require?
- How will this be explained to the woman and what information might she require?

- Extravillous cytotrophoblast invades the maternal circulation resulting in remodelling of the spiral arteries.
- Extraembryonic mesoderm, originating from the inner cell mass, invades the core of the villi and establishes the vasculature of the villi.
- The villi continue to grow and remodel throughout the pregnancy; the barrier to diffusion is reduced as fetal requirements increase.
- The placenta has specific transport mechanisms and a range of endocrine activities. It also has an important immunological role.
- Amniotic fluid, produced by the amniotic membrane, cushions and protects the fetus. It is also important in the development of the respiratory system.
- Inadequate maternal uteroplacental blood flow, described as placental insufficiency, is associated with the aetiology of pre-eclampsia and IUGR.
- Examination of the placenta is important in detecting any abnormality or retention of placental tissue.

decidua and fibrin between them. The clinical significance of the condition is uncertain but it may be a risk factor for antenatal haemorrhage and/or severe intermittent uterine contractions. It is more common in multigravidae and in women who have previously had a circumvallate placenta.

Case study 8.3 details an example of placental abnormality revealed by inspection.

Key points

- The placenta derives largely from the trophoblast layer of the embryo, which differentiates into two layers: the cytotrophoblast and the syncytiotrophoblast.
- The cytotrophoblast undergoes rapid mitosis and the syncytiotrophoblast aggressively digests and invades the maternal endometrial wall.
- Fragments of maternal blood vessels are engulfed forming lacunae and a framework for villi development.

Application to practice

The placenta has an important physiological role in supporting and maintaining pregnancy. Dysfunctioning of the placenta and its development results in abnormal conditions, which may be observed in pregnancy which may affect the health of the mother and baby before and after birth.

Knowledge of the gross anatomy and the variants in the placental structure is essential in the postnatal examination of the placenta and membranes.

ANNOTATED FURTHER READING

Benirschke K, Kaufmann P: *Pathology of the human placenta*, ed 5, New York, 2006, Springer.

A comprehensive reference text, which covers the structure of the placenta at birth, types of placenta, early development and cellular details.

Cudihy D, Lee RV: The pathophysiology of pre-eclampsia: current clinical concepts, *J Obstet Gynaecol* 29:576–582, 2009.

This is an overview of existing knowledge about pre-eclampsia, which can still be described as a 'medical mystery', which identifies and attempts to unify findings of past and current scientific investigation providing examination of the known risk factors, the epidemiologic trends, and recent research about the pathogenesis of the disease.

Desforges M, Sibley CP: *Placental nutrient supply and fetal growth, Int J Dev Biol* 54:377–390, 2010.

Detailed review of the mechanisms involved in placental transfer and how the capability of the placenta to supply nutrients affects fetal growth.

Fisk NM, Duncombe GJ, Sullivan MH: The basic and clinical science of twin-twin transfusion syndrome, *Placenta* 30:379–390, 2009.

Recent review about twin-to-twin transfusion syndrome which includes discussion on the underlying placental pathophysiology, the resulting fetal pathophysiology, fetal surveillance and recent therapeutic advances.

Harman CR: Amniotic fluid abnormalities, *Semin Perinatol* 32:288–294, 2008.

A clear and well-written description of the functions and dynamics of normal amniotic fluid volume and composition with detailed sections on oligohydramnios and polyhydramnios.

A review of placental development which also covers placental functions and transport mechanisms.

Huppertz B: The anatomy of the normal placenta, *J Clin Pathol* 61:1296–1302, 2008.

An excellent review describing the development of the placenta including the gross and microscopic anatomy and histology of the delivered placenta.

Arroyo JA, Winn VD: Vasculogenesis and angiogenesis in the IUGR placenta, *Semin Perinatol* 32:172–177, 2008.

A clearly written and well-illustrated description of placenta blood vessel formation in normal placental development

and in pregnancies complicated by intrauterine growth restriction.

Kaplan CG: Gross pathology of the placenta: weight, shape, size, colour, *J Clin Pathol* 61:1285–1295, 2008.

A comprehensive review of placental abnormalities, illustrated with photographic examples, which includes guidance on placental examination.

Kingdom J, Jauniaux E, O'Brien S: *The placenta: basic science and clinical practice*, London, 2000, Royal College of Obstetricians and Gynaecologists.

A comprehensive handbook covering scientific and clinical aspects of placental structure and function, placental pathology including growth restriction and pre-eclampsia), placental infection, preterm labour, placental malignancy, clinical assessment of the placenta and placental complications in labour.

Tyson RW, Staat BC: The intrauterine growth-restricted fetus and placenta evaluation, *Semin Perinatol* 32:166–171, 2008.

An excellent review which relates evaluation of the placenta to the pathophysiology underlying intrauterine growth restriction; includes an excellent table of the common gross and microscopic characteristics of the placenta in growth restriction.

REFERENCES

Achache H, Revel A: Endometrial receptivity markers, the journey to successful embryo implantation, *Hum Reprod Update* 12:731–746, 2006.

Aldoretta PW, Hay WW Jr: Metabolic substrates for fetal energy metabolism and growth *Clin Perinatol* 22(1):15–36, 1995.

Arroyo JA, Winn VD: Vasculogenesis and angiogenesis in the IUGR placenta, *Semin Perinatol* 32:172–177, 2008.

Benirschke K: Obstetrically important lesions of the umbilical cord, *J Reprod Med* 39:226, 1994.

Banerjee P, Fazleabas AT: Endometrial responses to embryonic signals in the primate, *Int J Dev Biol* 54:295–302, 2010.

Bischof P, Meisser A, Campana A: Paracrine and autocrine regulators of trophoblast invasion: a review, *Placenta* 21(Suppl A):S55–S60, 2000.

Brosens JJ, Pijnenborg R, Brosens IA: The myometrial junctional zone spiral arteries in normal and abnormal pregnancies: a review of the literature, *Am J Obstet Gynecol* 187 (5):1416–1423, 2002.

Burton GJ, Hempstock J, Jauniaux E: Nutrition of the human fetus during the first trimester: a review, *Placenta* 22(Suppl A):S70–S77, 2001.

Burton GJ, Woods AW, Jauniaux E, et al: Rheological and physiological consequences of conversion of the maternal spiral arteries for

uteroplacental blood flow during human pregnancy, *Placenta* 30:473–482, 2009a.

Burton GJ, Yung HW, Cindrova-Davies T, et al: Placental endoplasmic reticulum stress and oxidative stress in the pathophysiology of unexplained intrauterine growth restriction and early onset preeclampsia, *Placenta* 30Suppl A: S43–S48, 2009b.

Cai WQ, Bodin P, Sexton A, et al: Localization of neuropeptide Y and atrial natriuretic peptide in the endothelial cells of human umbilical blood vessels, *Cell Tissue Res* 272:175–181, 1993.

Calvano CJ, Hoar RM, Mankes RF, et al: Experimental study of umbilical cord length as a marker of fetal alcohol syndrome, *Teratology* 61 (3):184–188, 2000.

Carlson BM: *Human embryology and developmental biology*. St. Louis 1994, Mosby.

Cetin I, Corbetta C, Sereni LP, et al: Umbilical amino acid concentrations in normal and growth-retarded fetuses sampled in utero by cordocentesis, *Am J Obstet Gynecol* 162:253–261, 1990.

Cetin I, Alvino G: Intrauterine growth restriction: implications for placental metabolism and transport. A review, *Placenta* 30: Suppl A: S77–S82, 2009.

Chard T: Placental metabolism, In Chamberlain G, Broughton Pipkin F, editors: *Clinical physiology in obstetrics*, ed 3, Oxford, 1998, Blackwell, pp 419–436.

Demir R, Seval Y, Huppertz B: Vasculogenesis and angiogenesis in the early human placenta, *Acta Histochem* 109:257–265, 2007.

Desforges M, Sibley CP: Placental nutrient supply and fetal growth, *Int J Dev Biol* 54:377–390, 2010.

Edwards A, Megens A, Peek M, et al: Sexual origins of placental dysfunction, *Lancet* 355:203–204, 2000.

Evain-Brion D, Malassine A: Human placenta as an endocrine organ, *Growth Horm IGF Res* 13(Suppl A): S34–S37, 2003.

Firth JA, Leach L: Not trophoblast alone: a review of the contribution to the fetal microvasculature to transplacental exchange, *Placenta* 17:89, 1996.

Fowden AL, Forhead AJ: Endocrine regulation of feto-placental growth, *Horm Res* 72:257–265, 2009.

Fowden AL, Sferruzzi-Perri AN, Coan PM, et al: Placental efficiency and adaptation: endocrine regulation, *J Physiol* 587:3459–3472, 2009.

Hamilton-Fairley D, Johnson MR: The ovary. In Chamberlain G, Broughton Pipkin F, editors, *Clinical physiology in obstetrics*, ed 3, Oxford, 1998, Blackwell, pp 396–416.

Harman CR, Baschat AA: Comprehensive assessment of fetal wellbeing: which Doppler tests should be performed? *Curr Opin Obstet Gynecol* 15(2):147–157, 2003.

Harman CR: Amniotic fluid abnormalities, *Semin Perinatol* 32:288–294, 2008.

Hawfield A, Freedman BI: Pre-eclampsia: the pivotal role of the placenta in its pathophysiology and markers for early detection, *Ther Adv Cardiovasc Dis* 3:65–73, 2009.

Huppertz B: The anatomy of the normal placenta, *J Clin Pathol* 61:1296–1302, 2008.

Iles RK, Chard T: Human chorionic gonadotrophin expression by bladder cancers: biology and clinical potential, *J. Urol.* 145:453, 1991.

Jauniaux E, Gulbis B: Fluid compartments of the embryonic environment, *Hum Reprod Update* 6(3):268–278, 2000.

Jauniaux E, Jurkovic D, Campbell S, et al: Doppler ultrasonographic features of the developing placental circulation: correlation with anatomic findings, *Am J Obstet Gynecol* 166:585, 1992.

Jauniaux E, Gulbis B, Burton GJ: The human first trimester gestational sac limits rather than facilitates oxygen transfer to the foetus: a review, *Placenta* 24(Suppl A):S86–S93, 2003.

Jauniaux E, Poston L, Burton GJ: Placental-related diseases of pregnancy: involvement of oxidative stress and implications in human evolution, *Hum Reprod Update* 12:747–755, 2006.

Johnson MR, Bolton VN, Riddle AF, et al: Interactions between the embryo and corpus luteum, *Hum Reprod* 8:1496–1501, 1993a.

Johnson MR, Riddle AF, Irvine R, et al: Corpus luteum failure in ectopic pregnancy, *Hum Reprod* 8:1491–1495, 1993b.

Kaplan CG: Gross pathology of the placenta: weight, shape, size, colour, *J Clin Pathol* 61:1285–1295, 2008.

Kent A, Kitau MJ, Chard T: Absence of diurnal variation in urinary chorionic gonadotrophin excretion at 8–13 weeks gestation, *Br J Obstet Gynaecol* 98:1180, 1991.

Kingdom J, Sibley C: The placenta. In Hillier SG, Kitchener HC, Neilson JP, editors, *Scientific essentials of reproductive medicine*, Philadelphia, 1996, Saunders, pp 312–318.

Kingdom JCP, Awad H, Fleming JEE, et al: Obstetrical determination of

relative placental size, *Placenta* 14: A36, 1993.

Kingdom JCP, Sherlock J, Rodeck CH, et al: Detection of trophoblast cells in transcervical samples collected by lavage and cytobrush, *Obstet Gynecol* 86:283–288, 1995.

Knipp GT, Audus KL, Soares MJ: Nutrient transport across the placenta, *Adv Drug Delivery Rev* 38(1):41–58, 1999.

Knofler M: Critical growth factors and signalling pathways controlling human trophoblast invasion, *Int J Dev Biol* 54:269–280, 2010.

Lala PK, Chakraborty C: Factors regulating trophoblast migration and invasiveness, *Placenta* 24(1):575–587, 2003.

Learmont JG, Braude PR, Poston L: Flow induced dilation is modulated by nitric oxide in isolated human small fetoplacental arteries, *J Vasc Res* 31 (Suppl 1):26, 1994.

Meuris S, Nagy AM, Delogne-Desnoeck J, et al: Temporal relationship between the human chorionic gonadotrophin peak and the establishment of the inter-villus blood flow in early pregnancy, *Hum Reprod* 10:947, 1995.

Miller AWF, Hanretty KP: *Obstetrics illustrated*, ed 5, New York, 1998, Churchill Livingstone, pp 12, 99.

Miller J, Turan S, Baschat AA: Fetal growth restriction, *Semin Perinatol* 32:274–280, 2008.

Moore KL, Persaud TVN: *Before we are born: essentials of embryology and birth defects*, ed 5, Philadelphia, 1998, Saunders.

Murphy CR: Understanding the apical surface markers of uterine receptivity: pinopods-or uterodomes? *Hum Reprod* 15:2451–2454, 2000.

Myatt L, Brewer AS, Brockman DE: The comparative effects of big endothelin-1, endothelin-1, and endothelin-3 in the human fetal–placental circulation, *Am J Obstet Gynecol* 167:1651–1656, 1992.

Myatt L, Brockman DE, Eis ALW, et al: Immunohistochemical localization of nitric oxide synthase in the human placenta, *Placenta* 14:487–495, 1993.

Ray JG, Laskin CA: Folic acid and homocyst(e)ine metabolic defects and the risk of placental abruption, pre-eclampsia and spontaneous pregnancy loss: a systematic review, *Placenta* 20(7):519–529, 1999.

Schindler AE: First trimester endocrinology: consequences for diagnosis and treatment of pregnancy failure, *Gynecol Endocrinol* 18 (1):51–57, 2004.

Shiverick KT, Salafia C: Cigarette smoking and pregnancy I: ovarian, uterine and placental effects, *Placenta* 20(4):265–272, 1999.

Spencer K, Coombes J, Mallard SA, et al: Free beta human chorionic gonadotrophin in Down's syndrome screening: a multicentre study of its role compared to other biochemical markers, *Ann Clin Biochem* 29:506–518, 1992.

Stone S, Pijnenborg R, Vercruysse L, et al: The placental bed in pregnancies complicated by primary antiphospholipid syndrome, *Placenta* 27:457–467, 2006.

Ticconi C, Zicari A, Belmonte A, et al: Pregnancy-promoting actions of HCG in human myometrium and fetal membranes, *Placenta* 28:Suppl A:S137–S143, 2007.

Usadi RS, Murray MJ, Bagnell RC, et al: Temporal and morphologic characteristics of pinopod expression across the secretory phase of the endometrial cycle in normally cycling women with proven fertility, *Fertil Steril* 79:970–974, 2003.

Vitiello D, Patrizio P: Implantation and early embryonic development:

implications for pregnancy, *Semin Perinatol* 31:204–207, 2007.

Wenstrom KD, Owen J, Boots LR, et al: Elevated second trimester human chorionic gonadotropin levels in association with poor pregnancy outcome, *Am J Obstet Gynecol* 171:1038–1041, 1994.

Wilcox GR, Trudinger BJ: Fetal platelet consumption: a feature of placental insufficiency, *Obstet Gynecol* 77:616–621, 1991.

Wilcox AJ, Baird DD, Weinberg CR: Time of implantation of the conceptus and loss of pregnancy, *N Engl J Med* 340:1796–1799, 1999.

Wilson ME, Ford SP: Comparative aspects of placental efficiency, *Reprod Suppl* 58:223–232, 2001.

Chapter | 9 |

Embryo development and fetal growth

LEARNING OBJECTIVES

- To describe the formation of the bilaminar and trilaminar embryonic discs in weeks 2 and 3 of development.
- To outline the events involved in folding of the embryonic disc into the characteristic shape of the human embryo.
- To define key embryological terms: gastrulation, neurulation, primitive streak, somites and notochord.
- To outline events in development in the first 8 weeks.
- To describe developmental characteristics of the fetal organ systems.
- To discuss factors affecting fetal growth and the implications these have for future health.
- To relate the timing of development with sensitive periods and to appreciate the developmental factors limiting survival of a preterm baby.
- To briefly outline how common fetal abnormalities are related to abnormal embryonic development.

INTRODUCTION

During the 9 months of pregnancy, the single cell of the zygote divides to produce 6 billion cells of the mature fetus. On average, an adult cell is the product of about 47 cell divisions from the zygote, at least 40 of which occur before birth. The first 3 weeks of development are often described as the pre-embryonic period when the cells differentiate into germ layers from which all organs and tissues develop. The sequence of events in this stage, albeit with a different time course, is similar in all sorts of animals, including *Drosophila* (fruit fly), nematodes, amphibians and birds as well as mammals. The embryonic stage, embryogenesis or organogenesis, lasts from week 4 to week 8 in the human. During this time, the organ systems are established and the embryo develops distinct human characteristics. The fetal stage, from week 9 to birth, is largely a period of growth, during which time the systems become more refined and mature and the fetus gains weight, ready to function at birth. Fetal age is timed from fertilization, whereas pregnancy is dated from the first day of the last normal menstrual period. This means that the timing of the pregnancy is 2 weeks more than the true fetal age. The average length of pregnancy is 280 days (40 weeks) when the fetus is 266 days old (38 weeks). Understanding the key concepts of embryology and fetal development is important in monitoring the well-being of the fetus and developing appropriate healthcare programmes to promote better reproductive health outcomes. This field has important applications in prenatal diagnosis and treatments as well as prevention and management of infertility and birth defects. Pregnant women are also obviously interested in knowing how their baby is changing during the duration of the pregnancy. (Development in the first week after fertilization is described in Chapter 6.)

Chapter case study

Zara is 5 feet and 2 in. tall (155 cm) and, prior to pregnancy, wore size 8 clothes; she wears size 3 (European size 35.5) shoes. Her husband, James, is 6 feet tall (180 cm) and has quite a broad, muscular frame and has size 11 feet (European size 46). Zara has frequently discussed with her midwife her concerns that she will have

Continued

Chapter case study—cont'd

a big baby and problems in labour because James is tall and has a large frame.

- How can the midwife reassure Zara that the baby's growth is unlikely to be disproportionate to her size and what physiological measurements and observations can be made to support this?
- If Zara was found to be carrying a large baby how would the midwife be able to recognize this and what could be the possible explanations for this?
- How would having a large baby affect the plan of care for Zara; what are the potential concerns and how could they be mediated?

WEEK 2

By the end of the first week, the blastocyst has entered the uterine cavity, hatched out of the zona pellucida and started the process of implantation into the endometrial wall. Two types of cells are evident: the outer trophoblast (see Chapter 6) and the inner cell mass (or embryoblast). The inner cell mass gives rise to tissues of the embryo and also contributes towards some of the extraembryonic membranes. The undifferentiated cells from the blastocyst are called stem cells and have some potential therapeutic uses (see Box 9.1). At about day 7 after fertilization, the cells of the inner cell mass start to proliferate and

Box 9.1 **Stem cells, totipotency and pluripotency**

Stem cells are unspecialized cells that have the ability to self-renew and to differentiate into a number of cell types. This ability to produce a variety of differentiated cell types means that stem cells are a potential source of replacement cells that could be used to treat variety of diseases and repair damaged tissues. There are several categories of stem cells defined according to the variety of cells they are able to produce. Totipotent stem cells are able to produce all of the cells present in the fetus and adult together with those in the extraembryonic tissues such as placenta. Pluripotent cells are able to produce any cell in the body, multipotent cells can produce particular types of related cells, for example blood cells, whereas oligopotent (a few types of very similar cells) and unipotent (one cell type) have progressively more restricted lineages.

The zygote and cells from only the first few divisions are termed 'totipotent'. At the fourth cleavage division after fertilization, when the 8-cell embryo divided to form 16 cells, totipotency is lost. Genetic screening can be carried out at the 8-cell stage by the technique of pre-implantation genetic diagnosis by removing one of the eight cells for analysis. Since all cells at this stage are totipotent, the zygote will develop normally from the seven remaining cells. Also, if the cells are separated at this stage and allowed to implant, identical offspring will develop; this is a type of cloning. Following the loss of totipotency, the embryonic cells differentiate into pluripotent stem cells. These pluripotent cells can form any of the three types of germ cell layer (endoderm, mesoderm or ectoderm) and are therefore capable of becoming any cell in the body but cannot form a unique individual because they cannot form extraembryonic mesoderm and placental tissue.

There are a number of sources of stem cells which are usually classified as being embryonic (pluripotent) or adult (multipotent) stem cells. Embryonic stem cells (ESC) can be harvested from inner cell mass of the blastocyst (the trilaminar embryonic disc). Research using ESC is controversial because human ESC are taken from early embryos which are

destroyed. ESC can be obtained from a cloned embryo which would make them genetically compatible with the recipient and therefore avoid the issue of immune rejection. A potentially important and recent advance is to 'persuade' differentiated cells to return to the undifferentiated stem cell state by expression of specific genes, a technique referred to as induced pluripotency (iPS). This also offers the advantage that somatic cells from an adult can be converted into stem cells and then be used to treat diseases in the same person, again, avoiding the problem of tissue immune rejection.

Adult stem cells are derived from progenitor cell populations such as bone marrow cells which can be differentiated into liver, kidney, muscle and nerve cells as well as blood cells. Skin dermis cells can be transdifferentiated into many types of tissue including neurons, smooth muscle cells and fat cells. It is also possible that brain cells could be harvested from dead organ donors. A major concern of stem cell use is to control stem cell division to ensure that tissues are regenerated but tumours do not grow.

Most adult stem cells are multipotent but some stem cells from the umbilical cord and cord blood cells are pluripotent. It is possible to reprogram multipotent adult stem cells to become pluripotent. In some countries, parents are asked whether they would like to have their baby's cord blood cells frozen in case they can be used later in life to treat a disease. The blood is taken from the umbilical vein of the cleaned cord once the baby has been delivered; it is checked for infectious agents, tissue-typed and then stored in liquid nitrogen. Stem cells can be used either autologously (for the person they came from) or as an allogenic treatment, where the donor and recipient are different individuals. The information given to new parents suggests a much wider use of the stem cells harvested from their baby's umbilical blood but many of these applications are currently at the research stage. To date, stem cells have been used in humans to treat leukaemia and restore eyesight using limbal stem cell therapy. The treatment of type-I diabetes, spinal cord injuries, neurodegenerative and other diseases is an active area of research.

differentiate rapidly. The inner cell mass becomes flattened into a bilaminar embryonic disc with the cells forming two distinct layers (Fig. 9.1). The cells adjacent to the blastocyst cavity appear distinctly cuboidal. These form the hypoblast or primary endoderm layer, which gives rise

to the future gut and its derivatives. The upper layer of cells is formed of columnar epiblast cells, which will differentiate into the ectodermal layer. Some of the epiblast cells spread laterally to form the amnioblasts of the amniotic membrane that encloses the amniotic cavity. Cells from the hypoblast layer migrate forming a membrane called the exocoelomic membrane or Heuser's membrane which lines the cytotrophoblast so the blastocyst cavity is also enclosed. This is the cavity that will become the primitive (primary) yolk sac. There are two waves of endoderm cell remodelling of the blastocyst cavity, which form initially the primary yolk sac and then, at the beginning of the fifth week, the definitive (secondary) yolk sac (Fig. 9.2). The formation of the definitive yolk sac creates the chorionic cavity and the extraembryonic mesoderm, which gives rise to the vascular structures of the placenta (see Chapter 8). The definitive yolk sac synthesizes several proteins including alpha-fetoprotein (AFP). The bi-laminar disc lies between two fluid-filled cavities: the amniotic cavity on the epiblast (ectoderm) side and the yolk sac cavity on the hypoblast (endoderm) side. (The primitive yolk sac will shrink away from the cytotrophoblast in the fourth week, creating a new cavity called the chorionic cavity or extraembryonic coelom, which fills with fluid and becomes the largest cavity in the developing conceptus.)

At the end of the second week, a region of endodermal cells starts to thicken and become columnar, forming the prochordal plate (Fig. 9.3). This marks the cranial

7 days

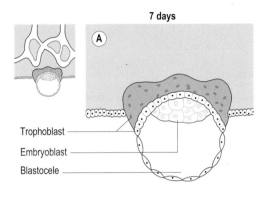

Trophoblast

Embryoblast

Blastocele

8 days

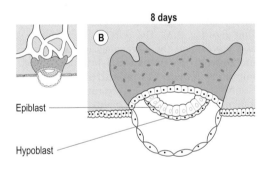

Epiblast

Hypoblast

9 days

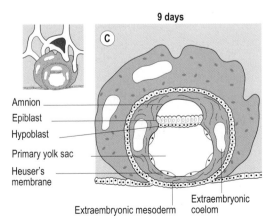

Amnion

Epiblast

Hypoblast

Primary yolk sac

Heuser's membrane

Extraembryonic mesoderm

Extraembryonic coelom

Fig. 9.1 Differentiation of the inner cell mass into the bilaminar disc: (A) 7 days; (B) 8 days; (C) 9 days. (Reproduced with permission from Fitzgerald and Fitzgerald, 1994.)

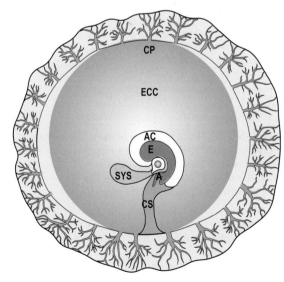

Fig. 9.2 First-trimester gestational sac about 3 weeks postfertilization, showing chorionic plate (CP) surrounding entire sac, extraembryonic coelom (ECC), amniotic cavity (AC) and embryo (E) with its secondary yolk sac (SYS) providing nutrients. (Reproduced with permission from Jauniaux et al., 2003.)

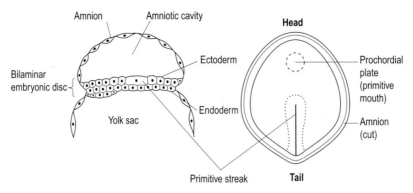

Fig. 9.3 Formation of the prochordal plate (future mouth) and primitive streak on the bilaminar and trilaminar embryonic discs.

Box 9.2 **Totipotency and pluripotency**

The zygote and cells of the early blastocyst are termed 'totipotent' which means that each cell has the ability to develop into all cells of the organism and form all the types of body tissue. At the fourth division after fertilization, when the eight cells present divide forming 16 cells, totipotency is lost. Genetic screening can be carried out by pre-implantation genetic diagnosis before the fourth division by removing one of the eight cells for analysis; the zygote will develop normally from the seven remaining cells. If the cells are separated and implanted, identical offspring will develop; this is a type of cloning. Following the loss of totipotency, the embryonic cells differentiate into pluripotent stem cells. These pluripotent cells can form any of the three types of germ cell layer: endoderm, mesoderm or ectoderm but cannot form a unique individual because they cannot form extraembryonic mesoderm and placental tissue.

WEEK 3

At this stage, when the woman may first realize she is pregnant, embryo development is rapid. A line of epiblast cells, starting from the caudal region (tail end) at the other side from the prochordal plate, undergoes very rapid cell division, forming the primitive streak in the midline (see Fig. 9.3). The cells of the primitive streak form a groove and then invaginate (move inwards) to spread between the epiblast and hypoblast layers. The bilaminar disc is therefore converted into a trilaminar disc consisting of three germ layers (ectoderm, mesoderm and endoderm), which give rise to specific tissues of the body (Fig. 9.4). The middle layer is the mesoderm, from which connective tissue, smooth muscle, the cardiovascular system and blood, the skeleton and the reproductive and

region (head end) and is the site of the future mouth. The prochordal plate is also important in influencing further development of the cranial region (Box 9.2).

By the second week, according to the embryologist's 'rule of twos', the following have taken place:

- two germ layers have formed: the endoderm and the ectoderm
- two trophoblastic layers have formed: cytotrophoblast and syncytiotrophoblast
- two waves of remodelling have occurred: that of the blastocyst into the primary and then the definitive yolk sac
- two novel cavities have formed: the amniotic cavity and the chorionic cavity
- two layers have formed from the extraembryonic mesoderm.

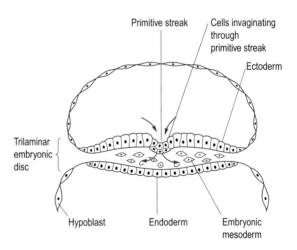

Fig. 9.4 The invagination of cells of the primitive streak between the ectodermal and endodermal layers creates a trilaminar embryonic disc. (Reproduced with permission from Fitzgerald and Fitzgerald, 1994.)

endocrine systems develop (Fig. 9.5). The epiblast becomes the ectoderm, which will develop into the epidermis, central and peripheral nervous systems and the retina. Therefore, the ectoderm, which will give rise to the skin, is in contact with the amniotic cavity from very early on in embryonic development. The hypoblast becomes the endoderm, from which epithelial linings and some glandular structures will form. The three germ layers interact, generating signals that induce cellular interactions and cause structural alterations and more complex interactions.

The endodermal prochordal plate is fused to the ectoderm forming the oropharyngeal membrane (future mouth). Below the primitive streak, there is another area of fusion between the ectoderm and endoderm; this is the cloacal membrane (the future anus). Rare birth complications such as imperforate anus may arise from abnormal development of the cloacal membrane. Some mesoderm cells migrate towards the prochordal plate forming a cord of adhesive cells (Fig. 9.6). This is the notochordal process, which develops a lumen forming the notochord canal. The notochord evolves into a cellular rod-like tube, which gives the trilaminar disc a degree of rigidity and defines the central head–tail axis of the embryo. If identical twins are going to develop, there are two parallel notochords.

If there are two notochords that cross, conjoined (Siamese) twins will result; on the position where the notochords cross dictates where the twins will be conjoined, for example twins with cephalic joining have a higher cross-over point of their notochords than twins who are joined at the hips (Spitz, 2005). The notochord establishes the development of the axial skeleton (bones of head and spinal cord) and the neural plate, which gives rise to the primitive nervous system. The vertebral column forms around the notochord and the notochord induces neurulation, the formation of the neural tube and early nervous system (see below). During the third week, aggregates of mesoderm on either side of the notochord form pairs of bead-like blocks called somites, which direct the segmented structure of the body and induce the overlying ectoderm to form structures of the nervous system.

The formation of the primitive streak, the three germ layers, the prochordal plate and the notochord is described as gastrulation. Gastrulation marks the beginning of morphogenesis, the emergence and development of body form and structure. It begins with the appearance of the primitive streak at day 14. The primitive streak defines the time when experimental manipulation of human embryos is legally obliged to stop under the terms of the UK Human Fertilization and Embryology Act of 1990 (amended

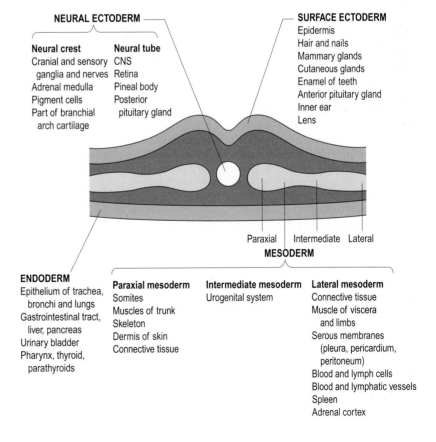

Fig. 9.5 The neural and surface ectoderm, the endoderm and the mesoderm will differentiate into future tissues of the body.

NEURAL ECTODERM

Neural crest
Cranial and sensory
  ganglia and nerves
Adrenal medulla
Pigment cells
Part of branchial
  arch cartilage

Neural tube
CNS
Retina
Pineal body
Posterior
  pituitary gland

SURFACE ECTODERM
Epidermis
Hair and nails
Mammary glands
Cutaneous glands
Enamel of teeth
Anterior pituitary gland
Inner ear
Lens

Paraxial   Intermediate   Lateral
MESODERM

ENDODERM
Epithelium of trachea,
  bronchi and lungs
Gastrointestinal tract,
  liver, pancreas
Urinary bladder
Pharynx, thyroid,
  parathyroids

Paraxial mesoderm
Somites
Muscles of trunk
Skeleton
Dermis of skin
Connective tissue

Intermediate mesoderm
Urogenital system

Lateral mesoderm
Connective tissue
Muscle of viscera
  and limbs
Serous membranes
  (pleura, pericardium,
  peritoneum)
Blood and lymph cells
Blood and lymphatic vessels
Spleen
Adrenal cortex

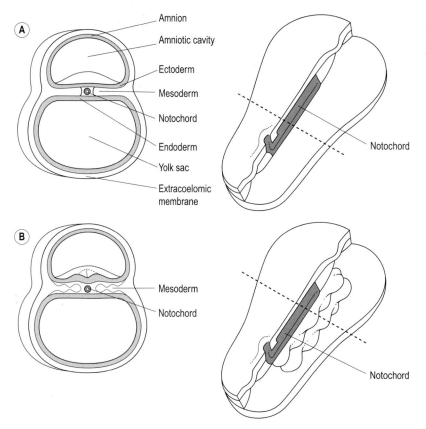

Fig. 9.6 Notochord formation: (A) 17 days and (B) 18 days. (Reproduced with permission from Goodwin, 1997.)

Labels for (A): Amnion, Amniotic cavity, Ectoderm, Mesoderm, Notochord, Endoderm, Yolk sac, Extracoelomic membrane, Notochord

Labels for (B): Mesoderm, Notochord, Notochord

2008). Gastrulation is a very sensitive stage of embryogenesis; the cell populations are very vulnerable to teratogenic insult at the beginning of the third week of development (Sadler, 2010). For instance, high levels of alcohol can kill cells in the craniofacial region of the embryonic disc affecting brain and face development. The very rare tumours of the neonate can be a result of remnants of primitive streak proliferating to form sacrococcygeal tumours. During the third week of development, as well as gastrulation, the primitive nervous system and cardiovascular system begin to develop.

Box 9.3 is a summary of the events taking place in weeks 1–3.

WEEKS 4–8: ORGANOGENESIS

During this period of embryonic development, the trilaminar disc folds into a C-shaped cylindrical embryo and all the major structures and organ systems are established. However, apart from the cardiovascular system, few of the systems function. Organogenesis, the development of the organ systems, is a critical period during which the

processes are susceptible to external influences that can cause disruption and subsequent serious congenital abnormalities. By the end of the eighth week, the embryo becomes known as the fetus and has a distinct human appearance (Fig. 9.7). Human development can be crudely classified as three types:

- growth: cell division
- morphogenesis: development of form, which involves movement of sheets and masses of cells
- differentiation: maturation of cells forming tissues and organs capable of specialized function.

Growth is achieved by hyperplasia (cell division) and hypertrophy (increase in cell size). Initially the cells are stem cells which are similar and not differentiated or specialized into any particular cell type. They differentiate into 1 of the 350 different types of cell found in the body in two phases. Before differentiation occurs, there is a stage of determination during which the cell becomes restricted in its capability to develop along different pathways. As the cells differentiate fully, they develop specific morphological and functional characteristics.

Differentiation is often orchestrated by the establishment of a signalling centre or polarizing region in a small

Week 1: fertilization to produce zygote

- Cleavage of zygote while travelling in uterine tube
- Cell division without increase in mass to form morula
- Fluid accumulation: hollow blastocyst formed
- 'Hatching' out of zona pellucida
- Blastocyst cells differentiate into trophoblast and inner cell mass
- Implantation in decidual wall

Week 2: inner cell mass forms bilaminar embryonic disc of hypoblast and epiblast

- Trophoblast differentiates into dividing cytotrophoblast and invasive syncytiotrophoblast (see Chapter 8)
- Lateral movement of cells from epiblast layer encloses yolk sac, forming the extraembryonic mesoderm
- Prochordal plate (mouth) develops at caudal end
- Day 14: primitive streak develops

Week 3: gastrulation

- Cells from primitive streak invaginate and migrate between the epiblast and the hypoblast forming the mesoderm
- Trilaminar disc of three germ layers: ectoderm (epiblast), mesoderm and ectoderm (hypoblast)
- Notochord forms, inducing development of the neural plate and giving rise to axis of development
- Somites become evident
- Neurulation begins

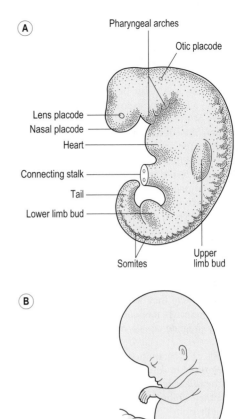

Fig. 9.7 (A) 4-week-old and (B) 8-week-old fetus. ((A) Reproduced with permission from Fitzgerald and Fitzgerald, 1994.)

bud of undifferentiated cells, as occurs in the development of the vertebrate limb. This process in which cells in one place influence the surrounding cells to develop in a specific way is known as induction. Induction involves the surrounding cells ('inducers') to produce cellular signals which have an effect on the responding cells ('responders') via cell receptors. Competence is the capacity to respond to the signal from an inducer which requires the responding tissue to be activated by a competence factor (Sadler, 2010). These interactions often involve epithelial cells, which are usually joined together forming tubes or sheets, and mesenchyme cells which are more dispersed. For instance, the epithelial cells forming the lining of the gut interact with the neighbouring mesenchyme cells to form the gut-associated organs such as the pancreas and liver and the epithelial tissue interacts with the limb mesenchyme cells to produce the initial limb buds. Continued signalling or 'crosstalk' between the different cell types allows differentiation to progress. The crosstalk occurs by the cells producing growth and differentiation factors which act at a paracrine (involving diffusible factors) or juxtacrine (involving non-diffusible factors) level.

Paracrine factors act by triggering a signalling transduction pathway in which a signalling molecule (or 'ligand') interacts with its receptor often conferring enzymatic activity to the receptor so it is able to initiate a cascade of protein phosphorylation changes that terminate with a transcription factor being activated. The transcription factor can then activate or inhibit gene expression. Juxtacrine factor signalling involves proteins on the surface of one cell or in the extracellular matrix interacting with the receptor on the surface of another cell or signals being transmitted from one cell to another via gap junctions. Differentiation can allow some plasticity. Branching morphogenesis is the formation of branched epithelial tubules which is essential to the development of several tissues including the kidneys, lungs, breasts and salivary glands.

One of the cornerstones of embryology is the concept that germ cells of the three layers of the developing embryo migrate to the final destinations (Horwitz and Webb, 2003). The migrating cells are thought to be polarized (have a front and back), to sense chemical signals and 'home' towards them by amoeboid movement. In gastrulation, cell migration leads to the formation of the three layers of the trilaminar disc which then migrate to targets where they differentiate. The muscle precursor cells migrate from the somites to their targets in the limbs. Failure of cells to migrate at all or to the correct location is thought to result in abnormalities or to have life-threatening consequences; for instance, congenital defects in brain development leading to mental disorders are ascribed to defects in neuronal migration. Cell migration also occurs in post-natal life and is central to homeostasis such as effective immune responses and repair of injured tissues in the wound healing process. Migration can also occur in pathological processes, including vascular disease and tumour metastasis, where some tumour cells migrate to new sites where they form secondary tumours. However, recent research has questioned whether germ cells do actually migrate at all during ontogeny (Freeman, 2003).

Apoptosis or programmed cell death is another mechanism important in embryonic development. Apoptosis involves the cells effectively autodestructing in a precisely timed manner. Embryogenesis also involves cell recognition and adhesion.

Folding

The disc-like arrangement of the germ layers is converted into a recognizable vertebral embryo by folding in the fourth week of development. Folding is due to a differential rate in growth of the different parts of the embryo. The embryo is in a contained space so as it grows, it curves and ridges of tissues form. The embryonic disc grows rapidly particularly in length, because of the growth of the brain and tail, so it has to fold. Although this is a momentous stage of development, relatively little is known about it. The yolk sac does not grow and, as the outer rim of the endoderm is attached to the yolk sac, the embryo becomes convex. Folding occurs at the cephalic (head) and lateral regions on day 22 and at the caudal (tail) end of the embryo on day 23 (Fig. 9.8). The cephalic, lateral and caudal edges of the embryonic disc are brought into apposition and the layers fuse along the midline, which converts the endoderm into the gut tube. Initially the foregut and the hindgut fuse, leaving the midgut open to the yolk sac. The folds cause a constriction between the embryo and yolk sac. The yolk sac gives rise to the primitive gut. The amnion expands, enveloping the connecting stalk and neck of the yolk sac, forming the umbilical cord. Folding is precisely coordinated and is controlled. Failure at this point results in

conditions such as omphalos and gastroschisis. The developmental pattern involves synchronized tissue communication and interaction. Adjacent tissues induce changes in the movement and behaviour of neighbouring cells. Signals integrating genetic and environmental influences control cell proliferation, migration and apoptosis (Bard and Weddon, 1996). These signals, which may be diffusible molecules or direct physical contact, direct the expression of particular genes in the responding cells. Although all cells have the same DNA in their nuclei, depending on the signal received, some will express certain genes but not others. So, for instance, a skin cell expresses the genes that control the behaviour of a skin cell because they are switched on by the signals skin cells receive. A liver cell has the same genes as the skin cell but expresses different genes.

The organization of the basic body plan

Techniques and concepts used to study molecular genetics (how the genetic code is expressed) in bacteria and *Drosophila* can be applied to mammalian embryogenesis, including human development. The DNA in the nucleus sets up a basic body plan, which establishes the pattern of the early embryo. The genes that control the basic body plan are the same in very diverse species. A highly conserved region of about 180 base pairs of DNA, known as the homeobox, is found in the genes that regulate the craniocaudal (head–tail) axis of embryonic development in almost all species studied (Murtha et al., 1991). The homeobox encodes a protein domain called the homeodomain which can bind DNA specifically. Homeobox genes encode transcription factors which switch on cascades of other genes, for instance all the ones needed to make a particular body part. Other morphogenic agents, signals and growth factors activate the homeobox genes. Hox genes are a particular subgroup of homeobox genes which are found in a special gene cluster, the HOX cluster. Hox genes determine the patterning of the body axis. They direct the identity of particular body regions, determining where limbs and other body segments will develop in the fetus. Limb abnormalities such as polydactyly may result from abnormal Hox genes. There appears to be a series of three sequential steps in the conversion of the oval trilaminar embryonic disc into the cylindrical configuration with the endoderm on the inside, the ectoderm on the outside and the mesoderm in between (Fig. 9.9) (Carlson, 2008). These steps result in segmentation of the embryo. Gap genes subdivide the embryo into broad regional domains. Pair-rule genes are involved in the formation of individual body segments and segment-polarity genes control the anterior–posterior organization of each segment (De Robertis et al., 1990). As the embryo develops, the segmental plan becomes less evident; remnants can be

Fig. 9.8 Folding of the embryonic disc into the fetal morphology: (A) 21 days; (B) 22 days; (C) 23 days; (D) 25 days. (Reproduced with permission from Goodwin, 1997.)

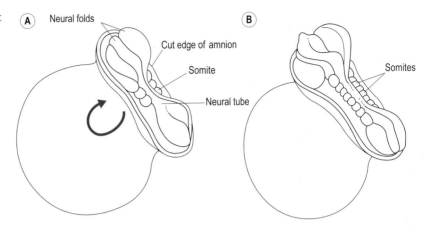

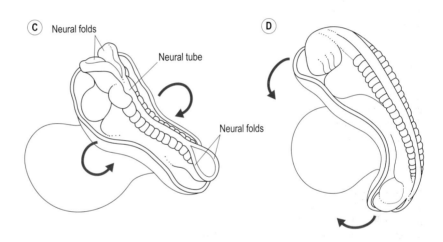

seen in the arrangement of the backbone and ribs and in the organization of the spinal nerves.

Box 9.4 summarizes the events taking place during weeks 4–8.

NINTH WEEK TO BIRTH: FETAL PERIOD

During this period, the body grows rapidly and the tissues and organs differentiate and mature (see below). The head growth rate becomes relatively slower so, by birth, the length of the head is about a quarter of the total length. Growth rate can be used to determine embryonic or fetal age (Box 9.5) and ultrasound examination can be used to examine developmental details (Box 9.6). With expert care, a fetus can be viable and may survive from 22 weeks.

Box 9.7 is a summary of the changes during the fetal period.

DEVELOPMENT OF ORGAN SYSTEMS

The central nervous system

Neurulation is the formation of the neural plate and neural folds and the closure of these folds to form the neural tube, which is the precursor of the brain and spinal cord. The neural tube is completed by the end of the fourth week. The developing notochord induces the overlying ectoderm to thicken forming the neural plate, a raised slipper-like plate of neuroepithelial cells. This will give rise to the central nervous system (brain and spinal cord) and other structures such as the retina. In the middle of the third week, the neural groove appears in the centre of the neural plate (Fig. 9.10). To each side of the groove are neural folds, which enlarge at the cranial end as the start of the developing brain. Marked development of

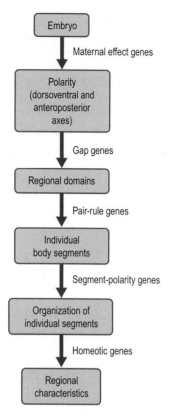

Fig. 9.9 Organization of the vertebrate body plan: three steps in the conversion.

the brain is a characteristic of embryonic development in primates; human brain growth exceeds that of other species, continuing into adulthood. At the end of the third week, the neural folds start to fuse forming the neural tube, which separates from the surface ectoderm. The neural crest cells, which detach from the lateral edges of the neural folds, give rise to the spinal ganglia and ganglia of the autonomic system as well as a number of other cell types (Box 9.8). The paraxial mesoderm, closest to the notochord and developing neural tube, differentiates to form prominent paired blocks of tissue, or somites. The first somites appear from day 20. There are about 30 pairs of somites by day 30 increasing to a total of 44 pairs, but the cranial ones begin differentiation as new somites are added at the caudal end. The somites differentiate into sclerotomes, myotomes and dermatomes, which give rise to the axial skeletal bones, skeletal muscles and the dermis of the skin, respectively. The number of somites indicates the age of the embryo. The limbs carry with them the nerves from the somites from which they developed. The somatic pattern of development is important in understanding referred pain (see Chapter 13).

Neural tube defects (NTD) are one of the most common congenital abnormalities (see Chapter 12), resulting from the failure of the neural tube to close during embryogenesis. Neurulation begins in the middle of the neural tube and proceeds cranially (towards the head) and caudally (towards the tail). Anencephaly (absent brain) results if the neural tube fails to close in the cranial region so the brain and spinal cord are fully exposed to the exterior; this condition is lethal and most cases are diagnosed by antenatal ultrasound scans and the pregnancies terminated. Failure of neurulation at the caudal end results in spina bifida. The extent to which spina bifida results in loss of neurological function depends on the severity of the lesion and its level in the spinal cord. The most common site for spina bifida is the lumbosacral region which suggests that close of the neural tube in this region is more susceptible to environmental and genetic influences. Neurulation is very sensitive to disturbances such as teratogenic drugs or lack of folate, which is required for DNA synthesis of the rapidly dividing cells (see Chapter 7).

Most neurons are formed between 10 and 18 weeks; this is therefore the critical window for brain development. Undernutrition or other insults in the first trimester often result in microcephaly (small cranial vault) (James and Stephenson, 1998). Congenital microcephaly is also associated with environmental factors such as cytomegalovirus, rubella (German measles), or varicella (chicken pox) virus infections and toxoplasmosis as well as genetic disorders such as trisomy 21. There is also evidence that microcephaly can be a genetic abnormality. Mutations of the gene for the abnormal spindle-like microcephaly-associated protein (ASPM) can cause microencephaly. It is thought that this gene is responsible for the evolution of an increase in the size of the human cerebral cortex (Ali and Meier, 2008); a novel allele of the gene arose about the same time as humans developed agriculture and cities and began to use written language. Although mental retardation can result from genetic abnormalities and exposure to teratogens such as viruses, the leading cause of mental retardation is maternal alcohol abuse.

In later gestation, undernutrition may result in blood flow being redistributed to the brain at the expense of other tissues. As brain size in humans is proportionately larger, the effects of protecting the brain from undernutrition may be exaggerated compared with other species (Barker, 1998). Glial cells begin to develop at about 15 weeks. In the second half of pregnancy, the glial cells hypertrophy and the axons and dendrites undergo marked growth. This rapid nervous system growth spurt continues until the second post-natal year and at a slower rate for at least the first decade, and is unique to humans (Johnson, 2001). The fetal response to impaired nutrition tends to 'spare' the brain at the cost of somatic growth, hence the asymmetric (disproportionate) growth patterns of babies born after intrauterine growth retardation (IUGR)

Box 9.4 **Summary of embryonic period: weeks 4–8**

4th week

- Neural tube fusing but neuropores open at rostral (anterior) and caudal ends
- Folding produces characteristic C-shaped curved embryo
- Otic pits present (primitive ear)
- Optic vesicles formed
- Upper limb buds appear, then lower limb buds
- Three pairs of brachial arches present
- Beating heart prominent
- Forebrain prominent
- Attenuated tail
- Rudiments of organ systems established
- Rostral neuropore, then caudal neuropore, close
- CRL 4–6 mm

5th week

- Rapid brain development and head enlargement (cephalization)
- Facial prominences develop
- Upper limb buds become paddle-shaped
- Lower limb buds are flipper-like
- Mesonephric ridges denote position of mesonephric (interim) kidneys
- CRL 7–9 mm

6th week

- Joints of upper limbs differentiate
- Digital rays (fingers) of upper limbs evident

- External ear canal and auricle (pinna) formed
- Retinal pigment formed so eye is obvious
- Head very large, projects over heart prominence
- Reflex responses to touch
- CRL 11–14 mm

7th week

- Notches between digital rays partially separate future fingers
- Liver prominent
- Rapidly growing intestines herniate out of small abdominal cavity into umbilical cord
- CRL 16–18 mm

8th week

- Digits of hand separated (but still webbed)
- Notches visible between digital rays of feet
- Stubby tail disappears
- Purposeful limb movements occur
- Ossification begins in lower limbs
- Head still disproportionately large (about half of total embryo length)
- Eye lids closing
- Ears are characteristic shape but still low-set
- External genitalia evident (but not distinct enough for sexual identification)
- CRL 27–31 mm

Box 9.5 **Estimation of embryonic/fetal age**

- Greatest length (GL) is used to measure embryos of about 3 weeks, which are straight
- CRL is sitting height, used to measure older, curved embryos
- Carnegie embryonic staging system uses external characteristics to estimate developmental stage
- Number of somites
- Fetal head measurements, such as biparietal diameter and head circumference
- Abdominal circumference
- Femur length and foot length

Box 9.6 **Ultrasound examination**

- Estimation of size and age of embryo
- Detection of congenital abnormality
- Evaluation of growth rate
- Investigation of uterine abnormality or ectopic pregnancy
- Guidance for CVS

where their heads seem disproportionately bigger. However, neither brain function nor neurology is perfectly protected; neuronal number tends to be reduced and myelination disturbed (Gluckman and Pinal, 2003). The IUGR brain also seems more vulnerable to asphyxia.

Human brain size is enormous compared to other primates. Bite muscles of the jaw are very strong and enclose the skull in non-human primates. It is suggested that early humans developed a single gene mutation that resulted in weaker jaw muscles (Stedman et al., 2004). The slacker jaw muscles relaxed their grip on the skull, allowing the human brain to grow and expand. Alternative explanations suggest that environmental changes forced humans to invent tools and develop manual dexterity, that natural

Box 9.7 **Summary of changes in the fetal period**

9–12 weeks

- Growth in body length and limbs accelerates
- Ears are low-set, eyes are fused
- Primary ossification centres develop in skeleton, notably skull and long bones
- Intestines return to abdominal cavity and body wall fuses
- Erythropoiesis (formation of red blood cells) decreases in liver and begins in spleen
- Urine formation begins
- Fetal swallowing of amniotic fluid

13–16 weeks

- Rapid growth
- Coordinated limb movements (not felt by mother)
- Active ossification of skeleton
- Slow eye movements
- Ovaries differentiated and contain primordial follicles
- External genitalia recognizable
- Eyes and ears closer to normal positions

17–20 weeks

- Growth slows down
- Limbs reach mature proportions
- Fetal movements felt by mother ('quickening')
- Skin covered with protective layer of vernix caseosa, held in position by lanugo (downy hair)
- Brown fat deposited

21–25 weeks

- Fetus gains weight
- Skin wrinkled and translucent, appears red–pink

- Rapid eye movements begin
- Blink-startle responses to noise
- Surfactant secretion begins but respiratory system immature
- Fingernails are present
- May be viable if born prematurely

26–29 weeks

- Lungs capable of breathing air
- Central nervous system can control breathing
- Eyes open
- Toenails visible
- Fat (3.5% body weight) deposited under skin so wrinkles smooth out
- Erythropoiesis moves from spleen to bone marrow

30–34 weeks

- Pupillary light reflex
- Skin pink and smooth, limbs chubby
- White fat is 8% of body weight
- From 32 weeks, survival is usual

35–38 weeks

- Firm grasp
- Orientates towards light
- Circumference of head and abdomen are approximately equal
- White fat is about 16% of body weight, 14 g fat gained per day
- Skin appears bluish-pink
- Term fetus is about 3400 g, CRL is about 360 mm

selection favoured bigger brains because they permitted more complex and supportive societies or that evolution in an environmental niche where marine food provided a good source of long chain fatty acids allowed marked brain development (Park et al., 2007). Impaired nutrition, particularly early in development, permanently affects brain size and cell number (assessed by head circumference); neurodevelopmental abnormalities occur at increased frequency in IUGR children.

Fetal sensory organs develop around the middle of gestation. At 24 weeks, the fetus responds to noise. As gestation progresses, the fetus exhibits increased sensitivity and responds to an increased range of sound frequencies. Babies are thought to enjoy being carried and cuddled because they can hear sounds of their mother's heart and digestive system, which they became accustomed to in utero.

Gastrointestinal system

The gut begins as a single tube running from mouth to anus. The mouth and anus are fused areas of endoderm and ectoderm (see above). The tube is therefore fixed at both ends so that when it grows it convolutes and loops (Fig. 9.11). Some parts of the tube dilate, such as the stomach and colon, and the gut rotates around other structures such as the developing liver. Between the sixth and eighth week of development, the proliferation of the epithelial cells lining the gut obliterates the lumen, which is then gradually recanalized. Early growth of the gut is extremely rapid so it extrudes into the amniotic cavity. If it is not withdrawn at about 10 weeks, the abdominal wall fails to close and the baby is born with exomphalos or gastroschisis. The incidence of gastroschisis is increasing;

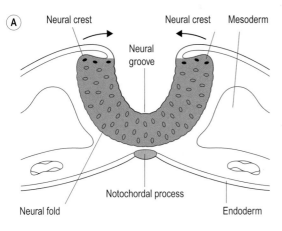

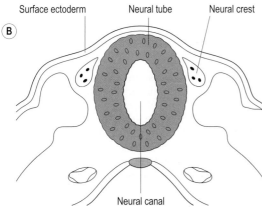

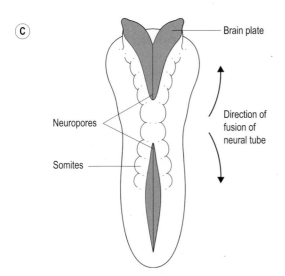

Fig. 9.10 The neural groove and neural tube fusion: (A) 21 days; (B) and (C) 23 days.

Box 9.8 **Tissues arising from cells of the neural crest**

- Spinal ganglia
- Ganglia of the autonomic system
- Adrenal medulla
- Thyroid gland
- Glial cells
- Schwann cells
- Melanocytes (pigmented)
- Pharyngeal arch cartilage
- Odontoblasts (of teeth)
- Pupillary and ciliary muscles of eye
- Dermis and hypodermis of neck and face
- Meninges

it is more common in infants born to young underweight mothers. Gastroschisis can be detected by ultrasound and by raised AFP levels in amniotic fluid and maternal serum. Normal fusion of the lateral body folds occurs at the linea nigra, the abdominal line that becomes pigmented in pregnant women (see Chapter 11). Normal growth of the gut depends on fetal swallowing. A fetus swallows about a third of the total volume of amniotic fluid per hour by the 16th week of development. Not only does amniotic fluid provide about 10% of the fetal protein requirements but it also seems to be associated with effective development of the gastrointestinal mucosa, liver and pancreas and promotion of growth.

The digestive enzymes are present from about 24–28 weeks, with the exception of lactase (see Chapter 16). Peristaltic coordination of the fetal gut is evident from the 14th week of development. By 34 weeks there is coordination of sucking, swallowing and peristalsis. As the gut matures, it produces mucus, which will eventually be required to lubricate the passage of food and faeces during transit. The mucus accumulates in the fetal gut as meconium. Adrenaline, produced in response to fetal distress, stimulates contractions of the gut and can lead to meconium-stained amniotic fluid. The liver reaches metabolic maturity relatively late in gestation, storing glycogen in the last 9 weeks. Inadequate placental transfer of amino acids will affect tissues with high protein turnover, such as the liver (James and Stephenson, 1998). The placenta is extremely metabolically active and extracts 40–60% of glucose and oxygen from the maternal circulation (Gluckman and Pinal, 2003), some of which transfers from maternal to fetal circulation and then is re-extracted from the fetal circulation. In IUGR, the rate of placental extraction from

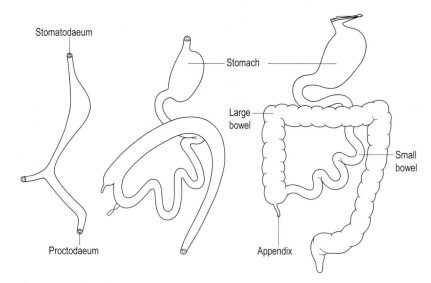

Fig. 9.11 Convolution of the primitive gut. (Reproduced with permission from James and Stephenson 1998.)

the fetal circulation increases and can lead to loss of lean body mass from the fetus and wasting. There is a hierarchy: the fetus may become catabolic to nourish the placenta and both fetus and placenta may be compromised in attempting to sustain maternal requirements. As hepatic stores of glycogen and fat are mobilized in IUGR, the liver is the first organ affected so the head:abdomen ratio is an important indicator of IUGR.

Case study 9.1 is an example of developmental abnormality of the gut.

The face and neck

The face is formed between weeks 5 and 12 from the brachial (pharyngeal) arches which are pouches and clefts of tissue. The endoderm of the pouches forms the parathyroid glands, thymus, tonsils and middle ear. The thyroid gland begins as epithelial cell proliferation of the tongue which descends towards the trachea. The nose grows downwards as a pillar of tissue (Fig. 9.12). The eyes, which are formed from a combination of nervous tissue and specialized ectoderm, are initially in a lateral position but move medially. The ears are initially low-set. Below the nose, maxillary and mandibular processes extend to form the floor of the nose and the roof of the mouth. The upper lip is formed from processes that extend to meet centrally. Inadequate fusion of the maxillary processes causes congenital malformations of the mouth, such as cleft lip or palate. Palatal fusion is complete by the 11th week.

The skeleton and skull

The skeleton develops the mesoderm layer and the neural crest. Most bones are formed initially from condensed mesenchyme tissue as cartilage which then undergoes ossification. The ribs and vertebral column develop from the sclerotome components of the somites. The skull develops from mesenchymal tissue around the brain. It is formed from the neurocranium, which protects the brain, and the viscerocranium, which forms the skeleton of the face. Each of these elements of the skull has membranous and cartilaginous components. Ossification is of the membrane rather than of cartilage and begins from the base of the skull.

The bones of the calvaria (cranial vault) have not completed development at birth. In the fetus, the flat bones of the calvaria are held together by soft fibrous sutures made of dense connective tissue, which allows some flexibility. The fetal head can mould to the shape of the maternal pelvis and distort as it passes through the birth canal. During delivery, the frontal bone becomes flat, the occipital bone is drawn out and the parietal bones overlap (this is described as 'moulding'). The head usually returns to a normal shape a few days after delivery. Six large

Case study 9.1

At 11 weeks of gestation, Julie has an ultrasound scan. She is asked to return for a further scan in 2 weeks as her unborn baby appears to have some gut tissue herniating into the umbilical cord. Julie seeks advice from her midwife.
- Is this normal?
- How might you reassure Julie that the ultrasonographer was just being cautious?
- If there were a pathological condition present, what two conditions are most likely?
- How would they be further investigated before Julie is advised upon the prognosis?

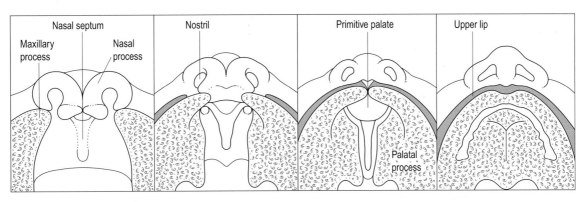

Fig. 9.12 Growth of the palate and nose between the sixth and ninth week. (Reproduced with permission from James and Stephenson, 1998.)

membranous fontanelles are formed where the sutures meet (see Chapter 13). The posterior fontanelles close at about 3 months after birth and the anterior ones close when the infant is about 18 months old. Raised intracranial pressure can be detected by palpating these fontanelles; a depression indicates dehydration.

The fetal skull is relatively large compared with the skeleton. The newborn skull has relatively thin bones compared with those in later life. The face is relatively small and has a characteristic neonatal roundish shape because the jaws are small. The paranasal sinuses (which give the individual shape of the face and resonance of the voice) are virtually absent and the facial bones are underdeveloped. After birth, brain growth is rapid so the calvaria increase markedly during the first 2 years. The calvaria continue to grow until the child is about 16 years old; the skull bones then thicken.

The muscles and limbs

The first skeletal muscles to develop are the back muscles from the paired somites. Bone formation is closely associated with muscle growth and the nervous connections from the spinal cord. The limbs become evident as buds or bulges associated with particular somites in the fourth week of development. The limb buds are formed from migration of muscle cells from the myotomes. The cells form pairs of muscle masses. Adhesive cells form a compacted region between the two muscle masses, which differentiates into cartilage. Cartilage is stiff but flexible, whereas bone is stronger but more brittle and able to fracture. Ossification, the conversion to bone structure, begins from about 8 weeks but is still not complete by birth. This preponderance of cartilage in the skeleton aids flexibility at delivery. The arms are slightly ahead of the legs in development because the fetal circulatory system gives an advantage to the upper body (see Chapter 15). Bones and muscles closest to the body develop first so the humerus and femur develop before the distal regions of the limbs. The differential timing of development means

that drugs such as thalidomide affect different limbs and parts of the limbs depending on time of exposure of the fetus to the teratogens (Box 9.9). By 41 days, the fingers and toes develop from paddle-like plates. The sculpting of the digits is due to apoptosis of the tissue between the digital rays. A common minor congenital defect observed at birth is a failure of separation of the digits. By 9 weeks, the body skeleton is almost complete, although the skull bones are still forming. Development of the limbs and digits can be impaired by amniotic bands (derived from tears in the amnion possibly as a result of infection or toxic insult) which encircle and constrict parts of the fetus.

Box 9.9 **Thalidomide**

Thalidomide was marketed in 1957 as 'Contergan', a sedative and antiemetic drug suitable for treating nausea and vomiting of pregnancy (morning sickness). Congenital malformations of the limbs and ears rose in parallel with sales of the drug with a lag of 7–8 months (Lenz, 1962; McBride, 1961). The drug was withdrawn in November 1961; 5850 infants were affected, of whom 40% died, leaving 3900 survivors. Thalidomide disturbs cartilage formation and the establishment of the nerve connections to muscles. It is teratogenic 20–36 days after fertilization. Limb development begins at 24 days. Early exposure to thalidomide caused unique birth defects including absence of arms; later exposure successively affected development of ears, legs and thumbs. Absence of limbs is called amelia and absence of long bones, so a hand or foot comes directly from the torso, is called phocomelia. Different species metabolize the drug differently; fetal development in the rodent test species (rats and mice) was not affected. Thalidomide and its analogues have effects on inflammation and blood vessel growth; it is currently used for treatment of complications of leprosy and has been used in clinical trials for a range of disorders including cancers and AIDS (Melchert and List, 2007).

The cardiovascular system

This is one of the first systems to develop; its function is important extremely early in development, unlike some of the other systems that do not have to achieve full function until after birth. This is because, as the embryo becomes larger, diffusion of oxygen and nutrients is no longer adequate.

The primordial vascular system develops by vasculogenesis (new vessel formation) and later development is by angiogenesis (new vessels branching off the existing vessels and remodelling). A few cells in the mesoderm of the yolk sac lose adherence and start to move, forming clusters called blood islands (Fig. 9.13). The haemocytoblasts (or haemangioblasts), the precursors of both blood cells and blood vessel endothelial cells, are nucleated and start to synthesize primitive forms of haemoglobin. The outer cells of the blood islands, angioblasts, develop characteristics of endothelial cells, the cells that line blood vessels. The blood islands fuse, forming vascular channels that eventually amalgamate to form a primitive vascular network with identifiable routes. Blood vessels form by vasculogenesis, where the vessels develop from blood islands, and by angiogenesis, where new vessels branch off existing vessels. The endothelial cells interact with pericytes, vascular smooth muscle cells, to form the vessel walls (Bergers and Song, 2005). The organization of the routes across the yolk sac is similar to the geographical organization of river deltas where little streams meander and combine, taking the route of least resistance.

Expansion and elastic resistance of the vessel walls, which become rhythmic generating a peristaltic pattern, propel the blood cells. Blood vessel differentiation and growth is orchestrated by a range of signals including cell adhesion molecules, transcription factors and angiogenic growth factors and their receptors (Breier, 2000). It is thought that abnormal molecular regulation of blood vessel formation is the cause of capillary haemangiomas, the most common tumours of the infant. Capillary haemangiomas are dense masses of capillary endothelial cells which are usually associated with craniofacial structures. They are usually benign and self-limiting but occasionally they may proliferate or ulcerate and bleed or may persist as 'port-wine stains'.

The primitive heart develops from a horseshoe area of embryonic mesoderm, anterior to the prochordal plate. It forms two tubes, one on each side of the foregut, which fuse to form a single heart tube. The primitive atrium forms where the flow from the umbilical veins from the placenta joins with the blood vessels from the head, generating the greatest volume of blood. The swirling vortex of blood leaving the primitive atrium induces the development of the primitive ventricle, which becomes the main source of pumping activity. The characteristic shape of the heart is generated by the flow of blood cells within the vascular channels; this causes the heart tube to form an S-shaped loop that will eventually take on the configuration of the heart (Fig. 9.14). By 21 days after fertilization, the cells surrounding the heart have become differentiated as myocardial cells capable of eliciting an organized response, so the heart, which consists of four chambers in series, begins beating.

The development of the outer layers of the vessel walls is stimulated by stress (Martyn and Greenwald, 1997). In areas where there is more turbulence, the vessel wall responds by developing more elasticity. Therefore, the heart and arterial structures develop thicker and more elastic walls. The mature organization of the chambers of the heart is achieved by the ingrowth of the septa towards the central atrioventricular endocardial cushion in the centre and apoptosis of excess tissue (Fig. 9.14). Abnormalities in the endocardial cushion development or excess apoptosis result in cardiac malformations including atrial and ventricular septal defects (known as a 'hole in the heart') and defects or transpositions of the great vessels. Abnormalities of the cardiovascular system are the more common human birth defect partly because they often allow normal fetal development and only become significant from birth. Most cardiovascular abnormalities have multifactorial causes due to the interaction of environmental and genetic factors. Cardiovascular teratogens include vitamin A, alcohol and some viruses and maternal gestational disorders such as hypertension and diabetes are associated with an increased risk. Many chromosomal abnormalities and genetic syndromes cause heart malformations probably because so many different genes are involved in the complex embryonic development of the cardiovascular system.

The growth of the fetal heart partially depends on afterload. If afterload is increased by factors leading to peripheral vasoconstriction or high placental impedance, the likely outcome is a growth-restricted baby with an enlarged heart (Veille et al., 1993). If the fetus receives less than adequate nutrition or oxygenation during its development then blood flow is diverted to the brain and heart. The decreased flow to the peripheral vessels results in the development of less elastic tissue, which is the hypothesis underlying the association of poor maternal nutrition with an increased risk of cardiovascular disease in adult life (Barker et al., 1993). The initial response to impaired nutrition is to increase placental growth; if this is not adequate, blood flow is diverted to the brain (and other essential organs such heart, adrenal glands and placenta). Therefore, adults, who were small at birth, but with relatively large placentas, have an increased risk of developing hypertension because less elastic tissue was established in their blood vessels during fetal development (Fig. 9.15). It is argued that impaired fetal nutrition also leads to fewer tissue stem cells being formed which leads eventually to early exhaustion of organ function and the development of chronic adult disease (Cianfarani, 2003).

The respiratory system

The trachea and major bronchi develop as outpouches of the primitive alimentary tract. The development depends on interaction between the endodermal bud from the developing foregut and the splanchnic mesoderm it

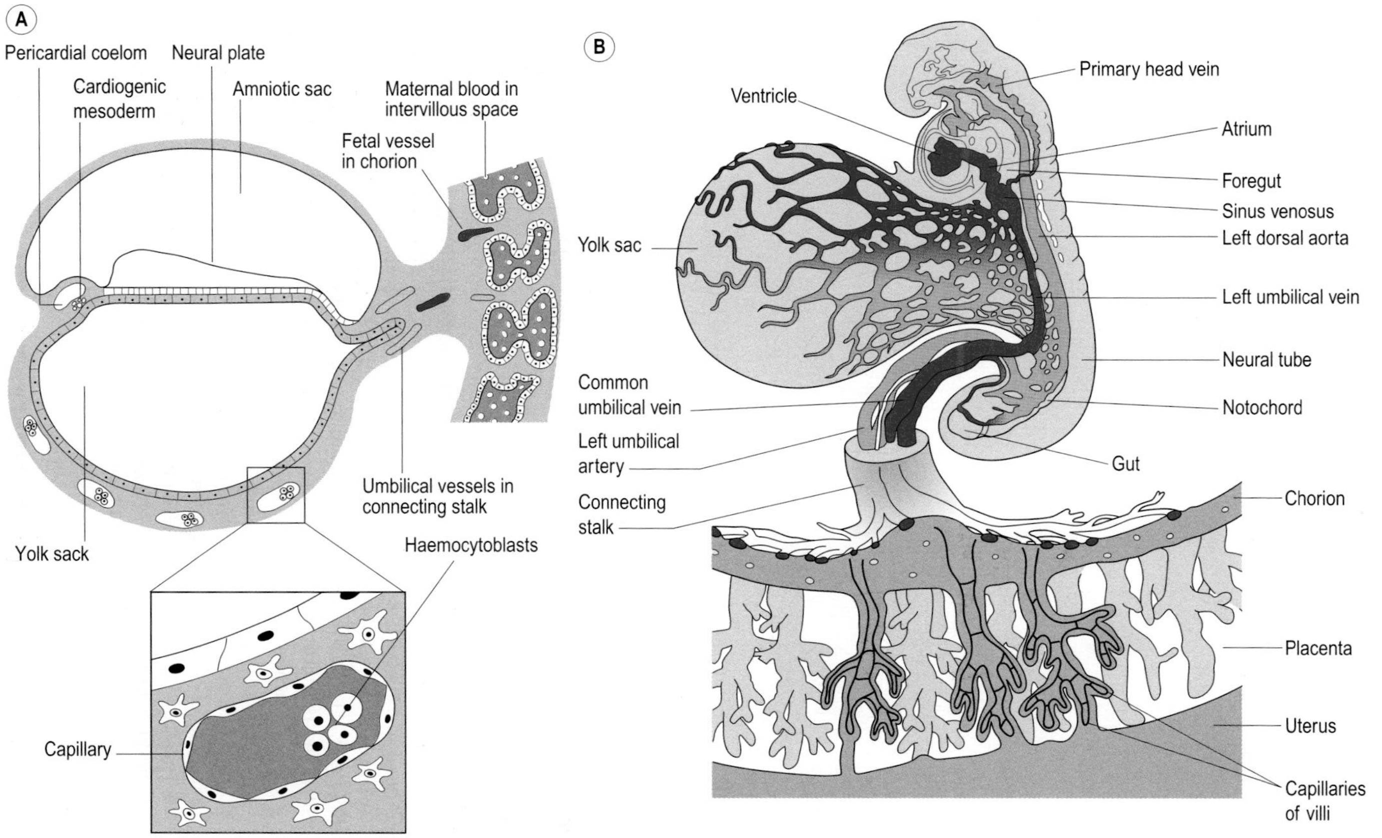

Fig. 9.13 Formation of the first blood vessels: (A) appearance of blood islands; (B) vessels at 24 days ((A) Reproduced with permission from Fitzgerald and Fitzgerald, 1994; (B) reproduced with permission from Goodwin, 1997.)

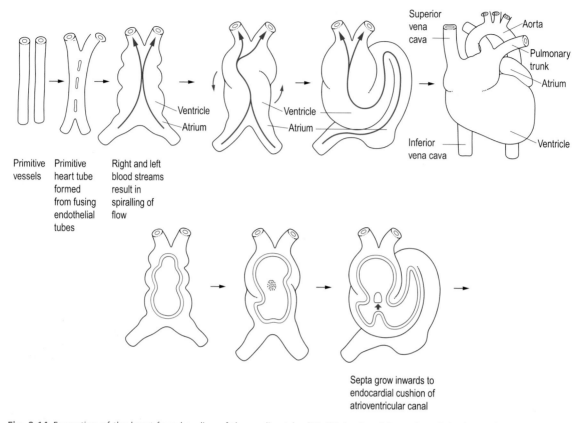

Primitive vessels

Primitive heart tube formed from fusing endothelial tubes

Right and left blood streams result in spiralling of flow

Ventricle

Atrium

Ventricle

Atrium

Superior vena cava

Aorta

Pulmonary trunk

Atrium

Inferior vena cava

Ventricle

Septa grow inwards to endocardial cushion of atrioventricular canal

Fig. 9.14 Formation of the heart from bending of the cardiac tube (21–35 days) and formation of the heart chambers.

invades at about day 22. The bud bifurcates between day 26 and day 28. In the fifth week of development, three secondary buds develop on the right branch and two on the left; these are the main bronchi and primitive lobes of the lung. There are four stages in the development of the respiratory system: the embryonic phase from weeks 3 to 5, the pseudocanalicular phase from 5 to 16 weeks, the canalicular phase from 16 to 26 weeks and the terminal sac phase from 24 weeks until birth (Fig. 9.16). One of the most critical stages in development is the production of phospholipid-rich surfactant from the type II pneumocytes, allowing efficient inflation and gas exchange following birth and therefore post-natal survival. Although the cells can be identified at about week 22, production of surfactant increases significantly after 30 weeks. The diaphragm starts to develop as the peritoneal membrane high in the neck and descends as the lungs and heart develop. This is the reason why diaphragmatic pain is often felt as referred pain in the shoulder. If the development of the diaphragm is incomplete, it results in a diaphragmatic hernia which allows the abdominal contents can protrude into the chest cavity. In severe cases, the abdominal contents can restrict growth and development of the lungs (causing pulmonary hypoplasia).

Fetal breathing movements (FBM) are a feature of normal fetal life and are used to assess fetal well-being. FBM oppose lung recoil and maintain the level of lung expansion that is essential for normal growth and structural maturation of the fetal lungs (Harding and Hooper, 1996). Normal development of the fetal lungs is very important as there is limited capacity for later recovery. FBM are inhibited by fetal hypoxaemia, hypoglycaemia, maternal alcohol consumption, maternal smoking, intra-amniotic infection and maternal consumption of sedatives or narcotic drugs. The absence of FBM is associated with lung hypoplasia, premature rupture of fetal membranes and oligohydramnios. Decreased amniotic fluid volume causes decreased lung growth and expansion, whereas tracheal occlusion, which prevents expulsion of lung fluid, can cause overgrowth of lung tissue (Nardo et al., 1998). At term, the infant has about 50 million alveoli, half the adult number; these continue to increase in the first 8–10 years of life.

The urinary system

The urinary and genital systems both develop from the intermediate mesoderm and are closely associated (see Chapter 5 for a description of genital development).

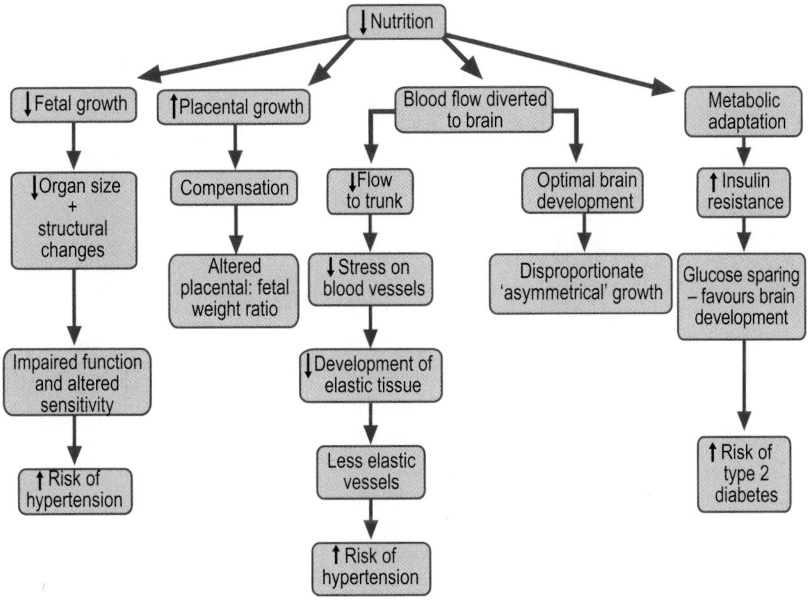

Fig. 9.15 The fetus adapts to suboptimal nutrition with strategies for survival. The slower growth rate reduces use of nutrients but affects final organ size and function. The redistribution of blood to the brain affects development of the blood vessels and predisposes to later hypertension. Altered metabolism and peripheral insulin resistance favours glucose availability for the developing brain but the 'thriftiness' predisposes to insulin resistance, obesity and type II diabetes if the individual experiences good or over-nutrition in later life.

During embryonic folding, urogenital ridges appear each side of the primitive aorta (Fig. 9.17). The nephrogenic ridge develops into the renal system of kidneys, ureters, bladder and urethra. Abnormalities of the kidneys and ureters affect 3–4% of newborn infants. Most of the abnormalities are harmless, such as variation in blood supply, abnormal position or shapes, and urinary tract duplications such as supernumerary kidneys. However, unilateral renal agenesis (one kidney failing to develop) affects 1 in 1000 liveborn babies. Bilateral renal agenesis or Potter's syndrome (inadequate development of both kidneys) affects 1 in 3000 fetuses and is incompatible with life. It is usually associated with oligohydramnios. Three pairs of kidneys develop during fetal development: the pronephroi, the mesonephroi and the metanephroi (singular: pronephros, mesonephros and metanephros). The pronephroi are transient non-functional structures that exist for only a few weeks. When they degenerate, their ducts are utilized in the next stage. The mesonephroi appear in the fourth week and function as intermediate kidneys until the end of the embryonic period, disgorging waste products into the remnants of the yolk sac. They degenerate and disappear in the eighth week, although parts of their structure persist as mesonephric or Wolffian ducts in males (see Chapter 5).

The permanent kidneys, or metanephroi, develop from the fifth week and begin to function about 4 weeks later.

The kidneys start development in the pelvis and appear to migrate upwards. In fact, this observation is due to continued downward growth of the embryo. As the kidneys 'ascend' out of the pelvic area, new arteries at successively higher levels supply them. During fetal life, the kidney is subdivided into lobes, which disappear in infancy as the nephrons grow. The main increase in size is due to elongation of the proximal convoluted tubules and loops of Henlé. Disruption of renal branching during development leads to renal dysplasia, the major cause of renal failure in children (Piscione and Rosenblum, 2002). Functional maturation of the kidneys occurs after birth.

Until 20 weeks' gestation, the skin is not keratinized so fluid can move through this semipermeable membrane. Essentially the outer barrier is the amnion. As the skin matures and lays down keratin, the rate of transudation decreases and the outer barrier of the fetus becomes the skin. The urine then becomes an important source of amniotic fluid. The fetus produces up to 600 mL of urine per day. Amniotic fluid is also produced by the amniotic membrane and the fetal lungs. The fetus swallows most of the amniotic fluid; the rest diffuses through the amniotic membranes to the maternal circulation.

The epidermis of the skin develops from the ectoderm, which is colonized from melanocytes from the neural crest and Langerhans cells from the bone marrow. The dermis is derived from the embryonic mesoderm.

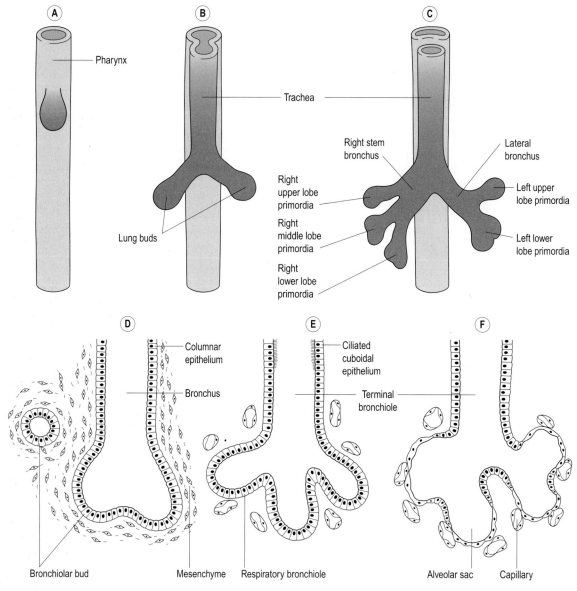

Fig. 9.16 Respiratory system development: (A) pharyngeal pouches (4 weeks); (B) 32 days; (C) 35 days; (D) pseudocanalicular phase (17 weeks); (E) canalicular phase (17–26 weeks); (F) terminal sac phase (26 weeks).

Fetal growth

At 4 weeks, the crown-rump length (CRL) is about 4 mm and increases by 1 mm per day up to 30 mm (Beck, 1996). Thereafter, between weeks 8 and 28, the growth increases markedly, to about 1.5 mm per day, so this period is recognized as the fetal growth period. The organs and tissues continue to grow and mature. Although growth is most rapid during this period (compared with any other time in life), factors affecting growth may have their origins earlier. In fact, environmental insults regulating growth appear to last for several generations. Fetal growth is due to interaction between the genetic drive for growth and the nutritional supplies in pregnancy to support it, which involves a dynamic interaction between fetus, placenta and mother.

There are characteristic differences between the different phases of growth during development (James and

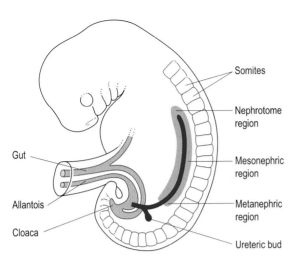

Fig. 9.17 The development of the renal system from the urogenital ridges.

Labels: Somites, Nephrotome region, Mesonephric region, Metanephric region, Ureteric bud, Gut, Allantois, Cloaca

Stephenson, 1998). Growth in the first trimester is principally through increased cell number. In the second trimester, cell division continues albeit at a slower rate and the cells increase in size. In the third trimester, cell division slows further and the increase in cell size continues. There is little variation in fetal growth up to about 16 weeks of gestation (Gluckman and Pinal, 2003), after which genetic and environmental influences have a more marked effect on outcome. Fat deposition, determined by nutrient availability and insulin levels, plays an important contribution in the final weight. There are 42 successive cell divisions between fertilization and birth, but only five more from birth to adult size (excluding mitotic cell division to replace dead cells).

All low-birthweight infants are potentially at some health risk. Low birthweight is traditionally defined as being less than 2500 g at birth. Low birthweight remains one of the great challenges to modern health care services; small size at birth can affect susceptibility to infection, rate of post-natal growth and neurocognitive development. Low birthweight is associated with increased fetal mortality as well as higher neonatal and infant morbidity and mortality with the most adverse outcomes arising in the most immature infants. A number of chronic adult diseases originate *in utero* as a result of fetal adaptation to suboptimal quality or quantity of nutrients in order to optimize survival (Langley-Evans and McMullen, 2010), including glucose intolerance, insulin resistance and type II diabetes mellitus, heart disease, hypertension, stroke, obstructive lung disease, hyperlipidaemia, hypercholesterolaemia, hypercortisolaemia, renal disease, osteoporosis, schizophrenia, obesity and reproductive disorders.

The use of low birthweight as the outcome measure of the success of a pregnancy is very widespread and it can be measured with precision and validity (Kramer, 1998). Infant mortality increases exponentially with lower birthweight. However, birthweight is a function of two factors (gestational length and rate of fetal growth) which have different aetiologies and different prognoses. The simple definition of a low-birthweight infant as one who weighs less than 2500 g at birth does not differentiate between infants who are growth-restricted (small at term) and infants who are born prematurely. Prematurity is often complicated by IUGR. Some small-for-gestational age (SGA) infants are constitutionally small rather than growth-restricted or growth-retarded. Growth in the first trimester of pregnancy affects birthweight; early growth restriction is associated with complications and increased risk of adverse outcomes (Bukowski et al., 2009).

Birthweight is a crude outcome measure of optimal intrauterine growth and development; suboptimal maternal body composition and nutrient intake can have a long-term effect on the offspring without necessarily affecting size at birth (Godfrey, 2001). Birthweight does not identify effects of nutrition on body composition and development of specific tissues and organs; a similar birthweight can be attained with different growth trajectories. Birthweight may not identify growth restriction. For instance, if an infant does not reach its potential birthweight but is born above 2500 g, it will not be classified as growth-restricted. Conversely, an infant with 'normal' birthweight, such as 3.4 kg, may be growth-retarded and have long-term health risks if it was destined to be bigger under optimal intrauterine conditions. Most infants born of low birthweight in developed countries are born prematurely rather than growth-restricted; in most cases, the cause(s) of preterm delivery is not known. Rates of low birthweight babies are higher in areas with a higher level of socio-economic deprivation; birthweight is also related to income level and accessibility to healthcare, education and housing.

A variety of factors affect fetal growth (Box 9.10). Chromosome and genetic disorders often cause fetal growth retardation; excluding these, the dominant cause of growth retardation is due to an inadequate supply of nutrients and oxygen (Gluckman and Pinal, 2003) related either to maternal supply or to placental transfer capacity.

Fetal factors

Male offspring are on average heavier than female offspring. The ovaries have limited capability to synthesize steroid hormones, whereas the testes produce testosterone, which has anabolic effects. Studies suggest that the Y chromosome and higher testosterone level positively promotes growth (James and Stephenson, 1998). There may also be sex-specific adaptation of the placenta which affects fetal growth (Clifton, 2010). Multiple pregnancies tend to result in smaller babies, probably because of the limited haemodynamic support in late gestation,

---

Box 9.10 **Factors affecting fetal size**

- Fetal factors
- Maternal size (lean body mass): maternal genetic effects
- Maternal weight gain and nutrition in pregnancy
- Maternal age extremes
- Maternal behavioural factors such as smoking, recreational drug use
- Multiple pregnancy
- Fetal oxygenation: affected by maternal anaemia and so on
- Maternal medical conditions such as hypertension, heart disease, infections and diabetes
- Placental sufficiency affected by pre-eclampsia, uterine blood flow and so on
- GHs such as insulin and IGFs

---

although overcrowding is also implicated. Aneuploidy is also a risk factor for IUGR (see Chapter 7). Parity affects birthweight; first-born infants tend to be slightly lighter than second and subsequent siblings (Shah, 2010a).

Maternal size

The classic experiments on horses showing that the size of offspring of hybrid crosses between small Shetland ponies and large carthorses was most closely related to maternal size demonstrated that maternal size is a critical determinant of birthweight (Walton and Hammond, 1938). However, final adult size is also affected by paternal genetics to different degrees in different species; in humans about 5% of the variability in size is attributed to paternal influences (Robinson and Owens, 1996). In the past, pregnant women were asked for their shoe size, which correlates with their pelvic size, and their husband's hat size, which was found to be related to the size of the baby; the relationship of the two sizes was used to predict the likelihood of difficulties in delivery. A small maternal size appears to impose a constraint on fetal growth, although factors such as immaturity, social circumstances, maternal behaviour (such as smoking and alcohol consumption), diseases and psychological stress all affect the outcome of the pregnancy. Shorter maternal stature is positively correlated with lower socio-economic status, malnutrition, chronic disease, increased levels of stress and large family size. The cycle of deprivation tends to repeat, as there is a correlation between maternal height and birthweight and between birthweight and adult size, which is not solely due to genetic influences.

Half-siblings who share the same mother have similar birthweights (Gluckman and Harding, 1994). The birthweights of babies born after ovum donation are more strongly related to the weight of the recipient mother than

to that of the donor woman (Brooks et al., 1995). These findings suggest that birth size is more strongly influenced by uterine environment than by genetics.

It is suggested that there is a conflict between the maternal and paternal genes governing fetal size (Moore and Haig, 1991). Paternal genes favour fetal growth and the transfer of nutrients to the parasitic fetus; if this happens at the expense of maternal health or life, the male can choose a different mate. Maternal genes limit transfer to the fetus to optimize survival of the mother and her children. The father's birthweight influences placental size. Birthweights of mothers correlate with their children's birthweights and even with their grandchildren's birthweights, suggesting that the maternal constraint on fetal growth is set very early (Barker, 1998). The paternal effect on the fetal growth trajectory is permitted by the lifting of the maternal constraint on growth. Therefore, fetal growth rate responds to, and is appropriate for, the prevailing nutrient availability. Maternal constraint is also a mechanism for limiting fetal growth to maternal pelvis size. Constraint of growth by maternal factors is important in preventing fetal overgrowth and dystocia which is risky for mother and infant (and survival of the species). There are paternal factors that influence birthweight; infants whose fathers are older or who were born of low birthweight themselves have an increased chance of having lower birthweight (Shah, 2010b).

Growth hormones

It has been suggested that growth in children from fetus through infancy and childhood to puberty follows a mathematical model on which three growth curves are imposed, forming a sigmoidal curve (Fig. 9.18; Karlberg et al., 1994). Phase 1, the infancy growth rate, begins in fetal life with a rapid deceleration until about 3 years of age. This is the phase of growth that seems to be regulated by insulin-like growth factors (IGFs; see Chapter 4); the effect of poor nutrition on growth may be mediated by IGFs. The childhood phase begins in the first year of life and is due to the effect of growth hormone (GH; see Chapter 3), provided thyroid hormone secretion is normal. During this period most of the growth is localized in the lower body (particularly leg length), as the long bones are very sensitive to GH. Children who have deficiency of GH or who are encephalic have normal birthweight and early infant growth; the deficiency usually becomes apparent only after 6 months of age. The final component of growth is the pubertal growth spurt, which is stimulated by the interaction of sex hormones with GH. Although levels of GH in the fetus are high, GH receptors are expressed at low levels in fetal tissues so GH has little effect. This is supported by observations that GH-deficient fetuses or young infants have almost normal linear growth. Fetal growth seems to be controlled rather by IGFs and their receptors (Robinson and Owens, 1996).

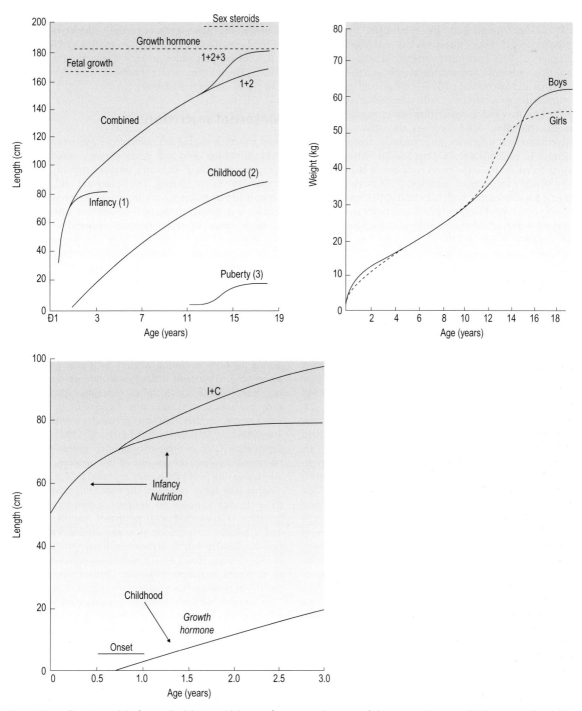

Fig. 9.18 Karlberg's model of growth: (A) sigmoidal curve from a combination of three growth curves; (B) the curve of weight increase; (C) the curve of increase in length. (Reproduced with permission from Karlberg et al., 1994.)

IGFs are mitogens (i.e. they stimulate cell division and differentiation) and are modulated by binding proteins, which control growth before and after birth (see Chapter 15). This mechanism can explain both the interaction of genetic drive and nutrient supply and the effects of maternal and paternal size. IGF-II is the primary growth factor influencing embryonic growth, whereas IGF-I, produced by the fetal liver and amniotic membranes, regulates growth in late gestation. IGF-I increases the efficiency of the placenta so fetal weight increases without a corresponding increase in placental weight. Fetal insulin, driven by fetal glucose availability, is the main regulator of IGF-I; IGF-I is very sensitive to maternal nutrition. IGF-I is also involved in fetal gut maturation. Both IGF-I and IGF-II have anabolic effects via the type I receptor. IGF-II also binds to the type II receptor, which effectively competes with the type I receptor for available IGF-II. IGF-II is paternally imprinted and expressed and promotes growth via the IGF-I receptor, whereas the type II receptor, which is hypothesized to be maternally imprinted, limits or controls growth by clearing or 'mopping up' the free IGF-II (Harding and Johnston, 1995). Overexpression of IGF-II leads to the Beckwith–Weidemann overgrowth syndrome. Fetal hyperinsulinaemia appears to inhibit the production of IGF-I-binding protein, thus lifting the restriction on IGF-I and contributing to macrosomia (Wang and Chard, 1992). Nutrient availability may promote IGF-I levels and fetal growth. Thus, a balance can be achieved between paternal genes promoting growth and maternal genes restricting and regulating growth.

Insulin itself has a growth-promoting effect in the fetus; it is a growth-promoting hormone which signals nutrient plenty. Its somatogenic (growth-promoting) actions are mediated via IGF-I but it has a direct effect on fat deposition. Maternal hyperglycaemia causes increased placental transfer of glucose to the fetus. The higher concentration of glucose stimulates the fetal pancreas to produce insulin, which facilitates cellular uptake of glucose, stimulating anabolic metabolism and fetal growth. Babies of diabetic mothers are often macrosomic owing to particularly large fat stores. The macrosomia tends to be somatic so the bodies of macrosomic infants are big so their heads can appear relatively small. Fetal insulin deficiency, which is rare, can occur with nutrient deprivation or pancreatic agenesis, and results in fetal growth retardation (symmetrical IUGR) and decreased levels of body fat and muscle development (Robinson and Owens, 1996).

Glucocorticoids affect fetal growth and maturation by altering production and secretion of hormones, regulating receptor density and altering the activity of enzymes involved in activating and deactivating hormones (see also Chapter 15). The fetus is usually protected from maternal glucocorticoids because they are inactivated by the placental enzyme 11β-hydroxysteroid dehydrogenase which effectively acts as a barrier. However, maternal undernutrition downregulates this enzyme so the fetus is exposed to increased glucocorticoids (Gluckman and Pinal, 2003), which leads to fetal growth maturation. However, the higher levels of cortisol enhance maturation of the lungs and other organs, promoting survival of the IUGR infant; premature delivery frequently accompanies IUGR. Thyroid hormones promote fetal development and signal energy availability.

Maternal nutrition

Fetal growth is related to maternal size (reflecting nutrient level during her own fetal development), maternal body composition (which indicates nutrient supply), nutrient availability in pregnancy and placental efficiency. If periconceptual maternal nutrition sets the growth trajectory early in gestation, the fetal growth rate is more likely to be accommodated by nutrient availability when its demands are high in later gestation. The fetus is able to adapt metabolically to undernutrition in pregnancy by altering its growth rate and sparing nutrients for certain tissues, like the brain. This can lead to disproportionate organ development and fetal growth patterns; fetal adaptations to undernutrition tend to be permanent (Barker, 1998).

Maternal nutrition stores correlate with birthweight. Pregnant women exposed to conditions of starvation during the famines during World War II were particularly susceptible to nutrient deficiency if they were subject to nutritional deficiency in the preconceptual period or in early pregnancy. Not only was the size of their babies significantly smaller, but the prenatal growth of their grandchildren was also affected (Lumey, 1992). Nutrient deprivation later in pregnancy affected birthweights and fat deposition, but the lengths of the neonates were not affected so much and the babies appeared to regain normal weights after birth. However, the metabolic adaptation in those fetuses exposed to nutrient deprivation late in gestation is associated with persistent insulin resistance and a marked trend to develop glucose intolerance and non-insulin-dependent diabetes mellitus (NIDDM) later in life (Phillips, 1996). Fetal nutrition is not directly related to maternal nutrition; placental dysfunction can limit transfer of nutrients from the mother to fetus (Sibley, 2009).

In humans, dietary intervention studies have had disappointing results, producing improvement in fetal growth only in severely undernourished women (see Chapter 12). Part of the problem may be the methodology and ensuring that supplements intended for pregnant women are not used as alternative sources of nutrition or to feed other members of the family. The timing of the nutritional supplements may also be important, as fetal growth trajectories may be set before the nutritional status of the mother is improved by the intervention. Women experiencing marginal diets and seasonal famine for generations appear to have evolved strategies to conserve energy by suppressing metabolic rate and acquiring little fat during the pregnancy (Durnin, 1987). The energy cost of pregnancy in affluent countries where food is plentiful may be met with little or no increase in energy intake, although economies in energy expenditure may offset the increased requirements (see Chapter 12). Prepregnant size (body fat levels) may direct the trajectory that sets fetal growth via leptin, the product of the *ob* gene (Rink, 1994). Appropriate conditions during pregnancy can then fulfil the requirements for this trajectory to be achieved. In experimental animals, the effect of moderate maternal malnutrition over a number of generations is decreased birthweight, which is maintained for a few further generations even when food supply is restored to a good level (Stewart et al., 1980). A plentiful food supply imposed after generations of malnutrition in these animals is associated with obstructed labour and poor fetal outcome.

Acute undernutrition in late gestation can cause premature delivery by stimulating signals which promotes cervical ripening and uterine contractility and cause early labour (see Chapter 13). Macronutrient balance at different stages of pregnancy may affect fetal growth (see Chapter 12). Micronutrient availability can affect the somatotrophic and insulin regulation of growth; zinc deficiency is associated with IUGR. Vitamin E and vitamin A affect insulin sensitivity and GH secretion, respectively. Folate status affects gene imprinting and methylation.

Maternal nutrition could also exert an effect on fetal growth even before fertilization. The nutritional support of follicular development prior to ovulation and fertilization may affect the growth trajectory of the embryo (see above). Nutrition of the embryo prior to implantation may be important, as demonstrated by *in vitro* fertilization (IVF). Sheep and cattle embryos from IVF that are cultured for a few days before being replaced in the uterus grow into significantly larger fetuses (James and Stephenson, 1998). It is not clear whether IVF affects human birthweight. However, some 'unexplained infertility' in humans appears to be related to an inadequately developed endometrial lining. Couples with a previous history of 'unexplained infertility' have a high rate of small-for-dates infants, which may be associated with poor conditions for implantation (Wang et al., 1994).

Maternal behaviour

Differences in birthweight across different socio-economic groups may be largely attributable to differences in cigarette smoking. The birthweight appears to fall by about 14 g multiplied by the average number of cigarettes smoked per day. Smoking is associated with a poorer diet and level of health care, although effects on oxygen transfer are probably compensated for by 2,3-bisphosphoglycerate (2,3-BPG), which improves the efficiency of oxygen–haemoglobin dissociation (see Chapter 1). Smoking causes nicotine-induced vasoconstriction of the uterine vessels, carbon monoxide inhibits oxygen diffusion and cyanide affects enzyme systems (James and Stephenson, 1998). Improving fetal oxygenation in conditions of maternal hypoxia has achieved an improved fetal outcome (Battaglia et al., 1992) but there is controversy about the effect of maternal iron deficiency on pregnancy outcome (Godfrey et al., 1991). Alcohol consumption in excess of 40 mL/day is associated with effects on growth; one of the common effects of fetal alcohol syndrome is growth retardation (Hannigan and Armant, 2000). The use of hard drugs, such as heroin and cocaine, in pregnancy is associated with low birthweight babies but again it is difficult to dissociate the use of the drugs from the other variables. Caffeine, whether from coffee or other sources such as soft drinks, has an effect on fetal growth (see Chapter 12).

Other factors affecting fetal growth

Medical complications of pregnancy or pre-existing maternal diseases can affect fetal growth. Mild maternal hypertension does not restrict growth but severe hypertension is associated with low birthweight particularly if it is complicated with renal disease. Pre-eclampsia is a major cause of low birthweight; it has been suggested that IUGR of unknown cause may be due to undiagnosed pre-eclampsia (see Chapter 8). Obese and overweight women appear to be at increased risk of delivering a preterm infant (McDonald et al., 2010a). Severe respiratory and cardiovascular problems and chronic renal disease are also associated with growth retardation. Fetal growth retardation has also been observed in women with congenital uterine abnormalities. Infants conceived by IVF are more likely to be preterm and of low birthweight even when multiple gestation is taken into account (McDonald et al., 2010b).

Fetal malformations, especially those due to chromosomal abnormality, are strongly correlated with impaired growth rates. Trisomies and Turner's syndrome have a marked effect on birthweight (James and Stephenson, 1998). Chorionic villus sampling (CVS) indicates that in 1–2% of conceptuses tested there is a degree of confined placental mosaicism (where one or more types of placental cells have nuclei with an abnormal number of chromosomes). Placental mosaicism is associated with an increased frequency of IUGR (Robinson and Owens, 1996).

Maternal and fetal infections, such as rubella and cytomegalovirus, also detrimentally affect growth. It is not clear whether HIV affects fetal growth as coexisting problems cannot be dissociated. In developing countries, malaria infection causes placental disease and affects fetal growth. The fetus is also at risk from certain types of anti-malaria drugs such as quinine taken by the mother. Placental supply of amino acids is close to the minimum required to support fetal protein synthesis. It is possible that the adverse circumstances limiting fetal growth do so by increasing levels of catabolic hormones, such as catecholamines, cortisol and β-endorphin (Robinson and Owens, 1996) or by altering the expression of the receptor for IGF-II (Haig and Graham, 1991).

Complications associated with SGA

Babies who are small for gestational age (SGA) have an increased risk of perinatal complications (Box 9.11). Although some catch-up growth may occur post-natally, some of the effects of IUGR may be irreversible (Barker, 1998).

Case study 9.2 details the example of a baby with low birthweight.

Box 9.11 Complications associated with SGA

- Increased mortality
- Short- and long-term pulmonary morbidity
- Intrapartum hypoxia
- Hypothermia
- Hypoglycaemia
- Necrotizing enterocolitis
- Ophthalmic morbidity
- Neurological morbidity
- Delayed psychomotor development
- Polycythaemia
- Infection
- Pulmonary haemorrhage
- Sudden infant death syndrome
- Adult-onset cardiovascular and metabolic disease

 Case study 9.2

Razia gives birth to a healthy female infant at term. The baby appears healthy and chubby although she weighs only 2.6 kg.
- Is the midwife right to assume that Asian babies are normally smaller than Western babies?
- What reasons would you give to argue for or against this assumption?

Key points

- During the second week of development, the inner cell mass differentiates into the bilaminar disc, consisting of two germ layers: the epiblast and the hypoblast. The definitive yolk sac is created and the amniotic and chorionic cavities are evident. The differentiated cells migrate and adhere and the genes are switched on and off.
- The embryonic period consists of cell growth (increased cell number and size), differentiation, organogenesis (organization of tissues into organs) and morphogenesis (development of shape). This is the period that is most susceptible to teratogens, which can cause major morphological abnormalities.
- Gastrulation is the major event of the third week. It begins with the appearance of the primitive streak, results in the conversion of the bilaminar disc into a trilaminar disc, consisting of ectoderm, mesoderm and endoderm and establishes the axis for further embryonic development. The neural tube, precursor of the nervous system, and the somites also appear in the third week.
- The trilaminar disc is converted into the characteristic vertebral structure by differential growth of the cell layers causing folding and fusion.
- Weeks 4–8 are the period of organogenesis, differentiation of the major organ systems.
- Fetal growth is influenced by genes and the environment, but limited by nutrient and oxygen supply. Paternal genes tend to favour fetal growth whereas maternal genes tend to constrain fetal growth to a growth trajectory that may be set by environmental influences prior to fertilization.
- The fetus can adapt to undernutrition by altering metabolism and blood flow to protect the brain, albeit at the expense of other organs.
- Stem cell collection and storage from cord blood samples obtained immediately after delivery is becoming increasingly popular. Careful consideration is required by all health professionals, if this is requested, to ensure all legal and ethical issues are considered. Currently, it is still unclear what the actual benefits of fetal stem cell storage; however, on-going research is progressing into exploring the possible advantages of this. It is possible that some genetic conditions may be treatable with donated stem cells extracted from cord blood such as metabolic, immune and haematological disorders.

Application to practice

- An understanding of fetal development is required in the explanation of congenital conditions.
- Many factors, some of which are modifiable and can be affected by advice and guidance of the midwife, for example maternal smoking, stress and nutrition, affect fetal development and growth.

- As pregnancy progresses, most women are keen to know how their baby is developing, so the midwife should be able to describe fetal development and growth in an appropriate way.
- A basic understanding of fetal development is important in recognising abnormal conditions in the physical examination of the newborn (see Chapter 15).

ANNOTATED FURTHER READING

Barker DJP: *Mothers, babies and health in later life*, ed 2, New York, 1998, Churchill Livingstone.

Epidemiological studies link a number of adult diseases with fetal development. This book examines the evidence that fetal adaptation to undernutrition irreversibly alters anatomic, physiological and metabolic development, and links the fetal origins hypothesis to health policy.

Burton GJ, Barker DJP, Moffett A: *The placenta and human developmental programming*, Cambridge, 2010, Cambridge University Press.

An edited textbook with contributions from scientific experts which explore the role of the placenta in developmental programming, how placental development can disrupt the placental supply of nutrients and how gene expression can be affected by environmental, immunological and vascular insults.

Carlson BM: *Human embryology and developmental biology*, ed 4, St. Louis, 2008, Mosby.

A well-illustrated textbook which covers the molecular basis of development, cellular aspects, developmental anatomy and the progression of development. Includes recent research findings, case studies, timeline information, review questions and useful end-of-chapter summaries.

Copp AJ, Greene ND: Genetics and development of neural tube defects, *J Pathol* 220:217–230, 2010.

An excellent up-to-date-review covering mammalian neurulation and congenital defects of neural tube closure in depth, including the underlying developmental mechanisms, how mutant genes disrupt

neurulation, gene-gene and gene-environment interactions, the mechanisms by which folic acid supplementation prevents neural tube defects and possible causes of folic acid-resistance.

Gluckman PD, Hanson MA: *The fetal matrix: evolutions, development and disease*, Cambridge, 2004, Cambridge University Press.

Written by two of the experts in this field, this book covers fetal programming, evolutionary mechanisms that promoted survival of our hunter–gatherer ancestors, the implications of nutritional transition, and directions for future research and treatment.

Gluckman PD, Hanson MA: *Developmental origins of health and disease*, Cambridge, 2006, Cambridge University Press.

A well-referenced edited book that describes the epidemiological studies and animal research work that led to the current understanding that subtle influences on the fetus and during early life have profound and irreversible consequences for adult health and the risk of a wide range of diseases; includes a review of the key concepts of evolutionary developmental ('evo-devo') biology.

Sadler TW: *Langman's medical embryology*, ed 11, Philadelphia, 2009, Lippincott Williams Wilkins.

An up-to-date text (supported by online resources), illustrated with excellent line-drawings and photographs which covers stages of human development in detail with timelines and sections on the interaction between genetics and human development;

links molecular aspects including cellular signalling and experimental principles to clinical correlates.

Moore KL, Persaud TVN: *Before we are born: essentials of embryology and birth defects*, ed 7, Philadelphia, 2007, Saunders.

This book covers normal and abnormal human development week by week from fertilization through the development of the major organs and physiological systems to birth.

Moore KL, Persaud TVN: *The developing human: clinically orientated embryology*, ed 8, Philadelphia, 2007, Saunders.

This book is a more detailed description of embryological development, targeted at clinicians, which covers new research findings and their clinical applications. It includes aspects of molecular biology, effects of teratogens and detection of fetal defects.

NIH National Institutes of Health: *Stem Cell Basics*, http://stemcells.nih.gov/, 2010, U.S. Department of Health and Human Services.

A useful primer about stem cells which describes the biological properties of stem cells, current research areas and the potential use of stem cells in research treating disease; includes a comprehensive glossary.

Nüsslein-Volhar C: *Coming to life: how genes drive development*, 2006, Kales Press.

A unique portrayal of developmental biology, by an inspiring Nobel prize winner, which covers the historical aspects of cell biology, embryonic development, genetic control, birth defects and ethical issues.

REFERENCES

Ali F, Meier R: Positive selection in ASPM is correlated with cerebral cortex evolution across primates but not with whole-brain size, *Mol Biol Evol* 25:2247–2250, 2008.

Bard JBL, Weddon SE: The molecular basis of mammalian embryogenesis. In Hillier SG, Kitchener HC, Neilson JP, editors: *Scientific essentials of reproductive medicine*, Philadelphia, 1996, Saunders, pp 261–273.

Barker DJP: *Mothers, babies and health in later life*, ed 2, New York, 1998, Churchill Livingstone.

Barker DJP, Gluckman PD, Godfrey KM, et al: Fetal nutrition and cardiovascular disease in adult life, *Lancet* 341:938–941, 1993.

Battaglia C, Artini PG, Dambrogio G, et al: Maternal hyperoxygenation in the treatment of intrauterine growth retardation, *Am J Obstet Gynecol* 167:430–435, 1992.

Beck F: Human embryogenesis. In Hillier SG, Kitchener H, Neilson JP, editors: *Scientific essentials of reproductive medicine*, Philadelphia, 1996, Saunders, pp 274–281.

Bergers G, Song S: The role of pericytes in blood-vessel formation and maintenance, *Neuro-Oncology* 7:452–464, 2005.

Breier G: Angiogenesis in embryonic development: a review, *Placenta* 21 (Suppl A):S11–S15, 2000.

Brooks AA, Johnson MR, Steer PJ, et al: Birth weight: nature or nurture? *Early Hum Dev* 42:29–35, 1995.

Bukovsky A, Caudle MR, Virant-Klun I, et al: Immune physiology and oogenesis in fetal and adult humans, ovarian infertility, and totipotency of adult ovarian stem cells. Birth Defects Research Part, *C. Embryo Today* 87:64–89, 2009.

Carlson BM: *Human embryology and developmental biology*, ed 4, St. Louis, 2008, Mosby.

Cianfarani S: Foetal origins of adult diseases: just a matter of stem cell number? *Med Hypotheses* 61 (3):401–404, 2003.

Clifton VL: Sex and the human placenta: mediating differential strategies of fetal growth and survival, *Placenta* 31 (Suppl):S33–S39, 2010.

De Robertis EM, Oliver G, Wright CVE: Homeobox genes and the vertebrate body plan, *Sci Am* 263(1):46–52, 1990.

Durnin JVGA: Energy requirements of pregnancy: an integration of the longitudinal data from the five-country study, *Lancet* ii:1131–1133, 1987.

Fitzgerald MJT, Fitzgerald M: *Human embryology*, London, 1994, Baillière Tindall, pp 23, 24,37, 42.

Freeman B: The active migrateon of germ cells in the embryos of mice and men is a myth, *Reproduction* 125(5):635–643, 2003.

Gluckman PF, Harding JE: Nutritional and hormonal regulation of fetal growth: evolving concepts, *Acta Paediatr Suppl* 399:60, 1994.

Gluckman PD, Pinal CS: Regulation of fetal growth by the somatotrophic axis, *J Nutr* 133(5 Suppl 2):1741S–1746S, 2003.

Godfrey KM: The 'gold standard' for optimal fetal growth and development, *J Pediatr Endocrinol Metabol* 14(Suppl 6):1507–1513, 2001.

Godfrey KM, Redman CW, Barker DJ, et al: The effect of maternal anaemia and iron deficiency on the ratio of fetal weight to placental weight, *Br J Obstet Gynaecol* 98:886–891, 1991.

Goodwin B: *Health and development: conception to birth*, Milton Keynes, 1997, Open University, pp 203–205, 209.

Haig D, Graham C: Genomic imprinting and the strange case of the insulin like growth factor II receptor, *Cell* 64:1045–1046, 1991.

Hannigan JH, Armant DR: Alcohol in pregnancy and neonatal outcome, *Semin Neonatol* 5(3):243–254, 2000.

Harding R, Hooper SB: Regulation of lung expansion and lung growth before birth, *J Appl Physiol* 81 (1):209–224, 1996.

Harding JE, Johnston BM: Nutrition and fetal growth, *Reprod Fertil Dev* 7:539–547, 1995.

Horwitz R, Webb D: Cell migration, *Curr Biol* 13(19):R756–R759, 2003.

James DK, Stephenson T: Fetal nutrition and growth. In Chamberlain G, Dewhurst J, Harvey D, editors: *Clinical physiology in obstetrics*, ed 3, London, 1998, Gower Medical, pp 467–497.

Jauniaux E, Gulbis B, Burton GJ: The human first trimester gestational sac limits rather than facilitates oxygen transfer to the foetus: a review, *Placenta* 24(Suppl A):S86–S93, 2003.

Johnson MH: Functional brain development in humans, *Nat Rev Neurosci* 2(7):475–483, 2001.

Karlberg J, Jalil F, Lam B, et al: Linear growth retardation in relation to the three phases of growth, *Eur J Clin Nutr* 48(Suppl 1):S25–S44, 1994.

Kramer MS: Maternal nutrition, pregnancy outcome and public health policy, *Can Med Assoc J* 159 (6):663–665, 1998.

Langley-Evans SC, McMullen S: Developmental origins of adult disease, *Med Princ Pract* 19:87–98, 2010.

Lenz W: Thalidomide and congenital abnormalities, *Lancet* i:45, 1962.

Lumey LH: Decreased birthweights in infants after maternal in utero exposure to the Dutch famine of 1944–1945, *Paediatr Perinat Epidemiol* 6:240–253, 1992.

Martyn CN, Greenwald SE: Impaired synthesis of elastin in walls of aorta and large conduit arteries during early development as an initiating event in pathogenesis of systemic hypertension, *Lancet* 350:953–955, 1997.

McBride WG: Thalidomide and congenital abnormalities, *Lancet* ii:1358, 1961.

McDonald SD, Han Z, Mulla S, et al: Overweight and obesity in mothers and risk of preterm birth and low birth weight infants: systematic review and meta-analyses, *BMJ* 341: c3428, 2010a.

McDonald SD, Han Z, Mulla S, et al: Preterm birth and low birth weight among in vitro fertilization twins: a systematic review and meta-analyses, *Eur J Obstet Gynecol Reprod Biol* 148:105–113, 2010b.

Melchert M, List A: The thalidomide saga, *Int J Biochem Cell Biol* 39:1489–1499, 2007.

Moore T, Haig D: Genomic imprinting in mammalian development: a parental tug of war, *Trends Genet* 7:45–49, 1991.

Murtha MT, Leckman JF, Ruddle FH: Detection of homeobox genes in development and evolution, *Proc Natl Acad Sci USA* 88:10711–10715, 1991.

Nardo L, Hooper SB, Harding R: Stimulation of lung growth by tracheal obstruction in fetal sheep: relation to luminal pressure and lung liquid volume, *Pediatr Res* 43:184–190, 1998.

Park MS, Nguyen AD, Aryan HE, et al: Evolution of the human brain: changing brain size and the fossil record, *Neurosurgery* 60:555–562, 2007.

Phillips DIW: Insulin resistance as a programmed response to fetal undernutrition, *Diabetologia* 39:1119–1122, 1996.

Piscione TD, Rosenblum ND: The molecular control of renal branching morphogenesis: current knowledge and emerging insights, *Differentiation* 70(6):227–246, 2002.

Rink TJ: In search of a satiety factor, *Nature* 372:406–407, 1994.

Robinson JS, Owens JA: Control of fetal growth.. In Hillier SG, Kitchener HC, Neilson JP, editors: *Scientific essentials of reproductive medicine*, Philadelphia, 1996, Saunders, pp 329–341.

Sadler TW: *Langman's medical embryology*, ed 11, Philadelphia, 2010, Lippincott, Williams & Williams.

Shah PS: Parity and low birth weight and preterm birth: a systematic review and meta-analyses, *Acta Obstet Gynecol Scand* 89:862–875, 2010a.

Shah PS: Paternal factors and low birthweight, preterm, and small for gestational age births: a systematic review, *Am J Obstet Gynecol* 202:103–123, 2010b.

Sibley CP: Understanding placental nutrient transfer – why bother?

New biomarkers of fetal growth, *J Physiol* 587:3431–3440, 2009.

Spitz L: Conjoined twins, *Prenat Diagn* 25:814–819, 2005.

Stedman HH, Kozyak BW, Nelson A, et al: Myosin gene mutation correlates with anatomical changes in the human lineage, *Nature* 428:415–418, 2004.

Stewart RJC, Sheppard H, Preece R, et al: The effect of rehabilitation at different stages of development of

rats marginally malnourished for ten to twelve generations, *Br J Nutr* 43:403–411, 1980.

Veille JC, Hanson R, Sivakoff M, et al: Fetal cardiac size in normal, intrauterine growth retarded, and diabetic pregnancies, *Am J Perinatol* 10:275–279, 1993.

Walton A, Hammond J: The maternal effects on growth and conformation in Shirehorse–Shetland pony crosses, *Proc R Soc Lond B* 125:311–335, 1938.

Wang H, Chard T: The role of insulin like growth factor-1 and insulin like growth factor binding protein-1 in the control of fetal growth, *J Endocrinol* 132:11–19, 1992.

Wang JX, Clark AM, Kirby CA, et al: The obstetric outcome of singleton pregnancies following in vitro fertilization/gamete intrafallopian transfer, *Hum Reprod* 9:141–146, 1994.

Chapter | 10 |

Overview of immunology

LEARNING OBJECTIVES

- To review the immune system, identifying the roles of innate and specific immunity.
- To recognize how pregnancy affects the maternal immune system.
- To discuss the reasons why the fetus is not rejected.
- To appreciate the importance of placental transfer of immunoglobulins.
- To demonstrate an understanding of Rhesus incompatibility and how it is prophylactically treated.
- To appreciate the immunological immaturity of the neonate and why this is relevant to midwifery practice.
- To describe the principles of neonatal immunization.
- To outline the effects of human immunodeficiency virus (HIV) infection on the functioning of the immune system.

INTRODUCTION

Knowledge of the immune system is important in midwifery for several reasons. First, implantation and the nurture of an immunologically foreign fetus presents some interesting questions as to the functioning of the immune system in pregnancy. Second, some causes of infertility may be related to the immunological rejection of the sperm or fetus. During pregnancy, the maternal immune system is modified so the fetus is not attacked, but maternal defences against infection still function. Pregnant women have enhanced immunological responses to bacterial infections. However, they seem to develop increased susceptibility to viral infections such as seasonal influenza, and human immunodeficiency virus (HIV)-related problems may increase during pregnancy. Pregnancy affects immune-related conditions in a variety of ways: some may temporarily improve during pregnancy, such as asthma (Bohacs et al., 2010), whilst others may worsen and cause serious complications such as systemic lupus erythematosus (SLE) which can increase the risk of maternal death of 20 times or more (Day et al., 2009). Maternal immune adaptations in pregnancy also seem to prepare for possible pathogenic contamination of the placental wound site, during the vulnerable period of the puerperium. Blood group incompatibility and the resulting immune response can compromise the well-being of the developing fetus. The neonate is born immunologically immature but receives some passive immunity, both during pregnancy and neonatally in breast milk.

 Chapter case study

Zara and James try and live a healthy lifestyle; they both have never smoked and have not drunk any alcohol for many years. They follow a vegetarian diet and prefer to have organic, fresh products that are unprocessed and rely on milk products, nuts and pulses as the main source of protein in their diet. What precautions do Zara and Steve need to take and what particular types of food do they need to avoid and what are the reasons for this?

As part of their preparation to work in Africa, both Zara and James underwent in-depth medical screening to ensure that they were fit enough to undertake this work. Zara has the blood group O Rhesus negative and James has the blood group AB negative.

- As they are both Rhesus negative, then Rhesus incompatibility is not going to occur, but what possible complications could arise in the pregnancy as a result

Continued

The immune system is a complex network of specialized cells and chemical signals, which interact to provide a defence against infectious organisms. A number of microorganisms are associated with the body. Some, described as commensal organisms, exist within or on their host without causing any harm. Others are beneficial, or symbiotic, like those inhabiting the skin and the gut. However, some organisms, including microbes (bacteria, viruses, fungi, etc.), and larger organisms like tapeworms, are potentially damaging and are described as pathogens because they cause disease. The immune system of man has evolved to detect and eradicate these pathogenic organisms. Pathogens are diverse and numerous and have a rapid rate of replication and therefore are constantly evolving their own mechanisms to combat the host's defence.

The role of the immune system becomes clearly evident when it is compromised such as in acquired immune deficiency syndrome (AIDS) when HIV causes breakdown of the immune system (Fig. 10.1). However, under less extreme conditions, both infections and poor nutrition can overwhelm the immune system. To some extent, both the pregnant woman and the neonate are immunocompromised, but the concept that pregnancy is a state of immunosuppression which increases susceptibility to infectious diseases is controversial. It does not make evolutionary sense for pregnancy to be dangerous from an immunological perspective. Reproduction is crucial for survival of the species; a paramount aspect of this is that the immune system, and therefore the survival of the mother and fetus, is strengthened by enhanced recognition, cell communication, trafficking and repair mechanisms (Mor and Cardenas, 2010). It is preferable to describe pregnancy as a state of immunomodulation. An alternative explanation to the apparent increased risk of infection in pregnancy is that the mother is more readily sensitized by the changes that occur in her immune system.

THE EVOLUTION OF THE IMMUNE SYSTEM

The detection of the presence of pathogens initiates the immune response in the host, stimulating a cascade of interactions, which culminates in a counter-attack on the

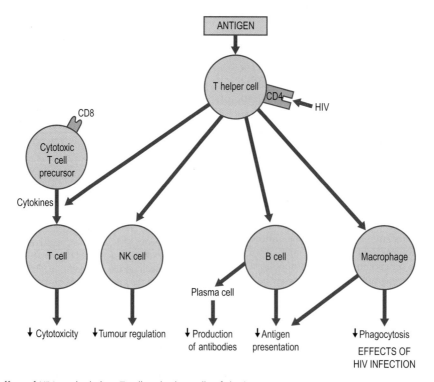

Fig. 10.1 The effect of HIV on the helper T cell and other cells of the immune system.

pathogen. There are two types of immunity: innate immunity and adaptive immunity.

Innate (natural) immunity pre-exists in an organism before any contact with pathogens; it is a collection of genetically encoded responses to foreign pathogens which does not change throughout the lifespan. Innate immunity occurs throughout the plant and animal kingdom, occurring in mammals, birds, sponges and worms. It evolved early and is particularly effective against bacteria, probably the earliest form of life on earth. It mounts an immediate non-specific response to an invading microorganism.

The second type of immunity, adaptive or acquired immunity, is facilitated by mechanisms that adapt to the presence of pathogens and becomes more effective with each exposure. As organisms became more complex and colonized new habitats, they were vulnerable to a broader range of more recently evolved pathogens such as viruses. Adaptive immunity occurs exclusively in higher multicellular organisms that have evolved relatively recently, such as mammals, birds and some fish (jawed vertebrates). It has evolved in response to increased pressure on survival and augments innate immunity; it is specific and effective at eliminating infection. The adaptive immune system ensures that, if an animal survives an initial infection by a pathogen, it is usually immune to further illness caused by the same pathogen; this response is exploited in medical vaccination programmes. Although the innate and adaptive systems operate differently, there are many common mechanisms and components. It has been hypothesized that the innate system, though more 'primitive', plays a critical role in viviparity and toleration of the fetal allograft (Sacks et al., 1999).

OVERVIEW OF THE IMMUNE SYSTEM

Innate immunity

Innate immunity is inherent and does not require contact with a pathogen for responses to occur. The defence is non-specific but not long-lasting. The responses are mobilized quickly and activated by receptors that generically respond to a broad range of pathogens. The first line of defence can be considered to be the physical and chemical barriers of the respiratory, reproductive and gastrointestinal systems and skin (Brostoff et al., 1991; Fig. 10.2). The skin is an impermeable barrier which is naturally acidic and undergoes continual desquamation. The gastrointestinal and respiratory tracts utilize peristalsis and cilia, respectively, to keep potentially infectious moieties moving. Commensal organisms on the skin or the epithelium of the respiratory and gastrointestinal systems create an environment which

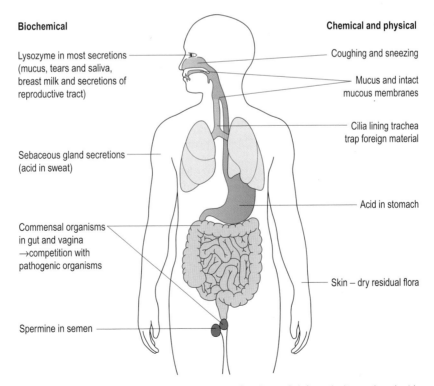

Biochemical

Lysozyme in most secretions (mucus, tears and saliva, breast milk and secretions of reproductive tract)

Sebaceous gland secretions (acid in sweat)

Commensal organisms in gut and vagina →competition with pathogenic organisms

Spermine in semen

Chemical and physical

Coughing and sneezing

Mucus and intact mucous membranes

Cilia lining trachea trap foreign material

Acid in stomach

Skin – dry residual flora

Fig. 10.2 The main physical and chemical barriers to infection (the 'first lines of defence'). (Reproduced with permission from Brostoff et al., 1991.)

is hostile to pathogens. In addition, various secretions such as sweat, tears and secretions in the respiratory and gastrointestinal systems contain antimicrobial substances. The chemical protective mechanisms of the innate immune system include that provided by lysozyme, the complement system, interferons and phagocytotic activity of the white blood cells (Table 10.1). The responses of the innate immune system, such as inflammation, generate cytokines (chemical signals) which recruit immune cells to the site of infection, resulting in identification and removal of dead cells and foreign substances and also communicate with the adaptive immune system via presentation of antigens.

Cells of the innate immune system express pattern recognition receptors (PRRs) which recognize pathogen-associated molecular patterns (PAMPs) which are unique molecular sequences expressed on the surface of pathogenic microorganisms (Koga et al., 2009). When PRRs of the immune cells bind to PAMPs on the pathogen, an inflammatory response is generated against the pathogen. One of the main families of PRRs is the Toll-like receptors (TLRs). Eleven types of TLRs have been identified in humans. TLRs are very specific to particular PAMPs that are molecules which are evolutionary conserved and critical to the pathogen's function (Koga and Mor, 2010). For instance, TLR4 recognizes gram-negative bacterial lipopolysaccharide and TLR2 recognizes bacterial lipoproteins, gram-positive bacterial peptidoglycans and fungal zymosan. TLRs also act with host cells which display 'danger signals', for instance, express different molecules on their surface when they are apoptotic or stressed or damaged, for instance, by reactive oxygen species.

Lysozyme

Lysozyme, which is sometimes described as 'the body's own antibiotic', is an enzyme that attacks the unique polysaccharide structure of bacterial cell walls. It is an abundant component of body secretions such as blood, sweat, tears, nasal secretion, breast milk and the mucous secretions of the reproductive tract.

The complement system

The complement system involves over 30 interacting proteins, mostly synthesized by the liver, and receptors which form an amplification cascade of defence, leading to cytolysis of bacteria, chemotaxis, opsonization and inflammation. As in the blood coagulation cascade, the components of the complement cascade exist in an inactive precursor form that can be triggered and activated. There are three pathways of activation: the classic pathway, which involves antibodies (or immunoglobulins), the alternative pathway, where the complement cascade is activated by the unique composition of an organism's cell wall (activator surfaces), and the mannan-binding lectin pathway. The outcome of complement activation is the formation of a membrane attack complex, cylindrical assembly of proteins that form a tube that perforates the plasma membrane of target cells. This perforation allows ions to enter cells so that fluid follows by osmosis and the bacterial cells swell and burst. The complement cascade stimulates the release of histamine and kinins from mast cells, recruits macrophages and neutrophils to the site and enhances phagocytosis by opsonization. The complement system may be a factor in a number of diseases such as multiple sclerosis, asthma, Alzheimer's disease, type 1 diabetes (Hewagama and Richardson, 2009) and autoimmune diseases such as SLE (Chen et al., 2010).

Interferons

Interferons are cytokines secreted by virally infected cells that carry out a non-specific defence which prevents viral replication. Viruses replicate by 'hijacking' protein synthesis in the host cells they have infected. Therefore, the cell is diverted to make viral mRNA, which is translated into viral proteins and assembled as viral particles. Interferons

Table 10.1 Defensive activity of the innate immune system	
Phagocytosis	Neutrophils and macrophages adhere to the surface of the target organism. Adherence is enhanced by opsonins, which form a bridge between the pathogen and the phagocyte. The phagocytic cells produce pseudopodia facilitating the engulfing of the pathogen into a cellular vesicle. Lysosomes fuse with the phagosome and degrade it
Cytotoxicity	Eosinophils and NK cells adhere to targets (opsonins increase efficiency). Eosinophils secrete chemicals, which damage the target cell membrane, causing cell death, and an inflammatory response, which is particularly effective against parasites. NK cells attack body cells expressing viral proteins in their membranes and some tumour cells. The NK cells adhere and release perforin, which penetrates the cell membrane causing cell death
Inflammation	The sequence of events is that the trigger (such as a bacteria signal) stimulates vasodilation and increased blood flow and delivery of blood cells (redness, heat and pain). Vascular permeability (swelling) occurs, which increases exudation and extracellular fluid (oedema), phagocyte invasion, promotion of fibrin wall enclosing infection and tissue repair

interfere with this production of new viral proteins; they damage the viral mRNA and inhibit protein translation, not just in the infected cells but in neighbouring uninfected cells as well, subsequently creating a barrier around the viral infection, which prevents the viral replication. Interferons also stimulate macrophages and natural killer (NK) cells; they can also up-regulate major histocompatibility complexes (MHCs). Interferons produced by genetic engineering are used therapeutically.

Leukocytes and lymphocytes

The cells of the immune system are leukocytes and lymphocytes. Although they are described as white blood cells, some of the cells spend very little time in the circulation, whereas others never enter the vascular system at all and remain in the lymphatic system, spleen or other tissues. Blood cells are derived from a single population of haemopoietic stem cells (HSCs) in the bone marrow. These precursor cells have the potential to divide into progenitor cells which can differentiate into all the cell types present in blood. After radiation for cancer treatment, the destroyed stem cells have to be replaced by a bone marrow transplant; very few cells need to be transplanted for regeneration of a mature population of cells.

Phagocytes

Neutrophils and macrophages are phagocytic white blood cells that can engulf and digest foreign cells and unwanted matter, such as the body's own dead and dying cells, through the processes of phagocytosis, cytotoxicity and the generation of an inflammatory response. The cells that mediate innate immunity are the granulocytes: neutrophils, monocytes, eosinophils and basophils. Neutrophils, also known as polymorphonuclear leukocytes, are the most numerous, forming about 40–70% of the circulating white blood cells. On entering the circulation, neutrophils, which have a lifespan of a few days, cease cell division. Neutrophils are motile and exhibit chemotactic behaviour, moving through a concentration gradient towards chemical messengers, such as those released from dividing bacteria, activated platelets or other phagocytotic cells, towards the site of infection. Neutrophils have multilobed nuclei which aid diapedesis (the amoeboid movement of the cells through the gaps between the capillary endothelial cells). Neutrophil phagocytosis is fast. Neutrophils usually reach the site of infection and begin phagocytosis within about 90 min of the initial stimulation; they surround the unwanted material and engulf it in a phagosome which merges with a lysosome containing substances that kill the engulfed bacterium or neutrophil granules to form a phagolysosome. The neutrophil can generate a vigorous and lethal respiratory burst releasing lethal reactive oxygen species or produce nitric oxide which kills both the phagocyte itself and the engulfed pathogen. Alternately, the bacterium is killed by myeloperoxidase from neutrophil granules which can generate hypochlorite (bleach) which is very toxic to bacteria; the green haem pigment of myeloperoxidase gives the greenish colour of bacterially infected mucous and 'pus'.

Adherence of the phagocyte to the target cell can be increased by opsonization. Opsonins include antibodies which bind specifically to an antigen on the pathogen surface and are then recognized by Fc receptors on phagocytes so that the pathogen is more efficiently recognized and phagocytosed. The complement component, C3, also binds to pathogens and is recognized by the complement receptor on phagocytes, thus increasing the efficiency of recognition and adherence of the phagocyte. Effectively, the opsonin acts as a bridge between the pathogen and the phagocyte, so promoting phagocytosis. Monocytes circulate for a short time in the bloodstream and then migrate to tissues and organs where they differentiate into macrophages and exhibit characteristics specific to their host tissue. Less than 7% of circulating white blood cells are monocytes, but 'resident macrophages' are abundantly distributed in the body tissues and are particularly dense around blood vessels, the gut walls, the genital tract and lungs. Macrophages are oestrogen-sensitive. Monocytes are the largest white blood cell and have a characteristic horse-shaped nucleus. They are also phagocytes and have a longer lifespan than neutrophils. Circulating monocytes respond more slowly than neutrophils, reaching the site of infection within about 48 h, but they have a greater capacity for phagocytosis, engulfing more material than neutrophils.

Many pathogens have evolved mechanisms to evade phagocyte activity; these include inhabiting niches like the skin where phagocytes cannot reach, suppressing inflammatory responses, interfering with the phagocyte recognition of pathogens or interfering with chemotaxis. In addition, some bacteria can block phagocytosis or survive within phagocytes or in the phagolysomes.

Natural killer cells

NK cells are cytotoxic lymphocytes which attack compromised host cells such as virally infected and cancerous cells. Although NK cells are lymphocytes, they are part of the innate immune system. NK cells kill cells which express low levels of MHC proteins, which is a common characteristic of both virally infected cell and some cancer cells. NK cells alter the target cell's plasma membrane by releasing proteases and perforins from their cytoplasmic granules so water and ions diffuse in; consequently, the virus-infected cell swells and lyses or dies by apoptosis. To recognize the body's own cells which are infected or behaving abnormally, NK cells have to be able to distinguish between self and altered-self state. Apoptotic cells are tagged by the phophatidylserine phospholipids of the cell membrane, which are usually orientated on the internal cytosolic face of the membrane, 'scrambling' to the exterior of the membrane which alerts phagocytotic cells.

Acquired or specific immunity

Lymphocytes, which constitute about 20–40% of the circulating white blood cells, coordinate the adaptive immune responses. These small cells have relatively little cytoplasm, few organelles and no granules. T lymphocytes (or T cells) have secretory vesicles containing perforins and granzymes. B lymphocytes are dominant in humoral responses, mediated by immunoglobulins (antibodies) which attack bacteria and viruses in body fluids. T lymphocytes are dominant in cell-mediated immunity (see Chapter 1). Small lymphocytes also circulate in the lymphoid system and spend much of the time resident in the organs of the lymphoid system. The lymphoid system is the main site of the adaptive immune responses. Fluid leaks out of the blood capillaries into the intercellular spaces. Some of the fluid re-enters the blood capillary (see Chapter 1) but some enters the lymphatic capillaries. This lymph fluid, therefore, has a similar composition to plasma, except that the protein component of plasma is retained within the blood vessels so lymph fluid has low protein content. Ultimately, the lymph fluid is transported through lymph vessels to the thoracic duct and back into the bloodstream. The small lymphocytes 'burrow out' of the small veins as they pass through the lymph nodes and so enter the lymphoid tissue. Each lymphocyte spends minutes in the bloodstream compared with hours residing in the lymphoid system. Lymphocytes have different levels of maturity; naïve lymphocytes which are mature but have not encountered the antigen they will recognize, effector cells which have been activated by an antigen and memory cells which have survived from past exposure to the antigen and could rapidly divide in response to subsequent exposure to the antigen.

Antigen recognition

The classical view is that cells of the immune system differentiate between self (body) and non-self (foreign) cells (and changed self in host cells which are infected by a virus), identifying foreign cells and pathogens which have evaded the innate immune system and attack them. It has been hypothesized that the immune system differentiates between dangerous and non-dangerous rather than between self and non-self or infectious or non-infectious (Gallucci and Matzinger, 2001). The surface of a pathogen displays a unique combination of antigenic determinants that can be recognized by the immune cells as 'foreign' or non-self. The whole cell that engenders an immune response is described as an antigen, although the cluster of antigenic determinants itself is called the epitope. Each antigen can be displayed by the pathogenic cell itself, or

can be secreted by a pathogen, for instance, bacterial toxins, or substances from non-pathogenic sources, such as plant pollens, resulting in allergic responses, or chemicals such as synthetic vaccines. Only certain parts of the entire antigen are immunogenic; these parts bind antibodies and activated lymphocytes. Most naturally occurring antigens have numerous antigenic determinants that can mobilize several different lymphocyte populations. Large chemically simple molecules (such as plastics) have little or no immunogenicity. Antigenicity depends on the ability of the host to identify the substance as an antigen; there are variations in individual responses.

Lymphocytes have high-affinity surface receptors that recognize antigens with very high specificity. Each lymphocyte has a single type of specific antigen receptor, unlike the cells of the innate (non-specific) immune system, which have many different types of receptor on each cell. These receptors differ between T lymphocytes (T-cell receptors) and B lymphocytes, the latter displaying on its cell surface copies of the specific antibody that each cell can secrete. Infective pathogens will normally display multiple antigens which are recognized as foreign by many different lymphocytes in the infected host. There are over 100 million pathogenic epitopes. Each person has, at birth, a population of lymphocytes consisting of clones, each of a few cells. A clone has a few identical lymphocytes, each of which has many copies of the same antigen receptor on its surface. The population of lymphocytes has the capability, described as its repertoire of receptors, to respond to a vast number of antigens, most of which are unlikely to be encountered in a lifetime. Initially, the number of cells expressing receptors for any particular antigen is small and this clone will remain small unless the antigen reacts. So, one of the first steps in mounting an effective immune response is to expand the clone by increasing the number of cells expressing the same antigen, a response termed 'clonal selection'.

There are far more antigen receptors than there are human genes encoded for by DNA (about 100 million epitopes and only approximately 25 000 different human genes). It is hypothesized, therefore, that each antigen receptor site is coded for by a few randomly selected genes. As there are several hundred possible genes involved, the random selection of a few genes that can be cut and spliced (somatic recombination) can produce enough combinations of antigen receptor gene segments to make all the 100 million epitope-binding sites. So, an individual can develop a huge number of diverse types of lymphocytes, each expressing a unique receptor for an antigen from a small family of genes. The gene segments recombine to form unique genes. This process is known as combinatorial diversification or V(D)J (variable, diverse and joining gene segment) recombination.

However, in the random production of antigen receptors, some lymphocytes will possess receptors for the body's own antigens. In the fetal thymus, clonal deletion takes place, which results in the destruction or deletion of self- or autoreactive T lymphocytes by apoptosis. This process is called central tolerance. Any T lymphocyte binding to specialized cells presenting self-epitopes on the surface will be stimulated to undergo apoptosis. Self-reactive B lymphocytes do not need to be destroyed because they require a signal from a T lymphocyte (helper T cell) before they can function. It seems that some of the self-reactive T cells escape central tolerance in all individuals (Weetman, 2010). These are prevented from causing autoimmune disease in healthy people by a range of peripheral tolerance mechanisms (Mueller, 2010). It is important that the immune system has self-tolerance and does not harm cells or molecules of the host that are recognized as antigenic; otherwise, the host would be damaged (as happens in autoimmune diseases).

Clonal selection and immunological memory

The immune response to a second and subsequent exposure to the antigen is faster and more effective than the first exposure (Fig. 10.3). The primary adaptive response, on the first exposure, is slow to develop, perhaps taking 7–14 days, and then builds slowly to a peak about 2 weeks later. The time for the response to become evident is termed the 'incubation period'. Then, symptoms become apparent until the immune response has become effective. The secondary adaptive response, when the host subsequently encounters the same antigen, develops sooner, lasts longer and is more effective so signs of infection or symptoms may be prevented. On first exposure, the small numbers of lymphocytes binding the antigen are stimulated to undergo rapid cell division. A single lymphocyte can divide fast enough to produce 64 000 daughter cells in 4 days. As the new cells, also bearing receptor sites specific to the stimulating antigen, are produced, they mature and differentiate. If B lymphocytes are activated, some members of the new population of lymphocytes are active in attacking the cells bearing the antigen. Most clone cells become antibody-secreting plasma cells. Others become memory cells, which have a long life and continue to circulate as a permanently enlarged clone of lymphocytes capable of recognizing specific antigens and mounting an immediate response. Effectively, the initial immune response is boosted by repeated exposure.

Individuals have immunity to an antigen if their immune system can mount a fast and effective specific response to that antigen. The role of a vaccine is to deliberately stimulate the immune response and increase the clonal size without causing the illness. Effective vaccines can be in the form of killed whole organisms, harmless organisms, organisms that have been modified or attenuated (as in most viral vaccines), fragments of organisms (as in many bacterial vaccines), substances with similar epitopes, synthetic epitopes or inactivated toxins

(Table 10.2). Some antigens are more effective at triggering clonal expansion, such as rubella (German measles) virus, which is highly antigenic; thus, after primary exposure, the host rarely acquires the infection again. Other pathogens, such as *Neisseria gonococcus* (causing gonorrhoea) and *Treponema pallidum* (causing syphilis), are only weakly antigenic; therefore, there are no effective vaccines available.

Passive immunity

Resistance to a specific pathogen, acquired by previous exposure or deliberate immunization resulting in clonal expansion, is active immunity. However, sometimes, the effect of infection can be disastrous before the immune system has time to mount a response. Passive immunization can overcome this by providing temporary resistance in the form of products from a donor source. Passive immunization causes destruction of the pathogenic cells without creating clonal expansion or making memory cells so its effects are not permanent. An individual who has no prior immunity but is exposed to antigens or a potentially dangerous disease is given preformed antibodies. Examples include treatment following a bite from a rabid dog or anti-D immunization following potential exposure to Rhesus-incompatible antigens (see below). The transfer of placental antibodies (IgG) to the fetus and consumption of antibodies (IgA) in colostrum and breast milk by the neonate are also examples of passive immunity.

Case study 10.1 looks at an example of exposure to German measles.

Lymphocytes

There are three types of lymphocytes: those that mature in the bone marrow, called B lymphocytes, those that mature in the thymus, called T lymphocytes and NK cells (see above).

B lymphocytes

B lymphocytes secrete antibodies which are responsible for the humoral immune response. On binding to an antigen, B lymphocytes undergo clonal expansion producing two types of daughter cells: memory B cells and plasma cells. The plasma cells are short-lived cells which synthesize and secrete large amounts of antibodies (immunoglobulins), which are specialized glycoproteins that bind specifically to the antigen that was recognized by the B lymphocyte. These antibodies bind to their target antigens and enable other components of the immune system, such as phagocytes and complement proteins, to attack the precise organism bearing the antigen rapidly and effectively. There are five classes of antibody (Table 10.3);

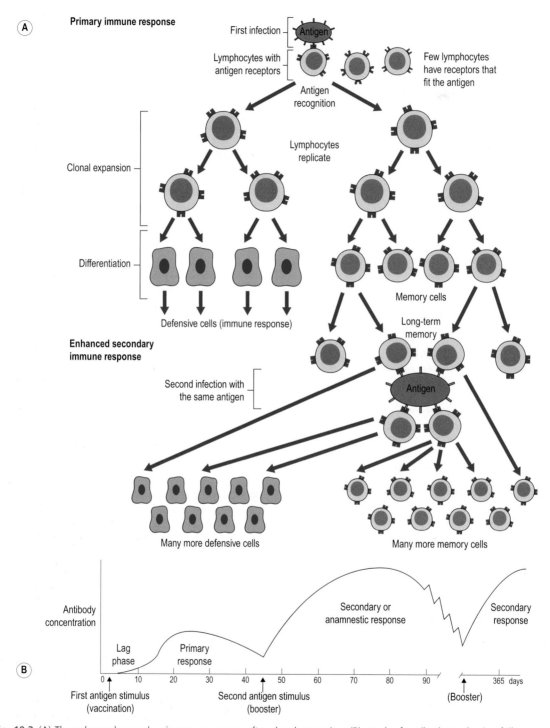

Fig. 10.3 (A) The enhanced secondary immune response after clonal expansion; (B) graph of antibody production following exposure to antigen. ((A) Reproduced with permission from Stewart, 1997.)

Table 10.2 Types of acquired immunity

ACTIVE NATURAL	ARTIFICIAL	PASSIVE NATURAL	ARTIFICIAL
Clinical or subclinical disease	Vaccines: dead or extract attenuated toxoids	Congenital (across placenta) colostrum	Antiserum antitoxin gamma globulin

Case study 10.1

Melanie is expecting her first baby. She attends the midwives' clinic at 11 weeks' gestation concerned over the welfare of her unborn baby. Her 3-year-old nephew, Michael, whom she sees regularly, has German measles.
- What factors would the midwife need to consider in advising Melanie over her concerns?
- Would there be any specific investigations to carry out?

If Melanie was susceptible to Rubella infection, how would this be recognized and what subsequent management and care be planned?

these differ in the structure of the 'Y'-shape of the tail, which affects whether the antibodies bind in groups or singly (Fig. 10.4). The antigen receptor on B lymphocytes is a surface immunoglobulin (sIg) closely resembling the structure of the antibody-binding site that will bind to the same antigen. The binding of the B cell to the epitope is relatively straightforward in that the antigen is intact or native, whereas T lymphocytes bind only to processed antigens. However, antigen binding by a B lymphocyte usually requires helper T-cell activity before clonal expansion can take place.

T lymphocytes

There are three subsets of T lymphocytes: helper T cells, regulatory T (Treg) cells (formerly called suppressor cells) and cytotoxic T cells. Unique glycoproteins on the cell surface, which are involved in mediating cell function, can be identified using monoclonal antibodies and used to distinguish different subpopulations of T lymphocytes. The system of nomenclature is based on the cluster of differentiation (CD) system. Cytotoxic T cells express CD8 protein markers in the plasma membrane and recognize and destroy cells that have become infected or cancerous. Some regulatory T cells also express CD8 but express other markers as well, including CD4 and CD25, which distinguish them from other T-cell types.

Table 10.3 Classes of antibodies

ANTIBODY	ROLE AND CHARACTERISTICS
IgG	Most abundant antibody (85% circulating antibody), found in blood and all fluid compartments including cerebrospinal fluid. Produced in large amounts at secondary adaptive response, therefore represent 'history' of past exposure to pathogens. Long lasting. Can diffuse out of bloodstream to site of acute infection and can cross placenta. Act as powerful opsonins bridging phagocyte and target cell. Important in defence against bacteria and activation of the complement system via the classic pathway
IgM	IgM molecules join in groups of five 'IgM pentamers', therefore tend to aggregate antigens into a clump that is a target for phagocytes and NK cells. Large molecules so cannot diffuse out of bloodstream. Very powerful activators of complement, important in immune responses to bacteria. First antibody produced when the body is confronted by a new antigen
IgA	Mostly in secretions such as saliva, tears, sweat and breast milk, especially colostrum. Link in groups of two to three. Protects body by adhering to pathogen and preventing its adherence to body cavity. Cannot activate complement or cross placenta
IgE	Tail binds to receptor on mast cells so involved in acute inflammation, allergic responses and hypersensitivity. Binding sites for antigens on larger parasites such as worms and flukes. Some people have IgE for common harmless environmental proteins such as pollen, fur, house dust mite and penicillin
IgD	Rarely synthesized; little is known about its functions. Large, found only in blood. May be involved in antigen stimulation of B cells

T helper cells express CD4 proteins, and are sometimes called CD4 + cells. Helper T cells interact with macrophages and produce cytokines, which activate and regulate other components of the immune system. Cytokines are soluble polypeptides with a short range and lifespan that are also synthesized by lymphocytes and macrophages. They can induce fever, stimulate lymphocytes, stimulate antigen expression and potentiate the destruction of tumour cells. Cytokines include interleukins, interferons, tumour necrosis factor (TNF) and some colony-stimulating factors

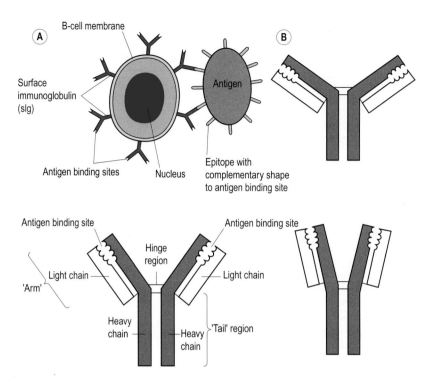

Fig. 10.4 (A) B-cell surface immunoglobulins are receptors for antigens; (B) the antibody molecule is a hinge-like structure that allows binding to two antigens. (Reproduced with permission from Stewart, 1997.)

(CSF). Helper T cells induce proliferation of lymphocytes, stimulate antibody production by B lymphocytes and enhance the activity of cytotoxic T lymphocytes.

The receptor for HIV is the CD4 protein expressed not only by T cells but also by macrophages and possibly other cells. HIV reduces the number of helper T cells by inducing apoptosis so none of the immune mechanisms work effectively. Infection of macrophages shifts the profile of cytokines produced, which contributes to wasting and acute respiratory distress syndrome. Macrophages can act as a reservoir of the virus.

T lymphocytes have antigen receptors on their surface, formed of two peptide chains that contain the binding site for a specific epitope. However, the T lymphocyte cannot bind to an epitope unless it is has been processed and presented to the T lymphocyte by one of the host's own cells. Although most nucleated cells have the capability of presenting an antigen and activating T lymphocytes, some cells generate a more efficient immunostimulatory response. These 'professional' antigen-presenting cells (APCs) are dendritic cells, B lymphocytes and macrophages that bind the antigen and phagocytose it, degrading its protein and then migrating to the lymph nodes. The resulting epitope fragments are displayed in the cleft of the MHC molecule (Box 10.1) on the surface of the APC (Fig. 10.5). Helper and Treg lymphocytes bind only to epitopes processed in this manner. Cytotoxic T cells

Box 10.1 The major histocompatibility complex

Each person has a unique configuration of MHC antigens or molecules on the surface of their cells (except monozygous twins who have identical MHC). MHC molecules are a marker of 'self' and are synonymous with human leukocyte antigen (HLA). MHC molecules present the antigens to T cells. There are different classes of MHC molecules, which present antigens with different effectiveness. MHC molecules restrict helper T cells to interact with immune cells that have already bound to the epitope for which the T cell also has an antigen receptor. It is these cells that are involved in rejection of transplanted tissue, as all MHC molecules are different. Tissue grafts have increased survival if there is some similarity in MHC structure between the donor and the recipient (hence the need for tissue typing) and if drugs are used to suppress the immune response.

recognize the epitopes of intercellular pathogens, such as viruses, that are incorporated into the cell membrane during cell replication of an infected cell harbouring the virus.

There are at least three forms of T helper cells: Th0, Th1 and Th2 cells, which are classified on the basis of

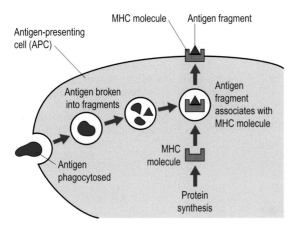

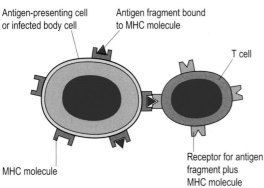

Fig. 10.5 Antigen processing by the APC. (Reproduced with permission from Stewart, 1997.)

their cytokine secretion. The dendritic cells present the antigen to T helper cells and direct them to differentiate into either Th1 or Th2 cells. When the resting T helper cells are initially activated, they become Th0 cells which have characteristics of both Th1 and Th2 cells; Th0 cells are then further activated and differentiate into either Th1 or Th2 cells depending on the type of threat. This pathway of differentiation is controlled by the cytokine secretion of the dendritic cell. Secretion of interleukins IL-12 and IL-10 by the dendritic cell drives the differentiation of Th1 and Th2 cells, respectively (Fig. 10.6).

The Th1 response tends to be initiated by viruses, cancer, yeasts and intracellular bacteria (e.g. *Mycoplasma pneumoniae* or Chlamydia). The outcome of the Th1 response is activation of cell-mediated immunity and the secretion of gamma-interferon (INF-γ), IL-2, lymphotoxin and granulocyte–macrophage colony-stimulating factor (GM-CSF). This activates cytotoxic T cells and NK cells to respond to target cells carrying intracellular pathogens or mutated proteins since these would not be responsive to

circulating antibodies. Body cells continuously turn over their protein and some of these protein fragments or peptides are displayed on the cell surface in association with MHC proteins which the cells of the immune system monitor. Virally infected or cancerous cells display peptides from viral or mutated proteins which are recognized as foreign by the immune cells and displayed by APCs to provoke an immune response. Following clonal expansion of the T lymphocyte that recognizes the non-self peptide, cytotoxic T cells seek out the virally infected or mutated cells and, on contact, produce toxic and perforating substances that induce apoptosis and then turn the immune response off when the antigen-expressing cells have been eliminated When the infection has resolved, most of the cytotoxic T cells die and are removed by phagocytosis; a small percentage of the T cells remain as memory cells.

Other bacteria, parasites, toxins and allergens predominantly trigger a Th2 response and secretion of IL-3, IL-4, IL-5, IL-6, IL-10 and IL-13 which activate eosinophils, leukocytes and B lymphocytes (which produce antibodies). The Th1 and Th2 systems suppress each other; the Th1/Th2 balance is important. For instance, some viruses produce proteins that mimic IL-10 and drive the differentiation of Th0 cells into Th2 cells which are less effective at attacking viruses so viral survival is enhanced. In pregnancy, the Th1/Th2 balance shifts in favour of Th2; this downregulation of Th1-induced cellular immunity and enhancement of Th2-induced humoral responsiveness in the maternal immune system in pregnancy is mediated by progesterone and is important in preventing fetal rejection (see below).

Regulatory T cells limit the activity of the immune cells and prevent damage to the body's own cells maintaining immune system homeostasis and tolerance to self-antigens (and are thus important in preventing autoimmune disorders) (Guerin et al., 2009). Treg cells are involved in maintaining peripheral tolerance. Treg cells accumulate in the lymph nodes draining the uterus and spleen in early pregnancy probably because they migrate towards human chorionic gonadotrophin (hCG) and chemokines produced by the trophoblast. Treg cells appear to be important in immune tolerance of the conceptus tissue (see below) and the sperm and oocytes.

Interaction of B and T lymphocytes

B lymphocytes and T lymphocytes interact (Fig. 10.7). The B lymphocyte binds to the native (intact) antigen via the sIg receptors on its cell surface. The antigen is then internalized by the B lymphocyte and processed so fragments appear on its cell surface associated with the MHC molecule. In this form, the T lymphocytes can recognize it so helper T cells are activated, producing the signal that allows the B lymphocyte to start cell division and differentiation.

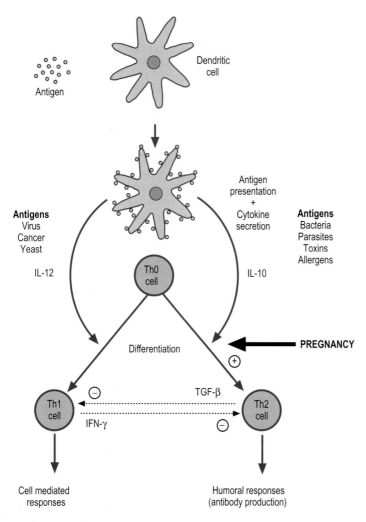

Fig. 10.6 The differentiation of T helper cells into either Th1 or Th2 cells depends on the type of antigen presented by the dendritic cells and the pattern of cytokine secretion. The outcome of the Th1 response is predominantly cell-mediated, whereas the Th2 response facilitates production of antibodies. The Th1 and Th2 responses are mutually suppressive. In pregnancy, the Th2 response is enhanced, which is important in preventing fetal rejection.

Interaction of the innate and adaptive immune systems

The innate system is an integral part of the immune response. It initiates an immune response by the macrophages, processing an antigen in association with the MHC and presenting it to lymphocytes; this is called signal 1. The full response requires adjuvants, such as endotoxin, which produce signal 2, pro-inflammatory cytokines or co-stimulatory surface molecules. This signal conveys the biological significance of the antigen and effectively instructs the adaptive system to respond (or not). Signals 1 and 2 stimulate T cells to become effector Th1 or Th2 cells. Macrophages secrete cytokines which activate other macrophages, NK cells and granulocytes.

THE IMMUNE SYSTEM IN PREGNANCY; ACCEPTANCE OF THE FETUS

Humans are 'outbred'. The genetic diversity resulting from sexual reproduction means that the fetus is phenotypically unique and immunologically distinct from both of its parents. The fetus has a unique combination of histocompatibility antigens. The fetus is classified as an allograft: foreign tissue from the same species but with different antigenic make-up. Half of the fetal antigens are derived from the father. There is a marked antigenic difference between the maternal tissues and the paternally inherited antigens

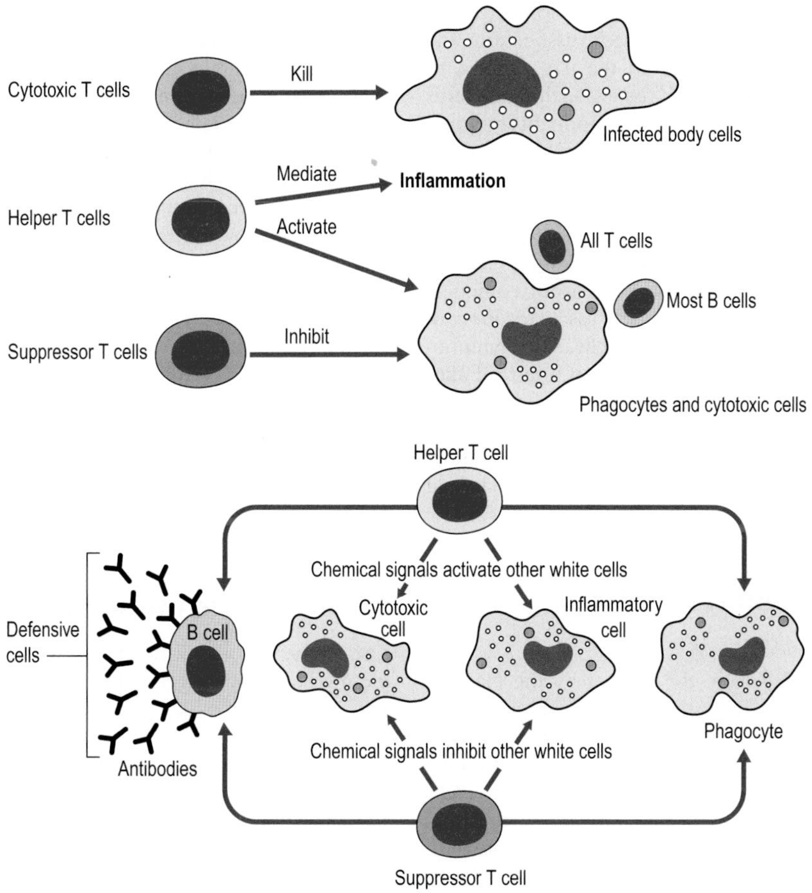

Fig. 10.7 The role of three different T cells and their interaction. (Reproduced with permission from Stewart, 1997.)

expressed by the fetus. If tissue from the offspring is grafted on to its mother, a strong maternal immune response is mounted and the tissue is rejected. It seems surprising therefore that the mother does not reject the fetus because of its foreign antigens. Medawar (1953) proposed several possibilities to explain why the fetus is not rejected: as fetal tissue is antigenically immature, it may not express normal antigens, the uterus may be a privileged site (or not in contact with fetal tissue) or pregnancy may affect the maternal immune system and normal immune responses. However, it is the placenta and not the fetus that is the 'transplant', and the placenta has very different characteristics than that of a transplanted tissue or organ, and the interaction of the trophoblast with the maternal immune system orchestrates cooperative modulation of the components of the immune system.

Fetal antigen expression

Fetal tissue is antigenically mature and does express antigens and immunocompetence from an early stage (Koga and Mor, 2010). MHC class I and II antigens, albeit in smaller amounts, are present on embryonic cells from the time of implantation throughout the pregnancy. The MHC antigens are the molecules that are normally recognized by a transplant-recipient's immune system and cause rejection of allografts (foreign tissue transplants), but trophoblast cells are an exception (Weetman, 2010). Paternal antigens are apparent at the eight-cell stage of the cleavage, and major histocompatibility antigens begin to be expressed at later stages of cell division. Dendritic cells from fetal skin are in contact with maternal blood and enter the maternal circulation; these cells express MHC antigens (Zenclussen et al., 2007). The zona pellucida and early trophoblast have glycoprotein coatings, which may limit the cell-mediated immune responses. Immunological problems are usually not a problem prior to implantation because the endometrium secretes immunosuppressive factors.

The uterus as a privileged site

Both the mother and other individuals reject grafts of fetal tissue because fetal tissue expresses antigens. Maternal responses to transplanted tissue remain competent in pregnancy; a pregnant mammal rejects tissue from the father of the fetus and tissue from the fetus grafted to areas other than the uterus. Some tissues, such as the testis and parts of the eye and brain, lack components required in immune responses or are not accessible to them (Mellor and Munn, 2008). These sites are immunologically privileged and can accept transplanted tissue with fewer problems. However, the uterus is not a privileged site as was suggested (Billingham, 1964); the development of ectopic pregnancies shows that the uterus is not a uniquely immunoprivileged site. The increased vascularization of the pregnant uterus allows efficient delivery of lymphocytes and other maternal immune cells so non-fetal allogenic tissue transplanted in the uterus is rejected (Beer and Billingham, 1974). Maternal and placental tissue are closely situated and in close proximity. There are a number of interfaces between maternal immune cells and placental cells that change as the pregnancy progresses.

The chorion and trophoblast as a barrier

The fetus is separated from the mother by the placenta and fetal membranes. It is suggested that the chorionic membranes are resistant to maternal rejection and can protect the fetus from maternal antibodies and immune cells. The placenta and chorion originate from cells derived from the fertilized zygote, which are therefore genetically and antigenically different to the maternal cells. Maternal blood bathes the chorionic villi (see Chapter 8) and is therefore in immediate contact with trophoblast cells which are derived from the zygote and thus have non-maternal antigens. This means that maternal blood containing immunologically responsive cells is in apposition with the syncytiotrophoblast (outer layer of non-mitotic cells; see Chapter 8).

Some cytotrophoblast cells (the dividing cells underlying the syncytiotrophoblast) penetrate the syncytiotrophoblast layer to form the cytotrophoblast columns, which anchor the villi to the maternal tissue. During implantation and placental development, other invasive trophoblast cells and fragments break away from the mass of placental tissue and enter the uterine veins and maternal venous system. It is this extravillous (non-villous) trophoblast that remodels the uterine spiral arteries to allow increased maternal blood flow to the intervillous space (see Chapter 8). This extravillous trophoblast layer of cells therefore makes extensive contact with the maternal tissue. Some of the cells breach the trophoblast and invade the maternal blood system, forming minute emboli which lodge in the pulmonary circulation where they are destroyed. However, even within the maternal circulation, the extravillous trophoblast cells do not appear to provoke a normal inflammatory or immune response (Johnson and Christmas, 1996). So, the trophoblast appears to provide an insulating barrier, protecting the fetus from the immunologically responsive maternal cells.

The trophoblast cells have low levels of expression of MHC class I antigens (HLA-A and HLA-B) and class II molecules are absent (Weetman, 2010) so they are not recognized by cytotoxic T lymphocytes. Non-trophoblastic placental cells, such as macrophages and stromal cells, do express fetal HLA antigens but are separated from the maternal cells by the HLA-negative trophoblastic barrier. Placental macrophages seem to have diminished ability to present antigens. Effectively, the trophoblastic tissue is presented to the mother's immune system as antigenically neutral. However, the expression of non-classical HLA-G antigen on the trophoblast cells protects the tissue from cytotoxic T lymphocyte activity and inhibits NK cells which recognize and lyze cells that are deficient in class I HLA expression. In addition, the trophoblast cells may actively contribute to maternal tolerance by secreting soluble factors which modulate the maternal immune response (Zenclussen et al., 2007).

The mother's immune response

The mother is tolerant to fetal antigens but it is not a single mechanism as suggested by Medawar but many local and systemic changes that cause tolerance. Different mechanisms operate at different stages of the pregnancy to mediate tolerance; some of the mechanisms operate locally at the placenta to prevent the fetal antigens being recognized and other mechanisms act on T cells to suppress fetal rejection. The mother does respond immunologically to fetal antigens on the trophoblast or on the fetal haemopoietic and stem cells that enter the maternal circulation. The placenta seems to be a site of active antigen-specific tolerance. Both lymphocytes and antibodies that recognize fetal antigens are present in maternal blood in pregnancy. In fact, an immune reaction by the mother to the paternal histocompatibility antigen seems to be essential for a successful outcome of pregnancy. During pregnancy, maternal T-cells become transiently and reversibly tolerant to paternal alloantigens both systemically and at the uteroplacental surface (Weetman, 2010). The maternal recognition of fetal antigens stimulates the generation of blocking antibodies (Johnson and Christmas, 1996). The blocking antibodies are asymmetrical so they mask the antigenic sites preventing maternal cells from binding to the antigens (Gutierrez et al., 2005). They bind fetal cells in the maternal circulation so they do not interact with maternal lymphocytes or cross the placenta to bind to antigenic sites. Progesterone, augmented by oestrogen and placental growth hormone, is important in both inducing the factor that pushes the helper T cells towards producing Th2 cytokines and up-regulating a number of other immunologically active molecules.

It is suggested that a lack of maternal immune response to the fetus could be harmful. The success of fertility and pregnancy is enhanced when the parents are genetically dissimilar (a concept described as 'hybrid vigour'). The incidence of pregnancy where the parents are closely related (consanguineous), as in incest, is far less frequent; thus, heterozygosity is promoted within the population. A close relationship between the parents means that the fetal antigens will be more similar to the maternal antigens so the maternal immunological response will be less.

Conversely, embryo implantation into a surrogate mother, where the embryo is less related to the mother than in a normal implantation, has a higher success rate. It has been suggested that some of the cases of unexplained recurrent pregnancy loss (RPL, also known as recurrent spontaneous abortion (RSA); more than three consecutive early pregnancy miscarriages) may be due to a failure of maternal cell immune responses and immunological adaptation (Kwak-Kim et al., 2009). Other known causes of RPL include chromosome and endocrine abnormalities, anatomical and haematological problems, and infections of the mother's reproductive system. It was controversially hypothesized that increased similarities of antigens between parents (described as HLA parental sharing) would result in the fetus having a high degree of antigen similarities with its mother. The mother would then not produce such a strong immune response to fetal cells, with perhaps fewer blocking antibodies, which would prejudice the outcome of the pregnancy. However, immunotherapy treatment for RPL where women are immunized with paternal leukocyte cells or antibodies has not been successful (Porter et al., 2006).

Fetal lymphocytes inhibit replication of stimulated lymphocytes in both the mother and unrelated individuals. This may account for the increased number and increased severity of maternal viral infections, especially in the later part of gestation. Trophoblastic cells express high levels of three membrane-bound complement-regulatory proteins that thwart potential complement-mediated damage to the trophoblast by either the classic or alternative pathways (Rooney et al., 1993).

The placenta is in contact with fluids containing high concentrations of progesterone, corticosteroids and hCG, which may act as local immunosuppressants and inhibit the effectiveness of immune cells. The uterine endometrium has extensive numbers of white blood cells, constituting up to a third of endometrial cells (Luppi, 2003). From early pregnancy, numbers and activity of monocytes and granulocytes progressively increase. The macrophages are highly activated and secrete substantial amounts of interleukin and IgE, which may play a vital role in immunosuppression and rapid non-specific anti-inflammatory activity. T lymphocytes are present but B lymphocytes are uncommon. Cytotoxic activity and interferon production by circulating or peripheral NK cells decreases; it seems that these cells migrate to the uterine tissue where they become known as uterine NK cells or uterine large granular leukocytes (uNK or uLGL or CD56+ cells). There seems to be two distinct populations of uNK cells, those associated with the endometrium and the more active uNK cells which are associated with the decidua underlying placental development. The uNK cells seem to be hormonally regulated as they occur in decidualized tissue in extrauterine ectopic pregnancies, and their association with the uterine tissue actually occurs before implantation during the secretory phase of the menstrual cycle (Manaster and Mandelboim, 2010). uNK have low cytolytic activity and are probably not involved in removal of damaged embryonic cells or regulation of trophoblastic invasion. However, they do produce cytokines, which are important in immunosuppression and growth regulation. The uNK cells may also be important in the protection against viral pathogens (Le Bouteiller and Piccinni, 2008). When uNK cells migrate to the endometrium, they proliferate and cluster around the spiral arteries where they are involved with both trophoblastic invasion and the first wave of remodelling of the uterine spiral arteries into the low-resistance vessels supplying the placenta (see Chapter 8). Progesterone stimulates the uNK cells to produce progesterone-induced blocking factor (PIBF) which is important in immunomodulation as it alters the profile of cytokine secretion by activated lymphocytes and keeps NK-cell activity low. IgA, secreted from the cells lining the uterine tubes, may also be important in protecting the uterine environment. It is suggested that a pregnancy-specific adjuvant, signal P, produced by the placenta, has opposing effects, activating components of the maternal innate immune system and suppressing the adaptive responses (Sacks et al., 1999). Signal P may also be responsible for the remission of autoimmune disease, such as rheumatoid arthritis and multiple sclerosis, in pregnancy. However, suppression of T-cell activity increases susceptibility to viral infections and to specific intracellular pathogens such as Listeria.

In summary, human pregnancy is a unique immunological situation. It takes place in the specialized environment of the uterus protected by the decidua. The immunological challenge intensifies very gradually and is moderated by hormones and cellular signals from maternal and fetoplacental sources which, together with fetal cells and DNA, can access the maternal compartment. The fetus avoids rejection because the trophoblast has limited expression of MHC class I or II molecules and the maternal adaptive immune responses are altered. So, the maternal immune system responds to the fetus which actively tolerizes the maternal immune response.

EFFECTS OF PREGNANCY ON THE IMMUNE SYSTEM

The maternal immune response is affected by pregnancy. Many of the cells of the immune system are affected by the hormonal changes. For example, macrophages and

T lymphocytes have oestrogen receptors. In pregnancy, the number of white blood cells, particularly neutrophils, increases and the cells respond more readily to challenges. hCG stimulates neutrophil production and response (Luppi, 2003). The high levels of oestrogen and progesterone decrease the number of helper T cells and increase the number of Treg cells. Yeast infections increase in pregnancy, possibly because of the effect of oestrogen on the flora of the reproductive tract. Women have a much higher incidence than men of autoimmune diseases, most frequently in child-bearing years. It is notable, however, that women who are not pregnant or who have never been pregnant still have a higher incidence of autoimmune diseases (due to the loss of self-tolerance—see above) than men. The exposure to female sex steroids is thought to drive this increased susceptibility (Hewagama and Richardson, 2009) so women experience a higher Th1-mediated response pattern. However, an alternative explanation is that the second X chromosome may create this genetic predisposition to autoimmune diseases.

Local concentrations of corticosteroids around the fetus and placenta suppress phagocytic activity, especially in response to Gram-negative bacteria. This means that pregnant women have a decreased ability to respond to Gram-negative infections of the reproductive tract such as gonorrhoea and Chlamydia (Hosenfeld et al., 2009) and *Escherichia coli*. Components of the complement cascade increase from the end of the first trimester so chemotaxis and opsonization are enhanced. Changes like this, which do not occur at the beginning of pregnancy, may be delayed to protect the fetus during implantation.

It has been suggested that the maternal immune response is important at all stages of pregnancy and may sense the reproductive fitness and compatibility of the male partner and the developmental competence of the conceptus to ensure biological benefits for the woman and her offspring (Robertson, 2010). This 'immune-mediated quality control' hypothesis proposes that the immune system expedites pregnancy loss if the pregnancy is not in the best interest of the female, for instance, because the conceptus is not developing appropriately or when external conditions do not favour the risk of investing maternal resources into pregnancy. The corollary is that pregnancy loss may not be pathological but may be a normal and beneficial part of optimal and healthy reproductive function.

NK cells and cytokines

Progesterone receptors on NK cells are upregulated as part of the immune responses to pregnancy. NK-cell activity around the uterus is suppressed by local increased concentrations of prostaglandin E_2 and other cellular signals (Dunn et al., 2003). This suppression of NK cells may be important in preventing rejection of the fetus. However, maternal resistance to intracellular pathogens such as

Toxoplasma and Listeria may also be reduced (Wegmann et al., 1993). The relative proportions of cytokines change in pregnancy. The association between chorioamnionitis and premature rupture of membranes may be related to cytokine-mediated stimulation of proteolytic enzyme released from neutrophils.

Theoretically, the fetus could be perceived by the maternal immune system as a tumour. The conceptus may secrete cytokines, which affect tissues locally, promoting trophoblast growth and fetal survival (Wegmann et al., 1993). Concentrations of cytokines that attack tumours, such as TNF, and stimulate NK-cell activity, such as IL-2, are suppressed. Local secretion of such cytokines may be important in protecting the fetus without compromising maternal immune function.

Toll-like receptors

TLRs are expressed by immune cells at the maternal–fetal interface and also in the non-immune cells of the trophoblast and decidua. Their expression in the human placenta is not constant and varies in a temporal and spatial manner (Koga and Mor, 2010). The expression of the TLRs increases throughout gestation, suggesting that the placenta in early pregnancy is less responsive to microbial challenges. It is suggested that pregnancy has three distinct immunological phases characterized by different immune responses and cytokine profiles (Mor and Cardenas, 2010). The first phase of implantation and placentation is an inflammatory phase (mediated by a Th1-dominant response) to ensure repair of the uterine endometrium and removal of cellular debris after the embryo breaks through and invades the maternal tissue. At this stage of pregnancy, the placental site has been likened to an 'open wound', with the cellular responses affecting the mother's well-being. The second phase is the period of rapid fetal development and growth and is an anti-inflammatory state (mediated by a Th2-dominant response) when the mother feels well. Then, the third phase is another inflammatory (Th1-dominant) state leading to uterine contraction, expulsion of the fetus and delivery or rejection of the placenta.

The other notable aspect is the relative lack of TLRs on the syncytial tissue compared to the villous cytotrophoblast and extravillous trophoblast, which suggests that the placental tissue only responds to bacterial and viral products that penetrate the outer layer of the placenta. It is suggested that the differential expression of TLRs is regulated by changing levels of sex steroids and that TLRs may be involved in tissue remodelling of the endometrium and preparation for implantation (Koga and Mor, 2010). Clinical observations and studies on animal models have demonstrated that TLRs are involved in a variety of pregnancy disorders, including spontaneous abortion, pre-eclampsia and premature labour. Activation of TLRs can inhibit trophoblastic migration which might be linked to the incomplete remodelling of the spiral arteries by trophoblastic cells in preeclampsia. TLRs are also important in identifying and responding to pathogens in amniotic fluid (Koga and Mor, 2010).

Antibodies and B lymphocytes

The levels of most antibodies do not change during pregnancy. However, IgG concentrations may fall. This fall may be due to haemodilution, increased loss in urine or placental transfer of IgG in the third trimester and it can increase the risk of streptococcal infection. Fetal secretion of cytokines may suppress cell-mediated immunity and enhance humoral responsiveness (Wegmann et al., 1993). SLE, an autoimmune condition causing tissue damage in the joints and kidneys, has an increased 'flare-up' frequency in pregnancy, which may be related to enhanced activity of B lymphocytes. This enhanced responsiveness by B lymphocytes may compensate for decreased T lymphocyte activity. B lymphocytes may also produce blocking antibodies which protect the fetus from attack by maternal T lymphocytes.

T lymphocytes

T lymphocytes are involved in graft rejection and could therefore pose a serious threat to the fetus. However, T-cell function is suppressed in pregnancy, especially in the first trimester (Koga and Mor, 2010). Circulating numbers of T lymphocytes are lower and they have decreased ability to proliferate, to produce IL-2 and to kill foreign cells. Ratios of helper and Treg cells change and the Th1/Th2 balance is shifted in favour of Th2, generating non-inflammatory responses, mediated by interleukins such as IL-4 and IL-10, which are compatible with trophoblast growth, survival of the fetus, fetal and infant growth and maintenance of pregnancy. IL-10 inhibits the activity of Th1 cells (Thaxton and Sharma, 2010). A Th1 reaction in the placenta generates inflammatory responses and is correlated with miscarriage; the cytokines secreted from Th1 cells are harmful in pregnancy as they inhibit embryonic and fetal development (Wegmann et al., 1993). A Th1 dominant pattern (upregulation of IL-2, IL-6, INF-γ and TNF-α) occurs in miscarriage; the inflammatory responses seem to mediate fetal rejection. An imbalance in the Th1/Th2 shift is also associated with preeclampsia and an inflammatory host response mediated by Th1 cytokines (Zenclussen et al., 2007). Trophoblastic production of cytokines promotes the change in Th1/Th2 balance as does progesterone and the decidual production of leukaemia inhibitory factor. Although the shift in the Th1/Th2 balance explains some of the changes in the immune system during pregnancy, the observations that Th2 knockout mice had normal pregnancies (Svensson et al., 2001) led to further scrutiny of the

hypothesis. Furthermore, uNK cells were shown to be necessary for successful pregnancy and INF-γ was shown to be critical in remodelling of the spiral arteries (Chaouat, 2007). So, the new model includes a new lineage of T cells, Th17 cells, which produce IL-17, a pro-inflammatory cytokine which induces inflammation and acknowledges the role of Treg cells in inhibiting proliferation and cytokine production from Th1, Th2 and Th17 cells (Saito et al., 2008). The number of Treg cells in the circulation and in the decidual tissue and the lymph nodes draining the uterus expand markedly in pregnancy (Leber et al., 2010). Initial expansion of the Treg cell population begins before pregnancy is established, probably in response to the presence of paternal allergens from sperm and seminal fluid in the female reproductive tract, although hormonal changes in the menstrual cycle may also play a role.

Rheumatoid arthritis, a cell-mediated autoimmune disease, frequently goes into remission during pregnancy, because of the suppression of T lymphocytes. The amelioration of symptoms in pregnancy led to the identification of glucocorticoids as anti-inflammatory agents (Hench, 1952). Hormonal changes in pregnancy may augment the suppression of T lymphocytes. As T lymphocytes are involved in the responses to viral infection, pregnant women are at increased risk of viral infections and may experience more severe viraemia.

The Treg cells are also involved in acceptance of paternal antigens expressed by the semi-allogenic fetus. The Treg population of cells are activated in very early pregnancy by paternal antigens, possibly when paternal antigens are present in the vagina even before fertilization (Zenclussen et al., 2007). The Treg cells undergo expansion and migrate to the lymph nodes and then to fetal–maternal interface after implantation. This Treg cell population which are specific for paternal antigens generates a tolerant microenvironment at the maternal–fetal interface throughout the pregnancy. Maternal and fetal cells are reciprocally recognized by each other's immune systems, which means that the mother can tolerate the fetal allograft and the fetus acquires a tolerogenic environment that helps to protect it against autoimmune diseases.

A number of the immune cells utilize and metabolize the essential amino acid, tryptophan. In response to inflammatory stimuli, the syncytiotrophoblast expresses and secretes indoleamine 2,3-dioxygenase (IDO), an enzyme which metabolizes tryptophan. As tryptophan is depleted, the T cells are starved, which promotes their differentiation into Treg cells (Mellor and Munn, 2008). So, IDO acts as a switch to promote the number of Treg cells; in the absence of IDO, Treg cells are reprogrammed to become pro-inflammatory Th17 cells. The products of tryptophan metabolism prevent T-cell and B-cell activation and proliferation. IDO also suppresses complement-mediated damage.

Susceptibility to infection

It has been suggested that as maternal immune responses are suppressed in pregnancy and the Th1/Th2 balance altered to favour acceptance of the fetus, pregnant women would have increased susceptibility to infection. Historically, pregnant women were observed to contract smallpox and poliomyelitis more readily. Today, viral hepatitis infections, particularly in developing countries, pose a major threat to pregnant women, who have 10 times the infection rate of non-pregnant women and experience higher morbidity and mortality rates. The prevention of vertical transmission

Box 10.2 Seasonal influenza

The immune changes in pregnancy mean that pregnant women who contract seasonal influenza (flu) are at increased risk of developing severe complications that can cause morbidity and mortality, especially during the third trimester. Physiological changes in the respiratory system probably contribute to the increased severity of respiratory complications. Flu viruses are classified as A, B or C types; types A and B are the main causes of mortality and type A is associated with pandemics (Toal et al., 2010). The surface antigens of flu viruses demonstrate 'antigenic drift' and change subtly so at-risk groups require annual vaccination. In the 1918 flu pandemic, one study of pregnancy showed that approximately half the women infected with influenza developed pneumonia and about half of these women with pneumonia died—a death rate of 27%. Surveillance of the swine flu pandemic in 2009/2010 showed that, like previous flu pandemics, pregnant women were at significant risk from the H1N1 virus (swine flu). Pregnant women who are colonized by bacteria such as methicillin-resistant *Staphylococcus aureus* (MRSA) and *Streptococcus pneumoniae* are at a higher risk of developing pneumonia if they are infected with the H1N1 influenza virus (Cheng et al., 2009). There is a higher rate of fetal abnormalities, premature delivery and stillbirths in pregnant women who contract influenza in early pregnancy which is probably caused by high fever; however, vertical transmission of flu virus has not been demonstrated. The presenting signs of seasonal flu are usually fever, cough, vomiting, breathlessness, myalgia, sore throats and chills. The World Health Organization advises pregnant women to have seasonal flu vaccines because of the high risks associated with pregnancy. Flu vaccines are fragmented, meaning that they contain parts of the virus and are not whole or attenuated (mild form of virus). The use of antiviral drugs such as neuraminidase inhibitors (oseltamivir and zanamivir) is also advocated in pregnancy because the risks associated with their use are outweighed by the risk of flu infection in pregnancy (Tanaka et al., 2009). Public health measures for containing infection include hand and domestic hygiene, cough etiquette and avoiding unnecessary travel and crowds if possible.

to the fetus or neonate is also an important consideration. Women who lack immunity and are exposed to primary cytomegalovirus have an increased susceptibility to infection in pregnancy, which is associated with fetal congenital abnormalities and is one of the most prevalent causes of mental retardation. Pregnant women have an increased susceptibility to listeriosis, influenza (Box 10.2), varicella (chickenpox), herpes, rubella (German measles), hepatitis and human papillomavirus. In addition, a number of latent viral diseases and other infections may be of greater severity. These include malaria, tuberculosis (TB), Epstein–Barr virus and HIV-associated infections (Wegmann et al., 1993), which can be reactivated in pregnancy. Pregnancy-induced suppression of helper T-cell numbers may be permanent so pregnancy can cause a progression of HIV-related disease. Pregnant women appear to have increased immunological responses to bacterial infection. However, increased incidences of urinary tract infections are probably related to anatomical changes rather than to altered immunological responses. Likewise, the increased severity of respiratory infections is usually associated with changes in diaphragm position which reduces secretion clearance and functional residual capacity. The immune changes in pregnancy may be responsible for the increased risk of breast cancer in the years immediately following pregnancy, particularly in women who are older at their first full-term pregnancy (Shakhar et al., 2007); however, a first full-term pregnancy at a younger age exerts a protective effect on lifetime risk of breast cancer. Some conditions, such as multiple sclerosis, improve in pregnancy because of the expansion of the Treg cell population. The postpartum period can also be an immunologically sensitive time, as the rapid reversal of the changes that occurred in pregnancy and a rebound of inflammatory responses can cause latent or quiescent infections to become full symptomatic diseases (Singh and Perfect, 2007). Thyroid autoantibody levels fall in pregnancy so conditions such as Graves disease are ameliorated, but the antibodies then peak in the postpartum period (Weetman, 2010) so postpartum thyroiditis and mild autoimmune hypothyroidism are relatively common in the first 6 months following delivery (see Chapter 12).

Microchimerism

For decades it has been assumed that maternal and fetal blood never mixes, but transplacental passage of a few cells appears to be normal. Microchimerism is the presence of a tiny number of cells or DNA within an individual, both in the circulation and in other tissues, that have come from another individual. The most common cause of microchimerism is fetal microchimerism, the trafficking of fetal cells in pregnancy; the cells could be blood cells or trophoblast cells which are continually shed during pregnancy (see Chapter 8). Fetal cells have been demonstrated to multiply and then persist in their mother's blood for decades after delivery (Sarkar and Miller, 2004) and, in some cases, a maternal cellular immune response against the fetal antigens is mounted. It has been suggested that fetal microchimerism might be associated with an increased risk of miscarriage (Lissauer et al., 2009) and that the higher incidence of autoimmune diseases in women is related to microchimerism, inducing a graft-versus-host disease. The transfer of cells is bidirectional and maternal cells are also transferred from the mother to the fetus, maternal microchimerism (Lissauer et al., 2009). Diseases thought to be associated with microchimerism include scleroderma, Sjögrens syndrome, Graves' disease and SLE. This hypothesis is applicable to men, children and women who have never been pregnant, because microchimerism can result from other sources such as transplantation and blood transfusion, and cells from a twin. Fetal microchimerism may have a protective function playing a role in tissue repair; in addition, studies have also implicated both an increased and a reduced risk of cancer associated with microchimerism (Lissauer, 2009). A recent and controversial hypothesis suggests that microchimerism offers evolutionary benefits (Apari and Rozsa, 2009); the mother benefits from receiving fetal cells, as their immune system will benefit from receiving paternal resistance alleles via the fetus and the fetus will benefit because the maternal immune system is thus strengthened.

FETAL AND NEONATAL PASSIVE IMMUNITY

The neonate's immune system is augmented by maternal transfer of immunoglobulins across the placenta to the fetus and in breast milk. The profile of immunoglobulins transported across the placenta and secreted into breast milk depends on specific transport mechanisms for the different classes of immunoglobulin (see Table 10.3). Maternal IgG crosses the placenta into the fetal circulation via a specific active transport mechanism, which is effective from around 20 weeks' gestation but markedly increases in activity from 34 weeks. The mother will produce an immune response to antigens she encounters by producing IgG, which can cross the placenta. Even if maternal levels of IgG are low, they will be transported across the placenta. This means that the fetus will receive passive immunization against prevalent pathogens likely to be in the environment from birth. This passive immunity provides essential temporary protection postnatally until the neonate's own immune system matures and produces its own antibodies. Preterm babies are at risk of transient hypoglobulinaemia because they receive less IgG and they are born with immune systems that are less mature than a term infant's. Placental dysfunction limits the transfer of IgG; therefore, SGA (small for gestational age) babies have lower levels of IgG. IgA, IgM and IgD do not cross the placenta but are supplied in high concentrations in the colostrum.

As well as beneficial IgG, potentially harmful IgG can cross the placenta. Maternal antibodies to fetal HLA will be generated as the maternal immune system encounters a few fetal cells. The maternal anti-fetal HLA antibodies will cross the placenta but do not cause any damage as they bind to non-trophoblastic cells in the placenta, which bear fetal HLA and can sequester maternal IgG (Johnson and Christmas, 1996). In autoimmune diseases, however, pathogenic maternal antibodies can be transferred across the placenta. For instance, antiplatelet antibodies can cross the placenta into the fetus of a mother with autoimmune thrombocytopenic purpura (Johnson and Christmas, 1996). The passive transfer of autoimmune antibodies may affect fetal growth and development and can potentially cause at least transient symptoms of the disease in the neonate. The resulting increased risk of haemorrhage in babies born to mothers with thrombocytopenia means that traumatic procedures, such as fetal blood sampling and instrumental delivery, are avoided. Some autoimmune conditions such as congenital heart block associated with SLE can cause irreversible damage to the neonate (Buyon et al., 2009).

Preterm babies are at a higher risk of vertical infection of group B streptococci if their mothers are group B streptococcus-positive, because they do not gain passive immunity from the placental transfer of immunoglobulins until after 34 weeks' gestation. Term babies do have some degree of protection from group B streptococci and this can be extended if the infant is breastfed. The use of antibiotics in the intrapartum period does reduce the number of group B streptococcal infections in the neonate, and so any mother who is found to be group B streptococci-positive at any time, not just during the pregnancy, may be offered antibiotic therapy in labour (RCOG, 2006). The antibiotics reduce the bacterial load and so the risk of infection is less, although a small number of neonatal infections may still occur (Royal College of Obstetricians and Gynaecologists, 2003).

The Rhesus factor and Rhesus incompatibility

In the last trimester, the placental transfer of maternal IgG will include IgG antibodies directed against the fetus's own antigens. Most of these are thought to bind to non-trophoblastic cells bearing fetal antigens within the placental villous tissue so they do not reach the fetal circulation. However, antibodies to the Rhesus antigen can cause severe complications. People who express the Rhesus antigen on their own red blood cell surface do not make antibodies against the Rhesus antigen. These people are described as Rhesus positive (Fig. 10.8). A mother who is Rhesus-negative does not have the Rhesus antigen

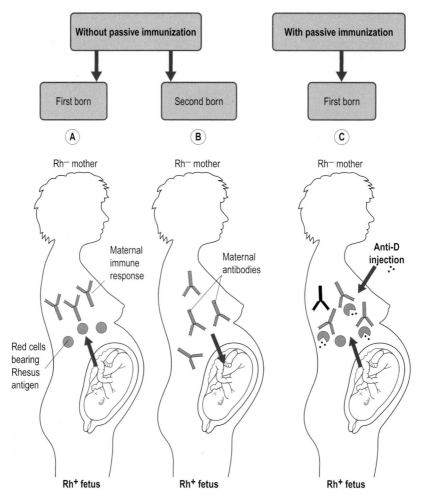

Fig. 10.8 (A) Rhesus-negative women can be sensitized when red cells from a Rhesus-positive fetus cross the placenta into her circulation. (B) Response comes after delivery of the first fetus, but in subsequent pregnancies, maternal antibodies can cross the placenta and damage the fetus. (C) Anti-D gamma globulin given to mothers immediately at delivery results in fetal Rhesus-positive cells not being recognized by maternal immune systems, so antibodies are not produced to endanger subsequent pregnancy.

on her own red blood cell surface, and her immune system has the capability of making Rhesus antibodies. About 10% of pregnancies in Caucasian populations are Rhesus-negative women with a Rhesus-positive fetus; in other ethnicities, there is a lower incidence of Rhesus-negative individuals.

The Rhesus antibody is not preformed (existing from birth) like the antibodies of the ABO blood grouping system. Rhesus antibodies are produced if the immune system is given the opportunity to recognize the Rhesus antigen as a foreign protein. In practice, this means that a Rhesus-negative mother could produce antibodies to the Rhesus antigen of fetal cells (which would recognize and attack the red blood cells of a Rhesus-positive fetus) if her immune system encountered it. The immune

response can be generated from exposure to red blood cells bearing the Rhesus antigen, for instance, from transplacental leakage of Rhesus-positive fetal cells or in rare instances from a Rhesus-positive blood transfusion (see Box 10.3 for conditions requiring anti-D administration).

The occasion when Rhesus isoimmunization is most likely to occur is at the time of the third stage of labour. During placental separation, there is the potential for a small amount of fetal blood (perhaps half a millilitre) to cross into the maternal circulation. Fetal blood can also enter the maternal circulation earlier in pregnancy, during therapeutic or spontaneous abortion, amniocentesis, abdominal trauma and in an ectopic pregnancy. If the fetal blood entering the maternal circulation is Rhesus-positive, it could stimulate the maternal immune cells to respond by clonal expansion, developing the capacity to produce large quantities of IgG. Once a woman makes antibodies to Rhesus antigens, she is isoimmunized for life. These IgG antibodies can then be transported across the placenta to the fetal circulation late in gestation of a subsequent pregnancy. The binding of maternal Rhesus antibodies to the Rhesus antigen on the surface of the fetal blood cells stimulates lysis of the red blood cells. Mild Rhesus incompatibility can cause mild anaemia and reticulocytosis (new immature red blood cells in the circulation). Severe Rhesus incompatibility is a cause of miscarriage, intrauterine death or hydrops fetalis (abdominal ascites, generalized oedema, polyhydramnios and enlarged placenta). In the neonate, Rhesus incompatibility can result in haemolytic disease of the newborn, where profound haemolysis causes anaemia, increasing the risks of heart failure, hyperbilirubinaemia (jaundice) and kernicterus (see Chapter 15).

Treatment

Prophylactic treatment has been practised since 1967 (Box 10.3) and severe Rhesus D alloimmunization is now rarely seen. Giving passive immunization prevents primary sensitization of the mother and the formation of cells that can produce IgG anti-Rhesus antibody. Although there is actually a complex system of Rhesus antigens, controlled by three pairs of genes (Cc, Dd and Ee), the Rhesus D antigen predominates in incompatibility between the mother and the fetus.

In accordance with national guidelines (see Annotated Further Reading), the majority of Rhesus-negative women are offered routine anti-D administration at either as two smaller doses at 28 and 34 weeks' gestation or one larger dose at around 28–30 weeks gestation. Following delivery of the baby to a Rhesus-negative woman, the Rhesus status of the infant has to be determined. If this proves to be Rhesus-positive, then a second test is performed to

estimate the amount of fetal blood in the maternal system (Box 10.4), as amounts greater than 4 mL may require more than the standard anti-D dose of 500 international units (i.u.). Although if both parents were Rhesus-negative, anti-D would not be required; the guidelines do not recommend testing of the father to identify his Rhesus status, because it is recognized that the apparent father might not be the biological father, which may create a difficult situation to manage. It is difficult to justify routine anti-D administration if the father is certain that he is Rhesus-negative; however, it is prudent to observe the infant for signs of early and excessive jaundice in case the conception occurred outside of the pair bond.

If a small volume (less than 4 mL) of fetal blood has entered the maternal circulation at delivery, the exogenous antibodies ('anti-D') will bind to the fetal Rhesus D antigen and cause cell lysis before the maternal lymphocytes have the opportunity to recognize the antigen and undergo subsequent clonal expansion. ABO compatibility exacerbates Rhesus isoimmunization so ABO incompatibility offers a degree of protection against Rhesus sensitization. If the fetal blood transfused is of a different ABO grouping, the existing natural maternal IgM anti-A or anti-B antigens will rapidly eliminate the fetal blood cells before an immune response can be mounted against the Rhesus D antigen.

Unnecessary administration of anti-D may be prevented by identifying the Rhesus state of the fetus early in pregnancy by isolating fetal DNA markers from maternal blood (Kolialexi et al., 2010). This will further minimize the risk of exposure to blood products by limiting administration to cases where it is required (and also better utilize the donor-dependent stock of anti-D).

Other antibodies

Most antibodies in the ABO system are IgM type so they do not cross the placenta. However, in successive ABO-incompatible pregnancies in group O mothers, a degree of neonatal haemolysis, causing mild neonatal jaundice, may occur. Haemolytic disease can potentially occur with other blood group incompatibilities such as the Kell and Duffy antigen systems. However, the density of these minor antigens on fetal red blood cells is so low that maternal IgG antibodies usually do not elicit a cytolytic effect. Women who require or have had multiple or large blood transfusions, for example, following postpartum haemorrhage, are at risk of developing antibodies to surface antigens which could potentially put their unborn babies at risk.

VULNERABILITY OF THE NEONATE

Neonates are born immunocompromised and are susceptible to infection. An intriguing idea is that the immaturity of the fetal immune system is an adaptive response which helps to protect it from premature rejection by its mother (Clapp, 2006), but the cost of this is the increased risk of infections of the newborn, particularly if born prematurely. The natural flora colonizes and protects the

external surfaces of the body, and those membranes that appear internal but come into contact with external pathogens, such as the upper respiratory tract, gut and urinary system. The natural flora may protect by competing with pathogenic microorganisms for resources or by altering the local environment, making it less hospitable to pathogens. The acid mantle of the skin promotes colonization of commensal microbes and restricts growth of pathogens (Behne, 2009). The neonatal skin is particularly vulnerable to change in pH through the use of detergents, resulting in atopic dermatitis raising the risk of skin infections in the neonate (Cork et al., 2009; see Chapter 15).

The fetus in the uterus is sterile because there is no route for colonization. Colonization takes about 6–8 weeks, which is similar to the time it takes for the resident flora of non-pathogenic bacteria to repopulate in NASA astronauts, who are made bacteriologically sterile before a space flight. As the bowel flora produces much of the body's vitamin K requirements, neonates have an increased risk of vitamin K deficiency until the resident flora is established. Colonization processes can be disrupted, for instance, by use of detergents, disinfectant swabs or antibiotic use. Colonization of the neonate begins at birth, with transfer of organisms from the mother's vagina, skin of her hands and breasts and the respiratory tracts of the baby's carers.

Neonatal skin is delicate and easily damaged, thus it can offer a route for opportunistic infection. The umbilical cord, which becomes necrotic, presents a locus for possible infection and offers a potential pathway to the liver. The neonatal defence mechanisms are further compromised by invasive procedures such as blood sampling or insertion of endotracheal or nasogastric tube or intravenous cannulae.

Infants have less efficient immune systems, especially if they are born prematurely or are small at birth. The cells of the immune system are immature and do not function as efficiently in early life; for instance, T lymphocytes have decreased responses and cytolytic function. The phagocytes exhibit decreased phagocytosis and bactericidal activity. Their function in severe illness, such as respiratory distress syndrome or meconium-aspiration pneumonia, is further limited. The complement cascade components at birth are 50–80% of the adult levels. Maternal mood in pregnancy may affect the development and functioning of the neonatal immune system following birth (Mattes, 2009).

Active immunization

The immature immune system of the neonate is supported by natural passive immunization from placental transfer of IgG and breast milk provision of IgA. It is also supported by programmes of deliberate immunization. Active immunization requires administration of an

Adjuvants

For example, aluminium hydroxide or phosphate: Increases antigenic properties of a vaccine that would otherwise produce only a weak immune response, for example, triple vaccine of diphtheria, tetanus and pertussis toxins.

Toxoid

Bacterial exotoxin treated so it does not cause a disease but still stimulates the immune cells. Examples include treatment of diphtheria and tetanus toxin with formalin.

Killed vaccine

Dead organisms such as pertussis, typhoid and paratyphoid: As with toxoid preparations, two or three doses and booster doses are required, as only a small number of antigens are introduced each time.

Attenuated vaccines

Live organisms that have been cultured to produce non-pathogenic strains: Very effective as organisms multiply within body mimicking a natural infection. Therefore, only one dose is required for full immune response (lifetime immunity), for example, smallpox, poliomyelitis, measles, rubella, TB.

antigen in a form that is inactivated and does not produce a disease (Box 10.5). IgG levels start to increase by 3 months so immunization is delayed after birth. However, some protection is required before the immune system is mature. Therefore, immunization programmes are often started when the baby is 3 months old. At about this age, many babies receive the 'triple' vaccine of pertussis (whooping cough), diphtheria and tetanus antigens presented appropriately. Diphtheria and tetanus elicit strong antigenic responses despite the infant's immature immune system, whereas children are given further doses of pertussis vaccine. Live polio vaccine is given orally at the same time as the 'triple' vaccine. Although theoretically, only one dose is required, there are at least three strains and the immune response may not be produced the first time. Measles vaccine is usually delayed until the infant is about 1 year old, as maternal IgG, which is present for the first 6–9 months of life, tends to destroy the attenuated organisms of the vaccine before the infant's immune system has time to recognize and respond to them.

Immunization using viral vaccines may be ineffective if the individual has had a recent viral infection, such as a cold. Levels of interferon persist after a viral infection so the virus in the vaccine preparation may not be able to reach concentrations adequate to stimulate the immune system. Therefore, immunization may not be effective until 2–3 weeks after a viral infection. Oral doses of vaccines may be ineffective if their absorption is compromised, for instance, with diarrhoea or vomiting. High levels of steroids suppress the immune response, so steroid therapy or overactive adrenal glands can limit the effectiveness of a live vaccine and compromise the immune response. Maternal antibodies in the neonate, for instance, from placental transfer of IgG, can abrogate the young infant's immune response to vaccination but subsequent booster vaccination usually surmounts this. Infants who are themselves HIV-negative but born to HIV-positive mothers may not respond efficiently to vaccines (Miles et al., 2010). Allergic reactions to vaccines can occur, especially to vaccines prepared in tissue culture or containing whole cells. Problems with allergic reactions are often associated with vaccines grown in egg-based tissue culture preparations or to which antibiotics have been added. Obviously, a severe reaction to a vaccine precludes its further use. Administration of live vaccines is not recommended in pregnancy. Immunization programmes benefit the health of the population unfortunately at the expense of the few individuals who may have an extreme reaction to a vaccine with irreversible effects.

OTHER IMMUNOLOGICAL ASPECTS OF PREGNANCY

Antisperm antibodies can be present in both men and women. In seminal fluid, they can cause immune infertility by inhibiting spermatogenesis or fertilization (Chiu and Chamley, 2003). However, the Sertoli cell protects the developing sperm and seminiferous tubules from antibodies and Treg cells secrete immunosuppressive cytokines in the epididymis. Some are coated with glycoproteins and lactoferrin, which may be why some antigen sites are evident only after sperm capacitation. Seminal fluid has potent immunosuppressive and signalling properties and can inhibit a range of immune responses (Robertson, 2005). The presence of antisperm antibodies in the secretions from the genital tracts, rather than in the blood, seems important particularly in male infertility. The risk of developing antisperm antibodies is increased with exposure to sperm that is excessive, as in prostitutes, or in an inappropriate site, as in homosexual men (Johnson and Christmas, 1996). A significant proportion of men have been shown to have antisperm antibodies associated with retention of sperm due to obstruction of the vas deferens or epididymis and so have retention of sperm, so the presence of antisperm antibodies is a useful predictor that obstruction is the primary cause of male infertility (Lee et al., 2009). Generation of antisperm antibodies may reflect a lack of immunosuppressive factors in the seminal fluid. It has also been proposed that exposure to semen can positively affect the maternal immune responses that promote the success of pregnancy (Robertson, 2005). Insemination might present a 'priming' event which induces maternal tolerance to paternal antigens in the semen, many of which will also be expressed by the developing conceptus.

Endometriosis, which is deposition of endometrial tissue at non-uterine sites, can be very painful if the tissue becomes inflamed. Severe endometriosis can cause infertility, but many women have extrauterine endometrial tissue that neither causes pain nor affects fertility. The cause of endometriosis is not known, but an autoimmune aetiology has been proposed (Tomassetti et al., 2006).

Preeclampsia, inadequate placental development following inadequate remodelling of the spiral arteries, is also suggested to have an immune component (see Chapter 8). The incidence of preeclampsia is higher in first pregnancies and in subsequent pregnancies with a new partner, which suggests an immunological mechanism. However, a change of partner is often associated with a longer inter-pregnancy interval which is more strongly correlated with preeclampsia (Redman and Sargent, 2010) as is a short interval between first coitus (exposure to the partner's sperm) and pregnancy. It appears that preconceptual exposure to antigens on sperm or in seminal fluid (or both) tolerizes the mother to the fetopaternal antigens and protects against preeclampsia. Barrier methods of contraception, artificial insemination with donor sperm and ICSI are all associated with increased risk. It is essential that there is maternal immune recognition of the fetopaternal allergens to ensure the success of implantation, placentation and placental growth.

The effects of HIV and AIDS in pregnancy are detailed in Box 10.6 and Case study 10.2.

Case study 10.2

Mary is 16 weeks' pregnant. She has no fixed abode and has not previously been seen by a health professional in relation to her pregnancy. Mary attends the local hospital antenatal clinic in a state of distress. She informs the midwife that she is an intravenous drug abuser and her best friend has just died from an AIDS-related illness.

- How prepared would you be, as the midwife, to counsel and advise Mary?
- What referrals and expert advice would you seek on her behalf?
- What considerations are needed in relation to the unborn child, in relation to both HIV transmission and Mary's general situation?

Box 10.6 **HIV and AIDS in pregnancy**

- HIV (human immunodeficiency virus) causes AIDS (acquired immune deficiency disorder).
- HIV is a retrovirus, which invades cells expressing CD4, including helper T cells, monocytes and neural cells.
- A retrovirus contains a single strand of RNA, which is incorporated into the host cell's DNA by an enzyme called reverse transcriptase.
- When the infected cell is activated, it will produce viral proteins, which can be released and infect other cells.
- HIV infection causes decreased numbers of helper T cells, which affect the organization of all the immune responses so the risk of opportunistic and pathogenic infection increases.
- In Britain, women usually acquire HIV from sexual exposure and intravenous drug use.

The biggest increase in HIV infection is heterosexual transmission in women.

HIV has to evade the mechanical, chemical and biological barriers of the female reproductive tract.

Progesterone-based contraception may accelerate HIV disease progression as progesterone inhibits cytotoxic T cells and NK cells; oestrogen may be protective.

Co-infections in the female reproductive tract which cause micro-ulcerations may increase HIV susceptibility.

Transmission of HIV is more efficient from men to women (compared to women to men) possibly because semen transforms the local environment of the female reproductive tract, for instance, increasing pH and upregulating pro-inflammatory cytokines.

- Pregnancy can mask some of the non-specific symptoms of HIV infection, such as fatigue, anaemia and dyspnoea.
- HIV can remain latent for years (estimated to be an average 11 years) before AIDS becomes evident.
- Progression to symptom development may be accelerated by pregnancy.
- HIV can be transmitted to the baby via the placenta, from exchange of body fluids at birth or from breast milk.
- Mothers with HIV may be advised to breastfeed their babies if the risk of fatal malnutrition is considered to be higher than the risk of HIV infection; lactoferrin is protective.

Key points

- Pregnancy enhances humoral immunity and suppresses cell-mediated immunity so responses to bacterial infection are enhanced, but there may be increased susceptibility to viral infections.
- Histoincompatibility, such as the differences in fetal and maternal antigen expression, would normally lead to tissue rejection.

- The trophoblast cells lack classic HLA antigens, which prevent an anti-fetal response, but express HLA-G, which prevents non-specific cytolysis.
- Fetal cells entering the maternal circulation are important in the generation of blocking antibodies, which block any immune response that does occur.
- Maternal IgG is transferred to the fetus late in gestation, which provides the neonate with passive immunization during the period of immunological immaturity. Harmful antibodies against fetal antigens are sequestered by non-trophoblastic tissue in the placenta.
- The birth of a Rhesus-positive baby to a Rhesus-negative woman can initiate an immune response. Prophylactic administration of anti-Rhesus-D immunoglobulin is therefore given after possible or actual exposure.
- The neonate is immunocompromised at birth. Immunization programmes seek to address this lack of immunity.

Application to practice

Pregnancy results in an alteration of the immune system, so normal non-pregnant white cell counts cannot be applied in pregnancy. An understanding of changes within the immune system will enable the midwife to explain the consequences of such changes to the pregnant women.

An understanding of rhesus incompatibility is necessary as this is a common potential problem.

Conditions that affect the maternal immune systems may complicate pregnancy, affecting not only the mother but also the fetus and the neonate. Such conditions require careful management and treatment to optimize outcomes for both the mother and the baby.

Midwives may be involved in the administration of some vaccines such as rubella and TB so an understanding of the immune system is required. The interaction of the maternal immune system and the baby is an important aspect of lactation and breastfeeding.

ANNOTATED FURTHER READING

Department of Health: *Immunisation against infectious disease—'The Green Book'* London, 2006, DoH, (updated 2010).

This a comprehensive reference guide on all types of vaccination for all healthcare professionals involved in immunization.

Druckmann R, Druckmann MA: Progesterone and the immunology of pregnancy, *J Steroid Biochem Mol Biol* 97:389–396, 2005.

A clear summary of the mechanisms by which the recognition of pregnancy upregulates progesterone receptors and alters cytokine production, thus suppressing the maternal immune responses to the fetus.

Gammill HS, Nelson JL: Naturally acquired microchimerism, *Int J Dev Biol* 54:531–543, 2010.

An in-depth and readable review of microchimerism which includes historical perspectives approaches to detect and confirm microchimerism and the relationship between persistent microchimerism and disease.

Kaushic C, Ferreira VH, Kafka JK, et al: HIV infection in the female genital tract: discrete influence of the local mucosal microenvironment, *Am J Reprod Immunol* 63:566–575, 2010.

A well-written description of the factors which affect HIV susceptibility to infection by heterosexual transmission.

Kitchen G, Horton-Szar D: Crash course: immunology and haematology, London, 2007, Mosby

This book presents the fundamental principles of haematology and immunology in an easy-to-understand format and is a useful introductory text for healthcare professionals.

Liu E, Laurin J: Viral hepatitis, A through E, in pregnancy. In Shetty K, Wu GY, editors: *Chronic viral hepatitis: diagnosis and therapeutics,* Washington, 2009, Humana Press, pp 353–373.

This chapter gives an overview of viral hepatitis infections in pregnancy including screening, treatments and outcomes.

McKibbin S, editor: *HealthScouter child immunization: childhood immunization schedule: parents guide for immunizations and vaccinations for children,* Brooklyn, 2009, Equity Press,

This is a useful guide for parents about the most common problems associated with immunization; includes hundreds of quotes, questions, and answers from patients themselves.

Mecacci F, Pieralli A, Bianchi B, et al: The impact of autoimmune disorders and adverse pregnancy outcome, *Semin Perinatol* 31:223–226, 2007.

A review outlining the issues for pregnant women affected by the more common

autoimmune connective tissue diseases: SLE, rheumatoid arthritis, scleroderma and Sjögrens syndrome.

National Institute for Clinical Excellence: *Routine antenatal anti-D prophylaxis for women who are RhD-negative,* 2008, NICE.

This review forms the basis of the current use of anti-D in the United Kingdom and provides a comprehensive and referenced guide to the use of anti-D.

Playfair JH, Chain BM: *Immunology at a glance,* ed 9, 2009, Wiley-Blackwell.

Covers a wide range of immunological topics using clear, well-labelled diagrams to summarize and simplify the mechanisms of immunological processes together with succinct written explanations on facing pages.

Price LC: Infectious disease in pregnancy, *Obstet Gynaecol Reprod Med* 18:173–179, 2008.

A thorough review of the main infectious diseases that can complicate pregnancies in the developed world and the screening, investigation and management principles.

Redman CW, Sargent IL: Immunology of pre-eclampsia, *Am J Reprod Immunol* 63:534–543, 2010.

A review of the relationship between the immune responses and preeclampsia which describes the early maternal adaptation to paternal/fetal antigens and the later non-specific, systemic inflammatory response which follows placental oxidative stress, thus explaining the first pregnancy preponderance and partner specificity of preeclampsia.

Royal College of Obstetricians and Gynaecologists: *Prevention of group B streptococcus (GBS) infection in newborn babies*, London, 2006, RCOG (amended 2007).

This leaflet gives a simple and concise explanation for the treatment of group B streptococcus; although primarily aimed at informing women, it provides a useful summary for healthcare professionals.

Sompayrac LM: *How the immune system works*, ed 3, 2008, Wiley-Blackwell.

Clearly explained textbook, illustrated with useful diagrams, which covers progressive development of immune concepts.

Toal M, Agyeman-Duah K, Schwenk A, et al: Swine flu and pregnancy, *J Obstet Gynaecol* 30:97–100, 2010.

This review provides a clear up-to-date summary of the current research and advice on the management of swine flu in pregnancy including the 2009 Department of Health and Royal College of Obstetricians and Gynaecologists' guidelines.

Wood P: *Understanding immunology (Cell & molecular biology in action series)*, ed 2, 2006, Prentice Hall.

A clear, well-illustrated introductory text which is written for students with little prior knowledge of immunology.

REFERENCES

Apari P, Rozsa L: The tripartite immune conflict in placentals and a hypothesis on fetal-maternal microchimerism, *Medical Hypotheses* 72:52–54, 2009.

Beer AE, Billingham RE: Host responses to intra-uterine tissue, cellular and fetal allografts, *J Reprod Fertil* 21:49, 1974.

Behne MJ: Epidermal pH, In Rawlings AV, Leyden JJ, editors: *Skin moisturization*, Portland, 2009, Informa Healthcare.

Billingham RE: Transplantation immunity and the maternofetal relation, *N Engl J Med* 270:720, 1964.

Bohacs A, Pallinger E, Tamasi L, et al: Surface markers of lymphocyte activation in pregnant asthmatics, *Inflamm Res* 59:63–70, 2010.

Brostoff J, Scadding GK, Male D, et al: *Clinical immunology*, London, 1991, Gower Medical.

Buyon JP, Clancy RM, Friedman DM: Cardiac manifestations of neonatal lupus erythematosus: guidelines to management, integrating clues from the bench and bedside, *Nat Clin Pract Rheumatol* 5:139–148, 2009.

Chaouat G: The Th1/Th2 paradigm: still important in pregnancy? *Semin Immunopathol* 29:95–113, 2007.

Chaouat G, Petitbarat M, Dubanchet S, et al: Tolerance to the foetal allograft? *Am J Reprod Immunol* 63:624–636, 2010.

Chen M, Daha MR, Kallenberg CG: The complement system in systemic autoimmune disease, *J Autoimmun* 34:J276–J286, 2010.

Cheng VC, Lau YK, Lee KL, et al: Fatal co-infection with swine origin influenza virus A/H1N1 and community-acquired methicillin-resistant *Staphylococcus aureus*, *J Infect* 59:366–370, 2009.

Chiu WW, Chamley LW: Human seminal plasma antibody-binding proteins, *Am J Reprod Immunol* 50:196–201, 2003.

Clapp DW: Developmental regulation of the immune system, *Semin Perinatol* 30:69–72, 2006.

Cork MJ, Moustafa M, Danby S, et al: Skin barrier dysfunction in atopic dermatitis. In Rawlings AV, Leyden JJ, editors: *Skin moisturization*, Portland, 2009, Informa Healthcare.

Day CJ, Lipkin GW, Savage CO: Lupus nephritis and pregnancy in the 21st century, *Nephrol Dial Transplant* 24:344–347, 2009.

Dunn CL, Kelly RW, Critchley HO: Decidualization of the human endometrial stromal cell: an enigmatic transformation, *Reprod Biomed Online* 7:151–161, 2003.

Gallucci S, Matzinger P: Danger signals: SOS to the immune system, *Curr Opin Immunol* 13:114–119, 2001.

Gutierrez G, Gentile T, Miranda S, et al: Asymmetric antibodies: a protective arm in pregnancy, *Chem Immunol Allergy* 89:158–168, 2005.

Hosenfeld CB, Workowski KA, Berman S, et al: Repeat infection with Chlamydia and gonorrhea among females: a systematic review of the literature, *Sex Transm Dis* 36:478–489, 2009.

Guerin LR, Prins JR, Robertson SA: Regulatory T-cells and immune tolerance in pregnancy: a new target for infertility treatment? *Hum Reprod Update* 15:517–535, 2009.

Hench PS: The reversibility of certain rheumatic and non-rheumatic conditions by the use of cortisone or of the pituitary adrenocorticotrophic hormone, *Ann Intern Med* 36:1, 1952.

Hewagama A, Richardson B: The genetics and epigenetics of autoimmune diseases, *J Autoimmun* 33:3–11, 2009.

Johnson PM, Christmas SE: Immunology in reproduction. In Hillier SG, Kitchener HC, Neilson JP, editors: *Scientific essentials of reproductive medicine*, Philadelphia, 1996, Saunders, pp 284–291.

Kleihauer E, Hildergard B, Betke K: Demonstration von fetlem Hamoglobin in den Erythrocyten eines Blutausstrichs, *Klin Wochenschr* 35:637, 1957.

Koga K, Aldo PB, Mor G: Toll-like receptors and pregnancy: trophoblast as modulators of the immune response, *J Obstetr Gynaecol Res* 25:191–202, 2009.

Koga K, Mor G: Toll-like receptors at the maternal-fetal interface in normal pregnancy and pregnancy disorders, *Am J Reprod Immunol* 63:587–600, 2010.

Kolialexi A, Tounta G, Mavrou A: Noninvasive fetal RhD genotyping from maternal blood, *Expert Rev Mol Diagn* 10:285–296, 2010.

Kovats S, Main EK, Librach C, et al: A class I antigen, HLA-G, expressed in human trophoblasts, *Science* 248:220–223, 1990.

Kwak-Kim J, Yang KM, Gilman-Sachs A: Recurrent pregnancy loss: a disease of inflammation and coagulation, *J Obstet Gynaecol Res* 35:609–622, 2009.

Le Bouteiller P, Piccinni MP: Human NK cells in pregnant uterus: why there? *Am J Reprod Immunol* 59:401–406, 2008.

Leber A, Teles A, Zenclussen AC: Regulatory T cells and their role in pregnancy, *Am J Reprod Immunol* 63:445–459, 2010.

Lee R, Goldstein M, Ullery BW, et al: Value of serum antisperm antibodies in diagnosing obstructive azoospermia, *J Urol* 181:264–269, 2009.

Lissauer DM, Piper KP, Moss PA, et al: Fetal microchimerism: the cellular and immunological legacy of pregnancy, *Expert Rev Mol Med* 11, e33, 2009.

Luppi P: How immune mechanisms are affected by pregnancy, *Vaccine* 21:3352–3357, 2003.

Manaster I, Mandelboim O: The unique properties of uterine NK cells, *Am J Reprod Immunol* 63:434–444, 2010.

Mattes E, McCarthy S, Gong G, et al: Maternal mood scores in mid-pregnancy are related to aspects of neonatal immune function, *Brain Behav Immun* 23:380–388, 2009.

Medawar P: Some immunological and endocrinological problems raised by the evolution of viviparity in vertebrates, *Symp Soc Exp Biol* 11:320–338, 1953.

Mellor AL, Munn DH: Creating immune privilege: active local suppression that benefits friends, but protects foes, *Nat Rev Immunol* 8:74–80, 2008.

Miles DJ, Gadama L, Gumbi A, et al: Human immunodeficiency virus HIV infection during pregnancy induces CD4 T-cell differentiation and modulates responses to Bacille Calmette-Guerin BCG. Vaccine in HIV-uninfected infants, *Immunology* 129:446–454, 2010.

Mor G: Inflammation and pregnancy: the role of toll-like receptors in trophoblast-immune interaction, *Ann N Y Acad Sci* 1127:121–128, 2008.

Mor G, Cardenas I: The immune system in pregnancy: a unique complexity, *Am J Reprod Immunol* 63:425–433, 2010.

Mueller DL: Mechanisms maintaining peripheral tolerance, *Nat Immunol* 11:21–27, 2010.

Porter TF, LaCoursiere Y, Scott JR: Immunotherapy for recurrent miscarriage, *Cochrane Database Syst Rev* CD000112, 2006.

Redman CW, Sargent IL: Immunology of pre-eclampsia, *Am J Reprod Immunol* 63:534–543, 2010.

Robertson SA: Seminal plasma and male factor signalling in the female reproductive tract, *Cell Tissue Res* 322:43–52, 2005.

Robertson SA: Immune regulation of conception and embryo implantation-all about quality control? *J Reprod Immunol* 85:51–57, 2010.

Rooney IA, Ogelesby TJ, Atkinson JP: Complement in human reproduction: activation and control, *Immunol Res* 12:276–294, 1993.

Sacks G, Sargent I, Redman C: An innate view of human pregnancy, *Immunol Today* 20:114–118, 1999.

Sarkar K, Miller FW: Possible roles and determinants of microchimerism in autoimmune and other disorders, *Autoimmun Rev* 3:454–463, 2004.

Saito S, Nakashima A, Myojo-Higuma S, et al: The balance between cytotoxic NK cells and regulatory NK cells in human pregnancy, *J Reprod Immunol* 77:14–22, 2008.

Shakhar K, Valdimarsdottir HB, Bovbjerg DH: Heightened risk of breast cancer following pregnancy: could lasting systemic immune alterations contribute? *Cancer Epidemiol Biomarkers Prev* 16:1082–1086, 2007.

Singh N, Perfect JR: Immune reconstitution syndrome and exacerbation of infections after pregnancy, *Clin Infect Dis* 45:1192–1199, 2007.

Stewart M: *Growing and responding*, Milton Keynes, 1997, Open University, pp 185, 188–191, 193, 200.

Svensson L, Arvola M, Sallstrom MA, et al: The Th2 cytokines IL-4 and IL-10 are not crucial for the completion of allogeneic pregnancy in mice, *J Reprod Immunol* 51:3–7, 2001.

Tanaka T, Nakajima K, Murashima A, et al: Safety of neuraminidase inhibitors against novel influenza A H1N1 in pregnant and breastfeeding women, *CMAJ* 181:55–58, 2009.

Thaxton JE, Sharma S: Interleukin-10: a multi-faceted agent of pregnancy, *Am J Reprod Immunol* 63:482–491, 2010.

Tomassetti C, Meuleman C, Pexsters A, et al: Endometriosis, recurrent miscarriage and implantation failure: is there an immunological link? *Reprod Biomed Online* 13:58–64, 2006.

Weetman AP: Immunity, thyroid function and pregnancy: molecular mechanisms, *Nat Rev Endocrinol* 6:311–318, 2010.

Wegmann TG, Lin H, Guilbert L, et al: Bi-directional cytokine interactions in the maternal–fetal relationship: is successful pregnancy a TH2 phenomenon? *Immunol Today* 15:15–18, 1993.

Zenclussen AC, Schumacher A, Zenclussen ML, et al: Immunology of pregnancy: cellular mechanisms allowing fetal survival within the maternal uterus, *Expert Rev Mol Med* 9:1–14, 2007.

Zipursky A, Hull A, White FD, et al: Foetal erythrocytes in the maternal circulation, *Lancet* i:451, 1959.

Chapter 11

Physiological adaptation to pregnancy

LEARNING OBJECTIVES

- To outline the roles of hormones mediating the physiological adaptation to pregnancy.
- To describe cardiovascular adaptations to pregnancy.
- To describe the respiratory changes in pregnancy.
- To describe the gastrointestinal adaptations in pregnancy.
- To discuss alterations in maternal carbohydrate metabolism in pregnancy.
- To discuss the need for iron supplementation in pregnancy.
- To relate physiological changes with signs, symptoms and discomforts of pregnancy.

Chapter case study

Zara is now in the third trimester of her pregnancy. She informs her midwife that she is not sleeping well, and James prefers to sleep in the spare room as Zara's loud snoring and frequent waking disturbs him. When Zara does sleep, she experiences vivid dreams that cause her to wake suddenly. Her sleeping is not helped by the fact she often wakes up feeling hungry and thirsty and is having to make increasingly frequent visits to the toilet. Zara has now stopped working and finds that the only way she can cope is to a have a rest in the afternoon. She often falls asleep sitting in front of the television for 3–4 h and says this afternoon sleep is less disturbed than the night time.
- What physiological changes could account for these changes in Zara's sleep pattern and what reasons would you give to reassure Zara that this is normal?
- Why do you think Zara is able to sleep more peacefully in the afternoon?
- Are there any advantages in these behavioural changes and might they be preparing Zara to care for her newborn baby?

INTRODUCTION

During the 279 days (40 weeks) of an average pregnancy (measured from the first day of the last menstrual period), maternal physiology changes remarkably to support the development of the fetus and to prepare the mother for labour and lactation. The changes begin in the luteal phase of the menstrual cycle, before fertilization and implantation, as progesterone secretion from the corpus luteum is initiated. If fertilization is successful, levels of progesterone and oestrogen progressively increase. Together, they orchestrate many of the changes to the maternal physiology in pregnancy.

ENDOCRINE CHANGES IN PREGNANCY

The physiological changes of pregnancy are controlled by an alteration in hormone secretion. The trophoblastic cells produce human chorionic gonadotrophin (hCG), which stimulates secretion from the corpus luteum, increasing ovarian steroid hormone production. As the placenta develops, it also produces oestrogen and progesterone. However, placental endocrine function is much broader as the placenta synthesizes a range of hormones and releasing factors that are similar to those originating from the hypothalamus and other maternal endocrine organs (see Chapter 8). Placental products may reach both the maternal and fetal circulation, thus regulating maternal physiology and fetal development.

Steroid hormones

Steroidogenesis depends on interaction and cooperation between the mother, placenta and fetus. The mother is the source of precursors for placental progesterone production and the fetus is the source of precursors for placental oestrogen production. Placental progesterone is used for fetal synthesis of testosterone, corticosteroids and mineralocorticoids. Progesterone is known as the hormone of pregnancy; it stimulates respiration, relaxes smooth muscle (of blood vessels, uterus and gut), increases body temperature, increases sodium and chloride excretion, and may act as an immunosuppressant in the placenta (Picciano, 2003). It is suggested that the repeated miscarriages might be associated with decreased progesterone levels due to stress (Arck et al., 2007). Stress affects the hypothalamic–pituitary–adrenal (HPA) axis and increases levels of the classical stress mediators, corticotrophin-releasing hormone (CRH) and glucocorticoids. CRH can inhibit GnRH and glucocorticoids can suppress pituitary luteinizing hormone (LH) secretion and thus affect steroid hormone production.

Progesterone levels increase gradually at first (Fig. 11.1). There is little change in progesterone concentration between the 5th and 10th week, but after the 10th week the levels increase more markedly as the placenta becomes the main site of steroid hormone synthesis. By the end of the first trimester, levels of progesterone are 50% higher than luteal levels and by term the levels have increased threefold. The syncytiotrophoblast uses maternal cholesterol as a substrate for progesterone synthesis. Placental production of progesterone is adequate by 5–6 weeks. A primate pregnancy can survive ovariectomy (oophorectomy, removal of ovaries), although the corpus luteum is essential in other mammalian pregnancies (Johnson and Everitt, 2000). Human corpus luteal production of 17α-hydroxyprogesterone decreases from 6 to 9 weeks as placental production increases. Measurement of the different progesterone metabolites was commonly used to assess placental function.

The primary oestrogen of pregnancy is oestriol. Early in pregnancy, oestrone and oestradiol levels increase but oestriol levels do not begin to rise until the 9th week when the fetal adrenal glands begin to synthesize the precursor dehydroepiandrosterone sulphate (DHEAS) from placental pregnenolone; DHEAS is the substrate for placental production of oestriol (see Chapter 3). Maternal and placental steroids are conjugated in the fetal liver and adrenal glands into water soluble, and thus biologically inactive,

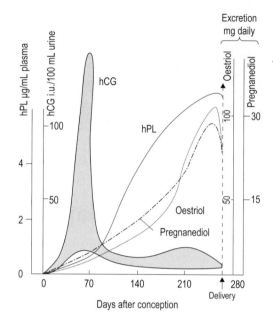

Fig. 11.1 Increasing concentrations of oestrogen and progesterone during pregnancy.

forms (so the fetus is protected from the effect of the steroids' precursors). As the 16-hydroxyl precursor originates only from the fetal liver, production of oestriol indicates fetal well-being. In 'at risk' pregnancies, decreased oestriol may indicate fetal distress and the need to induce premature delivery, although as an index of placental function and fetal well-being it has largely been replaced by Doppler investigation and biophysical profiling. Oestriol measurement is part of the Bart's (triple) test for Down's syndrome (see Chapter 7). Oestrone and oestriol levels increase about 100 times and oestradiol levels about 1000 times during the course of the pregnancy (Blackburn, 2007). The oestrogens promote the growth of the endometrium and breasts, enhance myometrial activity, increase sensitivity to carbon dioxide, increase pituitary prolactin secretion, promote myometrial vasodilation, stimulate fluid retention, alter the composition of connective tissue and increase the sensitivity of the uterus to progesterone in late pregnancy.

Human chorionic gonadotrophin

The main function of hCG is to maintain production of steroid hormones from the corpus luteum in early pregnancy until the placenta can take over. hCG has a very similar structure to that of LH – as well as follicle-stimulating hormone (FSH) and thyroid-stimulating hormone (TSH) – and acts on the LH receptors, prolonging the life of the corpus luteum. hCG is produced initially by the outer cells of the blastocyst which are the cells that differentiate into trophoblast cells and subsequently into the placenta. The syncytiotrophoblast, which evolves from the trophoblast (see Chapter 8), continues to produce hCG. It is secreted, and can be detected before implantation, in vaginal secretions and in the maternal circulation (see Fig. 11.1). As the lacunae begin to be formed by the invading syncytiotrophoblast, the hCG diffuses into the maternal blood and significant levels can be detected. Measurable urine values are present 2 weeks after fertilization; home pregnancy tests are very sensitive and specific. The presence of hCG confirms successful fertilization as, apart from very rare production by certain gut tumours, it is not produced by other tissues (Iles and Chard, 1991). hCG is produced in large amounts by hydatidiform moles (see Chapter 8); following evacuation of a molar pregnancy, urinalysis for the presence of hCG is continued for 2 years to exclude the development of choriocarcinoma.

Production of hCG is maximal at 8–10 weeks and then falls to a low plateau level that is maintained throughout the pregnancy. hCG levels, therefore, reflect the placental transformation from an organ of invasion to one of transfer. Persistently low levels of hCG are associated with abnormal placental development or ectopic pregnancy. If hCG is given to non-pregnant women, the corpus luteum is maintained and progesterone secretion rises. Alternatively, antibodies to hCG given to a pregnant woman cause the corpus luteum to regress. hCG, rather than LH, is used to induce ovulation in fertility treatment. By 4–5 weeks, the placenta and fetus are synthesizing significant amounts of steroid hormones and can assume endocrine control of the pregnancy. hCG has thyroid-hormone-stimulating properties, affecting appetite and fat deposition, and also affects thirst, release of antidiuretic hormone (ADH) and other osmoregulatory changes (Davison et al., 1990). It also promotes myometrial growth and inhibits myometrial contractility (Kornyei, Lei and Rao, 1993). The effects of hCG are summarized in Box 11.1.

Human placental lactogen

As hCG levels fall, there is increased secretion of human placental lactogen (hPL). The levels of hPL increase in parallel with the size of the placenta and correlate well with fetal and placental weight. hPL has a similar structure and properties to growth hormone and prolactin; it is a single polypeptide chain and is lactogenic and stimulates growth of both maternal and fetal tissues. hPL appears to protect the fetus from rejection, and low levels of hPL are associated with pregnancy failure and spontaneous abortion. hPL is antagonistic to insulin, resulting in increased maternal metabolism and utilization of fat as an energy substrate. This diabetogenic effect of pregnancy reduces glucose uptake by maternal cells, thus making more available for fetal use (see below). hPL is also called human chorionic somatomammatrophin.

> **Box 11.1 Effects of human chorionic gonadotrophin (hCG)**
>
> - Luteotrophic effect on corpus luteum that maintains synthesis and secretion of oestrogen and progesterone
> - Simulates placental progesterone production
> - Possesses thyrotrophic activity
> - May be responsible for nausea and vomiting
> - Stimulates maternal thyroid gland; increases appetite and fat deposition
> - Increases sensitivity to glucose
> - Decreases osmotic threshold for thirst and release of ADH
> - Suppresses maternal lymphocyte response thus preventing rejection of the placenta
> - Promotes myometrial growth
> - Inhibits myometrial contractility
> - Modulates trophoblastic invasion
> - Affects fetal nervous tissue development
> - Affects male sexual differentiation and stimulates fetal testes to produce testosterone
> - Stimulates fetal adrenal glands to increase production of corticosteroids

Relaxin

Relaxin is produced by the corpus luteum, and to a lesser extent by the myometrium and placenta. Levels of relaxin are highest in the first trimester. Relaxin has a role in the softening of elastic ligaments of pelvic bones and has been used clinically to enhance cervical ripening during induction of labour (see Chapter 13). Relaxin acts with progesterone to maintain uterine quiescence; it may also suppress oxytocin release and affect gap junction permeability. The softening and relaxation of the pelvic ligaments allow mobilization and growth of the uterus into the abdomen. Sometimes women experience low-back pain in pregnancy, which is associated with the stretching of these ligaments. For some women, this results in the pelvic joints becoming unstable and in severe cases results in symphysis pubis dysfunction (SPD), with severe pain on walking. Relaxin is also thought to be involved in endometrial differentiation during embryo implantation, wound healing and, possibly, tumour growth and progression (Ivell and Einspanier, 2002).

Adrenal and pituitary hormones

The adrenal gland increases in both size and activity during pregnancy. Oestrogen stimulates adrenal cortisol production by inhibiting the metabolism of cortisol and increasing the synthesis of cortisol-binding protein (transcortin). Progesterone increases tissue resistance to cortisol by competing at the receptor level and binding to the cortisol-binding protein; this also results in an increase in cortisol production. CRH from the hypothalamus affects the release of adrenocorticotrophin (ACTH), melanocyte-stimulating hormone (MSH) and β-endorphin from the anterior pituitary gland. ACTH stimulates the adrenal gland production of cortisol. Cortisol levels increase in response to stress, including increased cardiac output and decreased fasting glucose levels in the second trimester of pregnancy. Both CRH and ACTH are also produced by the placenta as well as by the maternal hypothalamic–pituitary axis; the placental hormones are subject to different feedback control mechanisms and may be important in initiating labour (see Chapter 13).

The increase in circulating levels of cortisol has a positive effect on certain conditions, such as rheumatoid arthritis and eczema. This observation led to the clinical use of exogenous cortisol as a treatment for these conditions. Both progesterone and oestrogen act synergistically to increase aldosterone production. Adrenal synthesis of androgens, oestrogen, progesterone and cholesterol increases in pregnancy.

The pituitary gland enlarges markedly during pregnancy. Much of the increase is due to increased number and activity of cells of the anterior pituitary gland. The gonadotrophs decrease in number as the raised oestrogen concentration inhibits release of FSH and LH, which are barely detectable for most of the pregnancy. However, under the influence of progesterone and oestrogen, the prolactin-secreting cells increase from 10% of the cell population to 50%. Prolactin levels increase progressively through the pregnancy to values 20 times higher than the prepregnant level. Production of ACTH increases, resulting in increased adrenal activity. MSH synthesis also increases so hyperpigmentation may occur (Elling and Powell, 1997). Pregnant women frequently observe that they tan more deeply or develop irregular pigmented patches. Towards the second half of pregnancy, oxytocin production from the posterior pituitary increases.

Thyroid hormones

The hypothalamic–pituitary–thyroid axis undergoes marked changes in pregnancy. Oestrogen, hCG and altered hepatic and renal function together act to change the levels of triiodothyronine (T_3), thyroxine (T_4) and thyroid-binding globulin (TBG); these changes are important to support the altered metabolism of pregnancy. Oestrogen stimulates hepatic synthesis of TBG by 50–100 times resulting in increased total amounts of T_3 and T_4, although free concentrations remain within normal physiological limits. hCG has mild TSH activity so it stimulates both the production of T_4 and the deiodination of T_4 to T_3 in the peripheral tissues. The high concentrations of hCG in the first trimester and the consequent increased secretion of thyroid hormones results in TSH release from the pituitary gland being

inhibited. This means that maternal circulating concentrations of free T_3 and free T_4 peak at the end of the first trimester (de Escobar et al., 2008) requiring an increased availability of iodine. If iodine is limiting, the maternal thyroid exhibits an autoregulatory response, increasing synthesis of T_3 (which requires 3 iodine atoms per molecule) at the expense of T_4 production. Thus there is no change in TSH but there will be less T_4 transported across the placenta to the fetus which could compromise neurodevelopment. Thyroid hormone receptors can be demonstrated in the fetal brain early in development (Bernal and Pekonen, 1984) suggesting early brain development requires maternal thyroid hormone input (later in gestation, both the maternal and fetal thyroid glands provide T_4). It should be noted that production of sufficient thyroid hormone requires a doubling of iodine intake compared to pregnancy requirement (which may mean potassium iodide supplements should be recommended – see Chapter 12).

Pregnancy mimics hyperthyroidism in a number of respects, for instance by increasing body temperature, and stimulating appetite and feelings of fatigue. In most pregnant women, the thyroid gland enlarges because thyroid activity increases and renal iodine loss is increased. Ancient Egyptians used the observation of pregnancy-induced goitre (thyroid gland hypertrophy) as confirmation of pregnancy (Glinoer and Lemone, 1992). The thyroid gland hypertrophies as it attempts to increase uptake of iodine for hormone synthesis. Nowadays, maternal goitre is rare in pregnancy partly because of better diets and iodine supplementation of table salt, but subclinical iodine deficiency can compromise fetal brain and central nervous system development resulting in neurological anomalies, reduced cephalic size (microcephaly) and reduced intelligence quotient (IQ). Many women are at the threshold of iodine deficiency and the demands of pregnancy can compromise them further, adding support for routine iodine supplementation in pregnancy (Perez-Lopez, 2007). Basal metabolic rate increases by 20–25% from the 4th month of pregnancy but much of the increase is related to the increased surface area of the mother and the increased work she has to do maintaining maternal and fetal tissue requirements. Nausea and vomiting have been linked not only to the changes in hCG (see above) but also directly to the rise in free T_4.

Hypothyroidism is common in women of reproductive age and in pregnancy can be associated with adverse maternal and neonatal outcomes including increased risk of pregnancy-induced hypertension, miscarriage, still-birth, postpartum haemorrhage, congenital malformation and fetal distress (Idris et al., 2005). Women with pre-existing thyroid deficiencies require close monitoring of thyroid function during pregnancy and often require increased doses of thyroxine due the altered metabolic demands of pregnancy.

THE REPRODUCTIVE SYSTEM

The blood vessels

The vasculature of the uterus undergoes a number of remarkable and unique changes during pregnancy. Uterine blood flow increases: the vessel diameter of the spiral arteries increases and vascular resistance falls (see Chapter 8). These essential changes accommodate the increased blood flow to the placenta, which is maintained under conditions of low blood pressure. The coursing of blood through the enlarged tortuous arteries produces a uterine 'souffle', which may be heard through a stethoscope or with a sonicaid. The enhanced blood supply to the uterus and the concomitant establishment of the maternal circulation to the placenta effectively diverts blood away from the legs (Burton et al., 2009).

The uterus

The uterus increases in all dimensions and also changes shape (see Chapters 2 and 13) during pregnancy. Uterine hyperplasia begins after implantation and is driven by oestrogen and growth factors (it occurs if the embryo is implanted in an extrauterine site; Blackburn, 2007). Early growth results in thickening of the uterine wall. The endometrium thickens into the decidua. The three layers of the myometrium become clearly defined as the uterine muscle undergoes initial hyperplasia (development of new fibres) and subsequent hypertrophy (increase in length and thickness of existing muscle fibres). Later uterine growth is mostly hypertrophy and hyperplasia of the myocytes and remodelling of connective tissue which is driven by distension as the fetus enlarges. The muscle fibres increase in length and width as the timing and speed of the myometrial action potentials change and the muscle cells increase their content of actin and myosin, gap junctions, sarcoplasmic reticulum and mitochondria.

In early pregnancy, the uterine isthmus increases from about 7 to 25 mm (Fig. 11.2). From 32 to 34 weeks, the isthmus forms the lower uterine segment (LUS). As effacement commences (at approximately 36 weeks), the external os is incorporated into the LUS (see Chapter 13). The blastocyst usually implants in the fundus (upper part) of the uterus. By 12 weeks, the fetus fills the uterine cavity and the fundus can just be palpated (felt) at the pelvic brim. By 20 weeks the fundus reaches the maternal umbilicus and by 8 months it reaches the sternum. As the uterus expands during pregnancy, it loses its anteverted and anteflexed configuration and becomes erect, tilting and then rotating to the right under the pressure of the descending colon. The uterus changes from its non-pregnant pear-shape and becomes spherical and then cylindrical. Abdominal measurement using the symphysis pubis as a reference point is often used to assess uterine size and fetal growth as pregnancy progresses.

Uterine quiescence is mediated by progesterone, relaxin, nitric oxide (NO) and prostacyclin (also known as prostaglandin PGI_2). The uterus is never completely quiescent and exhibits low-frequency activity throughout the pregnancy (as it does in the non-pregnant state). Braxton Hicks contractions are painless contractions that are measurable from the first trimester of the pregnancy. These contractions do not dilate the cervix but assist in the circulation of blood to the placenta. The contractions are usually irregular and weak, unsynchronized and multifocal in origin. The contractions of the circular muscles are less than those of the longitudinal ones (Blackburn, 2007). The uterine ligaments soften and thicken under the influence of oestrogen, resulting in increased mobility and capacity of the pelvis.

The cervix

The cervix increases in mass and width during the pregnancy. Oestrogen increases the blood supply to the cervix resulting in a lilac coloration and softer tissue

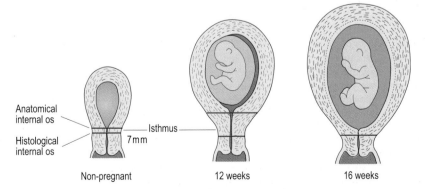

Fig. 11.2 The uterine isthmus increases from about 7 to 25 mm in the early part of pregnancy. (Reproduced with permission from Miller and Hanretty, 1998.)

texture; the water content of the cervix also changes. The collagen fibre bundles become less tightly bound (see Chapter 13). The cervical mucosa proliferates and the glands become more complex and secrete thickened mucus, which forms a plug or operculum protecting the cervix from ascending infection. The plug is held laterally by projections of thickened mucus in the mouths of the mucus-secreting glands. It is this plug that is released as 'the show' at the onset of labour when the cervix starts to be drawn up to form the LUS.

The vagina

Blood flow to the vagina increases likewise, resulting in softer vaginal tissue which is more distensible. The lilac coloration of the vagina and cervix was traditionally recognized as being an indicator of pregnancy (described as Jacquemier's sign). The increased blood flow means that the pulsating of the uterine arteries can be felt through the lateral fornices (Osiander's sign). The increased vascularization of the vagina can result in increased sensitivity and sexual arousal. Venous engorgement results in increased vascular transudation, which together with the increased cervical mucus production results in an increased vaginal discharge. The vaginal discharge (leucorrhoea) has a low pH (because of the effect of raised oestrogen levels on the vaginal flora) and is thick and white with an inoffensive odour. Oestrogen also stimulates the vaginal epithelial cell division so the cells acquire a distinctly boat-shaped appearance (which should not be mistaken for carcinoma cells). Early in pregnancy, the hypertrophied corpus luteum, which is about 3–5 cm long, distends from the ovarian surface; this may be palpated in some women or visualized during endoscopic examination in women undergoing egg retrieval for IVF (*in vitro* fertilization).

The breasts

In early pregnancy, vascularization of the breasts increases. This tends to result in a marbled appearance of the skin owing to the marked dilation of the superficial veins. The breasts, specially the nipple areas, may feel sensitive and tingle because of the engorgement of blood. (Changes to the breast in pregnancy are described in more detail in Chapter 16.) Pregnancy following diagnosis and treatment for breast cancer is becoming more common with earlier diagnosis and delayed childbirth. Although concerns have been raised about the possible promotional effects of raised oestrogen levels during pregnancy on residual metastatic disease, the majority of studies indicate no adverse effect on the outcome of pregnancy or on survival (de Bree et al., 2010).

The signs of pregnancy are summarized in Box 11.2.

Box 11.2 Signs of pregnancy

- Amenorrhoea
- Softening of vagina and cervix
- Increased blood flow to vagina and cervix causing lilac coloration (Jacquemier's sign)
- Pulsating of uterine arteries (Osiander's sign)
- Tingling and sensitive breasts with dilated superficial veins marbling surface
- Nausea and vomiting, possible changes in taste
- Increased frequency of urination as uterus compresses bladder
- Increased pigmentation of skin
- Bleeding gums
- Tiredness
- Increased appetite and thirst

THE CARDIOVASCULAR SYSTEM

The most notable physiological changes occur in the cardiovascular system in preparation for the increased demands of maternal and fetal tissues (Fig. 11.3). These changes are caused both indirectly by hormones (oestrogen, progesterone, prostaglandins and other vasoactive substances) and directly by mechanical effects and as a result of the increased load on the system. Marked haemodynamic adjustments take place in pregnancy; maternal blood volume and cardiac output quickly increase but paradoxically blood pressure falls because of the marked reduction in systemic vascular resistance and reduced blood viscosity due to haemodilution. Heart disease affects less than 1% of pregnancies and causes 10 deaths per million in England and Wales, but symptoms of heart disease (such as breathlessness, palpitations, fainting and oedema) are present in over 90% of pregnant women (de Swiet, 1998a). Superimposed on a pre-existing cardiac disease state, pregnancy may be dangerous and even potentially fatal. Measurement of cardiovascular system parameters is technically difficult and notoriously variable. Measurements obviously have to be indirect and are very sensitive to changes such as emotion, exertion and posture. In the research literature, there are many inconsistencies, some of which reflect differences in standardization of conditions (de Swiet, 1998a). In the last couple of decades there has been an increased incidence of myocardial infarction (MI) in pregnancy which reflects the increasing proposition of older women having babies (the risk of MI is 30-times higher in women over 40 years compared to women under 20 years; Curry et al., 2009) and increased obesity and pre-existing diabetes (Ward et al., 2007).

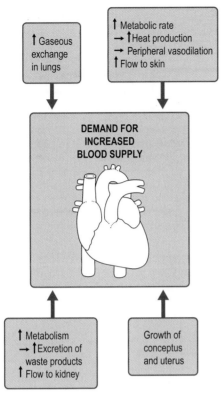

Fig. 11.3 The changed distribution of blood flow in pregnancy.

Blood volume

Total blood volume increases by 30–50%, more in multiple pregnancies (Brown and Gallery, 1994), resulting in a fall in plasma osmolality. The rise in blood volume correlates well with birth weight and, as it begins early in pregnancy, the mechanism of these early changes in the cardiovascular system is thought to be hormonally driven. It has been disputed whether the increase in volume (sodium and fluid retention) precedes the increased vascular space ('overfill' hypothesis) or whether the changes are stimulated by relative hypovolaemia (increased vascular capacity), known as the 'underfill' hypothesis (Schrier, 1992). The arguments for the 'underfill' hypothesis are supported by the observation that blood pressure falls before plasma volume expands (Duvekot et al., 1993). The consensus is that both mechanisms are important but the initial change is probably the decreased systemic resistance (Ward et al., 2007). Often in early pregnancy women feel faint, suggesting that the physiological compensation of the underfill has yet to occur.

Oestrogen stimulates angiogenesis (formation of new blood vessels and vascular beds) and increases the blood flow to the tissues. Oestrogen affects the distribution of

collagen in the tunica media of the large vessel walls, increasing venous distensibility. Oestrogen also stimulates endothelium-dependent vasodilatation, by increasing synthesis of NO (a potent vasodilator) and vasodilatory prostaglandins and inhibiting the release of endothelin-I (a vasoconstrictor). Production of both prostacyclin and NO increases in pregnancy (Morris et al., 1996). These signals affect placental blood flow, particularly remodelling of the spiral arteries (see Chapter 8).

Progesterone relaxes vascular smooth muscle causing systemic vasodilatation and decreased peripheral resistance, probably via vasoactive prostaglandins and enhanced nitric oxide (NO) production. The syncytiotrophoblast is an essential site of NO production which is important in maintaining vasodilation of the uterine blood vessels and ensuring a high flow and low resistance blood supply to the uteroplacental bed and fetus. The effect of the vasodilation is that the circulatory system increases its capacity and is relatively underfilled. One of the early effects of this is decreased glomerular arteriolar resistance which results in increased glomerular filtration rate (GFR) and renal blood flow (Ward et al., 2007). Relaxin production is stimulated by hCG and is also involved in renal vasodilation (Conrad et al., 2005). The decreased vascular tone in the blood supply to the kidneys causes renal compensatory mechanisms to increase plasma volume and cardiac output. In addition, both progesterone and oestrogen increase water retention by affecting the renin–angiotensin system (RAS) and oestrogen increases hepatic angiotensinogen production. This results in a rise in angiotensin II, which increases renal fluid resorption and stimulates the production of aldosterone. All components of the RAS increase in pregnancy but there is decreased sensitivity to vasoconstrictors such as angiotensin II and noradrenaline during pregnancy (so blood pressure does not rise). Renin is produced by the uterus, placenta and fetus, as well as the kidney. Levels of renin are two- to threefold higher than before pregnancy. These changes in the RAS may mediate the oestrogen-stimulated angiogenesis and increased cell growth and division. Relaxin increases production of ADH and oxytocin and modulates responses to angiotensin II. The increased ADH promotes water retention and thirst; the raised oxytocin promotes vasodilation and sodium excretion partly by increasing cardiac atrial natriuretic peptide production (Brunton et al., 2008).

Progesterone stimulates a 10-fold increase in the amount of circulating aldosterone. Progesterone is antagonistic to aldosterone but some progesterone is converted to deoxycorticosterone, which has mild aldosterone-like properties. Progesterone augments its effects on the circulatory volume by resetting the thirst centres in the hypothalamus and increasing thirst. Progesterone also lowers the sodium threshold for the RAS and blocks the vasopressive activity of angiotensin II in pregnancy (Blackburn, 2007). The net result of the changes in oestrogen and progesterone is an increase in vascular resistance followed by increased

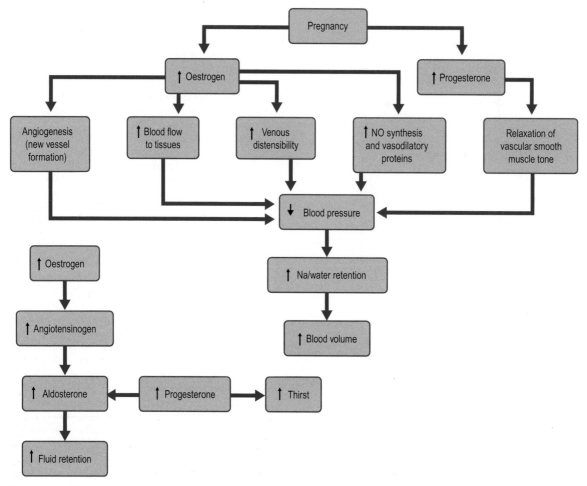

Fig. 11.4 The likely pathways for blood volume increase in pregnancy.

sodium and water retention and expansion of the circulating volume (Fig. 11.4).

Cardiac output

Blood volume and cardiac output increase in parallel (Fig. 11.5). Cardiac output increases by 30–50%, an average increase of 1.5 L/min from 4.5 to 6 L/min. Cardiac output rises quickly in the first trimester and is maintained throughout the pregnancy. The increase in cardiac output is greater in multiple pregnancies. Cardiac output is affected by posture: when the pregnant woman lies supine, her uterus impedes venous return from the inferior vena cava resulting in an apparent decrease in cardiac output. The measured drop in cardiac output in the third trimester, observed by a number of researchers, was most probably the result of measurements being made with the woman lying supine (Mabie et al., 1994). In labour, cardiac output increases by about 2.0 L/min.

Cardiac output is the result of two variables: heart rate and stroke volume (see Chapter 1). In pregnancy, both heart rate and stroke volume increase. Heart rate increases soon after implantation, by about 20% (an average of 15 beats more per minute) from about 70 to 85 beats/min. Stroke volume typically increases by about 10% from 64 to 71 mL. Steroid hormones and prolactin may affect the myocardium directly. Oestrogen stimulates an increased accumulation of components of the myocardial cells and increases contractility (Duvekot and Peeters, 1998). Heart rate is usually measured by the palpation of peripheral pulses and the increase in stroke volume means the pulse is easy to palpate in a pregnant woman. Heart rate is affected by many things; tachycardia (fast pulse) may be caused by excitement, stress, fear, medication, illegal use of drugs, etc. and so, in isolation, can be a poor indicator of physical problems such as sepsis and haemorrhage so needs to be considered in conjunction with other abnormal

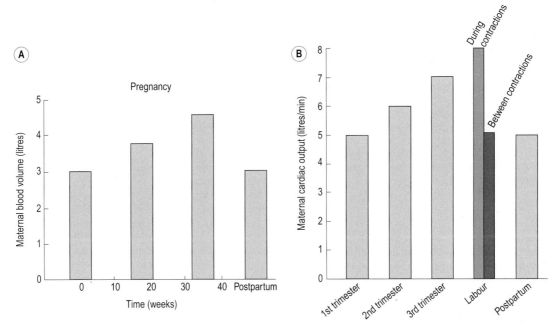

Fig. 11.5 The parallel increase in (A) blood volume and (B) cardiac output during pregnancy. Blood volume is increased up to 40%, thus increasing the load on the heart. (Reproduced with permission from Chamberlain et al., 1991. (B) After Whitfield, 1986.)

observations such as raised blood pressure, temperature, or respiratory rate.

Bradycardia is an abnormally slow heartbeat and is rare in pregnant women but can indicate heart block, raised intracranial pressure, medication and use of illegal drugs.

Heart

The early changes relating to the heart occur early in the pregnancy and are caused by hormonal changes. Later, the heart is displaced upwards by elevation of the diaphragm and is rotated forward so the electrocardiogram (ECG) changes and the location of the apex beat is directed forward to the anterior chest wall. The heart increases in size by an average of 70–80 mL (about 12%). This increase is due to increased filling and oestrogen-stimulated cardiac muscle hypertrophy (an increase in the size of pre-existing cardiomyocytes). The remodelling of the heart that occurs in pregnancy in response to increased blood volume and workload is an adaptive response analogous to the ventricular hypertrophy of an athlete's heart in continuous training. However, heart hypertrophy can lead to cardiac disturbances such as cardiac arrhythmias (Eghbali et al., 2006). The pregnant woman's heart is thus dilated and has increased contractility. Increased blood volume results in an increase in venous return and therefore increased atrial size. The heart sounds change because the mitral valve closes marginally before the closure of the tricuspid valve; thus the first heart

sound is louder with an exaggerated split. Many pregnant women (92–95%) develop innocent (non-significant) systolic murmurs in pregnancy. The increased blood flow through the mammary blood vessels may be perceived as a possible heart murmur; this is more common in lactation. The net result of increased contractility, increased venous return, cardiac hypertrophy, decreased peripheral resistance and increased heart rate is increased cardiac output. Women with known pre-existing cardiac disease must be carefully monitored during pregnancy as they may not have the physiological reserve to cope with this increased demand on the heart (see Case Study 11.1). Other conditions may also pose serious risk in pregnancy relating to increased cardiac output such as Marfan syndrome (see Box 11.3).

Arteriovenous (AV) difference

Increased cardiac output exceeds increased oxygen consumption (especially early in pregnancy when cardiac output increases considerably and oxygen consumption is relatively low) so more oxygen is returned to the heart from venous circulation compared with prepregnant values and the AV difference is smaller. The AV difference is 34 mL in mid-pregnancy rising towards term but is always less than the non-pregnant values of about 45 mL (de Swiet, 1998a). The higher return of oxygen to the heart suggests that the commonly measured decrease in haemoglobin concentration is not physiologically inadequate

Box 11.3 **Marfan Syndrome**

Marfan syndrome is a disorder of connective tissue and as a result has a high incidence of aortic aneurism due to the inherent weakness of the artery wall. Incidence of the disease is about 2 per 10 000 births and affects both men and women equally. As cardiac output is increased in pregnancy, the risk of aortic aneurism occurring is greatly increased and so the pregnant woman should have regular cardiac ultrasounds to optimize early detection of this potentially life threatening situation. If aortic aneurism occurs, emergency surgical intervention is required which involves the weakness of the aortic wall being strengthened by synthetic graft material.

and the relatively small increase in total haemoglobin (oxygen-carrying capacity) is more than sufficient to compensate for increased oxygen requirements. This supports the argument that the term 'physiological anaemia' is inappropriate (see p. 269). The increased AV difference, especially early in the pregnancy before increased oxygen consumption, means that early fetal development and organogenesis occur in an environment which is adequately oxygenated despite the maternal spiral arteries not connecting with the intervillous spaces in the early part of pregnancy (see Chapter 8).

Blood pressure

Normal pregnancy has relatively little effect on arterial blood pressure. Despite increased cardiac output and increased vascular capacitance, there is relatively little change in systolic pressure in pregnancy. However, diastolic blood pressure is lower in the first two trimesters and returns to prepregnant values in the third trimester. Both the development of new vascular beds and the relaxation of peripheral tone by progesterone result in decreased

Case study 11.1

Moira is a 23-year-old primigravida who, at the age of 19 underwent a heart and lung transplant as a result of cystic fibrosis. Moira and her partner had been well informed of the risks associated with a pregnancy, had planned not to have any children and so this pregnancy was unexpected.
- How should Moira's care be managed in relation to her transplant status and her pregnancy and what is the role of the midwife in this complex case?
- What are the possible complications and risks in this case and what would the midwife need to know and do to ensure early recognition, referral and intervention is optimized?

resistance to flow. This is augmented by a change in the profile of prostaglandins produced. The levels of the prostaglandin PGE_2 and prostacyclin, which stimulate vasodilation, rise early in pregnancy. NO (nitric oxide; formerly known as endothelium-derived relaxing factor, EDRF) also appears to play an important vasodilatory role (Palmer et al., 1987). The most important stimulator for NO production is shear stress such as that generated from a pulsatile blood flow (Maul et al., 2003). The increased difference between diastolic and systolic blood pressure means that for much of the pregnancy the pulse pressure is increased. Hypotension, particularly in early pregnancy, has been associated with fatigue, headaches and dizziness, which many women experience.

In pregnancy, changes in posture can cause acute haemodynamic changes (Blackburn, 2007). Blood pressure in normotensive women is higher when sitting and falls on lying, especially in the supine position (Box 11.4). Effects on venous pressure are relatively dramatic compared with the effects on arterial pressure. As there are no valves between the return from the femoral veins to the vena cava and heart, venous pressure in the legs is similar to the pressure in the heart so, if a pregnant woman lies in a supine position, the uterus can compress the aorta and, particularly, the thin-walled vena cava and iliac veins. (The aorta is compressed as well but to a lesser degree because it has a much thicker vessel wall.) Return of blood to the heart can also be impeded by the pressure of the fetal head on the iliac veins and by hydrodynamic obstruction due to outflow of blood from the uterine vessels. Most women experience a drop in blood pressure greater than 10% when they lie down; for some of these women this fall is extreme, reaching up to 50%. The effect of assuming the lithotomy position in labour is to decrease cardiac output significantly (Carbonne et al., 1996).

In late pregnancy, most women experience oedema of the lower extremities (see Case study 11.2) owing to the combined effects of progesterone relaxing the vascular tone, the impeding of the venous return by the gravid uterus and gravitational forces. The peripheral circulatory volume is increased by 500–600 mL/limb (de Swiet, 1998a). Oedema is further increased in hypertensive women and tends to increase with increased maternal age. Fluid drunk by the pregnant woman appears as increased leg volume and the expected diuresis is delayed until, she lies down, resulting in increased nocturia. Blood pressure is higher on the side of placental implantation and oedema may also be more marked in the leg on the side of placental implantation (de Swiet, 1998a). The effect of increased venous pressure is to increase the incidence and severity of varicose veins of the legs, vulva and haemorrhoids (Fig. 11.6).

The tendency to develop oedema is a also affected by the concentration of plasma proteins (see Box 11.5). The increment in plasma volume is not matched by an increase in plasma protein synthesis so there is decreased

Case study 11.2

It is the height of summer and Kathy, 38 weeks' pregnant, informs her midwife she feels fat and sluggish and cannot cope with the hot weather. Kathy's ankles are visibly swollen.

- Is the midwife right to assume that this is normal?
- What indicators would the midwife be able to use in an assessment to reassure Kathy that all is well?
- What factors may alert the midwife to suspect that all is not well?

Three days later Kathy presents to the midwives' clinic complaining of breathlessness and chest pain.

- What should the midwife do in response to Cathy's worsening symptoms?
- What are the possible causes of these symptoms?

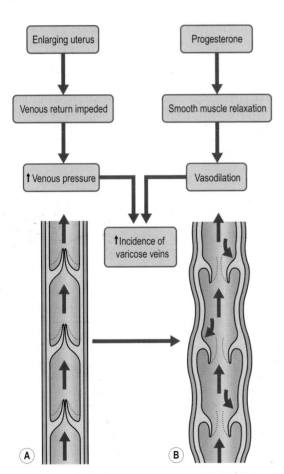

Fig. 11.6 The effect of increased venous pressure leading to increased incidence of varicose veins of the legs, vulva and haemorrhoids. (A) Normal vein with normal vascular tone; (B) varicose vein: the effects of progesterone on muscle tone cause incomplete valve closure, allowing the back-flow of blood.

Box 11.4 **Blood pressure monitoring**

As high blood pressure in pregnancy is a risk factor for serious maternal and fetal complications, it is important that blood pressure is measured accurately (NICE, 2008). Oscillometric (automated) blood pressure equipment is usually used however this is best used when serial monitoring is required such as in fulminating pre-eclampsia or eclampsia. Routine blood pressure monitoring should be undertaken with manual equipment (NICE, 2008). Important factors that affect the blood pressure reading include correct cuff size and the woman's position and posture, avoiding recent intake of caffeine or nicotine, taking the average of two readings, etc. The usual clinical definition of hypertension is:

(1) a single diastolic reading of 110 mmHg or above
(2) or a diastolic of 90 mmHg or above (but below 110) on 2 consecutive occasions at least 4 h apart
(3) and/or a systolic reading of 160 mmHg or above on 2 consecutive occasions at least 4 h apart.

Some women may not show the expected reduction in blood pressure in early pregnancy. This may be due to a degree of pre-existing renal disease or condition causing chronic hypertension but may also be an early indicator of hypertensive disease in pregnancy. Note that pre-eclampsia can be superimposed on chronic hypertension. A rise in blood pressure is often associated but not always present in pre-eclampsia. Other reasons for high blood pressure may be stress and anxiety, acute renal disease such as infection, raised inter-cranial pressure (the significance of this is increased with a slowing pulse). The blood pressure reading needs to be considered in the context of other risk factors. A drop in blood pressure may be caused by haemorrhage (significance is increased with the presence of tachycardia), advanced sepsis (septic shock), and drug induced.

Box 11.5 **Oedema and hypertension**

The pressures in the right ventricle, pulmonary arteries and pulmonary capillaries do not change but cardiac output increases. The higher pulmonary blood flow therefore has to be absorbed by decreased pulmonary resistance and dilatation of the pulmonary vascular bed so the volume of pulmonary circulation increases to match the increased cardiac output. Conditions where pulmonary resistance is increased or fixed have a poor maternal prognosis such as Eisenmenger's syndrome, which has a 30–50% mortality rate. Exercise presents an increased demand on the cardiovascular system (see Box 11.6).

plasma colloidal pressure. This, together with the increased venous pressure, means there is an increase in fluid loss from the capillaries. There may also be an increase in capillary permeability (Blackburn, 2007).

The effects of exercise on the cardiovascular system are summarized in Box 11.6.

Distribution of blood flow

Oestrogen increases blood flow to all tissues but the distribution of flow is affected by posture. Venous tone is affected by progesterone. The increased venous distensibility results in an increased incidence of varicose veins, venous thrombosis and thromboembolism. The uterus is the central target of the increased circulatory flow during pregnancy but distribution of flow to other organ systems, including kidneys, skin, lungs and breasts, increases as well. It is difficult to distinguish between blood flow to the increasing uterine tissue mass and that going specifically to supply the placenta because the uterine vessels are complex and inaccessible. AV shunts in the uterine vasculature have been identified; these allow a short circuit of the placental site after delivery of the placenta, rather than being important

Box 11.6 **Exercise in pregnancy**

Exercise affects maternal physiology because there is a hormonal response, weight is redistributed and heat is generated. Many women experience very good physical health especially early in pregnancy. However, the question is whether the adaptive response to exercise compromises fetal oxygenation and well-being. The ability to increase cardiac output in response to exercise progressively declines throughout pregnancy. Theoretically, redistribution of weight could affect the venous return and blood could be preferentially circulated to the skeletal muscles and to the skin for heat dissipation. Studies on animals suggest that uterine blood flow can be decreased substantially before fetal oxygen uptake or temperature regulation is compromised. It has been reported that over a third of the female medal winners in the 1956 Russian Olympic team were pregnant and the cardiovascular changes enhanced for their performance (de Swiet, 1998a). In practice, moderate exercise in normal healthy pregnancy is encouraged as maternal and fetal health seem to benefit. However, pregnant women are advised to avoid jumping and jerky movements because of joint instability. Vigorous exercise is not recommended during hot humid weather or if the mother has a fever. It is suggested that heart rate should not exceed 140 beats per minute, strenuous exercise should be done for less than 15 min at a time and a pregnant woman should not allow herself to become breathless. A pregnant woman should stop physical exercise if pain, vaginal bleeding or dizziness is experienced or there are known risk factors.

in increased flow during pregnancy. The increased flow to the uterus is about 500 mL/min more than that to the non-pregnant uterus but changes in uterine flow occur relatively late in pregnancy (de Swiet, 1998a). In rare situations of maternal cardiac arrest in late pregnancy, the altered blood flow will affect the ability of external cardiac massage to provide vital organ oxygenation. In such situations, immediate delivery of the infant must be considered either by perimortum caesarean section or an instrumental delivery if in the second stage of labour. Once delivered, the empty uterus will contract down enabling more blood to enter the central circulation improving oxygenation to the vital organs (Lewis, 2007).

Blood flow to the kidneys increases by about 400 mL/min from early pregnancy, facilitating elimination of waste products. Vasodilatory prostaglandins are implicated in the peripheral vasodilation, which is particularly evident in the vessels of the breasts, hands and face. Oestrogen and progesterone depress the normal response to angiotensin II and oestrogen abrogates the vasoconstriction mediated by the sympathetic nervous system. Blood flow to the lungs increases, reflecting the increased circulating blood volume and cardiac output. Distribution of blood to the skin is greatly increased (by about 500 mL/min) expediting heat loss. It is common for pregnant women to complain of being hot. Pregnant women usually have warm hands and feet and often complain that midwives' hands are cold. This vasodilatory effect is enhanced in smokers. Blood flow to the hands increases about sevenfold giving a very marked increase in skin temperature. The resulting peripheral vasodilation causes the capillaries to dilate and stimulates angiogenesis, and may give rise to the development of vascular spiders and palmar erythema, which is often associated with burning sensations (Henry et al., 2006). The increased blood flow means there is a decreased tendency to arteriolar spasm, and therefore conditions such as Raynaud's syndrome are abolished.

The increased blood flow to the skin stimulates the growth of nails and hair. The ratio of actively growing hair to resting (prior to falling out) hair is altered from 85:15 to 95:5 (de Swiet, 1998a). When this ratio returns to normal in the puerperium, vast amounts of hair can be lost. Mammary blood flow also increases (see Chapter 16). Coronary blood flow probably increases, reflecting the increased workload of the left ventricle, but it is thought that hepatic and cerebral blood flow do not significantly increase (de Swiet, 1998a).

In evolutionary terms, heat dissipation from the mucous membranes had been very important in mammals (this is best illustrated by dogs panting to lose heat). The increased flow to the mucous membranes in pregnancy can result in an increased congestion of the mucosa, which is demonstrated by an increased incidence of sinusitis, nosebleeds and snoring in pregnancy. It is suggested that elimination of waste products by the kidneys and heat by the skin is best fulfilled by an increased plasma volume rather than an increase in whole blood, which demonstrates the importance of the apparent physiological anaemia.

Haematological changes

The changes in maternal blood volume and composition increase the efficiency of the transplacental circulation and exchange mechanisms, thus benefiting fetal development. The haematological changes are also part of a maternal adaptive response that protects maternal homeostasis, including the ability to tolerate a sudden blood loss and to cope with placental separation. Thus, even women who have a degree of iron deficiency prior to pregnancy are protected from some decrease in haemoglobin levels at delivery. However, the adaptive responses to pregnancy potentiate the risks of iron-deficiency anaemia, thrombo-embolism and other clotting problems.

Plasma volume and blood cell mass/number

Pregnancy is a state of hypervolaemia. Blood volume increases in healthy pregnant women by about 1.5 L (30–50%, with a range of individual variation). Plasma volume increases initially rapidly from about 6 weeks' gestation and then the rate of increase becomes slower (Blackburn, 2007). The 40–50% increase in plasma volume is not matched by increased red blood cell mass and plasma protein production so there is a haemodilution (an apparent decrease) in haemoglobin and plasma protein concentration. Red blood cell mass increases by about 15–18% in women who do not take iron supplements and by about 25–33% in women supplemented with iron (Blackburn, 2007). The differences in plasma volume and red blood cell mass are accentuated by differential timing of the increases. Red blood cell mass begins to expand in the second trimester and the rate peaks in the third trimester. The maternal RAS may be involved; angiotensinogen competes for the erythropoietin receptors and may be a precursor of erythropoietin.

The increase in blood volume is higher in multigravidae and women who are obese, have multiple pregnancies or where the pregnancy is prolonged. The increment in plasma volume is positively correlated with birth weight and placental weight; pregnancies resulting in recurrent abortions, stillborn and low-birth-weight babies are associated with an abnormally low increase in plasma volume and an apparent increase (or no normal decrease) in haemoglobin concentration.

There is no reason for the relationship between plasma volume and blood cell mass, which are controlled by different mechanisms, to be retained throughout the pregnancy. The role of plasma is to fill the vascular space, maintaining the blood pressure, and to dissipate heat. Calculations suggest that the hypervolaemia is adequate to fill the increased vascular space of the pregnant uterus

and the enlarged vascular beds of the breasts, muscles, kidneys and skin and to provide a reservoir against the pooling of blood in the lower extremities. It will also decrease the effect of the haemoglobin lost in bleeding at delivery. The decreased viscosity of the blood lessens the resistance to flow and therefore the cardiac effort required to propel the blood. Observation of a 'normal' (prepregnant) or increased haemoglobin level (rather than a lower level seen in healthy pregnancies) may therefore represent an unsatisfactory increase in plasma volume rather than a true increase in haemoglobin concentration. Levels of haemoglobin are at their lowest between 16 and 22 weeks. The assertion that a degree of haemodilution is normal and a requisite adaptation to pregnancy, rather than indicating pathological anaemia, is supported by the increased AV difference (see above).

Most of the increase in blood cell mass is in the form of red blood cells. An initial depression of erythropoietin levels occurs, but progesterone, prolactin and hPL all stimulate erythropoietin synthesis and so promote red blood cell production; however, red blood cell mass correlates best with hPL levels. These influences result in mild hyperplasia of the bone marrow and an increased reticulocyte count. The function of red blood cells is oxygen transport; therefore red blood cell mass will increase physiologically at high altitude and decrease with prolonged bed rest. In pregnancy, the increment in red blood cells should reflect the need for more oxygen; the estimated increased requirement to supply the increased maternal tissues and conceptus is 15.0–16.5%, which is slightly lower than the measured rise of 18%.

Levels of 2,3-DPG (2,3-diphosphoglycerate) increase from early pregnancy so the oxygen–haemoglobin dissociation curve shifts to the right (see Chapter 1) thus facilitating oxygen unloading at the peripheral tissues. Red blood cells become more spherical, with an increased diameter and thickness, because plasma colloid pressure falls and thus more water crosses the erythrocyte membrane by osmosis.

Iron status

As plasma volume increases, haemoglobin concentration and haematocrit fall, reaching a lowest point at 16–22 weeks (Blackburn, 2007). The World Health Organization recommends that haemoglobin concentration should not fall below 11 g/dL at any point in pregnancy; others suggest it should not fall below 10 g/dL. If iron stores can be demonstrated not to be depleted, it would suggest that the decreased haemoglobin concentration is not attributable to iron deficiency. In pregnancy, the most accurate and appropriate method of determining iron status and anaemia is measurement of serum ferritin levels. Serum ferritin, the major iron-storage protein, becomes depleted before clinical indicators reveal anaemia. Serum ferritin is stable, is not affected by recent ingestion of iron and quantitatively reflects iron stores, particularly in the lower range. Serum ferritin levels of less than 50 g/L in early pregnancy indicate a need for iron supplementation and levels above 80 g/L are probably adequate to protect the woman from iron depletion. However, routine iron supplementation in pregnancy, of apparently healthy women with no apparent iron deficiency, results in red blood cells increasing by 30% rather than by 18% in unsupplemented women (Letsky, 1998). One method of assessing anaemia in non-pregnant subjects is by observing an increased red blood cell mass in response to increased iron supplementation (Yip and Dallman, 1996).

The need for routine iron supplementation in pregnancy is a controversial area (Haram et al., 2001). Letsky (1998) argues strongly that clinical indicators of anaemia are not sensitive enough to demonstrate iron deficiency in practice. Iron depletion causes a reduction in mean blood cell volume (MCV). However, increased erythropoiesis results in a higher proportion of young larger red blood cells, which tends to mask the effect of iron deficiency on cell volume even with established anaemia.

Although the amenorrhoea of pregnancy helps to conserve iron stores and absorption of dietary iron increases, the theoretical requirement of iron in pregnancy can probably be met only if the woman has good iron stores prior to conception. Letsky argues that, although pregnancy is a physiological state, many women enter pregnancy with insufficient iron stores to supply the high requirements particularly of the third trimester. However, maternal iron absorption increases by about fivefold in the second trimester of pregnancy and by about ninefold in the third trimester (Barrett et al., 1994) suggesting that absorption of iron increases in parallel with the increased requirement. Active transport of iron across the placenta is maximal in the last 4 weeks of pregnancy. The inadequacy of dietary iron may be related to the move away from the Palaeolithic iron-rich diet that was normal for most of human evolution to a cereal-based one with less meat and fish (Cordain et al., 2002). Although most of the body's iron is associated with haemoglobin, iron is also a component of the electron transport chain. Tissue enzyme malfunction occurs in the first stages of iron deficiency before significant anaemia is apparent and supplements can increase perceptions of well-being. Subclinical degrees of iron deficiency may adversely affect maternal exercise tolerance, cerebral function and well-being (Letsky, 1998). Offspring of iron-deficient mothers may have reduced iron stores and are at risk of infantile anaemia, which may affect their mental and motor development and have long-term consequences. Maternal iron-deficiency anaemia correlates with high placental fetal weight, suggesting fetal growth is impaired (see Chapter 9). Low birth weight and high placental fetal weight have been associated with hypertension in adult life (Godfrey et al., 1991), so iron-deficiency anaemia in pregnancy may have long-lasting and far-reaching effects. Concerns have been expressed about iron supplementation in early pregnancy (Weinberg, 2010) when iron demands are low because the embryo is so small and the increase in red blood cell mass can be met by iron 'savings' from menstrual loss having ceased. The placental circulation during the embryonic period creates an environment which is relatively hypoxic (see Chapter 8) so excess iron which can induce oxidative stress could potentially pose a teratogenic risk to the embryo at a period of maximum susceptibility. In addition, it is argued that iron loading could increase the risk of maternal gestational diabetes and pre-eclampsia (Weinberg, 2009).

Haemostasis

Pregnancy is a hypercoagulable state. Bleeding time in pregnancy decreases by about 30% because the ratio of clotting and fibrinolytic factors alters. There is an increase in fibrinogen and other clotting factors leading to an increased generation of thrombin and a decrease in fibrinolytic or anticoagulant substances (for instance protein S activity decreases and resistance develops to activated protein C). The number of platelets decreases slightly towards term but generally remains within the non-pregnant range. This response is variable; there may be increased platelet turnover and low-grade platelet activation (an increased number of aggregated platelets) as the pregnancy progresses, resulting in a larger proportion of younger platelets with increased volume. Low-grade chronic intravascular coagulation in the uteroplacental circulation may be part of the normal physiological response to pregnancy. Platelet count is further decreased in pregnancies with fetal growth retardation, and even in mild pre-eclampsia the lifespan of platelets is reduced.

Synthesis of antithrombin III (the main physiological inhibitor of thrombin and factor Xa) increases in pregnancy in parallel with the increased plasma volume. Levels decrease at delivery (thus increasing the tendency to thrombosis) and increase 1 week postpartum. There is a general increase in clotting factors, particularly in late pregnancy, as demonstrated in Von Willebrand's syndrome (an inherited clotting disorder), which improves with pregnancy. The change in amount of clotting factors seems to be compensatory in preparation for labour. The overall effect is hypercoagulability which is augmented by venous stasis of the lower limbs (Holmes and Wallace, 2005). The hypercoagulability is optimal in labour, meeting the demands of placental separation but can increase the risks of thrombosis and disseminated intravascular coagulation. At delivery, total blood loss can be as much as 500 mL. The normal blood flow of 500–800 mL/min is staunched within seconds (aided by myometrial contraction, which decreases blood flow and rapidly closes spiral arteries). A fibrin mesh then rapidly covers the placental site as 5–10% of the total circulating fibrinogen is deposited. Fibrinolytic activity decreases in pregnancy and remains low in labour. It returns to normal within an hour of delivery; the placenta produces inhibitors that block fibrinolysis. Most of the physiological changes in pregnancy are reversed quickly in the puerperium; however, the hypercoagulable state may exist for much longer (possibly over 6 weeks). This puts the woman in the early postnatal period at a higher risk of developing deep vein thrombosis and pulmonary embolism from changes that occur in the antenatal period.

Table 11.1 summarizes the haematological changes in pregnancy.

Table 11.1 Summary of haematological changes in pregnancy

	CHANGE IN PREGNANCY	NOTES
Plasma volume correlates	Increases by about 50% from 2600 to 3900 mL	More in second and subsequent pregnancies; with birth weight
Red blood cell mass	Increases by about 18%	Increase is greater with iron supplementation (to 30%)
Neutrophil count	Both cell number and metabolic activity increase	Initial increase occurs early in pregnancy and is similar to the response to other physiological stresses
Plasma proteins	Decrease	Decreased osmotic pressure predisposes to oedema
Clotting factors	Increase	Fibrinolytic factors decrease
Platelet count	Slight fall	Coagulability increases

THE RESPIRATORY SYSTEM

Maternal respiratory effort has to be increased in pregnancy to meet the increased metabolic demands of the maternal and fetal tissues. By the end of the pregnancy, 16–20% more oxygen is consumed. The respiratory system is also affected by the expanding uterine volume. In terms of physiological reserve, the stress put on the respiratory system by pregnancy is small compared with the increases that can be measured on exercise (Table 11.2). This contrasts with the much larger proportion of the cardiovascular physiological reserve required in pregnancy. The clinical implication of this is that patients with respiratory disease are much less likely to deteriorate in pregnancy than are those with cardiac disease.

Anatomy

Early in pregnancy, and therefore not secondary to pressure from the uterus, the diaphragm is displaced upwards by 4 cm (de Swiet, 1998b; Fig. 11.7). The respiratory excursion of the diaphragm increases and there is an increased flaring of the lower ribs (increasing the substernal angle from 68° to 103° by late pregnancy; Blackburn, 2007). This compensatory increase in the diameter of the thorax by about 2 cm (the circumference of the chest increases by about 15 cm) means that the volume of the thoracic cavity is about the same as that before pregnancy. The diaphragm performs the major work of respiration; the breathing is thoracic rather than abdominal. Hormonal influences cause the muscles and cartilage in the thoracic region to relax so the chest broadens. The subsequent decrease in chest wall compliance means the thoracic wall can move further inwards so there is less trapped air and the residual volume decreases. These anatomical changes probably do not completely reverse after the pregnancy (indeed it is said that the increased flaring of the rib cage is beneficial to opera singers after pregnancy).

Progesterone is a respiratory stimulant; it lowers the sensitivity of the peripheral and central chemoreceptors for carbon dioxide (Prabhakar and Peng, 2004). This means that respiratory drive is stimulated at lower carbon dioxide levels so pregnant women breathe more deeply. As

---

Table 11.2 Pregnancy and physiological reserve

PARAMETER	NORMAL	PREGNANCY	% INCREASE	EXERCISE	% INCREASE
Minute volume	7.5 L/min	10.5 L/min	40	80 L/min	1000
Oxygen consumption	220 mL/min	255 mL/min	16		
Cardiac output	4.5 L/min	6 L/min	30	12 L/min	

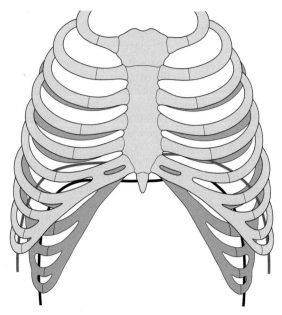

Fig. 11.7 Displacement of the diaphragm in pregnancy: the ribcage in pregnancy (light) and the non-pregnancy state (dark), showing the increased subcostal angle, the increased transverse diameter and the raised diaphragm in pregnancy.

progesterone increases during the pregnancy, the increased responsiveness to PCO_2 results in an increased tidal volume and therefore minute volume (Table 11.3). So hyperventilation (increased tidal volume) is normal in pregnancy. Oxygen consumption increases but arterial oxygen pressure does not change.

In pregnancy, the respiratory rate is unchanged but minute ventilation increases by 40% because tidal volume increases; this is apparent as early as 7 weeks. This hyperventilation exceeds the increased oxygen consumption. Efficiency of alveolar gas exchange is much more efficient when tidal volume is increased rather than respiratory rate (Fig. 11.8). Alveolar ventilation is further enhanced by the decrease in residual volume. About 150 mL of an inspired breath remains in the upper airways where no gas exchange takes place (this is known as the anatomical dead space). Although the dead space increases by about 60 mL in pregnancy because of dilatation of the smaller bronchioles, the net alveolar ventilation is increased. The increased tidal volume means that the functional residual capacity is reduced, thus an increased volume of fresh air mixes with a much smaller residual volume of air remaining in the lungs. Alveolar ventilation in pregnancy is thus increased by about 70% resulting in increased efficiency of mixing of gases, which facilitates gas exchange because the diffusion

gradient is bigger. The increased gradient of carbon dioxide concentrations between maternal and fetal blood aids transfer of carbon dioxide across the placenta and may be particularly important in adverse circumstances. Progesterone increases carbonic anhydrase levels in red blood cells (see Chapter 1) thus further increasing the efficiency of carbon dioxide transfer.

Maternal partial pressures of oxygen increase slightly (from 95–100 to 101–106 mmHg) and levels of carbon dioxide decrease (from 35–40 to 26–34 mmHg). The small increase in PO_2 has little effect on haemoglobin saturation. Posture, however, affects alveolar oxygen levels: a supine position in late pregnancy results in a lower alveolar oxygen pressure than when in a sitting position. This change in alveolar oxygenation is probably not significant for the fetus although it may be compensatory at high altitude. Air travel is associated with increased dyspnoea and respiratory rate. The decreased level of carbon dioxide in pregnancy results in a mild respiratory alkalosis. The change in pH affects levels of circulatory cations such as sodium, potassium and calcium, aiding transfer across the placenta and increasing provision for fetal growth. Metabolic compensation to the relative alkalosis occurs by increasing renal excretion of bicarbonate ions. The resulting fall in serum bicarbonate, which limits the buffering capacity in pregnant women, causes maternal pH levels to increase to the upper end of the normal physiological range, from 7.40 to 7.45. Maternal ability to compensate further for metabolic acidosis is therefore limited, which may create problems in prolonged labour or where there is inadequate tissue perfusion (see Chapter 13).

Progesterone has a local effect on the smooth muscle tone of the airways and the pulmonary blood vessels and decreases airway resistance. Diffusion capacity is the ease with which gases can cross the pulmonary membranes. In early pregnancy, diffusion capacity decreases probably because of the effects of oestrogen on the composition of the mucopolysaccharides of the capillary walls, which increases diffusion distance (de Swiet, 1998b). This effect may last for months after delivery. Increased water retention in the pulmonary tissues also results in a decrease in diffusion capacity. There is an increased closing volume suggesting that the calibre of the small airways is decreased; this may be due to increased lung fluid. The decreased efficiency of pulmonary gas transfer is partially compensated for by progesterone-induced relaxation of bronchiole smooth muscle, which decreases airway resistance. The decreased airway resistance means that air flow is increased. Prostaglandins also affect bronchiole smooth muscle. $PGF_{2\alpha}$, which increases throughout the pregnancy, is a smooth muscle constrictor; PGE_1 and PGE_2, which increase in the third trimester, are smooth muscle dilators. The work of breathing is

Table 11.3 Lung volumes and capacities

PARAMETER	DEFINITION	NORMAL RANGE	CHANGE IN PREGNANCY
Tidal volume (TV)	Volume of a normal breath at rest	500 mL	Increases by 150–200 mL (25–40%) 75% increase occurs within first trimester
Respiratory rate (RR)	Number of breaths per minute	12 breaths/min	Unchanged/slightly increased to 15 breaths/min
Minute volume (MV)	Total air taken in 1 min of respiration (= TV × RR)	6000 mL/min 6.5 L/min	Increased by about 40% 10 L/min
Inspiratory reserve volume (IRV)	Volume of air that can be inspired above the resting tidal volume	3100 mL	Unchanged
Expiratory reserve volume (ERV)	Volume of gas that can be expired in addition to the tidal volume	1200 mL	Reduces progressively from early pregnancy to about 1100 mL
Residual volume (RV)	Volume of gas remaining in the lungs after a maximal expiration	1200 mL	Decreases progressively
Total lung capacity (TLC)	Maximum volume of the lungs (= TV + IRV + ERV + dead space)	6000 mL	Unchanged
Vital capacity (VC)	Total volume of gas that can be moved in and out of the lungs (= TLC − residual volume)	4800 mL	Increased 100–200 mL in late pregnancy? (not apparent in obese women)
Inspiratory capacity	Total inspiratory ability of the lungs (= IRC + TV)	2200 mL	Increased about 2500 mL at term
Functional residual capacity (FRC)	Volume of gas remaining in the lungs after a resting breath (= ERV + RV)	2800 mL	Decreases progressively to 2300 mL – increases mixing efficiency
Residual volume (RV)	Volume of gas remaining after a maximal expiration (= FRC − ERV)	2400 mL	
Physiological dead space			Increases by ~60 mL
Alveolar ventilation	Difference between TV and volume of physiological dead space		Increased

probably unchanged as the decreased airway resistance compensates for the congestion in the bronchial wall capillaries.

Many pregnant women experience dyspnoea, causing discomfort and anxiety, often early in pregnancy before there are changes in intra-abdominal pressure. This correlates well with PCO_2 and may be due to hyperventilation (de Swiet, 1998b). Capillaries in the upper respiratory tract become engorged, which can create difficulties in breathing via the nose and aggravate respiratory infections. Laryngeal changes and oedema of the vocal cords caused by vascular dilation can promote hoarseness and deepening of the voice, and a persistent cough. In severe cases, these changes in laryngeal thickening may cause complications should endotracheal intubation be necessary, for instance in anaesthesia. Forced expiratory volume

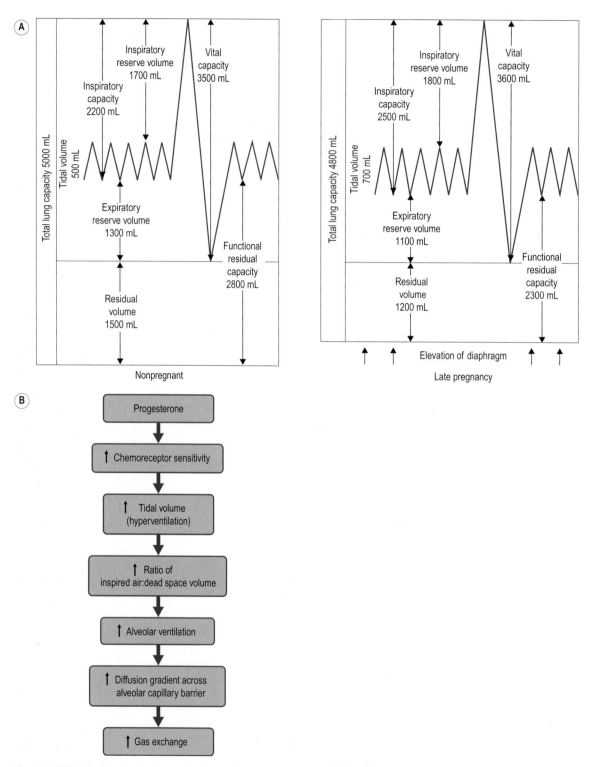

Fig. 11.8 (A) Alteration in alveolar gas exchange during pregnancy, and (B) its mechanisms.

over 1 s and peak flow rate are not usually affected in pregnancy.

In labour, pain causes an increase in tidal volume and respiratory rate (these effects are abolished by effective epidural anaesthesia). In the second stage, muscle demands result in metabolic acidosis (increased lactate and pyruvate production); this is countered to a degree by the respiratory alkalosis from hyperventilation (Blackburn, 2007). Pregnant and recently delivered women with identified respiratory risk factors or complications should have their respiratory rates monitored because increased respiratory rate can be an early indicator of physical deterioration. Oxygen saturation monitoring should not be used in place of observing respiratory rate because a drop in SaO_2 is usually a late sign of physical deterioration. SaO_2 will often be normal in the presence of a raised respiratory rate as this initial compensatory effect maintains adequate oxygenation. If the respiratory rate is raised, SaO_2 monitoring should be used so that interventions such as oxygen therapy are observed to be effective in preventing further deterioration (Lewis, 2007).

THE RENAL SYSTEM

Increased urinary frequency, leakage and nocturia are so common that they are considered a 'normal' part of physiological adaptation to pregnancy; urinary tract infections (UTIs) are also relatively common. The marked haemodynamic and hormonal changes in pregnancy cause renal function to be altered. During pregnancy, the kidneys increase excretion of waste products in response to the increase in maternal and fetal metabolism, and retention of fluid and electrolytes is altered in response to cardiovascular changes. It is generally accepted that the increased circulating blood volume and haemodilution in pregnancy are achieved by the kidneys increasing their tubular reabsorption rate of sodium. The retention of sodium is stimulated by deoxycorticosterone derived from progesterone. Fluid retention is facilitated by the action of angiotensin II (see above for description of the RAS). Oestrogen increases both angiotensinogen production and renin production. ADH secretion tends to be triggered at lower plasma osmolality during pregnancy, possibly affected by hCG levels (Blackburn, 2007). Likewise, the osmotic threshold for thirst decreases from early pregnancy.

The gross anatomy of the renal system is altered in pregnancy. The kidneys enlarge, by about 1 cm in length and by about 30% in volume, owing to an increase in renal blood flow and vascular volume (Jeyabalan and Lain, 2007). Alterations in both prolactin, prostaglandin and relaxin levels have effects on renal blood flow (Baylis and Davison, 1998). The increased renal blood flow, due to haemodilution and hormonal changes, results in an increased GFR from early pregnancy. The increased GFR results in more sodium, glucose and amino acids in the filtrate; however, tubular reabsorption also increases so most of the increased sodium load is reabsorbed. The sodium retention results in water accumulation. The increase in GFR also results in a fall in serum creatine and urea levels so a 'normal' non-pregnant level of serum creatinine (of 1 mg/dL) may indicate renal impairment in pregnancy (Maynard and Thadhani, 2009) or other conditions associated with a lack of plasma volume expansion such as pre-eclampsia (Jeyabalan and Lain, 2007). Assessment of proteinuria is also important in indicating pre-eclampsia and in the care of pregnant women with pre-existing kidney disease. Pregnancy is more becoming more common in kidney transplant recipients as fertility increases markedly after transplantation. The outcome of pregnancy in women with chronic kidney disease (CKD), who have mild renal impairment, little proteinuria and normal blood pressure, is good, though more severe CKD is a risk for preterm delivery and pre-eclampsia. Routine antenatal care includes dipstick protein testing of a random urine sample to monitor proteinuria. Although this screening method has a high incidence of false-negative and false-positive results, it is much less cumbersome than a 24-h urine collection which can be inaccurate if there is undercollection (Maynard and Thadhani, 2009).

The tendency for pregnant women to become insulin-resistant in the latter part of pregnancy results in increased blood glucose. This, together with the increased GFR, results in increased glucose concentration of the filtrate, which together with an increased tubular flow rate, can mean that the maximum capacity for glucose reabsorption in the tubules is exceeded causing some glucose to be present in the urine (glucosuria). This does not necessarily indicate diabetes. Likewise mild proteinuria is common and benign in pregnancy, although with coexisting hypertension it can indicate complications of pre-eclampsia.

There is a cumulative retention of sodium and potassium especially in the last trimester when fetal demands for sodium are high. Urinary excretion of calcium increases but free calcium levels remain stable as dietary absorption of calcium increases. Acid–base balance is also altered in pregnancy (Baylis and Davison, 1998). Hydrogen ions fall slightly primarily because of respiratory alkalaemia associated with hyperventilation. Although systemic blood pressure may be reduced, autoregulation (local control of glomerular blood pressure) maintains optimal renal function.

The calyces of the kidneys and the ureters become dilated and lose some of their peristaltic activity in pregnancy. The ureters elongate and become tortuous so they accommodate an increased volume of urine, which is associated with an increased risk of infection. It was generally accepted that this dilation of the ureters was primarily due to the action of progesterone on smooth muscle. However, the ovarian arteries and veins increase in size and compress the ureters, particularly on the right side where the vessels cross over the ureter almost at right-angles, whereas on the left they run approximately parallel to the ureter. This, together with the stress imposed on the ureters by the expanding uterus upon the pelvic brim, explains the extent of these morphological changes.

Bladder function is also affected in pregnancy. Urinary frequency and urgency increase early in pregnancy as the enlarging uterus in the pelvic cavity puts pressure on the bladder; fluid intake is also higher. At term, when engagement occurs, the presenting part of the fetus increases stress on the bladder. In the second trimester, the bladder is displaced upwards so urinary frequency is closer to prepregnant levels. Urinary incontinence is also relatively common in pregnancy (FitzGerald and Graziano, 2007) and may negatively affect quality of life. Under the effect of progesterone, bladder tone decreases during pregnancy so its capacity increases and may be up to a litre by term. The decreased bladder tone and displacement of the ureters by the enlarging uterus can affect competence of the vesicoureteral sphincters (valves created by the normal oblique angle of entry of the ureters into the bladder wall become compromised as the entry of the ureters tends to be perpendicular). The result is possible reflux of urine from the bladder into the ureters, which increases the chance of ascending urinary infection, which if severe, can cause infection of the kidney (pyelonephritis). Urinary retention is not common in pregnancy but classically it occurs at the end of the first trimester; there are several predisposing factors for urinary retention including a retroverted uterus, uterine fibroids, uterine anomalies and a contracted pelvis (FitzGerald and Graziano, 2007).

The walls of the bladder become more oedematous and hyperaemic, which increases the vulnerability to infection and trauma. The relatively lax walls of the bladder may also result in incomplete emptying of urine. This urinary stasis increases the risk of a UTI as the urine, which is richer in glucose and amino acids in pregnancy, remains in the bladder allowing the usually harmless number of bacteria in the urine to reach pathological levels. Women with UTI are thought to be at increased risk of premature labour. As the pregnancy progresses the effect of posture on renal function becomes exacerbated. The structural changes of the renal system persist into the puerperium (see Chapter 14) and women who have experienced a UTI during pregnancy are at increased risk of recurrent infection in the puerperium. Women who have a positive result for Group B Streptococcal B infection (colloquially known as 'strep B') during antenatal screening do not normally need antibiotic therapy in the antenatal period unless a UTI develops. A UTI in these circumstances indicates an exceptionally high bacterial load which increases

Case study 11.3

Penny is expecting her second child at 24 weeks' gestation and presents herself at the maternity day assessment unit. Two days previously, Penny noticed her frequency of micturition had dramatically increased. Since then she has felt lower central abdominal pain radiating from the groin round to the right side of her back. The midwife suspects that Penny may have a UTI. A provisional diagnosis is made on ward-based urinalysis that indicates the presence of leukocytes and nitrites.

- What is the significance of these findings and why do they indicate the presence of an infection?

The midwife instructs Penny on how to provide a midstream specimen of urine (MSU) and requests that the duty doctor examine Penny. Penny is prescribed a course of antibiotics with the proviso that this may be changed if the laboratory tests indicate that the antibiotic is inappropriate.

- How could the midwife describe to Penny the reasons why the UTI has occurred?
- What else besides taking the antibiotics could the midwife advise Penny to do to (a) help resolve the infection now and (b) avoid further infection in the future?
- What are the risks and possible consequences if the infection is not treated?

the risk of transmission to the fetus during birth so should be treated (RCOG, 2003).

Case study 11.3 details an example of a urogenital tract infection.

THE GASTROINTESTINAL SYSTEM

Maternal nutrition is very important in the outcome of pregnancy but disturbances of gastrointestinal function are the most common cause of complaints in pregnancy (Fig. 11.9). Over 50% of women experience an increased appetite (and consequent increased consumption of food) and even more an increased thirst. hCG affects the hypothalamus decreasing the osmotic threshold for thirst. The changes are most marked in the first half of pregnancy; subsequently they may decline although some persist, albeit to a lesser extent. Surveys have measured an increased intake of food and drink in pregnant women although not all of them are conscious of these changes (Hytten, 1991). Changes in maternal appetite do not directly reflect changes in fetal growth or maternal metabolism. Appetite tends to be increased in early pregnancy and may be promoted by several hormones including leptin. Leptin usually suppresses food intake but in pregnancy, leptin levels increase because hormonally induced central leptin resistance develops (Grattan et al., 2007).

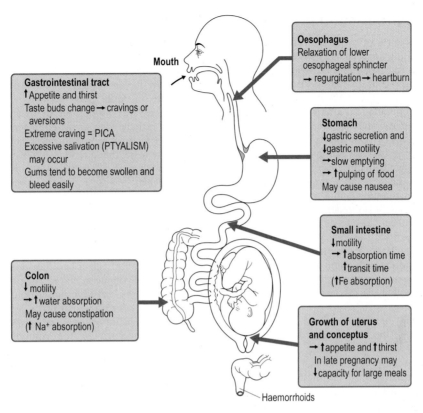

Mouth

Oesophagus
Relaxation of lower
oesophageal sphincter
→ regurgitation → heartburn

Gastrointestinal tract
↑Appetite and thirst
Taste buds change → cravings or
   aversions
Extreme craving = PICA
Excessive salivation (PTYALISM)
   may occur
Gums tend to become swollen and
   bleed easily

Stomach
↓gastric secretion and
↓gastric motility
→slow emptying
→ ↑pulping of food
May cause nausea

Small intestine
↓motility
→ ↑absorption time
   ↑transit time
   (↑Fe absorption)

Colon
↓ motility
→ ↑water absorption
May cause constipation
(↑ Na⁺ absorption)

**Growth of uterus
and conceptus**
→ ↑appetite and ↑thirst
In late pregnancy may
↓capacity for large meals

Haemorrhoids

Fig. 11.9 Gastrointestinal function in pregnancy.

This means that despite the raised levels of leptin, food intake and thus fat deposition are increased. In advanced pregnancy, both appetite and the capacity for food intake decline owing to upward gastric displacement and pressure from the gravid uterus. A pregnant woman can compensate for her limited capacity by increasing the frequency of consumption of small meals and snacks. Oestrogen suppresses appetite but progesterone stimulates it, causing a shift in the central control of energy balance. Decreased plasma glucose and amino acid levels, which are secondary to increased responsiveness to insulin, also stimulate appetite. Cyclical patterns of appetite are also observed during the menstrual cycle. Thirst is increased; progesterone resets the thirst threshold by 10 mOsm so plasma osmolarity falls. Increased angiotensin, prolactin and relaxin levels are also dipsogenic.

Food cravings and aversions

Changes in food habits can be deliberate, for instance avoiding fried or fatty foods that are considered less healthy. Two-thirds of pregnant women express marked food preferences as cravings or aversions. The commonest cravings are for fruit and highly flavoured foods such as pickles, kippers and cheese. It is suggested that the sensitivity of the taste buds is dulled in pregnancy (Bowen, 1992) so highly seasoned foods are more appreciated. Unsatisfied cravings are often thought to explain food-shaped birthmarks (King, 2000). Common aversions are to tea and coffee, meat, fried foods and eggs and to caffeinated drinks, alcohol and smoking. Food cravings and aversions need to be assessed as part of a full dietary assessment; they do not necessarily have an adverse effect on dietary quality. Usually cravings cause an increase in energy and calcium intakes and aversions frequently result in decreased intake of alcohol, coffee and animal protein.

Pica, an extreme craving usually for a non-nutritious substance, has been identified for coal, soap, disinfectant, toothpaste, mothballs and ice. Usually pica does not affect either maternal or fetal health. In the southern states of America, there seems to be a social tradition of Black women eating laundry starch, chalk and clay. Sense of smell may be enhanced; pregnant women are especially sensitive to noxious smells such as nicotine and coffee. The timing of the changes in taste and smell appears to reflect secretion of hCG.

Nausea and vomiting in pregnancy

Between 50% and 90% of pregnant women experience nausea and vomiting in pregnancy (NVP), usually in the first trimester although 20% of women experience NVP throughout gestation. It may be the first physical manifestation of pregnancy. NVP is more common in Westernized urban populations and is affected by ethnicity, occupational status and maternal age (Coad et al., 2000). The peak of NVP is usually at about 8–12 weeks; symptoms usually resolve by mid-pregnancy. Although about 50% of women suffering from NVP are affected to a greater extent in the morning, some women experience nausea and vomiting in the evening, in a biphasic pattern or throughout the day. It is thought that women who are underweight experience less severe symptoms of NVP compared to women with normal preconceptual weight (Huxley, 2000). NVP does not necessarily mean that nutrient intake is decreased. Some women eat more as continual snacking alleviates symptoms and others alter their diet in a way that usually improves dietary quality (Coad et al., 2002).

There are several theories about the causes of NVP. Serum hCG peaks in the first trimester but the relationship between NVP and hCG secretion is not clearly established. The effects of progesterone on gastric smooth muscle tone, particularly those on upper gastrointestinal tract motility, the patency of the lower oesophageal sphincter and delayed gastric emptying, suggest a possible role for steroid hormones. NVP is usually conservatively treated with rest and reassurance and advice to consume frequent small meals rich in easily digested carbohydrate and low in fat (King and Murphy, 2009). Meat and strong smells may aggravate NVP. It has been suggested that NVP is an evolutionary mechanism that protects the embryo by causing pregnant women to physically expel and subsequently avoid foods that might contain teratogenic and abortifacient chemicals (Flaxman and Sherman, 2000). An alternative explanation is that NVP has a functional role in stimulating early placental growth by reducing maternal energy intake and suppressing maternal tissue synthesis in early pregnancy so nutrient partitioning favours the developing placenta (Huxley, 2000). Although NVP may have a socioeconomic impact and create much misery, it is considered to be favourable prognostic sign and is associated with a positive outcome of pregnancy (Coad et al., 2002). Intractable and persistent nausea and vomiting causing dehydration, electrolyte imbalance (hypokalaemia), metabolic disturbances (ketonuria) and nutritional deficiencies is known as hyperemesis gravidarum (HG). This may require hospitalization to correct the electrolyte and fluid imbalances. Risk factors for HG include previous HG, hyperthyroid disorders, pre-existing psychiatric diagnosis, molar pregnancy, gastrointestinal disorders, and multiple gestation with a female and male twin (King and Murphy, 2009).

Mouth

Gums often become hyperaemic, oedematous and spongy. This is because of the effects of oestrogen on blood flow and connective tissue consistency. Gums therefore bleed more easily and are vulnerable to abrasive food and vigorous tooth brushing. Gingivitis and periodontal disease occur in a large proportion of pregnant women and are more extreme with increased maternal age and parity and where there are pre-existing dental problems. Contrary to folklore belief that a tooth is lost for every baby, there is no evidence of demineralization of dentine resulting from pregnancy as fetal calcium stores are drawn from maternal body stores (skeleton) and not from maternal teeth (Blackburn, 2007). However, there is an increase in the number of caries treated during pregnancy. This may be because gum changes result in an increased awareness of dental problems and many women receive free dental care in pregnancy. Saliva becomes more acidic in pregnancy, but the volume produced does not usually change. In rare instances, excessive production of saliva, termed ptyalism or ptyalorrhoea, may occur. It can occur in isolation or in association with HG, where swallowing of saliva induces extreme nausea and vomiting in an affected woman.

Oesophagus

Heartburn, a painful retrosternal burning sensation, is common in pregnancy, affecting 30–70% women. The effects of progesterone on the tone of the lower oesophageal sphincter mean its competence is impaired and regurgitation of gastric acid is more likely. Similar changes occur during the menstrual cycle and in women taking combined oral contraceptive pills. These changes are associated with increased progesterone levels. The risk of a hiatus hernia is increased; the sphincter is displaced and becomes intrathoracic instead of straddling the diaphragm. This usually begins in the second trimester and worsens as the pregnancy progresses. It is due to progesterone-induced relaxation of the lower oesophageal sphincter and a change in pressure gradients across the stomach. The enlarging uterus causes distortion of the stomach and changes the angle of entry of the oesophagus. Because the patency of the pyloric sphincter may also be impaired, both alkaline and acidic secretions may reflux into the oesophagus.

Heartburn is increased with multiple pregnancies, polyhydramnios, obesity and excessive bending over. Alcohol, chocolate and coffee all act directly on the lower oesophageal sphincter, reducing the muscle tone and exacerbating heartburn. Gastric reflux can be limited by advising more frequent intake of smaller meals, the avoidance of seasoned food, and of postural influences such as lying horizontally or bending forwards. Antacid preparations are associated with a number of undesirable side-effects:

aluminium salts may cause diarrhoea, magnesium salts are associated with constipation, phosphorus may affect the calcium/phosphorus balance and exacerbate cramp, sodium may affect water balance and long-term use of antacids is associated with malabsorption, particularly of drugs and dietary minerals.

Stomach

Studies on gastric secretion in pregnancy are not conclusive but suggest acid secretion tends to decrease, which may explain why remission of symptoms of a peptic ulcer is not an uncommon event. Secretion of pepsin also falls; this is probably secondary to the decreased acid secretion. Studies have shown that stomach gastric tone and motility markedly decrease in pregnancy. Thus in advanced pregnancy the stomach drapes loosely over the uterine fundus. This tends to delay gastric emptying especially following ingestion of solid foods. The delay of chyme released from the stomach may increase the likelihood of heartburn and nausea and can result in delayed absorption of glucose.

Intestine and colon

Progesterone-induced relaxation of smooth muscle decreases gut tone and motility and thus transit time in the gut increases which may enhance absorption (Blackburn, 2007). However, pregnant women may experience bloating and abdominal distension. Duodenal villi hypertrophy and increase in height, which expands absorption capacity. Absorption of several nutrients, such as iron, calcium, glucose, amino acids, water, sodium and chloride is increased (Blackburn, 2007); the increased absorption of iron in late pregnancy coincides with raised placental uptake and decreased maternal stores. However, progesterone may inhibit transport mechanisms for other nutrients such as the B group of vitamins.

The relaxation of the smooth muscle in the colon leads to increased water absorption and increases the incidence of constipation (Case study 11.4). The raised levels of angiotensin and aldosterone also increase sodium and water absorption from the colon in pregnancy. As the enlarging uterus compresses the colon, many women experience increased flatulence.

Case study 11.4

Josie is 14 weeks pregnant and is suffering from constipation. She is a vegetarian and normally consumes a high-fibre diet.
- What physiological changes may account for her constipation?
- What advice could the midwife give to help alleviate this problem?

Liver and gall bladder

Progesterone affects the smooth muscle tone of the gall bladder resulting in flaccidity, increased bile volume storage and decreased emptying rate. Water resorption by the epithelium cells of the gall bladder is decreased so the bile is more dilute and contains less cholesterol. There is a tendency to retain bile salts resulting in the formation of cholesterol-based gallstones in pregnancy. Cholestasis is a condition often observed in late pregnancy where women complain of itchy and irritable skin (though no rash is present) because bile salts are deposited in the skin.

In many species, pregnancy-induced liver enlargement results from increased circulation. In humans, however, morphological changes appear to result from hepatic displacement by the gravid uterus rather than an actual growth increase. Increased glycogen and triacylglyceride storage occurs in the hepatic cells. The raised level of oestrogen affects hepatic synthesis of plasma proteins, enzymes and lipids. The most marked changes are the fall in albumin (which is exaggerated by haemodilution), increase in fibrinogen (see above) and increased cholesterol synthesis. Synthesis of many binding proteins involved with placental transport of nutrients increases. Although epigastric pain is common in pregnancy due to reflux of gastric contents through the lower oesophageal sphincter, it may be a symptom of severe complications such as fulminating pre-eclampsia caused by hepatic oedema.

Changes in the liver and other physiological systems can affect drug kinetics. Changes in gastric secretion and gut motility can affect absorption and bioavailability of drugs. Changes in the cardiovascular system such as plasma volume and protein binding changes can affect the apparent volume of distribution and changes in the renal system can affect drug elimination particularly increased renal excretion of drugs unchanged. Hepatic metabolism of drugs catalysed by certain isoenzymes are increased during pregnancy. Therefore pregnant women may require different dosing regimes (changes in dose and timing of the dose) of various drugs (Pavek et al., 2009).

THE SKIN AND APPEARANCE

A number of changes can be observed in the appearance of a pregnant woman (Box 11.7). The increase in MSH means that there is a progressive increase in skin pigmentation, especially in women with dark hair and complexions. The nipple and the areola darken early in pregnancy. A dark line develops from the navel to pubis; this is the linea nigra showing the embryonic folding and fusion line of the abdomen. Facial chloasma (melasma) – irregular blotchy pigmentation usually in the shape of a butterfly mask ('mask of pregnancy') around the eyes and forehead – is common. Freckles and recent scars may darken and many

Box 11.7 **Top-to-toe observation of a pregnant woman**

- Hair: thicker and glossier
- Face: may have chloasma and/or oedema
- Hands: warm, may develop vascular spiders and palmar erythema
- Skin: warm, well-vascularized, hyperpigmentation (related to MSH production)
- Skin conditions, such as eczema, may improve
- Abdominal wall: pigmentation of linea nigra, lax abdominal muscles, striae gravidarum may be seen (related to cortisol production)
- Pruritus (localized itching usually of abdomen): occurs in about 20% of pregnant women in the third trimester, but earlier in pregnancy it may be a sign of pruritus gravidarum (intrahepatic cholestasis of pregnancy due to raised bile acids), which is associated with premature delivery, fetal distress and perinatal mortality
- Breasts: dilation of superficial veins, pigmentation of nipples and areola
- Legs: oedema may be evident around ankles; varicose veins may develop
- Posture and gait: lordosis, changed centre of gravity (related to effects of hormones on cartilage and connective tissue)

women tan more deeply in pregnancy. Pigmentation changes may remain after pregnancy in women with darker hair and skin, and chloasma may be exacerbated by exposure to the sun. Endocrine changes of pregnancy result in changes in the structure and function of the blood and lymph vessel structure of the skin and mucous membranes (Henry et al., 2006).

THE SKELETON AND JOINTS

Posture and gait change in pregnancy. The weight of the gravid uterus changes the woman's centre of gravity altering the angle of inclination of the pelvic brim to the horizontal plane. The lumbar spine is naturally anteriorly convex, but the combined effects of progesterone, relaxin and the weight of the uterus on the intravertebral discs exaggerate this curve. The resulting lordosis of the spine compensates for the shift in the centre of gravity but may result in muscle and ligament strain. By the end of pregnancy, many women adopt a typical posture where they stand and walk with their backs arched and the shoulders held backwards. Lordosis is increased by poor posture generally, obesity, skeletal disorders, tuberculosis and by wearing high-heeled shoes. Oestrogen and relaxin affect the composition of the cartilage and connective tissue of pelvic joints, which soften in preparation for labour. The large

diameter collagen fibres are remodelled via the action of elastin and collagenolysis to smaller diameter fibres (Ward et al., 2007) The symphysis pubis and sacroiliac joints become more mobile and flexible so the pelvis becomes wider resulting in a rolling unstable movement and waddling gait when walking. Pregnant women may, therefore, experience muscle and ligament strain and discomfort or pain. The incidence of backache increases particularly after the 5th month. Some women experience severe back pain, often with peak intensity at night.

Occasionally in late pregnancy the symphysis pubis may separate. This condition, described as diastasis or SPD, can cause the pregnant woman great discomfort when walking or when her legs are abducted. In severe cases, women are often observed to walk sideways as this tends to be less painfully when walking in a normal forward motion. The lower back is also affected by breast changes, stretching of the round ligament and decreased tone of abdominal muscles. In the third trimester, pressure of the uterus stretching or compressing nerves and blood vessels can result in numbness and tingling of extremities. Leg cramps, especially of the calf and thigh muscles, are common in the second half of pregnancy. They may be related to calcium/phosphorus metabolism and increased neuromuscular irritability. Raised phosphate levels are implicated and reducing dietary intake of milk is often beneficial. About 10% of pregnant women experience restless legs syndrome 10–20 min after getting into bed; the cause is unknown (Manconi et al., 2004). Calf pain is also associated with deep vein thrombosis which is not so common but there is an increase risk of this in pregnancy and so all calf pain needs careful investigation and monitoring.

Calcium metabolism

There is increased turnover of calcium early in pregnancy. Maternal calcium metabolism changes to facilitate calcium transport to the fetus. The placenta actively transports calcium from the maternal blood during the third trimester. Placental calcium concentrations are higher than maternal levels so the fetus is protected if maternal concentrations fall. Placental efficiency is much greater than the absorptive capability of a fetus's gastrointestinal tract; thus a baby born prematurely with immature gut function cannot absorb calcium efficiently and the skeleton is slower to mineralize. In the last 10 weeks of gestation, the fetus obtains 18 g of calcium and 10 g of phosphorus from the maternal circulation, which is equivalent to 80% of the mother's normal dietary calcium in that period. However, the 28–30 g of calcium accumulated by the fetus represents a very small fraction of the total maternal calcium.

hPL and prolactin stimulate vitamin D synthesis, which increases absorption of calcium. Gastrointestinal absorption of calcium increases throughout the pregnancy even in vitamin D deficiency (Fudge and Kovacs, 2010). hPL increases bone reabsorption of calcium. Oestrogen stimulates parathyroid hormone secretion, which increases calcium absorption, decreases urinary losses and increases release of calcium from bone. Calcitonin secretion is also increased; calcitonin inhibits mineral release from the maternal skeleton but allows the actions of parathyroid hormone on the gut and kidney. Maternal serum calcium levels fall progressively in pregnancy. Levels are related to haemodilution of albumin and increased urinary losses and transport across the placenta. Urinary excretion of calcium decreases after 36 weeks, which augments dietary sources of calcium.

Homeostasis, mediated by maternal hormones, means that the maternal skeleton is conserved. If dietary calcium is adequate, there is no marked change in maternal skeletal mass or bone density. There is no evidence that high parity is associated with increased fractures in later life. Calcium supplements tend to reduce blood pressure by a small amount and may be useful in the treatment of pre-eclampsia (see Chapter 12). Calcium requirements in pregnancy are probably overestimated; clinical deficiency is rarely observed. However, a low vitamin D intake in pregnancy and little exposure to sunlight is associated with osteomalacia, as demonstrated by Asian women in the UK who have lower plasma calcium and an increased incidence of maternal osteomalacia and neonatal rickets.

VISION

The changed hormonal profile of pregnancy influences the maternal nervous system. In the third trimester, mild corneal oedema is common; fluid is retained and the cornea becomes slightly thicker, which affects refraction. Tear composition changes; levels of lysozyme alter and tears often become greasy. This, together with altered corneal sensitivity, may cause blurring or intolerance to contact lenses. Progesterone, relaxin and hCG affect intraocular pressure, which can fall (which will improve glaucoma). Unless they experience problems, it is wise for pregnant women to delay new prescriptions for spectacles. Women with pre-eclampsia and retinal oedema, and those with diabetes, are particularly prone to visual complications which may also be associated with headaches at the back of the upper neck.

THE NOSE AND LARYNX

The nasal mucosa becomes hyperaemic and congested in pregnancy, causing nasal stuffiness and obstruction. This seems to be oestrogen-related and may interfere with sleep and sense of smell. It is associated with congestion of the Eustachian tubes (often described as blocked ears unrelieved by swallowing), which may cause a transient mild hearing loss. Many women will develop snoring during pregnancy (see above). Erythema and oedema of the vocal cords can lead to hoarseness, coughing and vocal changes. Softening of the cartilage within the larynx is not usually a problem but it may make tracheal intubation harder if required. Difficult intubation in pregnant women is further complicated by obesity and so it is good practice to ensure that intubation guidelines are present in all maternity units providing both routine and emergency surgical intervention.

SLEEP

Sleep patterns change in pregnancy. An increased desire for sleep and napping in the first trimester has been observed (Brunner et al., 1994). It is suggested that progesterone affects neuronal activity in the brain reducing the level of excitatory neurotransmitters (Smith, 1991). Oestrogen enhances this effect by increasing the number of receptors for progesterone. The amount of rapid eye movement (REM) sleep increases from 25 weeks, peaking at 33–36 weeks. Stage 4 non-REM sleep (deep sleep) decreases. It is this state that appears important for tissue repair and recovery from fatigue. In the second half of pregnancy, women tend to sleep less as they frequently are disturbed by nocturia, dyspnoea, heartburn, nasal congestion, muscle aches, stress and anxiety and fetal activity.

CARBOHYDRATE METABOLISM

Maternal metabolism changes in pregnancy to meet increased maternal needs, including the accumulation of maternal energy stores in readiness for labour and lactation, and to facilitate fetal growth and development (Fig. 11.10). Metabolism in pregnancy must also facilitate both the accumulation of fetal energy stores for the transition to extrauterine life (see Chapter 15) and maternal accumulation of fat stores in preparation for labour and lactation. Pregnancy is primarily anabolic: food intake and appetite increase and activity decreases. Pregnancy has been described as a 'state of accelerated starvation' (Frienkel et al., 1972) because there is an increased tendency to become ketotic. Pregnancy is a diabetogenic state; women acquire insulin resistance in later pregnancy which appears to represent a temporary excursion into metabolic syndrome.

Early pregnancy

Metabolism in the first trimester is predominantly anabolic with synthesis of new maternal tissues including deposition of maternal fat. It can be considered as a time

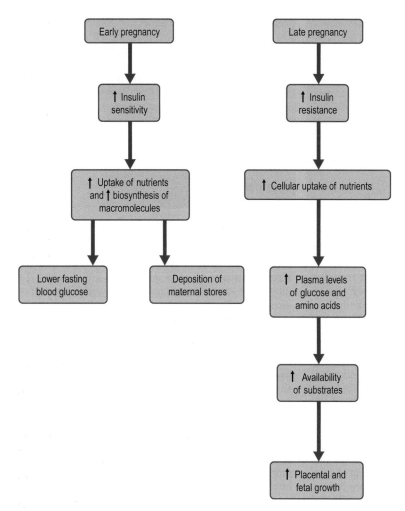

Fig. 11.10 Changes in maternal carbohydrate handling during pregnancy.

of preparation for the subsequent high demands of rapid fetal growth; over 90% of fetal growth occurs in the second half of pregnancy (King, 2000). Early in the pregnancy, there is an increased response to insulin so fasting blood glucose levels are lower than normal. The tissues exhibit increased sensitivity to insulin so there is increased uptake of nutrients and synthesis of macromolecules by cells which promotes maternal tissue growth. As the pregnancy progresses, most women develop insulin resistance so levels of glucose and amino acids in the blood rise, thus increasing the availability of substrates required by the fetus and placental uptake.

In the first trimester, increased insulin is produced in response to glucose. Early in pregnancy, the raised levels of oestrogen and progesterone orchestrate the changes in metabolism. Oestrogen stimulates pancreatic β-cell growth (hyperplasia and hypertrophy) and therefore insulin secretion. It also enhances glucose utilization in peripheral tissues and increases plasma cortisol. So the net effect is to decrease fasting glucose levels, improve glucose tolerance and increase glycogen storage. Hepatic metabolism of insulin may also be altered. Lowered glucose levels between meals increase the tendency to become ketotic. Placental transfer of amino acids, increased hepatic gluconeogenesis (conversion of amino acids, particularly alanine, to glucose) and raised insulin levels, which stimulate cellular uptake, together result in lowered maternal levels of amino acids. During the first half of pregnancy, the progressive increment in insulin levels, augmented by progesterone and cortisol, stimulates hepatic lipogenesis (triacylglyceride synthesis and storage) and suppresses lipolysis (fat breakdown). An increase in the numbers of insulin receptors on the adipocytes means there is enhanced removal of triglycerides from circulation. Increased fat storage in early pregnancy results in hypertrophy of adipose cells. During fasting, ketogenesis is increased as the triglycerides are utilized.

Later pregnancy

As the pregnancy progresses, the fetal placental unit grows and levels of placental hormones, which are antagonistic to insulin, increase. Therefore maternal tissues exhibit decreased sensitivity, or resistance, to insulin, which means that insulin is less effective at stimulating glucose uptake. Pregnancy-induced insulin resistance affects adipocytes to a lesser degree. The dominant effect in the second and third trimesters is related to the high levels of hPL, but human placental growth hormone, prolactin, cortisol and progesterone are also involved. Tumour necrosis factor α (TNFα), resistin and leptin may also be involved in the increased insulin resistance that develops in pregnancy. Levels of hPL increase markedly after 20 weeks. hPL is a very potent insulin antagonist with effects similar to those of growth hormone. Raised hPL results in decreased peripheral tissue responses to insulin and therefore increased circulating levels of glucose and amino acids, which are available for transport to the fetus. hPL increases lipolysis and nitrogen retention, decreases urinary potassium excretion and increases calcium excretion.

Progesterone augments insulin secretion, increasing fasting levels, but decreases peripheral insulin effectiveness. Cortisol inhibits glucose uptake and oxidation, increases liver glucose production and possibly augments glucagon secretion. Therefore, in later pregnancy, fasting results in mobilization of maternal triacylglyceride stores leading to a marked increase in levels of maternal fatty acids. This provides an alternative substrate for maternal metabolism so glucose is spared for central nervous system and fetal requirements. As tissue uptake of glucose is suppressed so levels of glucose are raised, which stimulate insulin release from the pancreas. Hyperinsulinaemia is a normal development in the later part of pregnancy; levels of insulin double by the third trimester. The raised level of insulin is important in stimulating protein synthesis. Raised insulin levels counteract the effect of the antagonistic hormones so maternal plasma glucose is maintained at levels similar to prepregnant levels. Insulin sensitivity rebounds after the delivery of the placenta. Women with insulin-dependent diabetes mellitus (IDDM) need to have a marked increase in insulin dose to compensate for the pregnancy-induced resistance to insulin.

In the postabsorptive states between meals, gluconeogenesis and fat mobilization provide substrates for maternal metabolism and placental transfer. Maternal cells metabolize the increased ketones and free fatty acids, thus sparing glucose and amino acids for placental uptake. As blood sugar increases in the pregnancy, it can exceed the transport maxima of the nephrons (i.e. the capacity to reabsorb the glucose from the glomerular filtrate) so some glucose is excreted in the urine. A degree of glucosuria is normal in pregnancy. As renal absorption of glucose is limited (so there are increased losses) and hepatic gluconeogenesis is decreased, hypoglycaemia, hypoalaninaemia and hyperinsulinaemia result.

Gestational diabetes mellitus

Gestational diabetes mellitus (GDM) is defined as carbohydrate intolerance that begins or was first recognized in pregnancy. It is the extreme end of the spectrum of normal physiological changes in pregnancy and is increasing with the increased prevalence of overweight and obesity in the population. Gaining excess weight during pregnancy also increases the risk of GDM (Morisset et al., 2010). GDM is due to the inability of the maternal pancreas to increase insulin secretion enough to counter the pregnancy-induced insulin resistance. Inability to produce adequate insulin at this stage of pregnancy is probably due to a limitation of the pancreatic β-cells (which may be related to the pregnant woman's own pancreatic development in utero). Inadequate secretion of insulin, and altered carbohydrate metabolism, may become evident again when there is further demand for insulin, as in a subsequent pregnancy or in later life, and is particularly associated with increased body weight (and therefore cell number). GDM (or delivery of an infant weighing more than 4.5 kg) is a risk factor both for future pregnancies and for prediabetes and type 2 diabetes mellitus. Indeed as GDM appears to represent an early stage in the progression to type 2 diabetes, it has been suggested that follow-up of women affected in pregnancy offers an opportunity to prevent type 2 diabetes and cardiovascular disease (Di Cianni et al., 2010). Infants of diabetic mothers and those with either macrosomia or microsomia also have an increased diabetogenic tendency and are more likely to develop obesity, metabolic syndrome and type 2 diabetes themselves (Reece, 2010). In women who develop gestational diabetes, strict dietary control is important in reducing adverse effects on the fetus. A moderate energy restriction (about 30% of total energy) can benefit glucose metabolism without causing ketonaemia in obese women with GDM (Metzger and Freinkel, 1987). If refractory to dietary treatment, some women with GDM may require insulin therapy as well. Diabetic women and women who require insulin therapy for GDM are at higher risk in pregnancy with problems associated with abnormal blood glucose levels such as increased risk of infection.

Case study 11.5 is an example of raised glucose levels in pregnancy.

Case study 11.5

Cathy is expecting her fourth baby. At 28 weeks' gestation, a random blood glucose revealed a blood glucose level of 11 mol/L. Cathy looks well and, as in all her other pregnancies, says she feels exceptionally healthy. Cathy is referred to the consultant clinic for further investigations. Her previous baby was delivered at 37 weeks' gestation weighing 4.960 kg.

- What is the provisional diagnosis and what investigations will be carried out to confirm this diagnosis?

- What physiological interactions between the mother and fetus are occurring that could explain this phenomenon?
- How can the midwife best explain these to Cathy and what advice should she be given?
- What are the possible consequences for Cathy and her baby if no further investigations are carried out and no treatment advised?

Key points

- The physiological adaptation to pregnancy is mediated by the increase of steroid hormone secretion. Steroid hormones are initially produced from the corpus luteum under the influence of hCG and subsequently from the placenta.
- The maternal endocrine system is affected by the increase in steroid hormones so other hormones augment the effects of oestrogen and progesterone. For instance, secretion of MSH and cortisol increases in pregnancy, affecting skin pigmentation and improving some pathological conditions such as eczema.
- Generally early physiological changes in pregnancy are regulated by hormonal changes, whereas later changes may be due to structural effects of the enlarging uterus.
- Reproductive system: under the influence of oestrogen, the uterus increases in size and vascularization, and spontaneous uterine contractions are suppressed. The breasts undergo development in preparation for lactation.
- Cardiovascular system: physiological changes are particularly marked in this system, meeting the increased demands of the maternal and fetal tissues. The vascular system expands as progesterone stimulates vasodilation of the vascular smooth muscle and oestrogen stimulates angiogenesis and increased blood flow. The RAS responds to the underfilled vascular system by increasing sodium and water retention; thus blood volume increases by about 40%. Plasma expansion is greater than blood cell increase leading to overall haemodilution.
- Cardiac output increases early in pregnancy, initially as a result of increased heart rate, which is subsequently followed by increased stroke volume. Myocontractility is increased throughout pregnancy, which stimulates a degree of ventricular hypertrophy.
- Blood pressure decreases in early pregnancy, reaching a minimum in mid-pregnancy, and then returns close to prepregnant values towards term. The effects of posture on blood pressure are marked in pregnancy.
- The dilution of plasma proteins increases the formation of oedema. The ratio of clotting factors changes so bleeding time decreases.
- Respiratory system: excursion of the diaphragm alters as the rib cage flares increasing the efficiency of inspiration. Progesterone affects the sensitivity of the chemoreceptors, which increases respiratory drive. Therefore, hyperventilation is normal in pregnancy and results in lower circulating carbon dioxide levels and higher concentrations of cations, which facilitate exchange across the placenta.
- Gastrointestinal system: progesterone stimulates appetite and thirst and affects the sensitivity of the taste buds. Progesterone also affects the smooth muscle of the gut, which alters motility and transit time. This can result in increased efficiency of absorption but may also cause nausea and constipation. Decreased tone of lower oesophageal sphincter may result in reflux and heartburn.
- Skin: the increase in MSH levels results in increased pigmentation of the nipple and areola, the linea nigra and possibly chloasma. Increased blood flow to the skin, which is important in heat regulation, affects growth of hair and nails and may cause congestion of the mucous membranes.
- Skeleton: posture is affected by changed weight distribution and altered composition of the cartilage and connective tissue resulting in an exaggerated curvature of the spine.
- Metabolism: maternal metabolism is affected by altered thyroid hormone secretion and altered responses to insulin. In the first half of pregnancy, increased sensitivity to insulin favours deposition of maternal fat stores. In the second half of pregnancy, insulin resistance results in raised levels of substrates in the maternal plasma, which favour placental transport and fetal growth. Extremes of insulin resistance result in gestational diabetes mellitus.

Application to practice

Women experience many changes within their bodies and naturally will seek explanations and reassurance from the midwife as the changes occur. The midwife should use her knowledge of the physiological changes to aid her in assessing whether the pregnancy is progressing normally.

ANNOTATED FURTHER READING

Blackburn ST: *Maternal, fetal, and neonatal physiology: a clinical perspective*, ed 3, Philadelphia, 2007, Saunders.

An excellent in-depth description of physiological adaptation to pregnancy and consequent development of the fetus and neonate that draws from physiological research studies. The chapters are clearly organized by physiological systems and link physiological concepts to clinical applications including the assessment and management of low- and high-risk pregnancies.

Calderwood CJ, Thanoon OI: Thromboembolism and thrombophilia in pregnancy, *Obstet Gyn Reproduct Med* 19:339–343, 2010.

A recent review of the risk factors and management of venous thromboembolism in pregnancy and the association between thrombophilias and adverse pregnancy outcomes.

Chamberlain G, Steer P: *Turnbull's obstetrics*, ed 3, New York, 2001, Churchill Livingstone.

A comprehensive textbook with a medical approach to obstetric principles and practice and the development of clinical protocols.

Creasy RK, Resnik RIJ: *Maternal–fetal medicine: principles and practice*, ed 5, Philadelphia, 2003, Saunders.

Covers all disciplines pertinent to obstetricians including genetics and genetic testing, fetal and placental growth and development, epidemiology, immunology, physiological adaptation to pregnancy as well as clinical applications and medical complications in pregnancy.

Freyer AM: Drug-prescribing challenges during pregnancy, *Obstet Gyn Reproduct Med* 18:180–186, 2008.

A brief but insightful discussion about challenges to drug-prescribing in pregnancy covering issues such as preconception counselling, compliance, evidence about drug safety, fetal and maternal changes affecting drug handling and the role of the placenta.

Gilbert ES, Harmon JS: *Manual of high risk pregnancy and delivery*, ed 5, St Louis, 2010, Mosby.

This book is an excellent reference for midwives who provide high-risk care in practice and it details many of the pathological problems that can arise during pregnancy and delivery.

Goland S, Barakat M, Khatri N, et al: Pregnancy in Marfan syndrome: maternal and fetal risk and recommendations for patient assessment and management, *Cardiol Rev* 17:253–262, 2009.

This paper provides a review of current clinical information and provides recommendations for the management of patients with Marfan syndrome during pregnancy.

McCarthy FP, Kenny LC: Hypertension in pregnancy, *Obstet Gyn Reproduct Med* 19:136–141, 2009.

A practice-based review covering the classification and diagnosis of hypertension and its management.

REFERENCES

Arck P, Hansen PJ, Mulac JB, et al: Progesterone during pregnancy: endocrine-immune cross talk in mammalian species and the role of stress, *Am J Reprod Immunol* 58:268–279, 2007.

Barrett JF, Whittaker PG, Williams JG, et al: Absorption of non-haem iron from food during normal pregnancy, *BMJ* 309:79–82, 1994.

Baylis C, Davison JM: The urinary system. In Chamberlain G, Broughton Pipkin F, editors: *Clinical physiology in obstetrics*, ed 3, Oxford, 1998, Blackwell, pp 263–307.

Bernal J, Pekonen F: Ontogenesis of the nuclear 3,5,3′-triiodothyronine receptor in the human fetal brain, *Endocrinology* 114:677–679, 1984.

Blackburn ST: *Maternal, fetal, and neonatal physiology: a clinical perspective*, ed 3, Philadelphia, 2007, Saunders.

Bowen DJ: Taste and food preference changes across the course of pregnancy, *Appetite* 19:233–242, 1992.

Brown MA, Gallery EDM: Volume homeostasis in normal pregnancy and pre-eclampsia: physiology and clinical implications, *Baillières Clin Obstet Gynaecol* 8:287–310, 1994.

Brunner DP, Münch M, Biedermann K, et al: Changes in sleep and sleep electroencephalogram during pregnancy, *Sleep* 17(7):576–582, 1994.

Brunton PJ, Arunachalam S, Russel JA: Control of neurohypophysial hormone secretion, blood osmolality and volume in pregnancy, *J Physiol Pharmacol* 58(suppl.8):27–45, 2008.

Burton GJ, Woods AW, Jauniaux E, et al: Rheological and physiological consequences of conversion of the maternal spiral arteries for uteroplacental blood flow during human pregnancy, *Placenta* 30:473–482, 2009.

Carbonne B, Benachi A, Léveque ML, et al: Maternal position during labor: effects on fetal oxygen saturation measured by pulse oximetry, *Obstet Gynecol* 88:797–800, 1996.

Chamberlain G, Dewhurst J, Harvey D: *Illustrated textbook of obstetrics*, London, 1991, Gower Medical/Mosby, p 104.

Coad J, Al Rasasi B, Morgan JB: New perspectives on nausea and vomiting in pregnancy, *MIDIRS Res Digt* 10:451–454, 2000.

Coad J, Al Rasasi B, Morgan J: Nutrient insult in early pregnancy, *Proc Nutr Soc* 61:51–59, 2002.

Conrad KP, Jeyabalan A, Danielson LA, et al: Role of relaxin in maternal renal vasodilation of pregnancy, *Ann N Y Acad Sci* 1041:147–154, 2005.

Cordain L, Eaton SB, Miller JB, et al: The paradoxical nature of hunter–gatherer diets: meat-based, yet non-atherogenic, *Eur J Clin Nutr* 56(Suppl. 1):S42–S52, 2002.

Curry R, Swan L, Steer PJ: Cardiac disease in pregnancy, *Curr Opin Obstet Gynecol* 21:508–513, 2009.

Davison JM, Shiells EA, Philips PR, et al: Influence of humoral and volume factors on altered osmoregulation of normal human pregnancy, *Am J Physiol* 258:F900–F907, 1990.

de Bree E, Makrigiannakis A, Askoxylakis J, et al: Pregnancy after breast cancer. A comprehensive review, *J Surg Oncol* 101:534–542, 2010.

de Escobar GM, Ares S, Berbel P, et al: The changing role of maternal thyroid hormone in fetal brain development, *Semin Perinatol* 32:380–386, 2008.

de Swiet M: The cardiovascular system. In Chamberlain G, Broughton Pipkin F, editors: *Clinical physiology in obstetrics*, ed 3, Oxford, 1998a, Blackwell, pp 33–70.

de Swiet M: The respiratory system. In Chamberlain G, Broughton Pipkin F, editors: *Clinical physiology in obstetrics*, ed 3, Oxford, 1998b, Blackwell, pp 111–128.

Di Cianni G, Ghio A, Resi V, et al: Gestational diabetes mellitus: an opportunity to prevent type 2 diabetes and cardiovascular disease in young women, *Womens Health (Lond Engl)* 6:97–105, 2010.

Duvekot JJ, Peeters LLH: Very early changes in cardiovascular physiology. In Chamberlain G, Broughton Pipkin F, editors: *Clinical physiology in obstetrics*, ed 3, Oxford, 1998, Blackwell, pp 3–32.

Duvekot JJ, Cheriex EC, Pieters FA, et al: Early pregnancy changes in hemodynamics and volume homeostasis are consecutive adjustments triggered by a primary fall in systemic vascular tone, *Am J Obstet Gynecol* 169(6):1382–1392, 1993.

Eghbali M, Wang Y, Toro L, et al: Heart hypertrophy during pregnancy: a better functioning heart? *Trends Cardiovasc Med* 16:285–291, 2006.

Elling SV, Powell FC: Physiological changes in the skin during pregnancy, *Clin Dermatol* 15:35–43, 1997.

FitzGerald MP, Graziano S: Anatomic and functional changes of the lower urinary tract during pregnancy, *Urol Clin North Am* 34:7–12, 2007.

Flaxman SM, Sherman PW: Morning sickness: a mechanism for protecting mother and embryo, *Q Rev Biol* 75:113–148, 2000.

Frienkel N, Metzger BE, Nitzan M, et al: 'Accelerated starvation' and mechanisms for the conservation of maternal nitrogen during pregnancy, *Isr J Med Sci* 8:426, 1972.

Fudge NJ, Kovacs CS: Pregnancy up-regulates intestinal calcium absorption and skeletal mineralization independently of the vitamin D receptor, *Endocrinology* 151:886–895, 2010.

Glinoer D, Lemone M: Goiter and pregnancy: a new insight into an old problem, *Thyroid* 2:65–70, 1992.

Godfrey KM, Redman CWG, Barker DJP, et al: The effect of maternal anaemia and iron deficiency on the ratio of fetal weight to placental weight, *Br J Obstet Gynaecol* 98:886–891, 1991.

Grattan DR, Ladyman SR, Augustine RA: Hormonal induction of leptin resistance during pregnancy, *Physiol Behav* 91:366–374, 2007.

Haram K, Nilsen ST, Ulvik RJ: Iron supplementation in pregnancy: evidence and controversies, *Acta Obstet Gynecol Scand* 80:683–688, 2001.

Henry F, Quatresooz P, Valverde-Lopez JC, et al: Blood vessel changes during pregnancy: a review, *Am J Clin Dermatol* 7:65–69, 2006.

Holmes VA, Wallace JM: Haemostasis in normal pregnancy: a balancing act? *Biochem Soc Trans* 33:428–432, 2005.

Huxley RR: Nausea and vomiting in early pregnancy: its role in placental development, *Obstet Gynecol* 95:779–782, 2000.

Hytten F: The alimentary system. In Hytten F, Chamberlain G, editors: *Clinical physiology in obstetrics*, ed 2, Oxford, 1991, Blackwell, pp 137–149.

Idris I, Srinivasan R, Simm A, et al: Maternal hypothyroidism in early and late gestation: effects on neonatal and obstetric outcome, *Clin Endocrinol (Oxf)* 63:560–565, 2005.

Iles RK, Chard T: Human chorionic gonadotrophin expression by bladder cancers: biology and clinical potential, *J Urol* 145(3):481–489, 1991.

Ivell R, Einspanier A: Relaxin peptides are new global players, *Trends Endocrinol Metabol* 13:343–348, 2002.

Jeyabalan A, Lain KY: Anatomic and functional changes of the upper urinary tract during pregnancy, *Urol Clin North Am* 34:1–6, 2007.

Johnson MH, Everitt BJ: *Essential reproduction*, ed 5, Oxford, 2000, Blackwell.

King JC: Physiology of pregnancy and nutrient metabolism, *Am J Clin Nutr* 71:1218S–1225S, 2000.

King TL, Murphy PA: Evidence-based approaches to managing nausea and vomiting in early pregnancy, *J Midwifery Womens Health* 54:430–444, 2009.

Kornyei JL, Lei ZM, Rao CV: Human myometrial smooth muscle cells are a novel target of direct regulation by human chorionic gonadotrophin, *Biol Reprod* 49:1149–1157, 1993.

Letsky E: The haematological system. In Chamberlain G, Broughton Pipkin F, editors: *Clinical physiology in obstetrics*, ed 3, Oxford, 1998, Blackwell, pp 71–110.

Lewis G, editor: *Saving Mothers' Lives: reviewing maternal deaths to make motherhood safer – 2003–2005*. The 7th report of the confidential enquires into maternal deaths in the United Kingdom, 2007, CEMACH.

Mabie WC, DiSessa TG, Crocker LG, et al: A longitudinal study of cardiac output in normal human pregnancy,

Am J Obstet Gynecol 170:849–856, 1994.

Manconi M, Govoni V, De Vito A, et al: Pregnancy as a risk factor for restless legs syndrome, *Sleep Med* 5:305–308, 2004.

Maul H, Longo M, Saade GR, et al: Nitric oxide and its role during pregnancy: from ovulation to delivery, *Curr Pharm Des* 9:359–380, 2003.

Maynard SE, Thadhani R: Pregnancy and the kidney, *J Am Soc Nephrol* 20:14–22, 2009.

Metzger BE, Freinkel N: Accelerated starvation in pregnancy: implications for dietary treatment of obesity and gestational diabetes mellitus, *Biol Neonate* 51:78–85, 1987.

Miller AWF, Hanretty KP: *Obstetrics illustrated*, ed 5, New York, 1998, Churchill Livingstone, p 34.

Morisset AS, St Yves A, Veillette J, et al: Prevention of gestational diabetes mellitus: a review of studies on weight management, *Diabetes Metab Res Rev* 26:17–25, 2010.

Morris NH, Eaton BM, Dekker G: Nitric oxide, the endothelium, pregnancy and pre-eclampsia, *Br J Obstet Gynaecol* 103:4–15, 1996.

NICE: *Antenatal care – routine care for the healthy pregnant woman*, 2008, National Institute for Clinical Excellence.

Palmer RMJ, Ferrige AG, Moncada S: Nitric oxide release accounts for the biological activity of endothelium-derived relaxing factor, *Nature* 327:524–526, 1987.

Pavek P, Ceckova M, Staud F: Variation of drug kinetics in pregnancy, *Curr Drug Metab* 10:520–529, 2009.

Perez-Lopez FR: Iodine and thyroid hormones during pregnancy and postpartum, *Gynecol Endocrinol* 23:414–428, 2007.

Picciano MF: Pregnancy and lactation: physiological adjustments, nutritional requirements and the role of dietary supplements, *J Nutr* 133:1997S–2002S, 2003.

Prabhakar NR, Peng YJ: Peripheral chemoreceptors in health and disease, *J Appl Physiol* 96:359–366, 2004.

RCOG: *Prevention of early onset neonatal group B streptococcal disease. (Green top guideline number 36)*, London, 2003, Royal College of Obstetricians and Gynaecologists.

Reece EA: The fetal and maternal consequences of gestational diabetes mellitus, *J Matern Fetal Neonatal Med* 23:199–203, 2010.

Schrier RW: A unifying hypothesis of body fluid volume regulation, *J R Coll Physicians Lond* 26:295–306, 1992.

Smith SS: Progesterone administration attenuates excitatory amino acid responses of cerebellar Purkinje cells, *Neuroscience* 42:309–320, 1991.

Ward C, Bushnell CD, James AH: The cardiovascular complications of pregnancy, *Prog Cardiovasc Dis* 50:126–135, 2007.

Weinberg ED: Are iron supplements appropriate for iron replete pregnant women? *Med Hypotheses* 73:714–715, 2009.

Weinberg ED: Can iron be teratogenic? *Biometals* 23:181–184, 2010.

Whitfield CR, editors: *Dewhurst's textbook of obstetrics and gynaecology for postgraduates*, 4th edn. Oxford, 1986, Blackwell Scientific.

Yip R, Dallman PR: Iron. In Ziegler EE, Filer LJ, editors: *Present knowledge in nutrition*, ed 7, Washington DC, 1996, ILSI, pp 277–292.

Chapter | 12 |

Maternal nutrition and health

- To review nutritional requirements and explain the role of the main nutrient groups in human health.
- To identify how and why nutrient requirements might change during pregnancy.
- To describe how the fetus adapts to low nutrient levels.
- To relate undernutrition to outcome of pregnancy.
- To discuss other factors that may affect weight gain in pregnancy and birth weight.
- To discuss how maternal diet and health affect the fetus in the short and long term.

INTRODUCTION

It is common for pregnancy to affect a woman's sense of well-being. Some aspects of health may be affected positively and others negatively. The role of nutrition, both before, during and after pregnancy, is important for the health of both the mother and fetus. Pregnant women are often receptive to advice and may make changes to their diet which may persist (Anderson, 2001). Maternal stressors, including perceived stress, chronic and acute stresses related to life events, work-related stress and pregnancy-related anxiety, as well as nutritional stress, are associated with adverse outcomes of pregnancy such as low birth weight (LBW), prematurity and intrauterine growth retardation (IUGR; Hobel and Culhane, 2003). Although stress, of all types, is a risk for preterm birth and premature labour, not all stressed women deliver prematurely suggesting that pregnant women (or their fetuses) have differing

vulnerability to the effects of stress. Optimal fetal nutrition is implicated in a range of health outcomes affecting birth weight, growth in infancy and childhood and the risk for later adult disease. The relationship between maternal and fetal nutrition is complex but the arguments that nutrient intake in pregnancy should be optimal seem well founded.

Chapter case study

Both Zara and James follow a vegetarian diet and try to lead a healthy lifestyle. At her first visit to the midwife, Zara was calculated as having a body mass index (BMI) of 24, which the midwife calculated from what Zara reported as her non-pregnant weight. During the pregnancy, Zara's baby appeared to be growing as expected and her midwife has measured Zara's uterine growth in centimetres using the symphysis pubis as the reference point; as expected, the fundal height has increased by 1 cm per week of pregnancy.

At 34 weeks' gestation, Zara is concerned that she only seems to have gained 4.5 kg over her non-pregnant weight unlike her sister who has put on over 10 kg and has been told by her midwife that her baby is a little bit on the small side.

- What factors could explain the differences in weight gain between Zara and her sister?
- What are the benefits of calculating the BMI of pregnant mothers and why is it preferable to calculate the BMI using the non-pregnant values if they are available?
- Does Zara's smaller weight gain give any cause for concern?
- What other reasons could explain why Zara's sister appears to have gained a lot more weight than Zara has?

OVERVIEW OF NUTRITION

Growth, development and optimal health rely on good nutrition and an adequate quality and quantity of nutrients for the cells. However, diet is influenced by many factors including wealth, religion, culture, and geographical and social factors. The insoluble macromolecules of food must be digested into soluble and absorbable subunits (see Chapter 1). The major components of the diet, or macronutrients, are carbohydrates, proteins and fats. Essential micronutrients are vitamins and minerals. Water is also an essential part of the diet.

Carbohydrates

Carbohydrates are the major energy source in the majority of human diets, but the amount and type of carbohydrate consumed varies amongst different population groups. With increased affluence in the Western world, there is a tendency to increase the proportion of fat in the diet at the expense of carbohydrate. There are two major types of carbohydrate: polysaccharides (or complex carbohydrates) and simple sugars (monosaccharides and disaccharides).

Monosaccharides, such as glucose, fructose and galactose, are not usually consumed in high quantities although they do occur in fruit. The major source of carbohydrate in the diet is usually starch from plant sources, plus some glycogen from animal liver and muscle. Dietary disaccharides include sucrose (table sugar), lactose (in milk) and maltose, which occurs in malt, beer and some sprouting seeds. Most starchy foods are high in carbohydrate and low in fat. With increasing affluence, added sugars tend to contribute more to the carbohydrate content at the expense of polysaccharides; soft drinks and sweet snacks may constitute a significant part of the carbohydrate intake.

Carbohydrates have differing effects on blood glucose levels and carbohydrate-rich foods can be compared using glycaemic index (GI) ranking. GI values for different foods are calculated by comparing their effect on blood glucose with the effects of a reference food (usually glucose or white bread). Carbohydrates with high GI are digested quickly and absorbed faster so the blood glucose response is fast. Carbohydrates that break down slowly, and result in a slow and sustained release of glucose into the circulation, have a low GI. Low GI foods prolong carbohydrate absorption, attenuate insulin secretion, increase the translocation of the insulin-responsive glucose transporter (GLUT4) to the cell membrane; they also result in more colonic fermentation of carbohydrate and beneficial short-chain fatty acid production High GI foods provide a rapid rise in blood sugar levels and are recommended for post-exercise energy recovery, whereas low GI foods release energy slowly and steadily and increase satiety and are appropriate for diabetics, dieters and endurance athletes. Health benefits of a low GI diet include reduced risk of obesity, diabetes and cardiovascular diseases and lowered incidence of colorectal cancers (Brand-Miller et al., 2009).

Many carbohydrate-rich foods contain indigestible non-starch polysaccharides (NSP or 'dietary fibre'). Dietary fibre is indigestible carbohydrate. Insoluble fibre promotes the formation of bulkier and softer faecal stools. Soluble fibre slows absorption of glucose and reduces blood cholesterol levels; it is associated with increased insulin sensitivity and decreased incidence of gut diseases. Soluble fibre forms a viscous gel with water and so protects against constipation as makes the faecal stools softer. Foods rich in complex carbohydrates include cereal grains, starchy vegetables, legumes, seeds and wholegrain cereals, all of which contain reasonable proportions (3–15%) of NSP. Most other vegetables, and most fruits, contain small amounts of both starch and NSP and variable amounts of sugars. Most foods that are not highly processed, with the exception of honey and dried fruits, do not contain much sugar, whereas most processed foods contain added sugars, usually sucrose.

Proteins

Proteins are made up of 20 types of amino acids linked together by peptide bonds. Indispensable or essential amino acids are those that cannot be synthesized from other amino acids in adequate amounts and, therefore, are required in the diet (Table 12.1). There are conditions,

Table 12.1 Amino acids		
ESSENTIAL AMINO ACIDS	**CONDITIONALLY ESSENTIAL AMINO ACIDS**	**NON-ESSENTIAL AMINO ACIDS**
Lysine	Cysteine	Alanine
Threonine	Tyrosine	Glutamic acid
Histidine	Arginine	Aspartic acid
Isoleucine	Citrulline[a]	Glycine
Leucine	Taurine[a]	Serine
Methionine	Carnitine	Proline
Phenylalanine		Glutamine
Tryptophan		Asparagine
Valine		

[a]Conditionally essential or essential only at certain ages or in certain conditions.

in which requirement is high or there is limited ability to interconvert amino acids, that result in an amino acid that can usually be synthesized from an indispensable amino acid being required in the diet. These amino acids are described as being conditionally indispensable, for instance premature babies with immature enzyme function or under conditions of stress may require amino acids that they will be able to synthesize when they are older.

Protein quality depends on the proportion of dietary protein that is absorbed across the gut (digestibility) and the ratio of the essential amino acids in the protein. A protein that is absorbed completely and utilized completely because the indispensable amino acids are in the optimum proportion for synthesis of new proteins is described as a high-quality protein, with a net protein utilization (NPU) value of 1.0 or 100%. Human milk and whole egg have an NPU of 1.0, whereas the overall protein availability in the Western diet is typically 0.7. The NPU of diets dependent on poor-quality proteins, such as those based on cassava (made from tapioca root), can be as low as 0.5.

In the absence of alternative sources of energy, protein can be metabolized as an energy source. Excess protein in the diet will also be used as a metabolic fuel. An adult is usually in nitrogen balance: protein intake is equal to protein breakdown so nitrogen in the diet is equal to excreted levels of nitrogen. Under conditions of growth and protein synthesis, there is a net accumulation of protein, and hence nitrogen, which is described as a state of positive nitrogen balance. States of growth, including pregnancy, result in positive nitrogen balance. Negative nitrogen balance usually indicates tissue breakdown or nutrient deficiency resulting in energy generation from protein sources. Illness and trauma cause negative nitrogen balance, although it also occurs with reduced activity and decreasing muscle mass and during uterine involution (see Chapter 13).

Fat

Fat is used for energy requirements. There is also a requirement for essential fatty acids, which cannot be synthesized by the body. These are the precursors of long-chain fatty acids and their metabolic products, prostaglandins and leukotrienes. Fat also provides the vehicle for absorption of fat-soluble vitamins. Most fat is present in the diet as triglycerides; a triglyceride is a glycerol molecule with three fatty acids (Fig. 12.1). There is a range of fatty acids of different chain length and degree of saturation, which is related to the number of double bonds in the fatty acid molecule. Saturated fatty acids have no double bonds, monounsaturated fatty acids have one double bond and polyunsaturated fatty acids have two or more double bonds. The body handles fatty acids differently depending on their length and the degree of saturation (Fig. 12.1C). Fats in foods are formed of triglycerides

containing a combination of different fatty acids, but are described by the predominant type. For instance, olive oil is particularly rich in monounsaturated fatty acids (with single double bonds).

Saturated fats are usually solid at room temperature and are usually of animal origin, although coconut and palm oils and cocoa butter have a high level of saturated fatty acids. Saturated fats become rancid very slowly so they store well. Unsaturated fats are usually liquid at room temperature and mostly of plant origin. The C=C double bond is not very stable so it oxidizes easily and the fat becomes rancid. In food processing, unsaturated vegetable oils are hydrogenated (have hydrogen atoms added to saturate the C=C bonds), which makes the fat harder and extends the shelf-life and flavour stability. Unsaturated fatty acids from vegetable and most animal sources naturally adopt a *cis* configuration, although ruminants produce some *trans* fatty acids which are thus found in low concentrations in milk and meat from ruminant animals. Positional isomerism, where the fatty acid has the same length and number and position of double bonds, but the hydrogen atoms either lie on the same side of the double bond (*cis* configuration) or on alternate sides (*trans* configuration) (Fig. 12.2). Hydrogenation and heating can convert the *cis* bonds to the *trans* isomeric forms. Many cellular processes depend on the fluidity of the membrane lipids which depends on the properties of fatty acid chains. Saturated fatty acids are more ordered and rigid. The double bonds of unsaturated fatty acids produce bends in the fatty acid which means that the fatty acids of the membrane pack less tightly together, thus conferring a greater degree of fluidity and flexibility to the cell membrane. *Trans* fatty acids are straighter and are more like saturated fatty acids in conformation even though they have double bonds. Cholesterol also inserts into the cell membrane bilayer and affects fluidity.

Diets high in saturated fat are associated with an increased incidence of atherosclerosis (damage to arterial blood vessels, causing hardening and plaque formation) and an increase in low-density lipoprotein (LDL) cholesterol levels which is a biomarker for heart disease. Diets higher in polyunsaturated fat are associated with increased high-density lipoprotein (HDL) cholesterol levels and an increased HDL:LDL cholesterol ratio which is associated with more favourable cardiovascular health. *Trans* fatty acids are implicated in increased risk of myocardial infarction and other cardiovascular problems. HDL levels are also increased by oestrogen (so they are higher in women) and by moderate alcohol intake and exercise.

There are two polyunsaturated fatty acids that are indispensable ('essential') in the diet as they cannot be synthesized by the body. These are linoleic acid (18:2, ω-6; chain length of 18 carbons and two double bonds, the first of which is at the carbon atom in the omega position 6 of the chain) and α-linoleic acid (18:3, ω-3; chain length

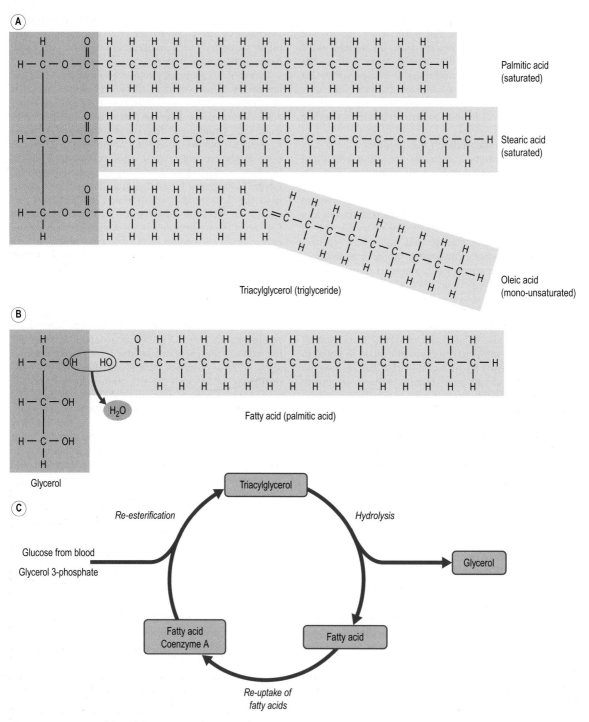

Fig. 12.1 Structure of fats: (A) a saturated fatty acid; (B) a triglyceride; (C) the fatty acid cycle.

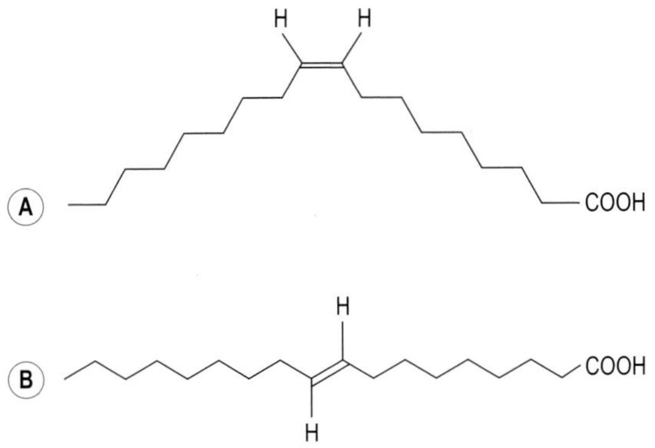

Fig. 12.2 (A) Cis and (B) trans isomerism of fatty acids.

of 18 carbons and three double bonds, the first of which is at the carbon atom in the omega position 3 of the chain). The body can further elongate and desaturate (lengthen and add more double bonds to) these essential fatty acids. However, there are two things to note. First, the fetus has limited ability to elongate and desaturate fatty acids so it is dependent on placental supply for both long-chain polyunsaturated fatty acids (LCPUFA) and the indispensable fatty acids. Second, the enzymes involved in the pathways of elongation and desaturation of the indispensable fatty acids into their longer chain metabolites are competitive. This means that the ratio of ω-6 fatty acids to ω-3 fatty acids is important for optimal development.

Vitamins

Vitamins are organic substances required in small amounts for metabolism, growth and maintenance; they are not synthesized by the body (either at all or in adequate amounts) and so are essential nutrients. Vitamins do not provide sources of energy but act as regulators of metabolic processes. They can be divided into water-soluble (Table 12.2) and fat-soluble vitamins (Table 12.3). The fat-soluble vitamins are more stable than water-soluble vitamins and are stored in the body, so when taken in excess they are more likely to cause toxicity than water-soluble vitamins. As B vitamins function as coenzymes in energy metabolism, requirement for B vitamins increases in parallel with increased energy consumption. Vitamins A, C and E function as antioxidants protecting cells from free-radical damage.

Minerals

Minerals regulate body function and are essential to good health. They are inorganic and become part of the body structure (Table 12.4). Excessive intake of minerals can be toxic or lead to illness indirectly because of the competitive nature of mineral absorption in the body. For example, excess iron can lead to zinc deficiency and excess zinc can lead to copper deficiency.

Table 12.2 Water-soluble vitamins

VITAMIN	ROLE	SOURCE
Thiamin (B_1)	Carbohydrate metabolism	Pork, wheat germ, yeast
Riboflavin (B_2)	Protein metabolism	Offal, milk, grains, legumes, eggs, vegetables
Niacin (B_3)	Production of energy from glucose; synthesis of fatty acids	Meat, nuts, legumes
Pyridoxine (B_6)	Synthesis and catabolism of amino acids; synthesis of antibodies and neurotransmitters	Pork, offal, grains, legumes, potatoes, bananas
Cyanocobalamine (B_{12})	Reactions preceding use of folic acid in DNA synthesis	Animal and dairy products, eggs, yeast
Folate	Formation of DNA	Liver, green leafy vegetables, kidney beans, oranges, melon
Pantothenic acid	Metabolism; synthesis of acetylcholine	Liver, egg yolk, milk, dried and spouting beans
Biotin	Synthesis of fatty acids, amino acids and purines (required for DNA and RNA)	Offal, egg yolk, tomatoes
C	Collagen formation, tissue formation and integrity, antioxidant, iron absorption	Citrus fruit, tomatoes, other fruit and vegetables

Table 12.3 Fat-soluble vitamins

VITAMIN	ROLE	SOURCE
A	Visual perception (rhodopsin synthesis); growth of epithelial tissue and bones, antioxidant	Liver, kidney, egg yolk
D	Hormone involved in bone mineralization and calcium homeostasis	Synthesized in skin, fish oils
E	Tissue growth + integrity of cell membranes; antioxidant	Vegetable oils, grains, milk, eggs, fish, meat
K	Synthesis of blood-clotting factors; bone metabolism	Gut flora, liver, green leafy vegetables

Table 12.4 Minerals

MINERAL	FUNCTION	DIETARY SOURCE
Sodium (Na)	Extracellular ion essential for the generation of action potentials; required in the active transport of small molecules into the cell	Table salt (NaCl)
Potassium (K)	Intracellular ion essential for the generation of action potentials; utilized by the cell to maintain ion concentration gradients	Meat, milk, fruits, vegetables
Calcium (Ca)	Bone and teeth structural component; essential for blood clotting, muscle contraction and nerve impulse conduction	Dairy products, fortified flour, cereals, green vegetables
Chlorine (Cl)	Cation in body fluids; gastric acid excretions	Salt (NaCl)
Phosphorus (P)	Structural component of bones and teeth; essential for formation of ATP for energy storage	Meat, dairy products cereals, bread
Magnesium (Mg)	Required by some enzyme activities; present in cells, body fluids and bone	Vegetables, milk, cereals, bread
Iron (Fe)	Transfer of oxygen in haemoglobin molecule; oxidation processes; electron transfer chain	Meat, vegetables, flour
Zinc	Enzyme activity; growth and development of the immune system; spermatogenesis; tissue growth	Oysters, steak, crab meat, red meat, milk products
Iodide	Thyroid hormones	Seafood, iodized table salt
Copper	Constituent of enzymes; energy production and release	Legumes, grains, nuts and seeds, offal
Manganese	Synthesis of urea; conversion of pyruvate in TCA cycle	Plant products
Fluoride	Essential to reduce decay in bone and tooth tissues	Fluoridated drinking water
Chromium	Carbohydrate and lipid metabolism	Unrefined foods, brewer's yeast, whole grains and nuts
Selenium	Antioxidant; catalyst for the production of thyroid hormone	Liver, shellfish, fish meat

PRECONCEPTUAL NUTRITIONAL STATUS

The sensitivity of the hypothalamus to environmental influences, such as nutrient availability, was probably of immense importance in promoting pregnancy in seasons when the fetus and infant had optimal chances of survival. Weight loss affects cyclical ovarian function in women. Anorexia nervosa disrupts the hypothalamic–pituitary–ovarian axis (see Chapter 4) and may cause amenorrhoea. Amenorrhoea related to inadequate nutrient intake is often reported in ballet dancers, competitive runners and other athletes (Frisch, 1990). It not only affects the ovulatory cycle but also can result in low levels of oestrogens, which reduce bone density and predispose to osteoporosis. It has been suggested that the menarche depended on women reaching a 'critical weight' (Frisch and McArthur, 1974). However, low body weight is not always associated with amenorrhoea. Conversely, dieting, high energy expenditure, nutrient restriction or erratic eating patterns (such as crash dieting and binging) can suppress normal reproductive cycles in women even if their weight stays within a normal range (Coad, 2003).

A minimal level of nutrient intake and fuel metabolism seem to be required to maintain reproductive functions, particularly the pulse generating secretion of gonadotrophin-releasing hormone (GnRH; see Chapter 4). Fluctuations in body fat can also disturb the transport and metabolism of the steroid hormones, which are fat soluble. Nutrient deficiency may itself suppress appetite. Studies in animals suggest optimal pregnancy outcome may depend on long-term nutritional status rather than a period of 'flushing' or short-term good-quality diet (Wynn and Wynn, 1991). Although restricted nutrient intake can suppress reproductive function, excess energy intake may also be disruptive. Obesity, in both men (Hammoud et al., 2008) and women (Zain and Norman, 2008), also affects fertility and conception rate. Polycystic ovary syndrome (PCOS), which often causes anovulation (see Chapter 6), is frequently associated with insulin resistance and hyperinsulinaemia even in the absence of obesity (Hirschberg, 2009). However, the symptoms and effects of PCOS on reproduction are more severe with increased body weight. In PCOS, increased obesity disrupts normal production of steroid hormones and affects carbohydrate handling.

A woman's weight, particularly if it is related to her height, indicates her nutritional status to some degree. Weight loss and nutrient fluctuation caused by self-imposed dieting, affecting reproductive function, may be the cause of infertility in a large proportion of the women seeking fertility treatment. Maternal nutritional status can be assessed by calculation of body mass index (BMI; Box 12.1). BMI is correlated to fat mass (and

---

Box 12.1 **The body mass index**

Body mass index (BMI) is used to indicate nutritional status and risk factors associated with obesity. It is a ratio of weight (measured in kilograms) against height (measured in metres squared).
  Calculation:

$$BMI = \frac{weight}{height} \left\{ \frac{kg}{m^2} \right\}$$

Interpretation:

Grade	BMI[a]	Definition
–	<20	Underweight
0	20–24.9	Desirable weight
I	25–29.9	Overweight
II	30–39.9	Mild obesity
III	40	Severe obesity

[a]*Normal*: 19.8–26.0.

A healthy shape is considered to be that usually associated with a BMI of 20–25 kg/m². Waist circumference and waist to height ratios are also used as indicators of healthy shape. A waist circumference of less than 80 cm is considered healthy in women and less than 94 cm in adult men, with waist circumferences above 88 and 102 cm, respectively, indicating risk. A waist:height ratio of less than 0.5 is also considered healthy with a ratio greater than 0.6 indicating risk to health.

---

health prognosis) but there are limitations to its use; BMI tends to overestimate fat mass in individuals who are active and have a high muscle mass and to underestimate fat in individuals who are sedentary. There are also racial differences in the correlation between BMI and fat mass; individuals from African and Polynesian races have less fat per BMI class compared with individuals from Caucasian races, whereas individuals from Asian races tend to have more fat. Whilst it is clear that the time to pregnancy is longer for underweight and overweight women, there is no consensus about the optimal BMI. A BMI of less than 18.5 kg/m² is not associated with good fertility or pregnancy outcome (Gesink Law et al., 2007). A BMI of greater than 30 kg/m² in a pre-pregnant woman is considered a considerable risk factor in the obstetric management of the pregnancy as well as affecting fertility (Lee and Koren, 2010). The higher incidence of obesity in the general population is reflected in the increased number of pregnant obese women who have more pregnancy-related complications such as hypertension, pre-eclampsia and gestational diabetes. Surgery for severe obesity is consequently becoming more commonplace. Bariatric (weight loss) surgery (such as gastric banding or gastric bypass) is an effective treatment for obesity which can restore fertility but as there may be initial nutritional compromise, it is recommended that women leave 2 years after the surgery before conceiving (Shah and Ginsburg, 2010).

Maternal protein intake affects gonadotrophin secretion and ovulatory maturation (Wynn and Wynn, 1991). Diets with abnormally high protein content and also those with very low protein content affect the menstrual cycle and fertility. It is possible that high-protein diets may cause one of the coenzymes involved in protein metabolism to become limiting. It is also suggested that low levels of B vitamins depress pituitary hormone secretion. Both embryonic development, especially early in gestation, and follicular development involve a rapid rate of protein synthesis and cell division, which are associated with a high energy and nutrient requirement. Preconceptual nutrient deficiency may retard development of the follicle and corpus luteum, affecting subsequent embryonic growth, even if the level of deficiency is not adequate to cause infertility. Excess intakes of some nutrients may increase mutation rate. Nutrient deficiency also affects male fertility, by altering DNA synthesis and rates of cell division. Selenium availability may be an important factor in male fertility.

Whether the mother enters pregnancy with high nutritional stores may affect the outcome of the pregnancy. Placental size in humans appears to be governed by genetic growth potential, anoxia and nutrient availability. In sheep, a period of poor nutrition early in gestation increases placental size, presumably as an adaptive mechanism to increase nutrient extraction (McCrabb et al., 1992). Provided this nutrient restriction is transient and the sheep are then returned to richer pasture, the increase in placental size is associated with an increase in lamb birth weight. In humans, an increased placental:fetal weight ratio is associated with poorer outcome and long-term health prognosis (Barker, 1998). However, larger babies have larger placentas but in proportion to their birth weight. Morning sickness may produce a period of poor nutrition in early pregnancy, which could stimulate placental growth (Coad et al., 2002). Provided the woman entered pregnancy with good nutrient stores and the effects on nutrient consumption were limited, nausea in pregnancy could promote placental enlargement and positively affect the fetal growth trajectory. An adequate interpregnancy interval may be important to allow replenishment of maternal stores, especially of vitamins such as folate.

Case study 12.1 looks at an example of assessing nutritional status in pregnancy.

NON-NUTRITIONAL FACTORS AFFECTING REPRODUCTIVE FUNCTION

Food can provide nutrition but it is also the source of a number of maternal infections (Box 12.2). Pregnant women are advised to be particularly careful about food

Case study 12.1

Fiona informs the midwife at the booking appointment that she has a healthy balanced diet.

- How can the midwife assess that this is an accurate statement?
- What observations can help the midwife assess Fiona's nutritional status?
- Are there any other factors that might affect Fiona's description of her diet?
- Are there any perceptions of what is a 'healthy balanced diet' that may actually be potentially harmful and if so what are they and why should they be avoided?

Box 12.2 **Food safety**

Listeriosis

- Caused by: bacterium *Listeria monocytogenes*
- Possible effects: miscarriage, stillbirth and neonatal death, brain damage, premature delivery, maternal mortality, meconium before 37 weeks gestation
- Sources: soil, soft cheeses, pate, raw seafood, cold meats, poultry, cook-chill food

Note: bacteria can multiply at low temperatures so women are recommended to thoroughly reheat refrigerated leftovers

Salmonellosis

- Caused by: *Salmonella enteric*
- Possible effects: maternal high fever, vomiting, diarrhoea and dehydration associated with food poisoning may increase the risk of preterm labour or miscarriage
- Source: raw meat, poultry and eggs, foods made from raw eggs such as mousses and sauces

Note: survives in soft-boiled eggs and mayonnaise, cross-contamination by uncooked foods or utensils is common

Toxoplasmosis

- Caused by: *Toxoplasma gondii*
- Possible effects: congenital mental retardation or blindness, neonatal convulsions, visual and hearing loss, haematological abnormalities, enlarged spleen and liver
- Sources: soil, raw or undercooked meat, cats' faeces and litter trays, goats' milk

Campylobacters

- Caused by: *Campylobacter jejuni* and *C. coli.*
- Possible effects: preterm delivery, intrauterine death
- Sources: undercooked poultry, unpasteurized milk

Box 12.3 **Factors affecting weight gain in pregnancy or birth weight**

- Maternal diet before and during pregnancy
- Maternal size, particularly lean body mass
- Age (younger women tend to gain more weight but pregnancy in adolescents is associated with an increased likelihood of an LBW baby)
- Birth order (first babies tend to be slightly smaller)
- Parity (multigravidae tend to gain less weight)
- Fetal sex (male babies tend to be an average of 150 g heavier)
- Nicotine (both smoking and tobacco chewing are associated with decreased birth weight)
- Alcohol (regular alcohol consumption is associated with lower birth weight)
- Hypoxia (high altitude and chronic maternal anaemia depress birth weight)

hygiene (Derbyshire, 2010). Although nutrient intake and weight gain are associated with clear effects on birth weight, a number of other factors have been shown to affect fetal size and growth potential (Box 12.3).

Age affects cell proliferation and gamete formation. Some diseases accelerate premature ageing of the germ cells. These include diabetes, parental gene mutation, multiple sclerosis, ulcerative colitis and Crohn's disease (Wynn and Wynn, 1991). Smoking, drugs, alcohol and radiation all affect cell division; indeed, smoking is probably the most important single factor influencing incidence of LBW babies in developed countries (Chiriboga, 2003). Viruses are mutagenic and have long been associated with abnormal fetal development. Sexually transmitted diseases (STDs) can cause pelvic inflammatory disease, which may affect fertility and pregnancy outcome.

Diseases caused by larger organisms, such as syphilis and gonorrhoea, are relatively easy to diagnose and treat. However, STDs caused by smaller microorganisms, such as chlamydia, papilloma, HIV, herpes and mycoplasmas, are difficult to eradicate. STD prevalence is associated with increased mobility of the population.

NUTRITIONAL REQUIREMENTS IN PREGNANCY

Energy requirements

The nutritional costs of pregnancy can be theoretically calculated by estimating the cost of the new maternal tissues (particularly maternal fat deposition) and the tissues of the conceptus (fetus, placenta, membranes and other tissues) – the 'capital gains' – and the metabolic costs of maintaining these growing tissues – the 'running costs' (Campbell-Brown and Hytten, 1998). Tissue accrued (based on an assumed body fat retention of 3.8 kg) accounts for about 185 MJ (50 000 kcal), and increased metabolism accounts for about 150 MJ (36 000 kcal), bringing the total specific cost of pregnancy to about 335 MJ (80 000 kcal) (Fig. 12.3). As more studies about nutritional requirements during pregnancy are performed, the recommended daily allowances of energy and other nutrients have progressively decreased. However, recommended allowances are intended to be a standard against which the nutritional status of a population, rather than that of an individual person, can be assessed.

Energy requirements during the pregnancy are highest in the middle (from 10 to 30 weeks) when maternal fat stores are being assimilated. During the last 10 weeks of the pregnancy, the rapid growth of the fetus has a high energy requirement but the rate of maternal fat storage is decreased (and often maternal intake is limited). In effect, the increased nutritional requirements of the pregnancy

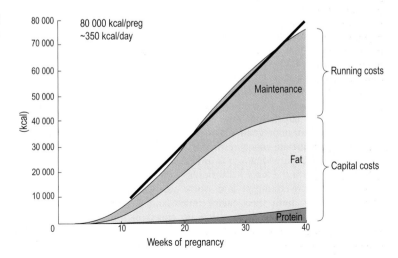

Fig. 12.3 The cumulative energy costs of pregnancy. (Reproduced with permission from Hytten, 1991.)

are spread fairly evenly over the later three-quarters of the pregnancy. The daily increase in energy requirement is calculated to be about 1.2 MJ (300 kcal) over the final three-quarters of pregnancy (Campbell-Brown and Hytten, 1998). This is calculated from the total cost of the pregnancy, estimated to be 335 MJ (80 000 kcal) divided by 270 days of pregnancy. The reported energy consumed in pregnancy by women 'eating to appetite' (with free access to food) is about 0.8 MJ (200 kcal) extra per day, less than the theoretical expected cost of the pregnancy. Many women, including those in developing countries and the poorer parts of affluent countries, successfully reproduce supported by energy intakes which appear to be well below the recommended levels. Some of this discrepancy is likely to be due to under-reporting of energy intake in pregnancy because of changed eating habits or subject fatigue in research studies.

Some of the additional energy requirements of pregnancy could be met by increased efficiency of maternal metabolism (decreased basal metabolic rate (BMR) or diet-induced thermogenesis (DIT) or the thermic effect of food (TEF)) and decreased activity-related energy expenditure (Forsum and Löf, 2007). However the BMR response to pregnancy is varied (while it is usually stimulated, it may be depressed or unchanged) and DIT (the increase in energy expenditure due to food consumption) probably remains unaltered. Decreased activity-related energy expenditure could make up a considerable proportion of the energy balance but women who are normally sedentary have little flexibility to further reduce their physical activity during pregnancy (Butte and King, 2005). Decreased energy expenditure in the second and third trimesters of pregnancy has been observed in the Five Country Study of pregnant women (Lawrence et al., 1987), which compared women living in Scotland, Holland, the Gambia, the Philippines and Thailand. Leisure activities and the rate at which heavy work was done decreased. Women who have a long history of poor nutrition, for instance those in subsistence farming communities, seem to be able to adapt more to sparing nutrients and economizing to support the cost of the pregnancy. This may be because these women are more physically active and so can decrease their energy expenditure by a greater degree. However many pregnant women living in developing countries are not able to reduce their activity. Physiological adaptation, for instance the lower resistance blood circulation, may alter the efficiency of energy metabolism in pregnancy (Forsum and Löf, 2007).

Dieting or deliberate energy restriction is not appropriate for most pregnant women; it is unlikely to be beneficial and may harm the fetus. Historically, women at risk of developing pre-eclampsia and obese women were recommended to limit their energy intake and weight gain. However, energy restriction has no effect on the development of pre-eclampsia; excessive weight gain is the result, not the cause, of the underlying clinical pathology. Inadequate energy intake, particularly in the first trimester, is associated with an increased incidence of LBW infants and congenital abnormalities (Carmichael et al., 2003). Excessive weight loss and fat mobilization in pregnancy can produce metabolites that can create metabolic stress and are detrimental to fetal development. Maternal health and later lactational capability may be compromised by dietary restriction in pregnancy. In obese women, energy restriction can be associated with lower infant birth weight (Merialdi et al., 2003). However, if obese women are motivated by their pregnant state to follow dietary recommendations and improve their diet, many will lose body fat.

Protein requirements

Protein requirements increase in pregnancy, to support maternal tissue synthesis and fetal growth. Metabolic adaptations enhancing the efficiency of protein synthesis are evident from early pregnancy onwards (Duggleby and Jackson, 2002). Low-protein diets are associated with an adverse outcome of pregnancy but low protein intakes are unlikely in affluent developed countries. Protein requirements for the growth of maternal tissues and the growth of the conceptus were calculated to be about 925 g (Campbell-Brown and Hytten, 1998) but have been reassessed to be closer to 500–700 g (Williamson, 2006). The increased protein synthesis, and therefore increased dietary requirement, in late pregnancy is about 6 g/day. In Britain and other developed countries, where the average NPU value is 0.7, this is equivalent to about 8–9 g of additional dietary protein being required to maintain nitrogen balance.

During the pregnancy, there is a fall in blood protein levels from about 70–60 g/L. Much of this fall is due to decreased plasma albumin concentration resulting from haemodilution. Albumin functions as a non-specific carrier of lipophilic substances such as some drugs, hormones, free fatty acids, unconjugated bilirubin and some ions. It has an important role in maintaining the plasma osmotic pressure. The fall in plasma colloid osmotic pressure increases movement of water out of the blood vessels (see Chapter 1), thus increasing lower limb oedema and affecting glomerular filtration rate (GFR). Plasma globulins increase in pregnancy.

Plasma levels of most amino acids fall in pregnancy. The most marked falls are observed in glucogenic amino acids, which can be used to form glucose, then those involved in the urea cycle and then the ketogenic branched-chain amino acids. Amino acids are actively transported across the placenta. The transfer of amino acids across the placenta is only just adequate for fetal protein synthesis so any factor adversely affecting amino acid transport mechanisms has the potential to limit growth. Imbalances in maternal amino acid concentration will be reflected by placental uptake. For instance, women with phenylketonuria (PKU) are advised to resume a low-phenylalanine diet (and take tyrosine supplements) prior to conception as high levels of phenylalanine can harm the fetus, even if the fetus does not have PKU. High phenylalanine levels in pregnancy are associated with fetal IUGR, congenital heart disease, microcephaly and mental retardation. The amino acid methionine is involved in folate metabolism; women who have higher dietary intakes of methionine seem to be at lower risk of delivering a baby with a neural tube defect (NTD; Shoob et al., 2001). Good sources of methionine tend to be foods such as animal proteins that are rich in other amino acids and total protein, iron, zinc and calcium.

The optimum birth weight in humans can be considered to be within the range of birth weights associated with the lowest incidence of perinatal mortality and morbidity, in the range 3500–4500 g (Wynn and Wynn, 1991). Mothers of babies in the optimal birth-weight range tend to eat more protein than women who give birth to babies with lower birth weight. Maternal intakes of B vitamins and some minerals, particularly magnesium, have been found to correlate well with birth weight (Wynn and Wynn, 1991). The main regulator of fetal growth seems to be availability of nutrients, which can affect growth directly by changing the availability of substrates required for growth, or indirectly by altering hormonal control of growth.

The normal protein intake of women in most developed countries, who regularly consume foods such as lean meat and poultry, fish, reduced-fat milk products, wholegrains and legumes as part of a balanced and varied diet, appears to be sufficient to provide the additional requirements of pregnancy. Vegetarian and vegan women must ensure a range of wholegrains and legumes are consumed daily to provide adequate protein. The U. S. Institute of Medicine (2002) recommends an additional 25 g of protein per day for pregnancy in addition to the recommended daily intake (RDI) of 46 g of protein per day (0.80 g/kg/day), a total RDI of 71 g of protein per day for pregnant women (or 1.1 g/kg/day). Women with twin pregnancies are recommended to consume an additional 50 g of protein per day together with an appropriate energy increment to optimize efficient utilization of the protein (Institute of Medicine, 2002). Women with very low energy intakes may be at risk of inadequate protein intake. The use of formulated protein supplements, powders or high-protein formulated beverages should be discouraged because clinical studies suggest they may be potentially harmful to the fetus (Kramer and Kakuma, 2003). Some popular weight-restriction diets have promoted high protein intake. However, the fetus has limited ability to detoxify ammonia and excrete urea, particularly during the vulnerable periods of organogenesis in the first trimester. In experimental animals, high protein intakes and apparent high levels of ammonia have been associated with increased rates of congenital abnormalities.

Fat requirements

In pregnancy, plasma lipids alter markedly. Levels of free fatty acids, triacylglycerides, cholesterol, lipoproteins and phospholipids transiently fall early in pregnancy and then rise (Butte, 2000). The changes in handling of lipids are orchestrated by hormonal changes and are associated with changed insulin resistance during the pregnancy (Robinson et al., 1992). The initial low maternal levels of fatty acids reflect maternal fat storage, which is highest early in pregnancy when maternal maintenance costs of pregnancy and fetal growth are relatively low (Campbell-Brown and Hytten, 1998). This appears to anticipate requirements later in pregnancy. In the later stages of pregnancy, when fetal requirements are maximal, maternal nutrient intake could be restricted by lack of availability of food or by restricted capacity for eating and gastrointestinal disturbances. Maternal fat stores, which are 3.5 kg on average, can subsidize a considerable part of the pregnancy. Oxidation of 3.5 kg of fat could theoretically produce 132 MJ (30 000 kcal).

During early gestation the fetus depends on placental transfer for fatty acid requirements (Herrera and Amusquivar, 2000). Lipids are transported across the placenta as lipoprotein complexes, classified by their density (Fig. 12.4). Triglyceride levels increase throughout gestation. Placental uptake of triglycerides occurs in the form of very low-density lipoproteins (VLDL). Placental lipase may hydrolyse VLDL, releasing the products for energy metabolism by the fetus (Robinson et al., 1992). The rising level of maternal fatty acids in the third trimester probably reflects mobilization of maternal fat stores. In later gestation, maternal fatty acids are predominantly used for maternal metabolism and ketone body synthesis. The more mature fetus can synthesis fatty acids de novo, using ketone bodies as fuels and lipogenic substrates.

LCPUFA requirements of pregnant women are particularly high, especially in the third trimester when fetal brain and nervous tissue growth is maximal; accretion of DHA into the developing nervous system and fetal brain is high. Arachidonic acid (20:4, ω-6) is essential for neonatal growth and is the precursor for eicosanoids, prostaglandins and leukotrienes, and docosahexaenoic acid (DHA; 22:6, ω-3) has a key role in fetal brain development and visual function. Therefore, fetal demand for indispensable fatty acids (linoleic acid, 18:2, ω-6; and α-linoleic acid, 18:3, ω-3) must be met from either maternal intake or be released from maternal adipose tissue. The placenta transports the indispensable fatty acids and their preformed long-chain derivatives, arachidonic acid and DHA from the maternal circulation to the fetus. Low maternal intake of these indispensable fatty acids is correlated with reduced neonatal growth (Herrera, 2002).

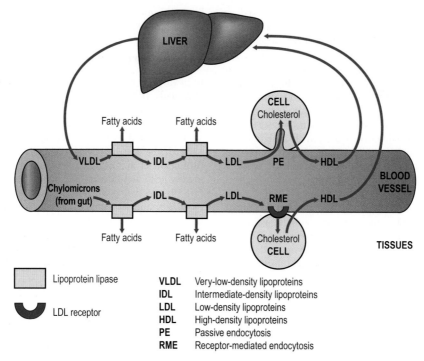

Fig. 12.4 Classification of lipoprotein complexes. (Reproduced with permission from Saffrey and Stewart, 1997.)

Oestrogen increases the conversion of essential fatty acids to long-chain fatty acids.

Consumption of fish, and therefore DHA, in pregnancy is associated with a reduced incidence of pre-eclampsia, LBW and preterm delivery (Makrides, 2009), probably because ω-3 fatty acids from marine sources inhibit ω-6-derived eicosanoids involved in cervical ripening and the initiation of parturition. Women who eat more marine foods also seem less likely to develop pregnancy-induced hypertension (Al et al., 2000). These positive effects of fish consumption on gestational duration and fetal development have generated much interest in requirements of LCPUFA for optimal outcome of pregnancy. However, it is not clear that supplementation with LCPUFA or fish oil might be beneficial as excess intake of LCPUFA can potentially increase the risk of oxidative damage (Herrera, 2002). The higher the content of PUFAs in the diet, the more likely damaging free radicals will be formed which are potentially toxic and can reduce antioxidant capacity.

Western diets are relatively rich in ω-6 fatty acids but poor in ω-3 fatty acids and intake of preformed DHA is low, so the supply of DHA to the fetus may be compromised. The ratio of ω-6 fatty acids to ω-3 fatty acids is estimated to be significantly higher than it was in the Neolithic era when the big brain of modern man evolved. Obese women with insulin resistance and thin women with little body fat are likely to be even more dependent on dietary DHA. Eating fish in pregnancy would increase DHA intake but much of the advice about fish liver oils containing vitamin A and not consuming an excess of fish in case of heavy metal contamination of fish has led pregnant women to avoid fish totally in pregnancy rather than increase their intake because they are pregnant.

A high fat intake is not recommended in pregnancy as there is an association between increased fat intake and the development of glucose abnormalities (Saldana et al., 2004). Ketonaemia appears to have a negative effect on fetal development and later intellectual performance (Rizzo et al., 1991). High-fat, low-carbohydrate diets are not optimal for pregnancy; it is suggested that a diet <30% fat and >50% carbohydrate reduces the risk of glucose intolerance and gestational diabetes.

Carbohydrate requirements

Adequate carbohydrate intake is important in pregnancy to ensure adequate glucose for maternal brain metabolism and transfer to the fetus but normal diets are usually rich in carbohydrates so there is no changed recommendation for pregnancy. Metabolism of carbohydrates and lipids alters, under hormonal influence, throughout pregnancy to ensure that the fetus receives a continuous supply of nutrients despite maternal intake being intermittent (Butte, 2000). Maternal glucose concentration is maintained at a significantly higher level in later pregnancy by increased hepatic glucose production in order to meet the increasing requirements of the placenta and fetus. The developing fetus utilizes glucose as its primary energy-producing substrate but it can also metabolize maternally derived ketoacids.

Maternal pre-existing diabetes (type 1 or type 2, but not gestational diabetes which develops later in pregnancy), high sucrose intake or prepregnancy obesity are all associated with an increased risk of NTD (Shaw et al., 2003). This is probably because the embryo does not have pancreatic function when the neural tube is developing and closing so it is unable to regulate excess of glucose at this time; high glucose levels lead to oxidative stress and embryonic depletion of inositol which can also affect neural tube development (Baker et al., 1990). The developing embryo may also be vulnerable to the effects of maternal hypoglycaemia following hyperglycaemia. Thus, good control of glucose metabolism in early pregnancy, which is more is likely to be achieved by a diet higher in foods with low GI, lowers the risk of congenital abnormalities. Gestational diabetes, because it becomes evident in the second half of pregnancy after embryonic development is completed, is not associated with an increased risk of congenital abnormalities but a high carbohydrate (low fat) diet with plentiful low GI foods is associated with a decrease in newborn macrosomia (Romon et al., 2001).

Adequate dietary fibre is particularly important in pregnancy because the high progesterone levels affect smooth muscle tone and result in a decreased rate of gastrointestinal transit. This has advantages for nutrient absorption as gut contents are in contact with sites of absorption for longer times but water is also absorbed to a greater extent, which often results in constipation. Recommending that pregnant women increase their intake of complex carbohydrates, such as wholemeal or wholegrain breads, cereals, legumes, fruit and vegetables, would provide carbohydrate with good sources of fibre. Promoting foods high in fibre helps to address problems of constipation as well as generally increasing carbohydrate intake. The other advantage of this is that many foods with higher fibre content also have a lower GI, which is particularly important for women who have, or are risk of developing, diabetes. Increasing intake of complex carbohydrate also has the positive outcome of displacing intakes of fat and added sugars.

Vitamins and minerals

It is thought that a range of micronutrient deficiencies might contribute to congenital malformations and the failure of human embryos to implant or survive (Keen et al., 2003). However, supplementation needs to be evaluated carefully as nutrient–nutrient interactions can be detrimental and some micronutrients are toxic in excess. Thus, both micronutrient deficiency and excess are associated with adverse pregnancy outcome. Levels of fat-soluble vitamins increase during pregnancy and levels of water-soluble vitamins fall. However, levels of vitamin A fall but levels of carotenoids rise. Fat-soluble vitamins cross the placenta more readily than water-soluble vitamins and their transport increases with gestational length; decreased levels of maternal plasma levels may be due to haemodilution rather than to increased uptake by maternal and fetal tissue. Thus, lower circulating levels of nutrients in pregnancy cannot be simply interpreted as indicating a deficiency. It is suggested that hormonal resetting of homeostatic mechanisms favours transfer of nutrients to the fetus (Campbell-Brown and Hytten, 1998). Low levels of nutrients in maternal plasma may limit maternal cell uptake while optimizing placental uptake. The placenta can extract nutrients from maternal plasma and transfer them to the fetus, maintaining transport against a concentration gradient. Thus, fetal concentration of vitamins may be 5–10 times the level in maternal blood. The 'pump' mechanisms of the placenta appear to be specific for vitamins; most minerals are not transported by similar mechanisms.

A good-quality maternal diet is probably able to provide the increased vitamin and mineral requirements of the pregnancy, particularly if energy intake is increased from a source of high-nutrient-density food. However, a poor-quality diet may adversely affect both fetal growth and the establishment of adequate stores for neonatal growth. Micronutrient requirements increase slightly in pregnancy but, unless the woman is at the threshold of a deficiency, most women consuming a varied and balanced diet should have adequate reserve. The possible exceptions to this generalization are iron and calcium nutritional status which should be assessed early in antenatal care. Periconceptual folate requirements are higher than can usually be provided by the diet. Vitamin A potentially presents some challenges in pregnancy, as both deficiency and excess are teratogenic. Certain subgroups within the population are at increased risk of vitamin D deficiency, such as Asian women.

Folate and folic acid

'Folate' is a generic term applied to dietary sources of related compounds that have the same biological activity in the body. Dietary folates are vulnerable to being broken down during food preparation. Folic acid is a synthetic form which is more bioavailable and more stable. Folate deficiency in early pregnancy is teratogenic and is associated with an increased incidence of NTDs; it can also cause megaloblastic anaemia of pregnancy, cervical dysplasia and atherosclerosis (Stover, 2004). There is a well-established protective effect of folic acid supplements that significantly reduce the incidence of NTDs and they may also reduce the incidence of other congenital abnormalities such as cleft lip. Poor folate intake is also associated with other negative pregnancy outcomes including LBW, abruptio placentae and increased risk of miscarriage.

Folate is involved in single-carbon transfer reactions in the metabolism of nucleic and amino acids, and hence the synthesis of DNA, RNA and proteins. Requirements for folate increase in pregnancy because the number of single-carbon transfer reactions increases, for instance for nucleotide synthesis and cell division. Blood folate levels fall in pregnancy, reflecting the high rate of DNA synthesis and cell division. Any factor that reduces DNA, RNA and protein synthesis increases the risk of congenital malformations, which are usually associated with a reduced cell number rather than a reduced cell size.

There is considerable interaction between folate and other vitamins, such as choline and vitamins B_6 and B_{12}, which also have a role in single-carbon methyl donation and, thus, recycling homocysteine to methionine. Deficiency of any of these vitamins can contribute to hyperhomocysteinaemia. Raised levels of homocysteine in pregnancy are associated with complications and adverse outcomes of pregnancy such as an increased risk of pre-eclampsia, NTDs and other congenital abnormalities, LBW and preterm delivery, placental abruption and spontaneous pregnancy loss (Holmes, 2003).

NTDs are the most common congenital abnormality resulting from failure of the neural tube to close effectively between 22 and 27 days postconception, which is usually before women realize they are pregnant. Increased intake of folic acid periconceptually overcomes unidentified abnormalities in folate utilization (Boddie et al., 2000) which are related to mutations of genes expressing enzymes in the folate metabolic pathways of genetically predisposed women. The incidence of NTD is 1.6 per 10 000 livebirths in England and 3.1 per 10 000 in Wales; NTDs are a clinical reason for offering termination of pregnancy so the actual incidence of pregnancies affected by NTDs is higher than the livebirth rate suggests.

Folic acid supplements, of 400 μg/day, are recommended for all pregnant women or women who might become pregnant. It is recommended that women who are at higher risk for pregnancy affected by NTD (because they have previously had an NTD-affected pregnancy, have a family history of NTD, have insulin-dependent diabetes, or are taking anticonvulsants known to affect folate metabolism) take a high-dose folic acid supplement (those who have already had one conception affected by a NTD should consume 4 mg folic acid per day to reduce the risk of recurrence). Although pregnant women seem aware of campaigns recommending increased folic acid consumption, many seem reluctant to take it (Health Education Authority, 1996). Possibly advice to supplement the diet with folic acid may appear to conflict with the usual health advice to avoid unnecessary drugs in pregnancy. Renaming folic acid as 'vitamin B_9' as is done in some parts of Europe might alter the perception of folic acid as a drug.

The levels of folic acid that are associated with reduced incidence of NTD are significantly higher than those that could be easily achieved from the diet. It is difficult to increase levels of folate-rich food to the level recommended (Cuskelly et al., 1996). Increased consumption of folate to reduce the risk of NTD is recommended 4 weeks before and 12 weeks after conception, which presents difficulties in many developed countries like the United Kingdom because about half of all pregnancies are unplanned.

The argument for supplementing a staple food, such as bread or flour, with folic acid (Wald and Bower, 1995) has been strengthened by the other advantages of increasing folate consumption. Folate is important in maintaining optimal levels of homocysteine; hyperhomocysteinaemia (accumulation of circulating homocysteine) is associated with cardiovascular disease, stroke, depression, Alzheimer's disease and some types of cancer. However, folic acid supplementation can mask the symptoms of pernicious anaemia due to low vitamin B_{12} intake which can delay the diagnosis of deficiency, increasing the risk of permanent neurological damage. Some drugs are folate antagonists and so increase the risk of NTDs (Pimentel, 2000). These include anti-epileptic drugs (such as carbamazepine and valproate), retinoids (used to treat acne) and some anti-tumour agents. Women who are pregnant with more than one fetus, breastfeeding women nursing more than one infant and those women with a high alcohol intake or are on chronic anticonvulsant or methotrexate therapy have increased requirement for folate.

Case study 12.2 looks at the issue of folic acid supplementation.

Vitamin A

Vitamin A (retinal) status in pregnancy is positively correlated with outcome of pregnancy in terms of infant size and gestational length. Requirements for vitamin A are highest in the third trimester of pregnancy when fetal

---

 Case study 12.2

Jane seeks preconceptual nutritional counselling. She has had a previous miscarriage and is keen to improve the quality of her diet. Jane expresses concern about taking drugs in pregnancy, including folic acid, and is adamant that the human race could not have evolved requiring nutrients that could not be provided by a healthy diet.

- How might a midwife summarize the characteristics of a balanced diet?
- What rich sources of folate could be identified and how might consumption be increased?
- Is the connection between a previous miscarriage and diet valid?
- How could Jane's fears about folic acid supplementation be addressed?

growth is highest. It is involved in vision, reproduction, gene expression, embryological development, growth, immune function, integrity of the epithelium and bone remodelling. Both deficiency and excess of vitamin A in pregnancy can cause fetal abnormalities. Low vitamin A status in pregnancy is associated with increased maternal mortality, decreased birth weight and increased risk of congenital abnormalities (Ramakrishnan et al., 1999). A high vitamin A intake is also associated with teratogenicity; this occurs in the first trimester and causes birth defects deriving from cranial neural crest cells such as craniofacial deformations (cleft lip and palate) and abnormalities of the central nervous system (not NTDs), heart and thymus.

Changes in animal husbandry, and increased use of growth-promoting agents and vitamin supplements given to animals, may make the livers of farmed animals considerably richer in vitamin A than they used to be. Birth defects in humans have been associated with the use of vitamin A analogues for treatment of acne. Women taking medications for the treatment of dermatological problems such as acne should check whether the medication contains large doses of vitamin A and, if so, discontinue its use prior to and during pregnancy. With some acne preparations, it is recommended that conception be avoided for a year after stopping treatment. Preformed vitamin A (retinal) is only available from animal-derived foods. Pro-vitamin A from carotenoids in coloured fruit and vegetables is not efficiently converted into retinal so pregnant women who avoid dairy products and meat need to consume at least five servings of fruit and vegetables per day and to select rich sources of carotenoids. No adverse effects of carotenoids from normal dietary levels of intake have been reported.

Vitamin D

Vitamin D maintains serum calcium and phosphorus concentrations within the range that optimizes bone health, by affecting the absorption of these minerals from the small intestine, their mobilization from bone and calcium resorption by the kidney. Vitamin D is synthesized in the skin; dietary requirements depend on exposure to sunlight. In pregnancy, vitamin D requirements increase substantially. Vitamin D deficiency in pregnancy is associated with decreased fetal growth and later increased risk of osteoporosis via the effect on maternal calcium homeostasis and increased neonatal vulnerability to rickets (Kovacs, 2008).

Dietary vitamin D is required for those individuals whose skin is not adequately exposed to sunlight (Hollis and Wagner, 2004). Women who are regularly exposed to sunlight are much less dependent on dietary sources of vitamin D. Risk factors for low vitamin D are low socioeconomic status, being covered or otherwise restricting access to ultraviolet light, and having a low educational level. Synthesis of vitamin D is affected by the season of the year and the amount of UV light. Less vitamin D is synthesized in the skin of dark-skinned people as melanin absorbs ultraviolet light. Being housebound or not exposing the face, hands and body to sunlight for cultural or religious reasons will limit vitamin D synthesis. Pregnant women who do not receive regular exposure to sunlight (estimated to be about 30–40 min of exposure of face and arms each day) are recommended to have a supplement of 10.0 μg (or 400 IU) of vitamin D per day by many authorities. However this level is under scrutiny and supplements at least 10 times this (which is possible to achieve naturally from sun exposure) are suggested as being optimal for long-term fetal health (including protection against auto-immune disorders) and to protect the mother against gestational diabetes, hypertension and pre-eclampsia (Hollis, 2007). It is prudent to recommend that exposure to sunlight is in the morning or late afternoon to reduce the risk of sunburn and excessive exposure to harmful UVR. It is not known to what extent the use of sunscreen affects vitamin D synthesis but pregnant women are encouraged to routinely use sunscreen during the middle of the day. Public health messages about sun avoidance to reduce the risk of melanoma have contributed to an increasing level of vitamin D insufficiency.

Vitamin K

Vitamin K is a coenzyme used in the synthesis of a number of proteins involved in bone metabolism and the blood coagulation cascade. Use of drugs that interfere with metabolism of vitamin K, such as warfarin, can increase the risk of fetal intraventricular haemorrhage, cerebral microbleedings, microencephaly and mental retardation. Anti-epileptic treatments can inhibit placental transport of vitamin K affecting fetal synthesis of clotting factors and increasing risk of haemorrhage. For this reason, it is recommended that pregnant women with epilepsy take a vitamin K supplement in the month before delivery and during labour. In addition, microbial synthesis of vitamin K may be compromised by the use of broad-spectrum antibiotic therapy (particularly if it is required for a prolonged period).

Vitamin B$_{12}$

Vitamin B$_{12}$ is a coenzyme involved in homocysteine-to-methionine conversion and for the reaction that converts L-methylmalonyl-coenzyme A to succinyl-CoA. Vitamin B$_{12}$ is involved in maternal and fetal erythropoiesis so requirements are increased particularly in the first two trimesters. Deficiency of vitamin B$_{12}$ increases the risk of neurological abnormalities in the fetus. Absorption of vitamin B$_{12}$ may increase in pregnancy; the fetus is dependent on maternal dietary intake (Allen, 2002). The placenta concentrates vitamin B$_{12}$ and then transfers it to the fetus down a concentration gradient so fetal levels of vitamin B_{12} are about double maternal levels. The placenta preferentially transports newly absorbed vitamin B_{12} rather than that from maternal liver stores, so transfer to the fetus may be compromised even though the mother shows no overt signs of deficiency.

Plants do not synthesize vitamin B_{12} so strict vegetarians and those people who consume low amounts of animal products are more likely to be deficient. Plant foods exposed to vitamin B_{12}-producing bacteria, or contaminated with soil, insects or other substances containing B_{12} or foods fortified with vitamin B_{12} are the only dietary sources for strict vegetarians. Fetal levels of vitamin B_{12} may be compromised even if the mother has only recently become a vegetarian. Pregnant women who are strict vegetarians need to take vitamin B_{12} supplements or eat foods that have been fortified with vitamin B_{12}, and continue doing so while they are breastfeeding. Infants are less tolerant to vitamin B_{12} deficiency than adults; breastfed infants may develop severe megaloblastic anaemia and neurological damage, even if their vitamin B_{12}-deficient mothers are not showing clinical signs of deficiency. The first symptoms of infant vitamin B_{12} deficiency are drowsiness, repetitive vomiting, swallowing problems, severe constipation and tremor (particularly involving tongue, face, pharynx and legs). Progression to unconsciousness, coma and, ultimately, death can be swift.

Vitamin C

Vitamin C is a water-soluble antioxidant and a cofactor for enzymes involved in the synthesis of collagen, neurotransmitters and carnitine. It is involved in the recycling of vitamin E and also enhances absorption of non-haem iron. Haemodilution in pregnancy results in plasma vitamin C concentration falling. Pregnant women have increased vitamin C requirements to ensure adequate transfer to the fetus and maternal needs are met. The placenta transports ascorbate from the maternal circulation, oxidizes it and transfers it to the fetus (Choi and Rose, 1989). Vitamin C deficiency is associated with premature rupture of the placental membranes (Siega-Riz et al., 2003), preterm delivery (Ramakrishnan et al., 1999) and infection (Casanueva et al., 1993). Intervention studies have shown reduced incidence of pre-eclampsia in at-risk women supplemented with vitamin C and vitamin E (Chappell et al., 2002). Additional vitamin C is recommended for pregnant women exposed to increased oxidative stress; these include smokers and women who use recreational drugs or consume significant qualities of alcohol or regularly take aspirin (Cogswell et al., 2003).

Calcium

Calcium requirements increase mostly in the third trimester when the fetal skeleton develops rapidly, incorporating a total of about 30 g of calcium. However, this is a tiny proportion of the calcium deposited in the maternal skeleton, which can act as a reservoir if dietary calcium is low. However, if the mother's own skeleton is still growing, as in adolescent pregnancy, there may be competition between the maternal and fetal skeletons for calcium. Young girls who become pregnant within 2 years of starting to menstruate are most at risk as demineralization of maternal bone may be particularly detrimental when peak bone mass is being accrued.

Vitamin D concentrations rise in pregnancy, resulting in increased intestinal calcium absorption, and calcium retention is increased; this occurs in advance of mineralization of the fetal skeleton. Calcium supplementation has been used therapeutically during pregnancy to prevent hypertensive disorders and related problems. Calcium is one of the main nutrients which need to be considered in the antenatal assessment; it is not uncommon for women of reproductive age to have an intake that is below the recommended intake. Pregnant adolescents are particularly at risk of inadequate intake of calcium as are women of all ages who do not consume dairy products. Pregnant women should be encouraged to consume at least three servings of calcium-rich foods a day. Although dietary sources of calcium are preferable, it may be necessary for women who avoid dairy produce and other calcium-rich foods to be prescribed a calcium supplement. Calcium supplementation in pregnancy for women who have a low calcium intake may protect against hypotensive disorders and pre-eclampsia (Hofmeyr et al., 2010). Women who are prescribed both iron and calcium supplements should avoid taking them at the same time of day to maximize absorption of both.

Iron

The requirements for additional iron in pregnancy remain controversial (see Chapter 11). First-trimester iron requirements are lower than for non-pregnant women due to menstrual savings but requirements are markedly higher by the third trimester (Hallberg, 2001). It is estimated that about 600 mg of iron are required for the fetus and placenta and blood lost at parturition (Campbell-Brown and Hytten, 1998). The expansion of maternal red blood cell mass accounts for about 290 mg of iron (Letsky, 1998), but this expansion probably accommodates for the blood lost at parturition. Amenorrhoea of pregnancy saves about 120 mg of iron, which is not lost in menstruation, and iron absorption increases.

Iron depletion (low iron stores) or deficiency (anaemia) appears to be common in pregnant women and the consequences are significant for both mother and fetus. Maternal anaemia increases risk of morbidity and mortality, and is associated with risk of heart failure, haemorrhage and infection. The risks of fetal death, perinatal mortality, preterm delivery and lower birth weight are also increased

(Scholl and Reilly, 2000). Maternal iron deficiency affects cognition, behaviour, motor development and activity of offspring (Allen, 1997), probably irreversibly. Infants of iron-deficient mothers are more likely to have low iron stores and be susceptible to iron deficiency themselves. Maternal iron deficiency affects the mother's physical work capacity and interaction with the infant.

There are two pathways of iron absorption; haem and non-haem iron absorption (Fig. 12.5). Haem iron from meat is highly bioavailable and affected to a negligible degree by other components of the diet. However, most dietary iron is non-haem iron, absorption of which varies with other dietary constituents, particularly those which influence the reduction of the insoluble ferric iron to soluble ferrous iron. Vitamin C and other organic acids significantly enhance dietary absorption of non-haem iron, as does the presence of meat, fish or poultry, though the mechanism is not clear. Inhibitors of non-haem absorption bind iron and render it less available; these include phytate (in legumes, grains and rice), polyphenols (in tea and coffee, grains, oregano and red wine) and vegetable proteins such as those in soybeans. Calcium inhibits absorption of both haem and non-haem iron with a dose-related effect. Non-haem iron is transported across the gut by the same divalent metal transporter which also transports other metals such as zinc and copper; this means that supplementation with one metal can affect the absorption of the others. The bioavailability of iron from meat is significantly higher than from plant-based foods, and the meat and other animal proteins enhance non-haem iron absorption, so individuals who consume omnivorous diets absorb more iron than do vegans or vegetarians.

Risk factors for iron deficiency in pregnancy include depleted iron stores prior to pregnancy (usually related to menstrual loss), not eating meat, chronic use of non-steroidal anti-inflammatory drugs (NSAIDs) such as aspirin (resulting in gastrointestinal lesions), low intake of factors which increase iron absorption (particularly vitamin C) and high intake of factors which decrease absorption. Iron deficiency is more likely with low socioeconomic status, poorer educational attainment and multiple gestation; adolescent women and those with a short interpregnancy interval are also at increased risk of iron deficiency. Use of oral contraceptives prior to pregnancy tends to result in a favourable iron status because menstrual loss is limited.

Pregnant women who are at risk of iron deficiency are usually prescribed iron supplements. Some women experience gastrointestinal effects in response to supplementary iron. Absorption of iron is best in the absence of other food (empty stomach) but may be associated with more side-effects. Low-dose supplements are associated with fewer side-effects and ferrous gluconate appears to be less irritating. However, iron is potentially toxic in excess; concerns focus on iron overload causing the generation of free radicals which can cause cellular damage and on the possible increased susceptibility to infection of women who are not iron deficient. Thus, iron supplementation should always be prescribed on the basis of biological criteria rather than being administered routinely.

Haemochromatosis is the most common genetic disorder affecting Caucasian populations (Heath and Fairweather-Tait, 2003); it is a recessively inherited disease resulting in iron overload. The clinical effects of haemochromatosis, due to deposition of iron in the liver, heart and pancreas, are not usually manifest or of concern in women of childbearing age as menstrual losses help to maintain iron balance. However, routine assessment of blood parameters

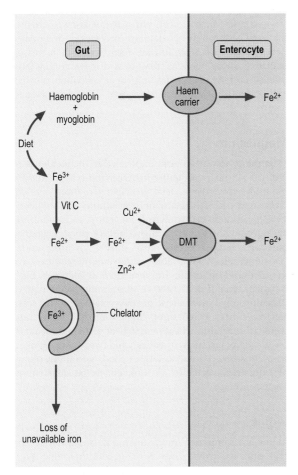

Fig. 12.5 Pathways of iron absorption. Haem iron from meat, poultry and fish is absorbed efficiently via the haem *tran* porter, whereas absorption of non-haem iron is affected by other dietary components. For instance, vitamin C enhances the conversion of Fe^{3+} (ferric iron) to the more soluble Fe^{2+} (ferrous iron) which is better absorbed. Some dietary components, such as phytate and polyphenols, bind to the iron and make it less available. Non-haem iron is transported across the gut wall via the divalent metal transporter (DMT). Zinc and copper can compete for transport by DMT and therefore inhibit iron absorption.

such as transferrin saturation in pregnant women could help to identify those women who might be at risk in later life.

To meet the additional requirements of pregnancy, women need to markedly increase their intake of iron-rich foods and the dietary factors that promote iron absorption. Nutritional assessment and dietary advice for pregnant women should take into consideration both sources of iron and the intake of factors affecting non-haem iron absorption. Timing of consumption of foods can influence nutrient–nutrient interaction. For instance, drinking fruit juice (high vitamin C content) with a good iron source will favour absorption, and drinking tea, which has a high tannin level, should be avoided with iron sources. Vegetarian and vegan women may find it difficult to meet their iron requirements solely from food sources; they should consume grains, vegetables and legumes, and have vitamin C-rich foods or drinks (raw fruits, fruit juice or vegetables) with meals. As adolescents have a higher iron requirement, this group is particularly vulnerable in being able to achieve an adequate iron intake particularly in the latter part of pregnancy and especially if they avoid meat. Supplementation may be necessary for those with low iron stores and/or low dietary iron intakes, but supplementation must always be given in conjunction with appropriate dietary advice, and under supervision from a health professional. There are concerns about excessive intake of supplementary iron and its potential effects on free-radical generation; also, the implications of iron supplementation on zinc and copper status need to be considered.

Zinc

Zinc is involved in cell proliferation, protein synthesis, protection from oxidative damage, apoptosis, hormone binding (by means of zinc fingers) and transcription, and is thus likely to affect embryonic and fetal development (Keen et al., 2003). Zinc deficiency in pregnancy is teratogenic; it is associated with increased risk of congenital abnormality (including NTDs) and other complications of pregnancy and delivery including haemorrhage, hypertension, pre- and post-term pregnancy and prolonged labour, growth retardation, retarded neurogenesis, neurobehavioural and immunological development and premature delivery (Mahomed et al., 2007). Iron supplementation can decrease zinc absorption, and zinc in excess may induce a secondary copper deficiency, as there is competition for the divalent metal transporters. Bioavailability of zinc in foods is particularly affected by high phytate content in foods such as cereal grains, legumes and nuts.

Selenium

Selenium forms part of the enzyme glutathione peroxidase, which metabolizes hydrogen peroxide formed from polyunsaturated fatty acids. Selenium is incorporated into proteins to make selenoproteins, some of which function as antioxidant enzymes preventing cellular damage from free radicals (natural by-products of oxygen metabolism). Other selenoproteins are involved in thyroid hormone metabolism (Thomson, 2004). The requirement for selenium is uncertain; a relatively low intake of selenium is required to prevent Keshan disease, a cardiomyopathy, but higher intakes of selenium may be protective against cancer and cardiovascular disease, by protecting against free-radical damage. Pregnant women have increased selenium requirements to allow for growth of the embryo and increased selenoprotein synthesis and tissue accumulation. The placenta actively transports selenium to the fetus (Hytten and Leitch, 1971), but it is not known whether maternal absorption of selenium increases in pregnancy. Requirements for selenium are increased with increased oxidative stress such as that caused by smoking and intense exercise. The main sources of selenium are fish and seafood, meat and poultry, eggs, dairy produce and bread.

Magnesium

Magnesium status has been implicated in the incidence of preterm labour (via uterine hyperirritability), pregnancy-induced hypertension, fetal growth retardation, cerebral palsy and mental retardation (Institute of Medicine, 1997). Studies of women from poor socioeconomic backgrounds, who have a higher risk of poor pregnancy outcome, have observed low intakes of magnesium (Doyle et al., 1989). Some intervention studies have found that magnesium supplementation increases birth weight (Merialdi et al., 2003). Magnesium forms part of the chlorophyll molecule so green vegetables such as spinach are rich in magnesium; other sources include nuts, seeds, wholegrains, wheat bran, wheat germ and breakfast cereals, dairy products, dried fruit and hard water. Women who consume a wide variety of foods including plenty of fruit and vegetables are unlikely to be deficient in magnesium.

Iodine

Iodine is a component of the thyroid hormones thyroxine (T_4) and its active form 3,3',5-tri-iodothyronine (T_3), which are important in growth and development and in energy production. Pregnant women have increased requirements for iodine as the fetus has a high requirement and maternal renal clearance is increased. The fetal brain is very vulnerable to maternal hypothyroidism; iodine deficiency is the major cause of preventable mental retardation worldwide. In pregnancy, severe iodine deficiency is associated with LBW and preterm delivery, congenital abnormalities, increased pregnancy loss, stillbirth, increased perinatal and infant mortality, psychomotor, speech and hearing defects, dwarfism, spastic diplegia, cretinism and mental retardation (Zimmermann and Delange, 2004). Mild-to-moderate iodine deficiency during pregnancy adversely affects both maternal and infant thyroid function and has implications for the mental development of the infant. Marginal iodine deficiency in pregnancy may be associated with impaired development but small effects on mental development such as IQ score reduced by a few points are difficult to assess, particularly as it is difficult to measure dietary iodine intake. Although iodized table salt is mandatory in the United Kingdom, individuals are consuming less salt for well-founded health reasons, consumption of commercially produced and processed foods which do not contain iodized salt has increased and there is reduced use of iodophors for cleaning equipment in the dairy industry. It has been proposed that pregnant women and women planning pregnancy should take an iodine-containing supplement of about 150 µg/day to optimise development of the fetus (Zimmermann, 2009) and these are becoming more available in many countries.

UNDERNUTRITION IN PREGNANCY

In experimental animals, maternal undernutrition in pregnancy usually leads to decreased birth weight. Maternal weight gain in human pregnancy is positively associated with birth weight and developmental outcome. However, in nutritional assessment it is important to determine prepregnancy weight from objective data and to assess the level of oedema. Women who are underweight have an increased risk of pregnancy loss and small babies that have increased morbidity and mortality. It is difficult to dissociate the effects of a poor diet in pregnancy from other variables. Women who consume a poor diet in pregnancy are likely to have consumed a poor diet before pregnancy and more likely to have had a poorer diet during their own growth and development. Many of them are shorter than average and a poor diet is associated with an increased incidence of smoking. Maternal shortness is also associated with a poorer social background, young maternal age and less formal education.

Diet quality

Although most nutritional studies have focused on energy requirements and consumption in pregnancy, the quality of the diet as well as the quantity may be important. In Britain, nutrient-deficiency diseases are rare but the quality of the diet varies markedly (see below). Mothers of LBW babies have not only low energy intakes but also diets of low nutrient density. Even in affluent countries, many women have daily intakes of B vitamins below the recommended level. Lifestyle changes, such as car ownership and less-active work patterns, mean energy requirements fall. However, nutrient requirements may not fall in parallel; indeed pollution and smoking increase requirements of certain nutrients. This means that, although energy consumption needs to fall to match reduced energy expenditure, the density of nutrients within the diet may need to increase to ensure that requirements are met.

Supplementation

Nutrient supplementation studies of the diet in pregnancy have produced inconsistent and inconclusive results. High-density protein supplementation depresses birth weight (Rush, 1989). Lower concentrations of protein have disappointingly small effects. Some of the studies are probably methodologically flawed and supplements may be used as alternatives rather than increasing nutrient consumption, or the target group may not consume them. Supplementation in the second and third trimesters of pregnancy may be too late to have an effect on birth weight; however, it may benefit maternal health and work potential and improve breastfeeding efficiency. Earlier supplementation may have a greater effect because nutrient support of early follicular development and maternal nutrient stores prior to conception may programme the fetal growth trajectory. More research studies investigating the effectiveness of supplements on the outcomes of pregnancy are needed particularly for those nutrients where intake is more likely to be compromised such as iodine, DHA, folate and choline (Zeisel, 2009).

Fetal adaptation to undernutrition

Subjected to inadequate substrate levels of either nutrients or oxygen, the fetus adapts by changing its metabolic activity in order to survive in utero and to optimize chances of surviving after birth in a nutritionally poor environment. Slowing of growth and reducing energy expenditure are part of this adaptation. Growth accounts for a large proportion of energy expenditure. Adapting to a lower growth trajectory means that nutrient requirement decreases and available nutrient levels may then be adequate. The placenta, which has a high nutrient and oxygen requirement itself, may also adapt. Although a number of adult-onset diseases are associated with impaired fetal nutrition (Fig. 12.6), they tend not to affect reproductive ability as they cause pathological problems late in life. Animal studies have demonstrated that marginal malnourishment for many generations requires optimal nutrition for several generations before normal size and behaviour are expressed (Stewart et al., 1980). This intergenerational effect may be one of the reasons why dietary supplementation in pregnancy has such a small effect on outcome.

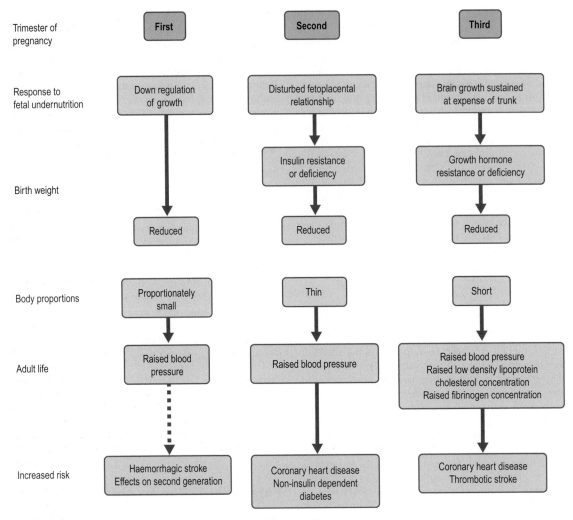

Fig. 12.6 Association of adult-onset diseases and impaired fetal nutrition.

Malnutrition

Interesting results come from studies looking at the effect of nutrient deprivation on previously well-nourished women. The Dutch Hunger Winter, from September 1944 to May 1945, was due to the Nazi blockade of food supplies exacerbated by very severe winter weather conditions. The severe nutritional deficiency affected fertility and birth weights and the birth rate fell dramatically, by about 50%, 9 months later (Lumley, 1992; Stein and Susser, 1975a). This was due both to effects on ovulation and an increased incidence of pregnancy failure. Congenital malformation rate increased among babies conceived during the famine and in the following 4 months, which demonstrates the importance of good preconceptual nutrition. However, many women were already pregnant at the time of the food shortage. If the women were deprived of energy in the second half of their pregnancy, the birth weight of their babies was reduced by 350 g on average. These babies were thin but of normal length. They appeared to develop and grow normally. However, in adulthood the male babies who had been exposed to deficiency late in development had lower rates of obesity compared with those who had experienced restricted nutrient levels early in development (Ravelli et al., 1976). Young women who had been exposed to nutrient deficiency early in gestation, but not later, had normal birth weights themselves. However, their babies were smaller than expected (Stein and Susser, 1975b). Adults of lower birth weight have increased risk of developing type 2 diabetes mellitus, heart disease, hypertension, obstructive lung disease, hypercholesterolaemia and renal disease (Godfrey and Barker, 2000). However, results from the longer, more severe, Leningrad siege do not show any association between intrauterine malnutrition and glucose intolerance and coronary heart disease in adulthood (Stanner et al., 1997).

Transient nutrient deficiency may alter fetal growth patterns without affecting final birth weight very much (Harding and Johnson, 1995). Birth weight is a crude outcome measure of optimal gestational growth and development. Suboptimal maternal body composition and nutrient intake can have a long-term effect on the offspring without necessarily affecting size at birth (Godfrey, 2001). Birth weight does not differentiate between the more subtle effects of nutrition on body composition and development of specific tissues and organs. It may not identify growth restriction; a similar birth weight can be attained with different growth trajectories. For instance, if an infant does not reach its potential birth weight but is born above 2500 g, it will not be classified as being of LBW even though its growth is not optimal. Nutrient deprivation before pregnancy or early in gestation affects brain growth and development in animals, which suggests that 'programming' of later brain growth is determined by nutrient availability before the demand for nutrients occurs. Lung growth is affected by later nutritional deficiency; lung weight and composition, muscle function, defence mechanisms and surfactant production are all susceptible to nutritional insult in late pregnancy.

MATERNAL OBESITY

Maternal obesity is associated with larger babies, macrosomia and increased perinatal mortality. Large-for-gestational-age babies are not longer in length but have increased deposition of adipose tissue. Routine antenatal care is more difficult in obese women, and labour is more likely to be prolonged and unsuccessful. Obese women are at higher risk of disorders such as hypertension, thromboembolism, pre-eclampsia and gestational diabetes. Obese women tend to have increased problems during delivery with more caesarean sections and associated problems; operative delivery is more complicated and there is increased risk in the puerperium (Yogev and Catalano, 2009). Maternal obesity is also associated with an increased incidence of congenital malformations (Prentice and Goldberg, 1996), particularly NTD. In obese women, folic acid seems to lose its protective effect.

LIFESTYLE ISSUES

Alcohol

Alcohol readily crosses the placenta so maternal alcohol levels determine alcohol levels in fetal blood and may affect embryonic development, growth, fetal brain function and later behaviour. Exposure of the fetus to alcohol can cause long-term behavioural and developmental problems; particular periods of embryonic development may be more vulnerable than others and patterns of drinking (such as regular or binge drinking) may determine the extent of the effect. Whether there is a 'safe' limit of alcohol exposure is uncertain; other dietary factors and genetics also play a role in the effects of alcohol. Therefore, it is prudent to advise all pregnant women to avoid alcohol completely if possible. Also, total abstinence is often found easier to adhere to.

Fetal alcohol syndrome, the most easily recognizable outcome of fetal alcohol exposure, is characterized by intrauterine and postnatal growth retardation, characteristic unusual facial features and adverse effects on brain function leading to mental retardation and/or behavioural disturbances. It occurs if the fetus is exposed to regular heavy alcohol intake or to very high alcohol concentrations at critical periods in development. However, fetuses exposed to lower amounts of alcohol may also be affected with fetal alcohol spectrum disorder which results in a range of symptoms that can be more difficult to diagnose definitively. These symptoms include attention deficit hyperactivity disorder (ADHD), inability to foresee consequences and learn from previous experience, inappropriate or immature behaviour, lack of organization, learning difficulties, poor abstract thinking, poor adaptability, poor impulse control, poor judgement and communication problems (Koren et al., 2003). Infants exposed to alcohol in utero may demonstrate withdrawal symptoms after birth such as hyperactivity, excessive crying, irritability, weak sucking, disturbed sleep, tremors and seizures.

Alcohol consumption is commonly under-reported and, in recent years, standard serving sizes and usual alcohol content of alcoholic beverages such as wine and lagers have increased making the recommendations based on alcohol units difficult to follow. It can be difficult to reassure women who have had a small amount of alcohol before realizing that they were pregnant and still maintain advocacy for abstinence (Koren et al., 2003).

Smoking

Although some women stop or reduce smoking when they become pregnant, a significant proportion continue to smoke throughout pregnancy. Smoking (and environmental or second-hand tobacco smoke) is associated with increased early spontaneous abortion and placental complications such as miscarriage placental abruption, sudden infant death syndrome, growth restriction and decreased birth weight, preterm delivery and long-term behavioural and psychiatric disorders (Shea and Steiner, 2008). The physiological mechanisms are not clear but both nicotine and carbon monoxide are vasoconstrictors and may affect blood flow to placental and fetal tissues. Nicotine can increase maternal blood pressure and heart rate which may compromise uterine blood flow. Carbon monoxide binds to haemoglobin forming carboxyhaemoglobin which can cause fetal hypoxia and is implicated in sudden infant death syndrome (Haustein, 1999). Cigarette smoke also contains lead, cadmium and thiocyanate all of which are potentially hazardous to the fetus. Cigarette smoke is a source of free radicals and oxidative stress. Smoking is also thought to affect absorption of micronutrients and to increase nutrient utilization (Cogswell et al., 2003). Thus, smoking increases maternal micronutrient requirements but may also decrease the appetite and food consumption. Smokers are more likely to consume alcohol and other substances which interact with nutrient metabolism and are less likely to take nutrient supplements. Many women who smoke in pregnancy or who quit smoking during pregnancy and resume in the postpartum period are influenced by weight concerns (Levine and Marcus, 2004). The most effective therapies for smoking cessation in pregnancy are behavioural interventions; more evidence is required about the effectiveness and safety of pharmacological treatment (Schneider et al., 2010).

Caffeine

Caffeine is a mild stimulant present in beverages, such as coffee, tea and cola, chocolate and medications such as cold remedies, allergy preparations, headache medications, diuretics and stimulants. Caffeine in pregnancy is associated with increased risk of fertility problems, congenital abnormalities, pregnancy loss, growth retardation and behavioural problems (Greenwood et al., 2010). Caffeine is readily transported across the placenta but the liver enzyme involved in caffeine metabolism is not expressed by the placenta or fetal liver (Olsen and Bech, 2008). In addition, some individuals metabolise caffeine more slowly. It is currently recommended that pregnant women limit their caffeine consumption to 200 mg/day. The caffeine content of tea and coffee ranges markedly but 200 mg caffeine is roughly equivalent to two mugs of instant coffee, one and a half mugs of filter coffee, four average mugs of tea, five cans of regular cola drinks, about two and a half cans of 'energy' drinks and 200 g of plain chocolate (caffeine in milk chocolate is about half that in plain chocolate).

Drug use, medication, herbs and 'smart' drinks

Most medications prescribed to pregnant or breastfeeding women will have been evaluated for safety and the maternal benefit weighed against the risk of the drug being transported across the placenta and affecting the fetus.

No drug is without side-effects (Shehata and Nelson-Piercy, 2000) and anxiety about birth defects is a major parental concern. Anti-anxiety drugs, antidepressants, and neuroleptic drugs may affect neurotransmitter function of the developing central nervous system. Many recreational drugs such as amphetamines, heroin, marijuana and hallucinogens are harmful in pregnancy. It is important that pregnant women discuss their condition with health practitioners including pharmacists.

Many women use herbs and herbal teas during pregnancy, possibly because they want to control their health without using other medication or because their midwife has recommended them (Low Dog, 2009). They are easy to access and are perceived to be safe; use of the internet has brought more information about their use into the public domain. A number of herbs have pharmacological actions and the safety and effectiveness of others are not known; there are also concerns about quality control and contamination. Some herbs are known to be unsuitable in pregnancy; for instance, raspberry leaf tea can stimulate contractions and is used to induce labour. Other herbs that should be avoided in pregnancy include black cohosh, pennyroyal, mugwort, Ma Huang or ephedra. Pregnant women are recommended to choose herbal teas made with ingredients that are a normal part of their diet such as mint, blackcurrant or orange extracts and avoid unfamiliar substances. Herbal teas should preferably be purchased from reputable sources.

Carbonated drinks are not harmful for pregnant and breastfeeding women *per se*; carbonation itself does not present problems. Carbonated drinks are usually not nutrient dense and may contribute only sugars; they may displace drinks which could provide more nutrients. Other ingredients in 'smart' drinks (also known as 'new age', 'designer' or 'energy' drinks) may be of concern. High levels of caffeine are commonly added to energy drinks. Guarana, a Brazilian berry extract, is a stimulant related to caffeine. Ginseng is not recommended for pregnant women. Many of the smart drinks also contain higher levels of amino acids and vitamins than are considered optimal for pregnant women.

Exercise

Pregnant women who exercise have reduced fat gain, more rapid weight loss after pregnancy, improved mood and improved sleep patterns (Kramer, 2002). It is suggested that labour progresses faster and more effectively in women who exercise, reducing the need for induction, pain relief and operative delivery (Olson et al., 2009). However, all women tend to decrease their activity as pregnancy progresses. Physiological adaptations to exercise during pregnancy protect the fetus, maintain placental and fetal tissue perfusion and oxygenation and facilitate nutrient delivery (Clapp, 2000). Exercise begun in early pregnancy enhances placental development and fetal growth, whereas initiating significant exercise programmes later in pregnancy may reduce fetoplacental growth (Clapp et al., 2000). Women should therefore be encouraged to begin or continue low-volume exercise throughout pregnancy but decrease exercise towards the end of gestation to optimize outcome.

The aim should be to maintain a good fitness level during pregnancy rather than to reach peak fitness or train for competitive events. Moderate aerobic and strength-conditioning exercises (such as swimming, yoga, stretching, biking and walking) as part of a healthy lifestyle are considered safe and beneficial for both healthy normal- and over-weight pregnant women (DeMaio and Magann, 2009). Exercise may also be useful in the prevention and treatment of maternal and fetal complications of pregnancy such as gestational diabetes and pre-eclampsia (Weissgerber et al., 2006). Activities which minimize the risk of loss of balance and fetal trauma are recommended (Davies et al., 2003), whereas activities that result in respiratory stress (hyperventilation) or hyperthermia should be avoided. Certain activities such as contact sports and walking or running on rocky or unstable ground should be avoided (as joint laxity and centre of gravity are affected by pregnancy). In late pregnancy, exercises that involve lying on the back are best avoided as the weight of the uterus can impede venous return to the heart and may cause postural hypotension (see Chapter 11). Women are advised to seek advice before starting an exercise programme in pregnancy and to seek immediate advice for any injury. Pregnant women with certain conditions such as a history of bleeding or preterm labour, placenta praevia (where the placenta is low in the uterus), anaemia, pre-eclampsia or hypertension, and medical conditions which limit cardiovascular reserve may be advised to avoid exercise programmes. Pregnant women taking part in physical activity should wear appropriate footwear, take frequent breaks and avoid exercising in extremely hot weather.

There are differences in physiological responses to exercise in pregnant women who are acclimatized to high altitude (live at high altitude) and pregnant visitors to high altitude (Entin and Coffin, 2004). Fetal oxygenation does not seem to be affected by air travel but exercise at high altitude may be associated with hyperventilation and pregnancy complications such as dehydration, bleeding and preterm labour.

Work and stress

Strenuous work and physical stress can potentially influence micronutrient status and outcome of pregnancy.

Women in employment may be at risk of compromised diets because they have less time for shopping and cooking. Peak energy expenditure, length of time spent standing (which has been shown to affect patterns of meals consumed) and type of activity (for instance, lifting may result in greater intra-abdominal pressure) may be more significant. Particular occupations, long and/or irregular working hours and shift work have been implicated in being associated with a poorer outcome of pregnancy (Shaw, 2003). Psychological stress can increase the risk of birth defects, early onset pre-eclampsia, preterm delivery and LBW (Triche and Hossain, 2007).

Key points

- The diet before pregnancy, as well as that consumed during pregnancy, can affect the nutrient status of the woman.
- The increased energy requirements of pregnancy can be met by a combination of increasing intake, decreasing activity and changing metabolism.
- A good-quality, nutrient-dense diet can supply the additional protein, vitamin and mineral requirements of pregnancy.
- Energy restriction and obesity affect reproductive function: both male and female fertility and fetal growth.
- Pregnancy-induced hormonal changes, including insulin resistance, affect transfer of nutrients to the placenta and fetus.
- Adaptation to poor nutrition in pregnancy results in changes in growth in utero and birth weight and may be linked to disease in adult life.

Application to practice

Advice on nutrition in pregnancy is important before and during pregnancy, and also for subsequent pregnancies.

Women who have a poor history of nutrition are at risk and the midwife needs to be aware of this to aid in the detection of problems associated with poor dietary intake.

Women with low body fat may have problems conceiving and so active weight gain may need to be encouraged to optimise conception.

Women with high body fat may also have problems conceiving (see Chapter 6). Obese women are at much higher risk from complications during pregnancy, delivery and the postnatal period.

ANNOTATED FURTHER READING

Barker DJP: *Fetal and infant origins of adult disease*, London, 1992, BMJ Books.

Describes the research underlying the fetal origins of adult disease (the Barker Hypothesis) in a compilation of the 31 key papers in this area.

Bhatia J, editor: *Perinatal nutrition: optimizing infant health and development*, 2004, CRC Press.

This book examines the role of maternal nutrition in fetal and infant growth and development and longer term health prospects, considering micronutrient supplementation and dietary recommendations.

Carlson S, Aupperle P: Nutrient requirements and fetal development: recommendations for best outcomes, *J Fam Pract* 56:S1–S6, 2007.

A good background to the roles and requirements for DHA in pregnancy which addresses issues related to supplementation in pregnancy and lactation and identifies research questions which need to be considered.

Langley Evans S, editor: *Fetal nutrition and adult disease: programming of chronic disease through fetal exposure to undernutrition*, 2004, CABI Publishing.

A research-based textbook which describes the epidemiological evidence, animal studies and likely biological mechanisms behind the hypothesis that maternal nutrition in pregnancy can be the cause of programming of lifelong disease risk such as heart disease, stroke, diabetes and hypertension.

Molloy AM, Kirke PN, Brody LC, Scott JM, Mills JL: Effects of folate and vitamin B_{12} deficiencies during pregnancy on fetal, infant, and child development, *Food Nutr Bull* 29: S101–S111, 2008.

An in-depth discussion about the importance of folate and vitamin B_{12} nutrition in pregnancy and lactation.

Symonds ME, Ramsay MM: editors: *Maternal-fetal nutrition during pregnancy and lactation*, Cambridge, 2010, CUP.

A detailed consideration of the nutritional requirements for each stage of fetal development and growth, and the implications if these are not met; a good synthesis of the underlying theory and scientific background with the clinical applications.

REFERENCES

Al MDM, van Houwelingen AC, Hornstra G: Long-chain polyunsaturated fatty acids, pregnancy, and pregnancy outcome, *Am J Clin Nutr* 71:285S–291S, 2000.

Allen LH: Pregnancy and iron deficiency: unresolved issues, *Nutr Rev* 55:91–101, 1997.

Allen LH: Impact of vitamin B-12 deficiency during lactation on maternal and infant health, *Adv Exp Med Biol* 503:57–67, 2002.

Anderson AS: Pregnancy as a time for dietary change? *Proc Nutr Soc* 60:497–504, 2001.

Baker L, Piddington R, Goldman A, et al: Myo-inositol and prostaglandins reverse the glucose inhibition of neural tube fusion in cultured mouse embryos, *Diabetologia* 33:593–596, 1990.

Barker DJP: Fetal origins of coronary heart disease, *Br Med J* 311:171–174, 1995.

Barker DJP: *Mothers, babies and health in later life*, New York, 1998, Churchill Livingstone.

Boddie AM, Dedlow ER, Nackashi JA, et al: Folate absorption in women with a history of neural tube defect-affected pregnancy, *Am J Clin Nutr* 72:154–158, 2000.

Brand-Miller J, McMillan-Price J, Steinbeck K, et al: Dietary glycemic index: health implications, *J Am Coll Nutr* 28(Suppl.):446S–449S, 2009.

Butte NF: Carbohydrate and lipid metabolism in pregnancy: normal compared with gestational diabetes mellitus, *Am J Clin Nutr* 71:1256S–1261S, 2000.

Butte NF, King JC: Energy requirements during pregnancy and lactation, *Public Health Nutr* 8:1010–1027, 2005.

Campbell-Brown M, Hytten FE: Nutrition. In Chamberlain G, Broughton Pipkin F, editors: *Clinical physiology in obstetrics* (ed 3), Oxford, 1998, Blackwell, pp 165–191.

Carmichael SL, Shaw GM, Schaffer DM, et al: Dieting behaviors and risk of neural tube defects, *Am J Epidemiol* 158:1127–1131, 2003.

Casanueva E, Polo E, Tejero E, et al: Premature rupture of amniotic membranes as functional assessment of vitamin C status during pregnancy, *Ann N Y Acad Sci* 678:369–370, 1993.

Chappell LC, Seed PT, Kelly FJ, et al: Vitamin C and E supplementation in women at risk of preeclampsia is associated with changes in indices of oxidative stress and placental function, *Am J Obstet Gynecol* 187:777–784, 2002.

Chiriboga CA: Fetal alcohol and drug effects, *Neurologist* 9:267–279, 2003.

Choi JL, Rose RC: Transport and metabolism of ascorbic acid in human placenta, *Am J Physiol* 257: C110–C113, 1989.

Clapp JF III: Exercise during pregnancy. A clinical update, *Clin Sports Med* 19:273–286, 2000.

Clapp JF III, Kim H, Burciu B, et al: Beginning regular exercise in early pregnancy: effect on fetoplacental growth, *Am J Obstet Gynecol* 183:1484–1488, 2000.

Coad J: Pre- and periconceptual nutrition. In Morgan JB, Dickerson JWT, editors: *Nutrition in early life*, Chichester, 2003, Wiley, pp 39–71.

Coad J, Al Rasasi B, Morgan J: Nutrient insult in early pregnancy, *Proc Nutr Soc* 61:51–59, 2002.

Cogswell ME, Weisberg P, Spong C: Cigarette smoking, alcohol use and adverse pregnancy outcomes:

implications for micronutrient supplementation, *J Nutr* 133:1722S–1731S, 2003.

Cuskelly GJ, McNulty H, Scott JM: Effect of increasing dietary folate on red-cell folate: implications for the prevention of neural tube defects, *Lancet* 347:657–659, 1996.

Davies GA, Wolfe LA, Mottola MF, et al: Exercise in pregnancy and the postpartum period, *J Obstet Gynaecol Can* 25:516–529, 2003.

DeMaio M, Magann EF: Exercise and pregnancy, *J Am Acad Orthop Surg* 17:504–514, 2009.

Derbyshire E: Food safety in pregnancy: conventional issues and future concerns, *Adv Food Hosp Tourism* 1:.

Doyle W, Crawford MA, Wynn AW: Maternal magnesium intake and pregnancy outcome, *Magnes Res* 2:205–210, 1989.

Duggleby SL, Jackson AA: Protein, amino acid and nitrogen metabolism during pregnancy: how might the mother meet the needs of her fetus? *Curr Opin Clin Nutr Metab Care* 5:503–509, 2002.

Entin PL, Coffin L: Physiological basis for recommendations regarding exercise during pregnancy at high altitude, *High Alt Med Biol* 5:321–334, 2004.

Forsum E, Löf M: Energy metabolism during human pregnancy, *Annu Rev Nutr* 27:277–292, 2007.

Frisch RE: The right weight, body fat, menarche and ovulation, *Baillières Clin Obstet Gynaecol* 4:3, 1990.

Frisch RE, McArthur JW: Menstrual cycles: fatness as a determinant of minimum weight necessary for their maintenance or onset, *Science* 185:949–951, 1974.

Gesink Law DC, Maclehose RF, Longnecker MP: Obesity and time to pregnancy, *Hum Reprod* 22:414–420, 2007.

Godfrey KM: The 'gold standard' for optimal fetal growth and development, *J Pediatr Endocrinol Metab* 14(Suppl. 6):1507–1513, 2001.

Godfrey KM, Barker DJP: Fetal nutrition and adult disease, *Am J Clin Nutr* 71:1344S–1352S, 2000.

Greenwood DC, Alwan N, Boylan S, et al: Caffeine intake during pregnancy, late miscarriage and stillbirth, *Eur J Epidemiol* 25:275–280, 2010.

Hallberg L: Perspectives on nutritional iron deficiency, *Annu Rev Nutr* 21:1–21, 2001.

Hammoud AO, Wilde N, Gibson M, et al: Male obesity and alteration in sperm parameters, *Fertil Steril* 90:2222–2225, 2008.

Harding JE, Johnson BM: Nutrition and fetal growth, *Reprod Fertil Dev* 7:539–547, 1995.

Haustein KO: Cigarette smoking, nicotine and pregnancy, *Int J Clin Pharmacol Ther* 37:417–427, 1999.

Health Education Authority: *Awareness, attitudes and behaviour towards folic acid amongst women: a report by the HEA*, London, 1996, HEA.

Heath AL, Fairweather-Tait SJ: Health implications of iron overload: the role of diet and genotype, *Nutr Rev* 61:45–62, 2003.

Herrera E: Lipid metabolism in pregnancy and its consequences in the fetus and newborn, *Endocrine* 19:43–55, 2002.

Herrera E, Amusquivar E: Lipid metabolism in the fetus and the newborn, *Diabetes Metab Res Rev* 16:202–210, 2000.

Hirschberg AL: Polycystic ovary syndrome, obesity and reproductive implications, *Women's Health* 5:529–540, 2009.

Hobel C, Culhane J: Role of psychosocial and nutritional stress on poor pregnancy outcome, *J Nutr* 133:1709S–1717S, 2003.

Hofmeyr GJ, Lawrie TA, Atallah AN, et al: Calcium supplementation during pregnancy for preventing hypertensive disorders and related problems, *Cochrane Database Syst Rev* 8: CD001059.

Hollis BW: Vitamin D requirement during pregnancy and lactation, *J Bone Miner Res* 22(Suppl. 2): V39–V44, 2007.

Hollis BW, Wagner CL: Assessment of dietary vitamin D requirements during pregnancy and lactation, *Am J Clin Nutr* 79:717–726, 2004.

Holmes VA: Changes in haemostasis during normal pregnancy: does homocysteine play a role in maintaining homeostasis? *Proc Nutr Soc* 62:479–493, 2003.

Hytten FE: Nutrition. In Hytten F, Chamberlain G, editors: *Clinical physiology in obstetrics*, (ed 2), Oxford, 1991, Blackwell, p 153.

Hytten FE, Leitch I: *The physiology of human pregnancy*. Oxford, 1971, Blackwell Scientific Publications.

Institute of Medicine: *Dietary reference intakes for calcium, phosphorus, magnesium, vitamin d and fluoride. Standing Committee on the Scientific Evaluation of Dietary Reference Intakes, Food and Nutrition Board, Institute of Medicine*, Washington DC, 1997, The National Academy of Sciences.

Institute of Medicine: *Dietary reference values for energy, carbohydrates, fiber, fat, protein and amino acids (macronutrients). Standing Committee on the Scientific Evaluation of Dietary Reference Intakes, Food and Nutrition Board, Institute of Medicine*, Washington DC, 2002, The National Academy of Sciences.

Keen CL, Clegg MS, Hanna LA, et al: The plausibility of micronutrient deficiencies being a significant contributing factor to the occurrence of pregnancy complications, *J Nutr* 133:1597S–1605S, 2003.

Koren G, Nulman I, Chudley AE: Fetal alcohol spectrum disorder, *Can Med Assoc J* 169:1181–1185, 2003.

Kovacs CS: Vitamin D in pregnancy and lactation: maternal, fetal, and neonatal outcomes from human and animal studies, *Am J Clin Nutr* 88:520S–528S, 2008.

Kramer MS: Aerobic exercise for women during pregnancy, *Cochrane Database Syst Rev* CD000180, 2002.

Kramer MS, Kakuma R: Energy and protein intake in pregnancy, *Cochrane Database Syst Rev* CD000032, 2003.

Lawrence M, Lawrence F, Coward WA, et al: The energy requirements of pregnancy in the Gambia, *Lancet* ii:1072, 1987.

Lee CY, Koren G: Maternal obesity: effects on pregnancy and the role of pre-conception counselling, *J Obstet Gynaecol* 30:101–106, 2010.

Letsky E: The haematological system. In Chamberlain G, Broughton Pipkin F, editors: *Clinical physiology in obstetrics*, (ed 3), Oxford, 1998, Blackwell, pp 71–110.

Levine MD, Marcus MD: Do changes in mood and concerns about weight relate to smoking relapse in the postpartum period? *Arch Womens Ment Health* 7:155–166, 2004.

Low Dog T: The use of botanicals during pregnancy and lactation, *Alt Ther Health Med* 15:54–58, 2009.

Lumley LH: Decreased birthweights in infants after maternal in utero exposure to the Dutch famine of 1944–45, *Paediatr Perinat Epidemiol* 6:240, 1992.

Mahomed K, Bhutta Z, Middleton P: Zinc supplementation for improving pregnancy and infant outcome, *Cochrane Database Syst Rev* CD000230, 2007.

Makrides M: Is there a dietary requirement for DHA in pregnancy? *Prostaglandins Leukot Essent Fatty Acids* 81:171–174, 2009.

McCrabb GJ, Egan AR, Hosking BJ: Maternal undernutrition during mid-pregnancy in sheep: variable effects on placental growth, *J Agric Sci* 1189:127–132, 1992.

Merialdi M, Carroli G, Villar J, et al: Nutritional interventions during pregnancy for the prevention or treatment of impaired fetal growth: an overview of randomized controlled trials, *J Nutr* 133:1626S–1631S, 2003.

Olsen J, Bech BH: Caffeine intake during pregnancy, *BMJ* 337:a2316, 2008.

Olson D, Sikka RS, Hayman J, et al: Exercise in pregnancy, *Curr Sports Med Rep* 8:147–153, 2009.

Pimentel J: Current issues on epileptic women, *Curr Pharm Des* 6:865–872, 2000.

Prentice A, Goldberg G: Maternal obesity increases congenital malformations, *Nutr Rev* 54:146–152, 1996.

Ramakrishnan U, Manjrekar R, Rivera J, et al: Micronutrients and pregnancy outcome: a review of the literature, *Nutr Res* 19:103–159, 1999.

Ravelli GP, Stein ZA, Susser MW: Obesity in young men after famine exposure in utero and early infancy, *N Engl J Med* 295:349, 1976.

Rizzo T, Metzger BE, Burns WJ, et al: Correlations between antepartum maternal metabolism and child intelligence, *N Engl J Med* 325:911–916, 1991.

Robinson S, Viita J, Learner J, et al: Insulin insensitivity is associated with a decrease in postprandial thermogenesis in normal pregnancy, *Diabet Med* 10:139–145, 1992.

Romon M, Nuttens MC, Vambergue A, et al: Higher carbohydrate intake is associated with decreased incidence of newborn macrosomia in women with gestational diabetes, *J Am Diet Assoc* 101:897–902, 2001.

Rush D: Effects of changes in protein and calorie intake during pregnancy on the growth of the human fetus. In Chalmers I, Enkin M, Kierse MJNC, editors: *Effective care in pregnancy and childbirth*, (vol. 1), Oxford, 1989, Oxford University Press, pp 255–280.

Saffrey J, Stewart M, editors: *Maintaining the whole. SK 220 Human biology and health, Book 3*, Milton Keynes, 1997, Open University Press.

Saldana TM, Siega-Riz AM, Adair LS: Effect of macronutrient intake on the development of glucose intolerance during pregnancy, *Am J Clin Nutr* 79:479–486, 2004.

Schneider S, Huy C, Schutz J, et al: Smoking cessation during pregnancy: a systematic literature review, *Drug Alcohol Rev* 29:81–90, 2010.

Scholl TO, Reilly T: Anemia, iron and pregnancy outcome, *J Nutr* 130:443S–4437S, 2000.

Shah DK, Ginsburg ES: Bariatric surgery and fertility, *Curr Opin Obstet Gynecol* 22:248–254, 2010.

Shaw GM: Strenuous work, nutrition and adverse pregnancy outcomes: a brief review, *J Nutr* 133:1718S–1721S, 2003.

Shaw GM, Quach T, Nelson V, et al: Neural tube defects associated with maternal periconceptional dietary intake of simple sugars and glycemic index, *Am J Clin Nutr* 78:972–978, 2003.

Shea AK, Steiner M: Cigarette smoking during pregnancy, *Nicotine Tob Res* 10:267–278, 2008.

Shehata HA, Nelson-Piercy C: Drugs to avoid in pregnancy, *Curr Obstet Gynaecol* 10:44–52, 2000.

Shoob HD, Sargent RG, Thompson SJ, et al: Dietary methionine is involved in the etiology of neural tube defect-affected pregnancies in humans, *J Nutr* 131:2653–2658, 2001.

Siega-Riz AM, Promislow JH, Savitz DA, et al: Vitamin C intake and the risk of preterm delivery, *Am J Obstet Gynecol* 189:519–525, 2003.

Stanner SA, Bulmer K, Andres C, et al: Does malnutrition in utero determine diabetes and coronary heart disease in adulthood? Results from the Leningrad siege study, a cross sectional study, *Br Med J* 315:1342–1349, 1997.

Stein Z, Susser M: Fertility, fecundity, famine: food rations in the Dutch famine 1944/5 have a causal relation to fertility and probably to fecundity, *Hum Biol* 47:131, 1975a.

Stein Z, Susser M: The Dutch famine 1944–45 and the reproductive process. 1. Effects on six indices at birth, *Paediatr Res* 9:70, 1975b.

Stewart RJC, Sheppard H, Preece R, et al: The effect of rehabilitation at different stages of development in rats marginally malnourished for ten to twelve generations, *Br J Nutr* 43:403–412, 1980.

Stover PJ: Physiology of folate and vitamin B_{12} in health and disease, *Nutr Rev* 62:S3–S12, 2004.

Thomson CD: Selenium and iodine intakes and status in New Zealand and Australia, *Br J Nutr* 91:661–672, 2004.

Triche EW, Hossain N: Environmental factors implicated in the causation of adverse pregnancy outcome, *Semin Perinatol* 31:240–242, 2007.

Wald NJ, Bower C: Folic acid and the prevention of neural tube defects, *Br Med J* 310:1019–1020, 1995.

Weissgerber TL, Wolfe LA, Davies GA, et al: Exercise in the prevention and treatment of maternal-fetal disease: a review of the literature, *Appl Physiol Nutr Metab* 31:661–674, 2006.

Williamson CS: Nutrition in pregnancy, *Nutr Bull* 31:28–59, 2006.

Wynn M, Wynn A: *The case for preconception care of men and women*, Bicester, 1991, AB Academic.

Yogev Y, Catalano PM: Pregnancy and obesity, *Obstet Gynecol Clin North Am* 36:285–300, viii, 2009.

Zain MM, Norman RJ: Impact of obesity on female fertility and fertility treatment, *Womens Health Lond Engl* 4:183–194, 2008.

Zeisel SH: Is maternal diet supplementation beneficial? Optimal development of infant depends on mother's diet, *Am J Clin Nutr* 89:685S–687S, 2009.

Zimmermann MB: Iodine deficiency in pregnancy and the effects of maternal iodine supplementation on the offspring: a review, *Am J Clin Nutr* 89:668S–672S, 2009.

Zimmermann M, Delange F: Iodine supplementation of pregnant women in Europe: a review and recommendations, *Eur J Clin Nutr* 58:979–984, 2004.

Physiology of parturition

LEARNING OBJECTIVES

- To describe uterine changes in pregnancy and its preparation for labour.
- To discuss theories of the initiation and timing of parturition in humans.
- To relate factors thought to be involved with initiation of labour to methods for inducing labour, possible causes and treatment of preterm labour.
- To describe the effects of labour on maternal and fetal physiology.
- To outline the physiology of pain in relation to childbirth and the rationale for choice of pain relief.

INTRODUCTION

The success of pregnancy and, ultimately, the survival of the species, depend on the baby being born healthy and mature enough to survive. In pregnancy and labour, the uterus has to fulfil two very different functions. It has to grow but remain quiescent during pregnancy to allow fetal development and then, at the appropriate time, commence the powerful and coordinated contractions which result in the birth of the infant. However, parturition also requires the maturation of the fetal systems essential for extrauterine survival. The mother also needs to be physiologically prepared for lactation. Therefore, the maturation of the fetus and the onset of labour need to be synchronized. Asynchrony leads to preterm birth (≤ 37 weeks gestation).

Most human infants are capable of surviving birth and are born at term (defined as between the end of the 37th week and 42 weeks of pregnancy). Preterm birth rates are increasing and in 2005, 9.6% of all births (12.9 million) worldwide were preterm (Beck et al., 2010). 85% of preterm births occurred in Africa and Asia. The highest rates of preterm births occur in Africa (11.9% of all births) and North America (10.6%); Europe has the lowest rates (6.2%). Modern practices such as women giving birth at a later age and fertility treatment (and subsequent multiple gestation) have increased the incidence of preterm birth (Lawn et al., 2009). Low socio-economic status, being of certain ethnicities or having low body mass index, bacterial vaginosis or other infections including periodontal disease, inflammation, vascular disease, uterine overdistension, stress, smoking and a history of preterm delivery and abortion are all risk factors for spontaneous preterm birth (Goldenberg et al., 2008). The causes of preterm birth are not well understood which limits effective obstetric and neonatal care. Therapeutic approaches currently focus on arresting established preterm labour; early diagnosis, treatment or primary prevention of preterm birth are surprisingly unsuccessful.

 Chapter case study

While working in Africa, Zara had been able to assist several of her African friends during childbirth, all of which had occurred at home and attended by mostly female relatives who had informed Zara that they would only call the local midwife if they felt things were going wrong. All her friends had had uncomplicated deliveries and Zara felt quite privileged to have witnessed childbirth in such a different way to how it is presented within most modern Western societies.

Continued

Chapter case study—cont'd

Zara is keen to have a waterbirth at home and wants to avoid all forms of pain relief. She also wants her sister and some of her close friends who are also heavily pregnant to be present if possible. As Zara has had all her antenatal care from her midwife, she particularly wants her midwife to care for her in labour, especially as her midwife has extensive experience of waterbirth.

- What factors do you think will be a positive influence on enabling Zara to have a normal birth?

Preterm birth is the predominant cause of perinatal morbidity and mortality in developed countries. Most early neonatal deaths, that are not associated with a lethal deformity, are associated with prematurity and preterm infants have an increased risk of complications not just in the neonatal period but in the long-term (Saigal and Doyle, 2008). Long-term consequences include cognitive and motor neurodevelopment disabilities that include cerebral palsy, mental retardation, deafness, blindness, learning disabilities, chronic lung disease and possibly an increased risk of disease in adult life. The shorter the gestation, the poorer the prognosis is. Even though very low-birth-weight babies (i.e. those born below 1000 g) may now survive, it is generally associated with rates of morbidity and much emotional stress for their parents, as well as a high financial burden on neonatal intensive care units. There are also long-term health and education costs associated with physical and mental handicap and neurodevelopmental complications. It can be argued that one of the principal objectives of obstetrics is to reduce preterm labour. The survival rate of premature infants born alive with borderline viability has improved over the last decade (Field et al., 2008), however improved survival rates have not been matched by a proportional decrease in the incidence of disability (Stephens and Vohr, 2009).

There are three categories of causes of preterm birth: iatrogenic or indicated, where complications of pregnancy such as eclampsia, pre-eclampsia or intrauterine growth retardation, enforce obstetric intervention and the deliberate induction of premature delivery (30–35% of cases); preterm premature rupture of (fetal) membranes (PPROM), which may be associated with infection (25–30% of cases); and spontaneous or idiopathic preterm labour (40–45% of cases; Goldenberg et al., 2008). The failure of spontaneous labour is also not well understood; prolonged pregnancy (gestation >42 weeks or 294 days) is also associated with increased fetal morbidity and mortality.

The factors controlling the transition from one state to the other are not well understood but are very important both in determining the possible causes of preterm labour and in understanding how to induce labour successfully without eliciting fetal distress. The control of the onset of human (and primate) parturition remains elusive.

There are marked differences between human and other mammalian species in the cascade of factors leading to parturition. Humans have a very high rate of premature birth compared with other species. For most domestic and laboratory animals the duration of gestation is remarkably constant; for example, there is less than 1% variation in sheep (Jenkin and Young, 2004). Theoretically, the length of gestation does not matter to the mother. The crucial aspect is that the baby can survive from birth. It seems plausible, therefore, that the fetus controls the length of gestation. Certainly, in some experimental animals, for example sheep, there is proven fetal involvement in the timing of labour but it is difficult to obtain such evidence in humans.

In other species, it seems that the same signal controls fetal maturation and triggers the onset of labour so parturition is synchronized. In humans, the two pathways seem to be separable (Fig. 13.1). The human fetus appears to undergo lung maturation 4–6 weeks before labour, unlike other species in which the signals initiating labour also stimulate fetal organ maturity. It is not clear why the events leading to parturition should be so complex in the human; however, it seems plausible that a variable length of gestation is advantageous. The complexity of control of parturition in humans might allow a transfer of control from mother to fetus. Thus, in early pregnancy, it may be physiologically expedient for the mother to terminate the pregnancy if it is harmful for her long-term health to continue. Spontaneous termination of a pregnancy that is unlikely to be completed, for example because maternal nutrient intake is insufficient, prevents needless maternal investment. Later in gestation, once the fetus is mature enough to survive, fetal control of parturition would allow the fetus to remain in the uterus if the environment was favourable. The fetus could respond to stress by switching from cell division and growth to accelerated maturation and earlier initiation of parturition. This would suggest that intrauterine growth restriction is part of an adaptive response to fetal stress which increases survival as long as the stressor is not too early or too severe. It is not surprising, therefore, that many of the signals involved in parturition are also involved in physiological stress responses. Midwifery and obstetric management of women in labour is often interventionist. This chapter covers the physiology of parturition; for information about clinical management, readers are referred to midwifery texts in the list of further reading.

STAGES OF LABOUR

From a clinical point of view, labour is often divided into three stages (Fig. 13.2). However, physiologically there is no abrupt transition between stages. The events leading to the onset of labour are gradually and inconspicuously initiated earlier in the pregnancy, and the three stages overlap. The first stage is that of progressive cervical

Fig. 13.1 The two distinct pathways controlling parturition and fetal development in the human.

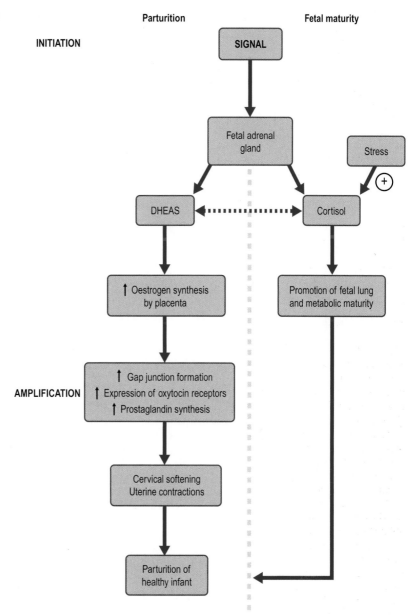

dilatation, timed from the onset of regular coordinated contractions accompanied by progressive effacement (thinning) and dilatation of the cervix. The end of this stage is marked by the full dilatation of the cervix as the uterine contractions pull the entire tissue of the cervix upwards until it becomes incorporated into the lower uterine segment, continuous with the uterine walls. This stage lasts an average of 12–14 h in primigravidae, but tends to be shorter in multigravidae. The second stage is fetal expulsion, from full cervical dilatation until the delivery of the baby. The contractions are strong and aided by the respiratory muscles. The second stage may take over an hour in primigravidae and as little as a few minutes in multigravidae. The third stage of labour involves separation and complete expulsion of the placenta and membranes, and control of bleeding from the uteroplacental circulation. The return to the prepregnant state is described as the puerperium (see Chapter 14).

From a physiological point of view, it is useful to think of labour being related to phases of uterine myometrial activity. For most of pregnancy, the uterus is in phase 0, the quiescent phase. Under the influence of progesterone

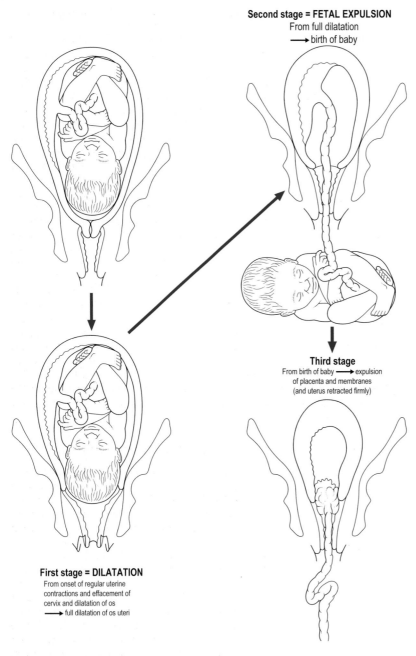

Second stage = FETAL EXPULSION
From full dilatation
⟶ birth of baby

Fig. 13.2 Stages of labour.

Third stage
From birth of baby ⟶ expulsion
of placenta and membranes
(and uterus retracted firmly)

First stage = DILATATION
From onset of regular uterine
contractions and effacement of
cervix and dilatation of os
⟶ full dilatation of os uteri

(the literal meaning of progesterone is 'pro-gestation', i.e. promoting and sustaining pregnancy), the uterus is relatively quiet and non-responsive to stimuli. Other factors involved in quiescence are prostacyclin, nitric oxide, relaxin, parathyroid hormone-related peptide, calcitonin gene-related peptide and vasoactive intestinal peptide (Terzidou, 2007). All these factors act to increase cAMP (or cGMP) and thus inhibit the release of intracellular calcium that is required for myometrial activity. In late pregnancy, the uterus changes from being quiescent (having a low level of muscle activity) to being activated; this is known as phase 1, the activation phase. This transition to activation is the initiation of labour; labour results from activation and then stimulation of the myometrium. The receptors and signalling pathways are modulated so they respond to contractile stimuli. Activation is partially stimulated by mechanical stretch of the uterus together with changes in signalling via endocrine and paracrine pathways, possibly resulting from an increased activity of the fetal hypothalamic–pituitary–adrenal (HPA) axis. Increased levels of oestrogen and CRH lead to an up-regulation of genes involved in contraction including genes for connexin 43, prostaglandins and oxytocin receptors. The increased production of oestrogen may be due to increased availability of fetally derived precursors. In the third phase of parturition, phase 2 - stimulation, the acti-vated uterus is spontaneously excitable and responsive to uterotonins such as prostaglandins, oxytocin and CRH; it develops coordinated, effective and forceful contractions. The activation of the uterus in this stimulation phase is the start of a positive feedback loop whereby the initial signals become further amplified and the uterus becomes fully sti-mulated allowing progression of the first and second stages of labour. This phase is accompanied by inflammatory-like biochemical changes. There is increased synthesis of prosta-glandins and cytokines and an influx of neutrophils which produce proteases which are involved in remodelling and ripening of the cervical tissue. The uterus is able to perform a remarkable mechanical effort to expel its contents – the baby, placenta and associated membranes and fluids – through the birth canal (Fig. 13.3). The final phase is the uterine involution phase.

THE UTERUS AT TERM

Uterine growth in pregnancy

The uterine muscle undergoes exceptional growth through-out pregnancy to accommodate the growing fetus. The prepregnant weight of the uterus is about 50 g in a

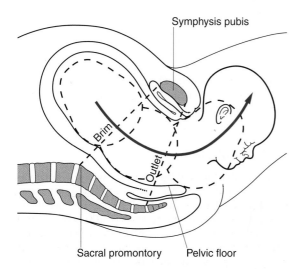

Fig. 13.3 Expulsion through the birth canal.

nulliparous woman and about 60–70 g in a multiparous woman with a capacity of about 10 mL. During pregnancy, uterine size increases 20-fold, to about 800–1200 g and a capacity of about 5 L. Initially, the uterus grows by hyper-plasia (increasing cell number). This is under the influence of oestrogen and, unlike later growth, occurs regardless of the site of implantation. By the 4th month, the uterine wall has thickened from 10 to 25 mm. Subsequent growth is due to hypertrophy and stretch stimulated by uterine distension. The uterine wall thins and the smooth muscle cells increase markedly in length (from 50 to 500 μm long and from 5 to 15 μm wide) as they accumulate contractile proteins. The increased overall size is accompanied by a change in uterine shape from a sphere to a cylinder. By term, the organization of the myometrial cells allows coordinated, strong and effective contractions to develop. The uterine muscle is innervated by adrenergic, cholinergic and peptidergic fibres, which are more abundant in the cervix and uterine tubes. The uterus also has many sensory nerves. By the third trimester, the uterine wall is thin, about 5–10 mm by term; the fetal movements are visible and the fetus can be palpated through the uterine wall (Blackburn, 2007). The uterus almost reaches the liver and displaces the stomach and intestine. The blood vessels in the non-pregnant uterus are extremely tortuous and coiled (see Chapter 2); this allows them to adapt to the increased requirements of the expanding uterine tissue. Uterine blood flow increases in pregnancy as the blood vessel diameter increases and resistance to flow decreases.

Uterine muscle organization

The uterus is predominantly comprised bundles each of 10–50 myometrial (smooth muscle) cells separated by connective tissue, formed of collagen and elastin. The dis-tribution of the smooth muscle varies throughout the length of the uterus. The smooth muscle density is highest in the fundus of the uterus (an approximate ratio of smooth muscle fibres:connective tissue of 90:10) and gradually declines until the cervix where the ratio is 20:80. Associated with the myometrium are leukocytes which produce cytokines. Pro-contractile proteins such as oxytocin receptors and connexin 43 are preferentially expressed in the fundal region of the uterus. The isthmus, which forms the lower segment of the uterus, has lower smooth muscle content. The lower segment forms at about weeks 28–30 of pregnancy. Caesarean sections late in gestation are usually via the lower segment of the uterus (lower-segment caesarean section, LSCS), whereas the incision in an emergency 'classic' caesarean section earlier in pregnancy usually is on the midline of the uterus and is likely to dictate the method of delivery in future deliveries. Contractile strength is related to the proportion of smooth muscle (Petersen et al., 1991). Therefore, the upper part of the uterus contracts strongly and the lower

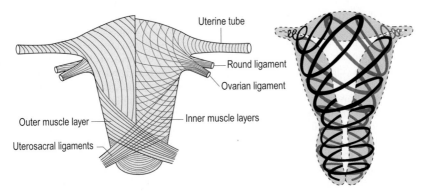

Fig. 13.4 Uterine muscle layers: (A) the inner and outer muscle layers; (B) spiral organization of central smooth muscle fibres. (Reproduced with permission from Sweet and Tiran, 1996.)

segment, which has a diminishing proportion of muscle, contracts weakly and passively (see Fig. 13.10, p. 338).

The uterine muscle forms three distinct anatomical layers, which are more evident with the hypertrophy of the uterus that occurs in pregnancy (Fig. 13.4). The innermost layer has muscle mostly in a longitudinal orientation. The myometrium has more muscle fibres in the inner layer than it does in the outer layers (Terzidou, 2007). The outermost layer has longitudinal and circular fibres. The middle layer of uterine muscle has spiralling fibres and is particularly well vascularized. It is this middle layer that ensures the blood vessels in the uterus are occluded in the third stage of labour as the spiralling fibres contract around the blood vessels. The lower uterine segment has a high expression of CRH receptor type I which is involved in relaxation and of the enzymes involved in cervical ripening.

The myometrium

The myometrium is formed of myometrial cells embedded in a collagen-rich connective tissue matrix which has blood vessels interspersed within it. The cytoplasm of the myometrial cells or myocytes is packed with long random bundles of actin and myosin. Compared with skeletal muscles, the concentration of actin is higher and the myosin has longer filaments, which increases the maximum shortening of the contractile cells. Myosin is both a structural protein and an Mg-ATPase, an enzyme that can hydrolyse ATP and utilize the energy for movement. When ATP is hydrolysed (broken down), actin and myosin cross-bridges form so actin and myosin slide past each other, shortening the cell so that the muscle contracts (Fig. 13.5). Myosin is made up of two heavy chains forming the ATPase and two light chains, which bind calcium and undergo phosphorylation. Phosphorylation is the incorporation of a phosphate group catalysed by a kinase, in this case myosin light-chain kinase (MLCK) which effectively activates the protein. Factors that negatively

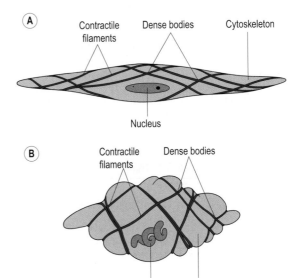

Fig. 13.5 Cell shortening and myosin contractile elements in myometrial muscle contraction: (A) relaxed; (B) contracted.

affect myometrial contractility may be important in maintaining uterine quiescence through pregnancy; those that increase contractility may be important in facilitating the progression of labour.

The role of calcium

Muscle contraction is triggered by a rise in the intracellular concentration of calcium ions. Electrical activity, calcium ion influx and development of myometrial tension are precisely synchronized (López Bernal, 2003). Calcium ions bind to the calcium-binding protein calmodulin (CAM) which regulates the activity of many of the intracellular enzymes generating a cascade of reactions leading to binding of actin and myosin (Wray et al., 2003).

Binding of calcium to CAM forms a Ca–CAM complex which activates MLCK. MLCK is inhibited when calcium levels are low. The activated MLCK undergoes a conformational change which exposes the catalytic site so the MLCK can be phosphorylated and will interact with actin, initiating contractions. Removal of calcium results in dephosphorylation of myosin by myosin light-chain phosphatase and causes muscle relaxation. Smooth muscle contraction can therefore be increased either by activating MLCK or by inhibiting myosin phosphatase.

Calcium enters the myometrial cell from the extracellular fluid or is released from intracellular binding sites and organelles including the sarcoplasmic reticulum of the myometrial cells. Calcium released from the sarcoplasmic reticulum can prime contractions that need to be sustained by calcium influx. Voltage-operated calcium channels regulate contractility by allowing calcium entry. Calcium-activated potassium channels set the threshold of activation of the cell membrane. There is a good correlation between intracellular calcium concentration and the muscular force developed with ionized calcium (Ca^{2+}) concentration increasing from approximately 100–500 nm during contraction. Uterotonins (substances that stimulate myometrial contractility), such as prostaglandins and oxytocin, increase calcium influx and mobilize intracellular calcium stores, therefore increasing intracellular calcium concentrations and MLCK phosphorylation and increasing myometrial activity. Agents that inhibit myometrial activity, such as progesterone, β-mimetics, relaxin and prostacyclin, decrease intracellular Ca^{2+} by promoting calcium uptake into the intracellular stores such as the sarcoplasmic reticulum so free calcium levels decrease and the uterine muscle relaxes. Calcium channel blockers, such as nifedipine, prevent calcium entry into the cells promoting relaxation of the uterus.

The control of myometrial contractions

Intracellular calcium levels (and myometrial activity) are controlled by various receptors on the myometrial cell surface. Most hormones that affect myometrial contractility bind to receptor sites that are coupled to one of two G-proteins: $G_\alpha s$ or $G_\alpha q$ (see Chapter 3; Bernal et al., 1995). The G-proteins act as transducers between the receptor and the effector regulating the cellular response by coupling the receptor to different signal-generating enzymes within the cell. These enzymes, in turn, generate an amplifying cascade of second messengers. The G-proteins allow the myometrial tissue to respond to a large number of agonists with a limited number of effects, either relaxation or contraction (Fig. 13.6). One of the G-protein pathways ($G_\alpha q$) is linked to the inositol phosphate pathway. Binding of agonists (uterotonins) to receptors coupled to this G-protein activates phospholipase C (PLC), generating inositol triphosphate and diacylglycerol. Inositol trisphosphate stimulates the release of

calcium ions from the sarcoplasmic reticulum and diacylglycerol activates the enzymes protein kinase C and phospholipase A. The latter releases arachidonic acid from membrane phospholipids; arachidonic acid is the precursor of prostaglandins. The result is a rise in intracellular calcium and therefore smooth muscle contraction. The other G-protein pathway ($G_\alpha s$) activates adenylate cyclase, an enzyme that generates cyclic adenosine monophosphate (cAMP) and inhibits release of calcium. Agonists that stimulate this pathway, such as β-adrenergic receptor agonists and prostacyclin, will cause decreased release of Ca^{2+} from intracellular Ca^{2+} stores and dephosphorylation of myosin (so MLCK cannot bind Ca–CAM) and thus uterine relaxation (Yuan and López Bernal, 2007).

Gap junctions

The onset of regular uterine contractions is gradual. As pregnancy progresses, the resting potential of the myometrial cells falls so that action potentials are generated with greater ease. Initially spontaneous uterine contractility is inhibited but becomes significant by mid-gestation. At about 20–24 weeks, hardening (or 'tightening') of the uterus can be felt as muscle contractions start. Initially, uterine activity is mostly of low amplitude and high frequency, with peak activity at night. This circadian rhythm stops at about 3 weeks before delivery, and may be mediated by cortisol (Germain et al., 1993). At first, small groups of myometrial cells contract together causing small fluctuations in intrauterine pressure. As pregnancy progresses, adjacent cells begin to contract synchronously so the contractions become more coordinated. This increased coordination results from cell–cell coupling and is due to the formation of intercellular gap junctions.

Gap junctions are formed from bundles of proteins, called connexins, that align forming pore-like symmetrical channels protruding through adjacent cells, so allowing contact and communication. Gap junctions exist in other tissues that act together in a coordinated fashion, such as cardiac muscle and pancreatic islets. In the open state, gap junctions allow rapid transmission of signals such as electrical stimuli and second messengers such as calcium and inositol trisphosphate (Fig. 13.7). This means that depolarization and smooth muscle contraction in one cell are quickly communicated to adjacent cells so there is a spread of excitation and a synchrony of contractions.

There is an increase in the synthesis of gap junctional protein connexin 43 and the number of gap junctions increases during gestation to about 1000 per myometrial cell. Physiological regulation of connexins and formation of gap junctions is by prostaglandins and steroid hormones; oestrogen and some prostaglandins increase and progesterone and nitric oxide suppress gap junction formation (Garfield et al., 1988). Gap junction density can be determined by measuring electrical resistance of tissue.

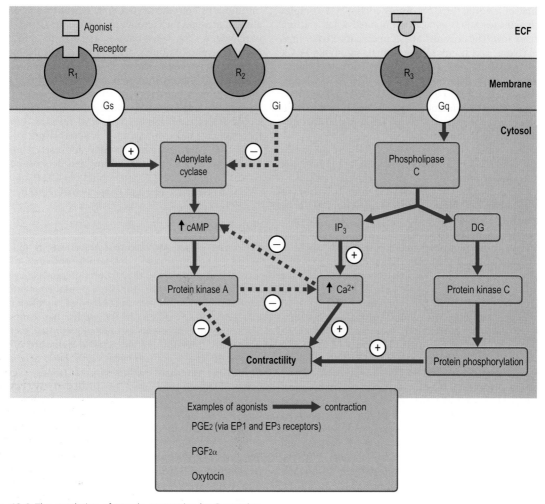

Fig. 13.6 The regulation of muscle contraction by G-proteins.

The resistance of human myometrium at term is about half of that in the non-pregnant uterus and much less than that in other smooth muscle (for instance bladder and stomach), which indicates that the cells of the pregnant myometrium are very well coupled. Gap junction formation increases prior to spontaneous labour, resulting in synchronization and coordination of high-amplitude high-frequency myometrial contractions so increased intrauterine pressure is generated (Neulen and Breckwoldt, 1994). This is why palpation especially near to term, can stimulates uterine tightening; palpation initiates the first stimulation of the uterus which then spreads throughout the myometrium. Often fetal movements will trigger uterine tightening for the same reasons. Suppression of gap junctions may be important at the time of implantation and in early pregnancy (Grummer and Winterhager, 1998).

Uterine contractions and quiescence

The uterus exhibits spontaneous contractility. A biopsy specimen of uterine tissue, placed in a physiological solution, will contract involuntarily every 2–5 min without stimulation. During the menstrual cycle, three patterns of uterine contractility have been described (De Ziegler et al., 2001). At the beginning of the cycle (menstruation), all layers of the myometrium contract exerting antero-grade (from fundus to cervix) expulsive forces; these contractions may be associated with painful cramps (dysmenorrhoea). During the receptive window, in the late follicular phase, uterine contractility involves only the inner layers of the myometrium and is gentle and not perceived by women; this facilitates retrograde (cervix to fundus) transport of sperm towards the uterine tubes where fertilization usually takes place (see Chapter 7).

Fig. 13.7 The gap junction.

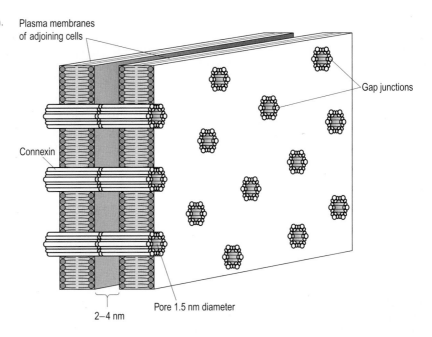

Plasma membranes of adjoining cells

Gap junctions

Connexin

Pore 1.5 nm diameter

2–4 nm

As progesterone levels rise after ovulation, the uterus reaches a stage of quiescence. In pregnancy, progesterone continues to increase and to suppress the rhythmic activity of the uterus. Progesterone decreases the expression of genes for contraction-related proteins, stimulates the relaxant pathways and suppresses the stimulatory pathways of the myometrium and inhibits the binding of oxytocin to its receptors (Mitchell and Taggart, 2009). Other inhibitors of uterine contractions early in pregnancy include relaxin, prostacyclin and nitric oxide, all of which increase intracellular cAMP and/or decrease intracellular calcium levels. It is also suggested that human chorionic gonadotrophin (hCG) inhibits myometrial contractility (Slattery et al., 2001).

However, the uterus is never completely quiescent. From about 7 weeks, the contractions, or 'contractures', are irregular, not synchronized and focal in origin; they have a very high frequency and a very low intensity (Wray, 1993). From mid-gestation, the contractions increase gradually in intensity and frequency until about 6 weeks before term when their intensity increases more markedly. The early Braxton Hicks contractions can be perceived but, although strong, they are not normally painful as the cervix remains closed. In labour, the contractions become synchronized, regular and more intense with increased duration. In primate models, in the few days before delivery, uterine contractions become synchronized during the night and disappear during the day until delivery. This pattern has not been observed in humans but women do have periods of active contractions which then cease suggesting there is also a degree of reversibility in the early stages of human labour (Smith, 2007).

The characteristics of the myometrium change markedly during pregnancy (Shynlova et al., 2009). In early pregnancy, there is a proliferative phase when the expression of IGF proteins is increased and an anti-apoptotic pathway is up-regulated. This is followed by a synthetic phase of growth and remodelling involving cellular hypertrophy and increased synthesis of extracellular matrix proteins. In the third phase the myometrial cells develop a contractile phenotype exhibiting increased excitability and sensitivity to calcium, spontaneous activity and enhanced responses to agonists. In the final phase of pregnancy, the myometrial cells are highly active and committed to labour. The cells are more excitable, there is increased connectivity between the cells and there are changes in the contractile proteins. In this phase, the myometrial cells actively participate in the inflammatory process by producing pro-inflammatory cytokines. There is a further stage of postpartum uterine involution (see Chapter 14).

The cervix

The consistency of the cervix changes in pregnancy to become softer and compliant in preparation for labour. For most of pregnancy, the cervix is a rigid cylindrical structure about 4–7 cm long which forms a closed canal (Mitchell and Taggart, 2009) though in women who have had a previous vaginal delivery, the cervix may be slightly shorted with an internal diameter of about a centimetre. The cervix consists mostly of collagen fibrils, elastic connective tissue and blood vessels with some smooth muscle fibres. Connective tissue changes affect the whole uterus but are more evident in the cervix. The uterine contractions imposed on the softened cervix result in it changing shape. During the pregnancy, the role of the cervix is to act as a closure for the uterus containing its contents and protecting them from ascending infection. Prior to the delivery of the baby, the cervix loses its structural rigidity and is pulled by the uterine contractions so it changes from being a tubular closure to becoming a wide-funnelled canal with very thin edges that is continuous with the rest of the uterine structure. In primigravida women, this shape change occurs in two distinct stages.

The first stage of cervical change is effacement, where the cylindrical shape is transformed into a funnel, but the internal sphincter, or os, is still patent and closed. The longitudinal muscle fibres of the cervix shorten. The differential localization of the fibres means that the outer margins of the cervix develop more tension so maximum uptake of the cervix occurs at the lower end and the external os and softer cervical tissue move upwards into the lower uterine segment (Gee and Olah, 1993). During vaginal examination, a midwife might feel an 'effacement ridge' of the cervical tissue undergoing effacement (Fig. 13.8) the ridge is the dissipating form of the external os.

The second stage begins when full dilatation is reached (the edges of the internal os can no longer be felt); the uterus and vagina form one continuous 'sleeve' opening for the exit of the fetus. In multiparous women, the transition from one stage to the other is far less abrupt so effacement and dilatation occur simultaneously. Dilatation is due to the retraction or shortening of the upper part of the uterus, rather than pressure from the descending presenting fetal part. Therefore, if there is no effective presenting part, as in a transverse lie, cervical dilatation still occurs. The dramatic changes in the cervix result from a combination of structural changes in the tissue and forces exerted by the uterine contractions.

The cervix is predominantly composed of fibrous connective tissue plus some smooth muscle and fibroblasts together with blood vessels, epithelium and mucus-secreting glands. The rigidity of the cervix is related to its high content of collagen, particularly type I and type III collagen. There are two elements to cervical softening: increased vascularity and water content, and structural changes in the connective tissue. At term, 90% of the weight of the cervix is water. Connective tissue is formed of collagen fibres and elastin held together by an extracellular matrix, or ground substance. The ground substance is predominantly composed of proteoglycans, which coat the collagen fibres and modify their physical properties, determining the water content of the tissue. Hormones that promote cervical softening affect the composition of the ground substance. Prior to the onset of labour, there is increased expression and activity of matrix metalloproteinases (MMP) which leads to a progressive breakdown of the collagen matrix; the composition of the proteoglycans changes so that dermatan sulphate decreases and hyaluronic acid and glycosaminoglycans increase.

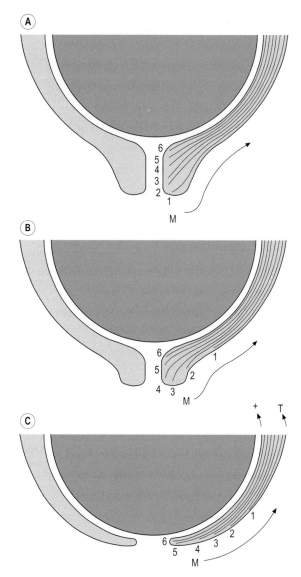

Fig. 13.8 The differential movement of tissue planes at the time of cervical effacement and early dilatation. M, direction of movement of collagen bundles; T, differential tension across the myometrium. (Reproduced with permission from Sweet and Tiran, 1996.)

Dermatan sulphate binds collagen fibrils tightly, whereas hyaluronic acid has a lesser affinity for collagen and attracts water. Although the proteoglycans are a minor constituent of the cervix, they have an amazing ability to bind water: 1 g of hyaluronic acid can bind about 1 L of water (Uldbjerg and Malstrom, 1991). The increased level of hyaluronic acid may act as a signal to activate resident macrophages and neutrophils to secrete interleukins. Interleukins increase prostaglandin activity and neutrophil migration and degranulation (releasing collagenase and elastase). Two other glycoproteins are also involved in cervical changes. Decorin binds and immobilizes the collagen fibres thus stabilizing the structure of the extracellular matrix in early pregnancy. Concentrations of decorin fall in late gestation. Fibronectin binds dermatan sulphate and collagen, protecting collagen from collagenase and stabilizing the extracellular matrix. Hyaluronic acid weakens the interaction of collagen with fibronectin.

The mechanical strength of the ground substance changes as the water content increases and the number of cross-links between elements of the connective tissue diminishes. The collagen increases in solubility and becomes disorganized and weakened (like a fraying rope) so it is more vulnerable to enzymatic digestion. Collagen is resistant to most proteases except collagenase from fibroblasts and neutrophil elastase. Amounts of neutrophil elastase in the cervix significantly increase at term. The association between intrauterine infection and premature labour may be linked to neutrophil infiltration and activation. The effects of oestrogen on cervical ripening are suggested to be mediated by insulin-like growth factor I (IGF-I; Stjernholm et al., 1996). Collagenolysis is a complex balance between availability of free collagenase and the inhibitory proteins. Connective tissue in the body of the uterus also changes at term altering uterine compliance. The level of elastin increases throughout the pregnancy. It provides the elastic recoil that coordinates the contraction–retraction cycle and is important in the return of the uterus to its normal shape after delivery.

Although the cervix has relatively little smooth muscle tissue, it may have an important functional role as a sphincter. The cervix constricts with uterine contractions in early labour (Olah, 1994). It is suggested that this coordinated muscular activity is important in the maintenance of cervical integrity during Braxton Hicks contractions before labour (Steer and Johnson, 1998).

Cervical ripening is predominantly an inflammatory process. Macrophages and neutrophils infiltrate the cervical tissue towards term. They produce cytokines and elastases and collagenases which digest the extracellular matrix proteins.

Assessment of cervical effacement

In practice, the cervix can be assessed by using a simple scoring system, the Bishop's score (Table 13.1). This is particularly useful prior to induction of labour and for monitoring the changes in the cervix as the induction progresses.

If the cervix is soft, effaced and has started to dilate, induction may be implemented by artificial rupture of the membranes, which augments endogenous prostaglandin production. If the cervix is less favourable, prostaglandin E_2 (PGE$_2$) is administered into the posterior fornix of the vagina to facilitate effacement. However, PGE$_2$ should

Table 13.1 Bishop's score			
BISHOP'S SCORE	**0**	**1**	**2**
Station of presenting part	−3	−2	−1
Position of cervix	Posterior	Mid	Anterior
Consistency	Firm	Soft	Very soft
Length	3–4 cm	1–2 cm	<1 cm
Dilation of cervix	0	1–2 cm	>2 cm
Total=	(Bishop's score)		

be used with caution in multiparous women because they have a greater sensitivity to it.

The cause of these structural changes in the cervix is not clear. It is thought to be hormonally controlled. Relaxin has been shown to be important in cervical ripening in rodents and has been used clinically to promote cervical ripening in humans. However, the levels of endogenous relaxin in pregnant women seem to be highest at the beginning of the second trimester. Oestrogen affects the synthesis of connective tissue components *in vitro* but has limited success when used pharmacologically as an induction method. PGE$_2$ causes cervical softening or 'ripening' and is produced naturally by both the cervix and the fetal membranes. PGE$_2$ appears to act by increasing collagenolytic activity rather than by changing the composition of the ground substance, which probably precedes prostaglandin use in successful induction of labour. Following delivery, glycoproteins that bind strongly to collagen are re-formed so the rigidity of the cervix is re-established; however, it never completely regains its original form (see Chapter 14). Damage to the cervix may have long-term consequences (Box 13.1).

Box 13.1 **Clinical issues relating to the cervix**

Longitudinal fibres allow full dilatation of the cervix to be achieved without the pressure of a presenting part, for instance in the case of a transverse lie. Artificial dilatation of an unprepared cervix may damage the collagen fibres. This can result in the cervix failing to remain intact during subsequent pregnancies, resulting in habitual spontaneous abortion, usually in mid-trimester. Preoperative preparation to avoid this involves the administration of a prostaglandin derivative, which induces cervical softening and aids artificial dilatation of the cervix. This method is used prior to procedures involving exploration of the uterine cavity such as termination of pregnancy, evacuation of retained products of conception, surgical ablation of the endometrium and investigation of infertility.

INITIATION OF PARTURITION

Animal models of parturition

Parturition in sheep has been studied in detail. Based on the assumption that mammals are likely to share similar physiological mechanisms for the onset of labour, clinical procedures derived from understanding the mechanisms of parturition in sheep were developed, both for inducing labour and for inhibiting preterm labour in humans. Progesterone is essential for pregnancy maintenance in sheep and the fetal lamb plays a crucial role in the timing of labour. Initiation of labour in sheep is driven by the maturation of the fetal brain; the effect is that progesterone falls resulting in increased uterine activity. Expression of pro-opiomelanocortin (POMC), the precursor of adrenocorticotrophic hormone (ACTH), progressively increases in the pituitary from mid-gestation as the fetal brain matures (Challis et al., 2000). Regulation of secretion of pituitary ACTH in the fetal lamb is by antidiuretic hormone (ADH, also known as vasopressin) and corticotrophin-releasing hormone (CRH). Thus, the first indicator of impending labour in sheep is a sharp rise in fetal cortisol levels due to mature secretion of ACTH from the pituitary gland and increased adrenal sensitivity to ACTH. Removal or abnormal development of the fetal lamb pituitary gland prevents the onset of labour. Infusion of ACTH, cortisone or dexamethasone (a cortisol analogue, frequently used as an anti-inflammatory drug) into the sheep fetus induces labour. Fetal stress such as hypoxia and undernutrition can stimulate preterm birth in sheep (Warnes et al., 1998) by increasing fetal HPA maturation.

The effects of raised cortisol levels are naturally efficient and both promote fetal organ maturity (functional maturation of the fetal lungs and other systems) and initiate labour. Cortisol induces 17α-hydroxylase activity in the placenta that promotes the conversion of C21 steroids to C18 steroids. Thus 17α-hydroxylase converts progesterone to oestrogen so that the progesterone:oestrogen ratio alters in favour of oestrogen. This increases prostaglandin ($PGF_{2\alpha}$) synthesis by the placenta and myometrium. The alteration in oestrogen and progesterone levels can be measured prior to the onset of labour. Exogenous oestrogen induces labour and infusion of progesterone inhibits labour in the sheep. Increasing oestrogen or decreasing progesterone levels stimulates the synthesis of $PGF_{2\alpha}$. Prostaglandins increase myometrial sensitivity to oxytocin. $PGF_{2\alpha}$ is important in cervical softening and increases uterine contractility. A positive feedback mechanism, known as the Ferguson reflex, amplifies the signals. The pressure of the fetal presenting part on the cervix activates a neurohumoral reflex whereby afferent nerves from the cervix impinge on the hypothalamus and increase oxytocin release from the posterior pituitary gland. Oxytocin stimulates uterine contractions and causes further release of $PGF_{2\alpha}$ from the uterus. However, initiation of labour in the human is different in a number of respects from that in the sheep. Note that pregnancy in some species, such as goats, rabbits and rodents, depends on progesterone secretion from the corpus luteum because the placenta is not the source of progesterone. Luteolysis, mediated by $PGF_{2\alpha}$, causes a fall in progesterone and initiation of parturition in these species. The fetus does not seem to play such an important role in the timing of parturition in these species as it does in sheep.

Initiation of parturition in humans

The mean length of human gestation is 39.6 weeks and the majority of births occur between 38 and 42 weeks (Steer and Johnson, 1998). Such a wide range of gestation times in normal pregnancy suggests the timing mechanism is not precise, possibly because it is affected by a number of factors including external influences. The fetus seems to maintain the pregnancy actively. Labour invariably ensues after fetal death has occurred, although it might be delayed by a few weeks (and therefore be pre-empted by mechanical removal of the products of conception). Labour occurs sooner if placental damage has occurred. The critical events permitting extrauterine survival are adequate maturation of the fetal lung and nervous system. The fetal brain may monitor this maturation and control the timing mechanism. Mothers of fetuses with brain abnormalities still progress into labour spontaneously but with a much wider range of gestation (see below). This suggests the fetal brain affects the precise timing of labour in humans, rather than controlling the exact length of gestation.

Hormonal changes associated with parturition in humans

The role of the fetal pituitary–adrenal axis

In sheep, maturation of the fetal HPA initiates parturition. Human fetal malformations such as anencephaly (no cerebrum), malformed pituitary glands or hypoplasia of the adrenal glands are associated with an increased range of gestation length (both longer and shorter) but women still undergo spontaneous labour (Steer and Johnson, 1998). In sheep, similar fetal malformations, either accidental or deliberate, result in significantly prolonged gestation which adversely affects the fetus. This implies that the fetal–adrenal axis has a supportive rather than a direct role in parturition, acting to fine tune the gestational length in humans, rather than functioning as the 'on–off switch' for the initiation of labour, as seen in sheep.

Cortisol

It is evident that the human fetal anterior pituitary gland undergoes maturational changes in the last weeks of gestation as the profile of hormonal release changes. However, there are no defined changes measurable in the maternal circulation prior to the onset of labour. The raised cortisol levels in the cord blood of infants, who have experienced a spontaneous delivery rather than an induced one, or delivery by caesarean section, are maternally derived and are secondary to maternal pain. Labour itself, whether spontaneous or induced, causes stress and therefore an increased production of cortisol, which can cross the placenta. It is possible to differentiate between cortisol of maternal origin and cortisol of fetal origin by comparing the levels in umbilical cord arterial blood with those in the cord vein. Blood in the vein flows from the placenta to the fetus so if cortisol levels are higher in the vein than in the arteries this suggests the source of cortisol is maternal.

Exogenous corticosteroids (such as dexamethasone and betamethasone) given to a pregnant woman at 24–34 weeks to promote fetal lung maturity (see Chapter 15) do not initiate parturition, although oestrogen and cortisol levels fall. Pharmacological doses of glucocorticoids introduced into the amniotic fluid increase uterine activity and induce labour; however, this effect is not observed with physiological doses. Most researchers have not been able to measure an increase in cortisol prior to the onset of labour, nor an effect on placental hormone production. Therefore, it now seems unlikely that cortisol is important in initiating labour in humans, although it has a vital role in the maturation of fetal lungs and other organs. Several factors may affect physiological responses to cortisol; these include corticosteroid-binding protein (CBP) which would influence the relative concentration of free cortisol, metabolism of cortisol to inactive cortisone by 11β-hydroxysteroid dehydrogenase and modification of corticosteroid receptor expression.

Progesterone:oestrogen ratio

In most animal models, progesterone withdrawal is the trigger for parturition. In the sheep, fetal cortisol affects steroidogenesis so progesterone levels fall and oestrogen levels increase. This is a result of increased expression and activity of placental 17α-hydroxylase (see above). Across almost all species, the fall in plasma progesterone concentration is a common endocrine event leading to parturition. However, progesterone levels do not fall prior to labour in humans. In humans, the placenta does not express inducible 17α-hydroxylase activity and therefore cannot convert progesterone to oestrogen. However, increases in free oestriol levels have been observed in saliva of women before the onset of labour, both preterm and at term (Goodwin, 1999).

High progesterone levels inhibit myometrial activity during implantation and favour uterine quiescence throughout the pregnancy. This suppression of myometrial activity is essential to the maintenance of pregnancy, although parturition begins without a measurable decrease in maternal peripheral progesterone levels. Large doses of progesterone are relatively unsuccessful in inhibiting preterm labour in humans. However, mifepristone, the progesterone receptor antagonist previously known as RU-486, inhibits progesterone so it blocks the effect of progesterone and induces labour (Thong and Baird, 1992). Mifepristone is used clinically as an effective abortifacient. It also has anti-glucocorticoid activity and can cause ripening of the cervix and increase sensitivity to contractile prostaglandins.

It is possible in humans that there could be a functional progesterone withdrawal such as local changes in progesterone concentration or receptor binding which, even in the absence of a fall in progesterone concentration in peripheral blood, may affect myometrial activity. As the uterus enlarges during the pregnancy, the part of the uterine wall distal to the site of implantation, and therefore furthest away from the major source of progesterone production, may re-establish uterine contractions and trigger the onset of labour (Challis et al., 2000). Measurement of absolute progesterone levels may therefore be misleading as the biological effects will be altered by receptor density, levels of binding proteins or postreceptor changes. The fetal membranes and maternal decidua can both metabolize progesterone and produce cortisol. Cortisol is antagonistic to progesterone and can increase the synthesis of CRH (Karalis et al., 1996). Fetal membranes, therefore, offer a mechanism for local control of progesterone concentration. Alternative mechanisms have been suggested for the apparent lack of progesterone withdrawal prior to human parturition. These include sequestration of progesterone, another progesterone-like steroid being involved as a natural antagonist or local inactivation of progesterone, for instance progesterone is converted into an inactive metabolite that competes for receptor sites (Challis et al., 2000). For instance, before labour, the major products of the paracrine steroid hormone synthesis could be progesterone and oestrone (a weak oestrogen) and following the onset of labour the major products could be less active progesterone metabolites and biologically active oestradiol (Mitchell and Wong, 1993). It has also been suggested that in humans there is a regionalization of uterine activity and high progesterone levels are important in promoting relaxation of the lower uterine segment while contractions in the fundal area facilitate the descent of the fetus (Challis et al., 2000). Changes in progesterone receptor expression could potentially act as a functional progesterone block and thus control myometrial progesterone responsiveness (Mesiano, 2004). The altered progesterone receptor profile is postulated to modulate oestrogen effects (and hence oxytocin responses) via expression of oestrogen receptors. The human progesterone receptor exists in several isoforms produced from a single gene. PR-B is the full-length isoform which is the major mediator of progesterone effects whereas PR-A lacks the N-terminal part of the protein that contains one of the functional domains so it tends to have effects that oppose those of PR-B. There are also PR-C and two other truncated isoforms. It seems that the expression of PR-A may increase significantly before the onset of labour at term so that the ratio of the two forms changes during gestation thus affecting the response of the uterine tissue and the ability of progesterone to suppress myometrial activity (Goldman and Shalev, 2007). The increased synthesis of PR-A may be mediated by inflammatory factors and Toll-like receptors (Smith et al., 2007); this pathway may be increased in some cases of preterm labour associated with infection.

The interaction of progesterone with its receptors requires specific co-activators; these co-activators are less abundant towards the onset of labour (Smith, 2007). Progesterone metabolites may also interact with the progesterone receptors in a different way to progesterone (Mitchell and Taggart, 2009). Progesterone bioactivity could also be regulated at the post-receptor level.

Human placental production of oestrogen increases throughout labour and the rate seems to increase in the latter part of gestation. In sheep, increased oestrogen causes increased contraction-associated proteins (CAPs) and up-regulation of prostaglandin synthase and consequent increased synthesis of PGE_2, promoting a positive feedback on myometrial contractility. However, spontaneous labour in humans can occur in the absence of measurable changes in oestrogen concentration. Exogenous oestrogen infusion in humans causes a transient increase in uterine activity and decreases the oxytocin threshold of the uterus but does not induce premature delivery or fetal membrane changes (Challis et al., 2000).

Synthesis of placental oestrogen depends on fetal cooperation in the provision of the precursors, and could thus potentially provide an opportunity for the human fetus to manipulate the progesterone:oestrogen ratio and uterine activity. The fetal adrenal gland in humans and higher primates is a relatively large percentage of body mass compared with the adult and has three zones: the outer adult zone produces mostly aldosterone, the unique fetal zone produces dehydroepiandrosterone sulphate (DHEAS) and the transitional zone produces mostly cortisol. This large fetal zone of the adrenal gland disappears in the neonatal period and may be regulated by hCG levels. DHEAS is the fetal adrenal C19 steroid precursor for placental oestradiol-17α and oestrone synthesis, which are implicated as having a role in labour. DHEAS is converted to oestrogens by placental sulphatase, aromatase and other enzymes (see Chapter 3). Production of DHEAS is controlled by ACTH from the anterior pituitary, which is itself regulated by hypothalamic CRH. CRH of placental origin can also stimulate production of DHEAS from the fetal zone (see below). However, women who have placental sulphatase or aromatase deficiencies and produce very little placental oestrogen can have normal pregnancy and labour (López Bernal, 2003). Thus, the changing ratio of oestrogen to progesterone may facilitate effective uterine contractions but is probably not critical for the induction of labour (Steer and Johnson, 1998).

Corticotrophin-releasing hormone

Hypothalamic CRH controls the function of the pituitary–adrenal axis in response to stress. CRH stimulates the anterior pituitary gland to produce corticotrophin which then stimulates the cortex of the adrenal gland to release cortisol. However, even in the presence of significant stress, levels of CRH are relatively low compared to the levels reached in pregnancy. CRH is expressed abundantly in the syncytiotrophoblast cells of the human placenta (but not in non-primate placentas) and CRH-receptors are expressed in the primate placenta and myometrium. Placental CRH seems to have an important role in the initiation of parturition in higher primates and humans. CRH is synthesized by the placenta predominantly into the maternal circulation though some enters the fetal circulation (Smith, 2007). Levels of CRH steadily increase in the maternal circulation from mid-term (about 90 days before the onset of labour) until about 35 weeks when levels sharply rise and are usually particularly high in pregnancies ending with premature labour (Wolfe et al., 1990) and those complicated by pre-eclampsia (Smith and Nicholson, 2007). CRH activity is attenuated by CRH-binding protein (CRH-BP), which is synthesized by the liver, placenta and brain so most CRH is in the bound (inactive) form during pregnancy. However, towards term, when levels of CRH increase, levels of CRH-BP simultaneously fall and the capacity of the CRH-BPO is saturated so circulating levels of physiologically active, free CRH markedly increase. The maternal adrenal CRH receptors are down-regulated so the ACTH response to CRH is blunted in late pregnancy; this protects the maternal pituitary-adrenal axis from over-stimulation.

The stress hormone, cortisol, normally has a negative feedback effect to inhibit CRH secretion and thus ACTH and cortisol secretion as part of the HPA axis. The opposite situation occurs with placental CRH where cortisol has a positive feedback effect to further increase CRH release by the placenta. This positive feedback is further augmented by increased prostaglandin production (Petraglia et al., 1995), which also increases placental synthesis of CRH. Fetal stresses such as hypoxia and hypoglycaemia result in increased CRH concentrations. CRH is a vasodilator in the placental vascular bed (Clifton et al., 1994) so increased CRH should result in increased blood flow and abrogation of the fetal insult. However, if the insult persists, then CRH would increase fetal ACTH secretion and increase DHEAS production thus increasing oestrogen synthesis which leads to myometrial activation.

Thus, CRH appears to be a mechanism by which a compromised fetus can precipitate labour when intrauterine life becomes unfavourable. The pathway by which CRH in the fetal circulation increases pituitary corticotrophin production which subsequently stimulates cortisol secretion by the fetal adrenal gland is important in the maturation of the fetal lungs and other organs particularly the central nervous system and gut (see Chapter 15). The maturing fetal lungs increase their production of surfactant proteins which can then enter the amniotic fluid; these surfactant proteins together with phospholipids and inflammatory cytokines are thought to stimulate inflammation in the fetal membranes and underlying myometrium and contribute to the amplification of the signals leading to labour (Smith, 2007).

It has been suggested that the ratio of placental CRH and CRH-BP acts as a placental 'clock' which controls the length of gestation and allows a distressed fetus to 'wind-on' the clock to initiate premature labour (Smith, 2007). CRH receptors can couple to different G-proteins in different tissues and at different stages of pregnancy (Karteris et al., 1998). So for most of pregnancy, CRH is coupled to the G-protein ($G_\alpha s$) involved in increasing cAMP levels. It therefore has a 'protective' role and promotes myometrial quiescence via the generation of cAMP and cGMP, and up-regulation of nitric oxide synthase expression. Near term, the expression of CRH receptors changes to the form that couples to the other G-protein pathway ($G_\alpha q$) so that CRH now activates PLC and mobilizes Ca^{2+} from intracellular calcium stores thus promoting increased myometrial contractility and labour (Hillhouse and Grammatopoulos, 2002). The involvement of a physiological stress pathway in the onset of labour could explain the relationship between maternal stress and reproductive failure (Nakamura et al., 2008) and the interesting possible relationship between maternal periconceptional nutritional status and the timing of parturition (MacLaughlin and McMillen, 2007). Maternal stress would stimulate the maternal pituitary-adrenal axis resulting in increased maternal cortisol production which would stimulate placental CRH release (Smith et al., 2007). Myometrial contractility is also enhanced by up-regulation of oxytocin receptor expression and cross-talk between the oxytocin and CRH receptors.

Other factors

It is argued that an alternative pathway for initiation of labour is the switching off of mechanisms that cause relaxation (see above; López Bernal, 2003). Cyclic nucleotides (cAMP, etc.) promote myometrial relaxation and β_2-adrenergic agonists are effective tocolytic agents (see Table 13.2). The enzyme adenylyl cyclase catalyses the production of cAMP from ATP. Coupling of receptors to adenylyl cyclase may be responsible for uterine quiescence. As progesterone inhibits activity of the phosphodiesterase which breaks down cAMP, thus terminating its action, progesterone sustains the effect of cAMP and promotes uterine relaxation during pregnancy.

Labour is an inflammatory process but the relationship between the immune system and parturition is not clear. It is clear that significant intrauterine infection can trigger parturition and cause preterm birth. Proinflammatory cytokines such as interleukin 1β (IL-1β), IL-6 and tumour necrosis factor-α (TNF-α), may have an important role in parturition (Mitchell and Taggart, 2009).

Signal amplification

Once labour has been initiated and the myometrium is activated, there is a positive feed-forward stimulation of myometrial activity. This signal amplification is mediated by prolabour factors, known as CAPs or uterotonins. These include prostaglandins and prostanoid receptors, oxytocin and oxytocin receptors, gap junctions and ion channels. It has not been easy to discriminate between those hormones and signals that initiate labour and those that amplify the triggering signals.

Prostaglandins

Prostaglandins (PGs) of the 2-series are known to be important in the feed-forward signal amplification and progression of labour; they promote myometrial contractions, cervical dilatation and membrane rupture. Prostaglandins are present in the circulation in low concentrations and are cleared in the pulmonary circulation so they are difficult to measure as they have paracrine activity and a short half-life. Prostaglandins can be formed as a consequence of tissue trauma (including labour itself and any manipulative or tactile stimuli). In late pregnancy, prostaglandin synthesis is readily stimulated by minor local stimuli, such as coitus, vaginal examination, sweeping the membranes or amniotomy, which are associated with inducing labour. Exogenous prostaglandins can be used therapeutically to ripen the cervix and to induce uterine contractions and labour. Mid-trimester abortion can be induced by procedures, such as intra-amniotic injection of hypertonic saline, that result in the increased synthesis and release of prostaglandins. Increasing DHEAS or oestrogen concentration and decreasing progesterone concentration increase production of prostaglandins (Challis et al., 2000). An increase is myometrial expression of prostaglandins receptors, particularly the receptor of $PGF_{2\alpha}$, is implicated in the causes of some preterm labour (Olson et al., 2003).

Prostaglandins are synthesized in the fetal membranes, decidua, myometrium and cervix; levels fall abruptly following placental separation. The rate-limiting step of prostaglandin production may be important in initiating labour. Activity of phospholipase A_2 (PLA_2) may regulate the level of arachidonic acid, which is the precursor

Table 13.2 Intervention in labour

DRUG/TREATMENT	EFFECT	NOTES
Treatment of preterm labour (tocolytic agents)		
Progesterone and related compounds	May relax uterus or block inflammatory pathways	Possibly reduce late preterm birth but not associated with reduced perinatal mortality or morbidity
β-Adrenergic agonists (betamimetics or 'β-agonists'), for example ritodrine, terbutaline, fenoterol	Inhibit uterine contractions	Effects often short-lived; unpleasant side-effects (cardiovascular, metabolic and neuromuscular)
Magnesium sulphate	Inhibits myometrial contractility by competing with calcium entry and inhibiting actomyosin interaction	Limited usefulness as a tocolytic agent but useful as cerebroprotective agent
Oxytocin receptor antagonists, for example atosiban, barusiban	Competitive inhibition of oxytocin	Clinical trials taking place; potentially useful as oxytocin receptors have limited distribution. Some side effects as acts on vasopressin receptors
Prostaglandin synthase inhibitors, for example indomethacin	Inhibit preterm contractions Reduce connectivity between myocytes	Serious neonatal complications in infants born <30 weeks Adverse effects on fetal renal function, associated with oligohydramnios
Calcium-channel blockers, for example nifedipine	Decrease intracellular calcium, cause uterine relaxation	May affect placental and uterine blood flow; cardiovascular side-effects (hypotension and tachycardia); nonsteroidal anti-inflammatory agents
Alcohol		Risk of aspiration, intoxication, depression and incontinence
Treatment of post-term labour (methods of induction)		
Oxytocin	Used to augment labour; oxytocin has little effect on unripe cervix	Production of endogenous oxytocin can be increased by nipple stimulation
PGF_2 agonists, for example dinoprostone, Cervidil, Prepidil	Cervical ripening, induction of labour	Effects depend on expression of receptors
Misoprostol (Cytotec)	Synthetic PGE_1 analogue; used to reduce acid in the stomach	Can cause the uterus to contract; nausea and diarrhoea
Mifepristone (RU-486; Mifegyne)	Antiprogestin	Primarily used to induce first trimester abortion

of prostaglandins (see Chapter 3). Increased oestrogen (or decreased progesterone) stimulates the release of PLA_2 from decidual lysosomes and therefore increases free arachidonic acid and subsequent prostaglandin synthesis. Arachidonic acid can also be produced indirectly via phospholipase C activity. Alternatively, the activity of cyclooxygenase (COX) may be rate-limiting (Aitken et al., 1990). The chorion produces prostaglandin dehydrogenase (PGDH), the enzyme which inactivates prostaglandins (Smith, 2007). In late pregnancy, chorionic PGDH activity decreases so the levels of PGE_2 rises.

The two most important prostaglandins in labour appear to be $PGF_{2\alpha}$ and PGE_2. At term, concentrations of PGE_2 and $PGF_{2\alpha}$ are higher in the decidua and myometrium (but these tissues are subject to tissue trauma so some authors believe raised prostaglandin levels are caused by increased uterine activity). PGE_2 is involved in cervical ripening, by mediating the release of MMP, and is metabolized by the myometrium to produce $PGF_{2\alpha}$. However, women with extrauterine pregnancies go into labour at term and experience painful uterine contractions even though there are no fetal membranes in contact with the uterus.

Maintenance of human pregnancy may depend on the synthesis of PGE_2 being inhibited and this inhibition of prostaglandin synthesis being attenuated at the onset of labour. Prostaglandin concentrations in the pregnant uterus are very low (about 200 times lower than at any stage in the menstrual cycle), but increase sharply in the maternal circulation from 36 weeks' gestation probably in response to the increasing level of CRH (Hertelendy and Zakar, 2004). Arachidonic acid, the precursor, is plentiful but synthesis of prostaglandins is inhibited, even if the pregnancy is extrauterine. Progesterone or the fetus may directly or indirectly moderate synthesis or metabolism of prostaglandins. Endogenous inhibitors of prostaglandin synthesis have been identified in maternal plasma; levels fall towards the end of gestation. Inhibitors of the COX enzymes, such as aspirin and indomethacin, block prostaglandin synthesis and are used therapeutically to treat preterm labour. Prostaglandin synthesis is up-regulated by cortisol (and dexamethasone), oestradiol, CRH and the inflammatory cytokines interleukin 1β (IL-1β) and tumour necrosis factor α (TNFα; Bowen et al., 2002).

Low doses of prostaglandins, particularly $PGF_{2\alpha}$, increase myometrial responsiveness to prostaglandins and oxytocin possibly by increasing the formation of gap junctions. In vitro, PGE_2 has a biphasic effect, stimulating at nanomolar concentrations and inhibiting at micromolar concentrations. It also has a dual action: when its effects are mediated by the EP_1 and EP_3 receptors, PGE_2 increases intracellular calcium concentration, but the EP_2 receptor is coupled to adenylate cyclase so PGE_2 acting at this receptor decreases intracellular calcium and favours relaxation. Variations in regional prostaglandin synthesis may occur (Wilmsatt et al., 1995).

Prostacyclin (PGI_2) is synthesized in the myometrium and cervix. It promotes myometrial quiescence. It has an important role in maintaining uterine blood flow in labour; it causes vasodilation of smooth muscle and inhibits platelet aggregation, potentially inhibiting thromboembolic complications. Myometrial relaxation between uterine contractions in labour prevents occlusion of the uterine vessels and hypoxia which could lead to uterine dystocia (Hertelendy and Zakar, 2004). Placental thromboxane (TxA_2) has opposing effects to PGI_2 and is important in the closure of the fetal ductus arteriosus and haemostasis after delivery. In pre-eclampsia, levels of prostacyclin are low and levels of thromboxane are high. This is the rationale for aspirin treatment of pre-eclampsia. Aspirin-like drugs, by inhibiting the COX enzymes and thereby prostaglandin synthesis, restore thromboxane levels in pre-eclampsia. Trials using aspirin caused a slight prolongation of gestation and diminution of uterine contractions, but also increased the risk of premature closure of the ductus arteriosus and postnatal bleeding problems in the mother.

Prostaglandins are metabolized by the enzyme PGDH which is located in the fetal membranes. Deficiency of PGDH is associated with preterm labour. Expression of PGDH is up-regulated by progesterone and IL-10 and suppressed by cortisol (and dexamethasone), oestradiol, CRH, IL-1β and TNFα. Parturition is, therefore, essentially an inflammatory process. The association between infection and preterm labour is thought to be due to the release of phospholipases from bacterial organisms (Romero et al., 2003), which cause an increase in arachidonic acid release and so prostaglandin synthesis. Decidual macrophages respond to bacterial products by releasing pro-inflammatory cytokines. Bacterial endotoxins, such as lipopolysaccharide, can either increase prostaglandin release directly or further stimulate release of cytokines which then increase prostaglandin synthesis. Lipopolysaccharide also contributes to premature rupture of the membranes.

Prostaglandins also have an important role in the establishment of a neonatal circulatory pattern (see Chapter 15). Respiratory distress syndrome is associated with high levels of $PGF_{2\alpha}$ in the infant's circulation, and patent ductus arteriosus with high PGE_2 levels. PGE_2 can prevent the ductus arteriosus from closing and inhibitors of prostaglandin synthesis can promote its closure. There is indirect evidence (i.e. fetal breathing movements, FBM, stop) that PGE_2 increases in the fetal circulation 48–72 h before the onset of labour (Thorburn, 1992). It is possible that this is mirrored by a local increase in PGE_2 concentration in uterine tissue, which initiates labour.

Oxytocin

Oxytocin is a peptide synthesized by the hypothalamus and released from the posterior pituitary gland (see Chapter 3). A synthetic form (Oxytocinon or Syntocinon) is used extensively for induction and augmentation of human labour and can prevent postpartum bleeding or haemorrhage. Endogenous oxytocin production can also be stimulated, for instance by nipple stimulation, with a favourable outcome. However, it is not certain whether oxytocin is important in the initiation of labour. As oxytocin receptors are generally localized to the uterus, mammary glands and pituitary, oxytocin antagonists and agonists have few systemic effects. Maternal oxytocin levels are very low and do not change very much before labour. Maternal pituitary production of oxytocin dramatically increases in the first stage of labour. However, focusing on circulating levels of oxytocin may be misleading. The concentration of oxytocin receptors in the myometrium and decidua rise dramatically (by 100–200 times) during late pregnancy so the sensitivity of the uterus increases (Fuchs et al., 1984). This means the uterus can be stimulated by low concentrations of maternal oxytocin levels that previously had no effect. Therapeutic doses adequate to augment labour are very variable, which probably reflects individual differences in receptor number. If used to augment labour infusions of Oxytocinon should commenced on low dosage which is gradually increased until regular, strong contractions (around 3 in every 10 min time period) are present to ensure hyperstimulation of the myometrium is reduced. The pattern of oxytocin release changes at the onset of labour, with an increased frequency of pulses (Fuchs et al., 1991). It may be important that maternal oxytocin levels stay low during the pregnancy so the sensitivity of the uterus to oxytocin is maintained. Oxytocin antagonists, such as atosiban, have been used to inhibit uterine contractility in preterm labour (see Table 13.2) but not always effectively. Atosiban is useful in slowing down preterm labour so that steroids can be administered to facilitate fetal lung maturity however it can also cause raised blood glucose levels so should be used with caution with diabetic women (Berkman et al., 2003). Note that all tocolytic medications have side effects some of which can be extreme and potentially life-threatening (Blumenfeld and Lyell, 2009).

Exposure of decidual cells to oxytocin increases the release of prostaglandins. Vaginal examination in late pregnancy stimulates the Ferguson reflex so oxytocin is released from the posterior pituitary, which stimulates uterine prostaglandin production. Earlier in pregnancy, this response does not occur, presumably because there are inadequate oxytocin receptors. Women who go into preterm labour seem to have an increased expression of oxytocin receptors and higher myometrial sensitivity to oxytocin. Failed induction of labour is associated with a reduced number of oxytocin receptors. Therefore the initiation of labour depends on mechanisms that induce the expression of oxytocin receptors in the myometrium rather affect the oxytocin level itself. Both oestrogen and prostaglandins increase uterine responsiveness to oxytocin.

Oxytocin is also synthesized by the decidua and may act locally (Miller et al., 1993). The fetal posterior pituitary produces both oxytocin and ADH (vasopressin). Exogenous Oxytocinon can cause uterine contractions in sheep and women carrying an anencephalic fetus (Honnebier et al., 1974); however, the physiological relevance of this is not clear as maternal oxytocin secretion does not rise until labour has been initiated. In spontaneous labour, fetal secretion of oxytocin is high and transferred across the placenta at levels comparable to those used to induce

uterine activity (Husslein, 1985). The increment in oxytocin levels is greater in the umbilical arteries than in the umbilical vein and is much higher than maternal levels, suggesting it is synthesized by the fetus and transferred across the placenta. Initiation and maintenance of human labour may therefore be influenced by fetal oxytocin production. ADH (vasopressin) is produced at even higher concentrations than oxytocin and may regulate prostaglandin production.

Relaxin

Relaxin is a polypeptide hormone produced by the corpus luteum, and decidua and placenta in pregnancy, which promotes tissue remodelling during reproduction (Bani, 1997). It has been found to inhibit myometrial contractility and promote vasodilation, via nitric oxide synthesis, until late pregnancy. It also appears to promote cervical ripening at parturition. Concentrations of relaxin appear to be highest in the first trimester and then fall. A very early fall is associated with preterm labour. Histologically, the number of cells staining positively for relaxin is much less after spontaneous delivery compared with caesarean section. Relaxin may inhibit PGE_2 production during pregnancy but favours its production in labour. It may act synergistically with progesterone during the pregnancy, maintaining uterine quiescence and inhibiting oxytocin release.

The maternal endocrine system

Ovaries are not necessary for the initiation of labour. Hypophysectomized women (who have no pituitary glands) and women with diabetes insipidus (a posterior pituitary defect) go into labour at term. However, the posterior pituitary stores oxytocin, which is synthesized in the hypothalamus. In the absence of a functional pituitary gland, oxytocin is probably secreted directly by the hypothalamus. Adrenalectomized women on corticosteroid maintenance therapy go into labour spontaneously but women with Addison's disease tend to have prolonged pregnancy.

The maternal nervous system

There is a higher density of adrenergic and cholinergic innervation towards the cervix. The non-pregnant uterus contracts in response to both adrenaline and noradrenaline but, at term, noradrenaline increases uterine contractions and adrenaline causes relaxation. α-Receptor antagonists, such as phentolamine, decrease uterine activity and inhibit the response to noradrenaline so adrenergic drugs are used to suppress contractions in preterm labour; β-receptor antagonists, such as propranolol, increase uterine activity. Catecholamines both stimulate and inhibit uterine activity, acting via the α_2-receptors and β_2-receptors respectively.

The α_1-receptors increase intracellular calcium concentrations and promote contractile activity. However, labour occurs normally in paraplegic women (who have no nervous input to the uterus), suggesting that the onset and progress of labour is under hormonal, rather than nervous, control. Neural control appears to modulate uterine activity but is subordinate to hormonal control.

Stretch

In a normal pregnancy, growth of the uterus keeps pace with the growth of its contents and the limit of stretchability is probably not reached. In fact, mechanical stretching of the uterine wall by the growing fetus induces smooth muscle hypertrophy and increases its tensile strength. However, overstretching, for instance with multiple pregnancy and polyhydramnios, is associated with a shorter gestation period. The probable mechanism is that stretching of the muscle fibres increases their excitability and that mechanical stress can increase responsiveness to uterotonins. In most smooth-muscle containing tissues in the body, stretching leads to reflex contraction. Multiple gestation and polyhydramnios are associated with over-distension of the uterus and a higher incidence of preterm labour. Distension of the uterus causes myometrial stretching and also stretching of the fetal membranes which line the inner surface of the uterus.

THE TIMING OF PARTURITION

In some mammalian species there is a clear seasonal influence on ovulation and delivery. There are obvious advantages to ensuring the young are born at the optimal time of year when there is a plentiful food supply and less threat from predators. In these species, the length of the daylight period, mediated by night-time secretion of melatonin, appears to play an important role. The human fetus possibly has the potential to survive birth as early as the 24th week of gestation. Most babies are delivered after the 37th week of gestation. However, there is a range of gestational periods producing healthy babies capable of survival. It is suggested that this variation in apparently normal gestation could allow changing environmental conditions to influence the precise timing. One suggestion is that the time of the lunar month could affect the timing after 37 weeks. Other suggestions are that gestational length may be linked to the length of the individual woman's ovarian cycle or may have a familial pattern. Women with longer menstrual cycles may have a lower level of oestrogen, which could affect the initiation of parturition (see above).

Mammals tend to labour most effectively during the period of the day in which they normally rest. They usually seek isolation and privacy and protection from terrestrial predators. Nocturnal species tend to give birth during the day and diurnal species tend to give birth at night (Rosenberg and Trevathan, 2002). This timing may be because the effect of the parasympathetic nervous system is then dominant; labour is inhibited by sympathetic stimulation. Both the start of labour and the actual time of delivery occur more frequently at night and in the early hours of the morning (Honnebier and Nathanielsz, 1994). Circadian rhythms occur in several variables including pregnancy-associated hormones and prelabour myometrial activity. Uterine activity and oxytocin levels are higher at night until about 3 weeks before delivery. The maternal circadian system probably entrains fetal cooperation. Circadian rhythms do not occur in sheep (Apostolakis et al., 1993).

THE EVOLUTIONARY CONTEXT OF HUMAN LABOUR

Humans have large and complex brains and are the only living mammal that habitually walks on two legs. They have a complicated mechanism of labour and routinely seek assistance when they give birth. The development of bipedal locomotion has resulted in a changed pelvic structure and physiology. One suggestion is that eye contact in sexual intercourse has led to the vagina forming a right-angle with the brim of the pelvis and uterus, presenting a laborious passageway in childbirth (Stewart, 1984). The relatively straight cylindrical pelvis of our forebears has evolved into a tilted conical birth canal. Pelvic size has decreased to enhance adaptation to the upright posture and swift movement.

It is thought that the upright stance of human ancestors led to thickening and lengthening of the pelvic bones and the forward curvature of the sacrum (Stewart, 1984); this stance imposes extra pressure on the pregnant cervix. Humans have a particularly high concentration of cervical collagen compared with other species. Unlike most other animals, where the cervix remains firmly closed until just before delivery, there is usually some degree of cervical softening relatively early in human pregnancy (Fig. 13.9); partial dilatation of the cervix occurs much earlier in gestation (Leppert, 1995). Because there is such a wide variation in the cervical changes among pregnant women, cervical assessment in isolation of other signs is an unreliable indicator of the imminence of labour. Towards the end of the first stage of labour, the changing shape of the cervix means that its tissue becomes integrated with the rest of the uterus (Fig. 13.8; see below).

The evolution of the human brain resulted in cephalization, the marked enlargement of head size in relation to overall body mass (Stewart, 1984). This creates the potential problem of obstructed labour, which occurs at a much higher rate in humans compared to other animals. The fetus has to negotiate rather than simply pass through

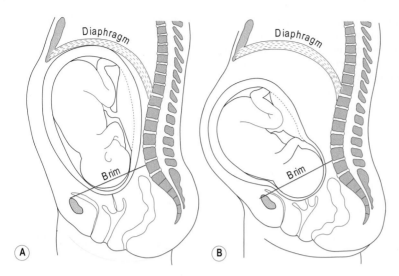

Diaphragm

Diaphragm

Brim

Brim

(A)

(B)

Fig. 13.9 (A) Prior to lightening: the fundus is in close proximity to the diaphragm and the lower uterine segment is still firm so the fetal head remains high. (B) After lightening (2–3 weeks before the onset of labour): the lower uterine segment has softened and dilated so the fetal head descends and the fundus sinks below the diaphragm, easing breathing. (Reproduced with permission from Bennett and Brown, 1999.)

the pelvic cavity. It seems that humans have adapted by the fetus completing *in utero* development at a relatively early stage, and being born at a much smaller proportion of the adult weight. Cephalization has resulted in secondary altriciality, the infant being born at an immature and helpless state of development. Human infants are born with a smaller proportion of adult brain size than other primates. This has significant implications for parental behaviour and social relationships as well as placing a higher emphasis on the importance of nutrition in providing for development of the nervous system in the postnatal year.

Humans are not the only animals that have difficulty in childbirth (Rosenberg and Trevathan, 2002). The smaller bodied primates, such as monkeys and gibbons, have similar cephalopelvic constraints; the neonate at birth has a head size that is close to the size of its mother's birth canal. Monkeys usually deliver in a squatting position away from other members of the social group, who may observe from a distance. The mother monkey may wipe mucus from the infant's mouth and nose and guide the infant, who is usually dexterous with developed motor skills, out of the birth canal towards the nipples (Rosenberg and Trevathan, 2002). Because of mechanical differences in the birth process, however, the human fetus has to rotate within the pelvic cavity and is usually born in an occipitoanterior position (head facing away from the maternal pubic bones, in the opposite direction from the mother). In this position, it is difficult for the mother to reach to clear a breathing passage or remove the umbilical cord from the infant's neck. Thus, human mothers actively seek assistance in childbirth and birth is a social rather than a solitary occurrence.

Whereas most primates squat during delivery, unless women are used to squatting, the semi-upright positions of kneeling and sitting are thought to be optimal (Rosenberg and Trevathan, 2002). The upright position (standing, squatting or sitting) results in a shortened second stage of labour and more favourable maternal and infant outcomes. Being upright allows maternal effort to be aided by gravity. The presenting part bears the force of the neonate. The occiput has well developed cranial plates and is best able to withstand the stress (Rosenberg and Trevathan, 2002).

It is suggested that the physiological control of birth is mediated by hormones that are derived from archaic brain structures such as the hypothalamus and pituitary gland (Odent, 2001) and that labour is facilitated by an environment that promotes these primitive pathways. The neocortex, on the other hand, is thought to inhibit the primitive pathways. The neocortex responds to bright light and to language. Thus, it is suggested that bright lights, feelings of being observed (and use of cameras and monitoring equipment) and use of language which stimulate neocortical activity might interfere with the primitive physiological processes and impede the progress of labour. This may explain why relaxation techniques may progress labour. Often women appear to become detached from their surroundings indicating that neocortex activity is suppressed as they inwardly focus on their body activity and dampening down their responses to external stimuli. Fear is an archaic emotional response; women often cry out and express emotional fear in advanced labour suggesting the archaic brain activity is dominant. Maternal levels of catecholamines peak towards the end of labour which increases maternal awareness and alertness as the baby is born. This is suggested to be an evolutionary advantage, promoting maternal behaviour and protectionism, even aggressiveness (Odent, 2001).

THE FIRST STAGE OF LABOUR

Uterine contractions in labour

If softening of the cervix has taken place, the coordinated uterine contractions exert a steady pull thus stretching the cervix. This effacement of the cervix often takes place before the contractions become completely regular so it may occur a week or so before labour. As the cervix effaces, the presenting part of the fetus, usually the head, descends into the cavity of the pelvis. The fetal position alters so that it fits well; this is described as engagement.

Contractions are involuntary and will therefore occur in an unconscious woman. However, they can be temporarily abolished by emotional disturbances (including moving from home to hospital and by a change in staff shifts). The frequency and strength of the contractions can be increased by enemas, prostaglandins and oxytocin preparations, and by stretching of the cervix or pelvic floor by the presenting part. Contractions are regular and intermittent. The intermittent nature is important as it allows recovery of both the uterus and the labouring woman and a resumed oxygen supply to the fetus.

Contractions begin to feel painful once the cervix starts to dilate. Backache often precedes cervical dilation. The pain is due to ischaemia in the muscle during the contraction because the uterine blood vessels are compressed. Similar pain occurs for the same reason in spasmodic dysmenorrhoea. Uterine pain is analogous to myocardial pain in angina when blood flow in the coronary arteries supplying the cardiac muscle is restricted. Baseline tone in labour is about 10–12 mmHg (Blackburn, 2007). An increase in intrauterine pressure of about 10–20 mmHg can be palpated abdominally and perceived by the women at 15–20 mmHg. Pain is often perceived when the pressure rises above 25 mmHg. Pressures may rise to 50 mmHg in the first stage and to 75–100 mmHg in the second stage. Weak contractions have a shorter duration with longer intervals between each contraction. The sensation of pain is related not just to the strength of contraction and the interval between each contraction but also to the well-being of the mother and position of the fetus. An anxious or tired woman experiences pain at lower uterine pressure intensity (see below). Maternal position and use of analgesics may influence the strength and timing of contractions. A woman whose baby is in a posterior position which commonly presents with a deflexed head (often described as an abnormal attitude or military position) also tends to have greater backache as there is increased pressure on the sacral bones and posterior joints of the pelvis.

Contraction waves

The uterus is also analogous to the heart in another respect in that it appears to exhibit pacemaker activity, although specific pacemaker cells have not been localized. Specific areas that depolarize more rapidly have not been identified, although it was believed that they were each side of the fundus, near the uterotubal junctions or cornuae. All myometrial cells have spontaneous pacemaker activity. The contractions tend to originate from cells near the fundus and spread as a wave, as the electrical activity moves through the gap junctions of the muscle fibres (Fig. 13.10). The waves are strongest at the fundus, which has the highest density of muscle fibres, and take about 15–30 s to travel down the length of the uterus (Blackburn, 2007). There is a polarity of wave contraction with rhythmic coordination between the upper segment, which contracts for longer and retracts, and the lower segment, which contracts slightly later, to a less extent and dilates. This is described as fundal dominance; it is similar to the peristaltic waves generated by smooth muscle in other viscera. If the wave pattern is abnormal, for instance if the lower part contracts first or more strongly, the waves become erratic and uncoordinated and labour does not progress efficiently. This is described as 'incoordinate uterine activity'.

The uterus relaxes between contractions, which is important for oxygenation of the fetus and myometrium. The upper part of the uterus does not relax fully between contractions but retracts instead. This means that the muscle fibres do not return fully to the original length but progressively and gradually get a little bit shorter and thicker with each contraction (Fig. 13.11). This means that the less active lower segment is pulled up towards the shortening upper part of the uterus. (If the uterine muscle relaxed completely following each contraction, the uterus would remain the same size and labour would not progress.) The weakest points are the os and cervix which are effaced and dilated, enlarging the opening of the uterus.

Formation of hindwaters and forewaters

As the lower segment stretches and the cervix starts to efface and change its position, the chorion becomes detached from the uterine wall. The operculum tends to become dislodged from the receding cervical canal. The loss of this mucus closure (or 'show'), which may be blood-streaked (caused by the rupture of tiny superficial blood vessels during detachment of the mucous plug), indicates the external os has started to dissipate and that active dilatation of the internal os is imminent. The membranes are extruded through the opening cervix by the pressure of the amniotic fluid (Fig. 13.12). The head of

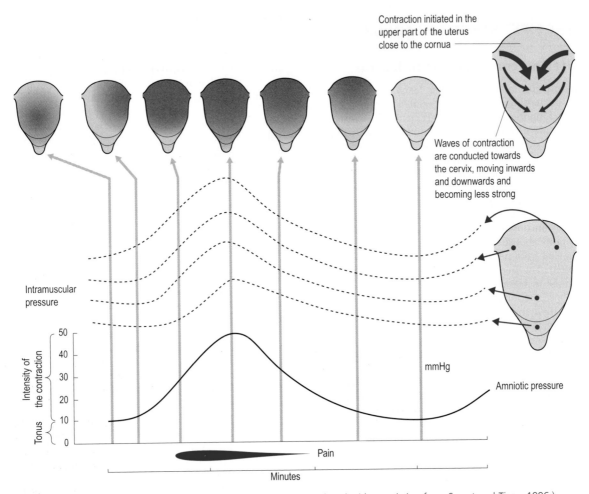

Contraction initiated in the upper part of the uterus close to the cornua

Waves of contraction are conducted towards the cervix, moving inwards and downwards and becoming less strong

Intramuscular pressure

Intensity of the contraction

Tonus

50
40
30
20
10
0

mmHg

Amniotic pressure

Pain

Minutes

Fig. 13.10 Contraction and retraction of uterine muscle cells. (Reproduced with permission from Sweet and Tiran, 1996.)

the fetus tends to act as a ball-valve separating the amniotic fluid pushing through the cervix (forewaters) from the remainder of the fluid (hindwaters). The forewaters transmit the pressure generated from the waves of contraction, spreading the force evenly over the cervix, which aids its further effacement and dilatation. The hindwaters help to cushion the fetus from the contraction pressures. As the fundus presses on the upper aspect of the fetus (usually breech) during contractions, the pressure is transmitted through the fetal body to the lower segment and cervix (this is known as the fetal axis pressure). As uterine contractions progress, the pressure of the fluid in the forewaters rises and the membranes tend to rupture. When the fetus is in an abnormal position (for example in a breech or posterior and deflexed cephalic position), the pressure of the forewaters is not as great because the presenting part does not plug the cervix as effectively. This explains why a 'soft and floppy bag' of forewaters is associated with abnormal presentations.

Membrane rupture

As well as an increase in the pressure of the forewaters, the fetal membranes may also rupture when the contractions cause the presenting part to distend them. There is a loss of lubricant between the chorion and amnion leading to increased shear force and cell rupture (Blackburn, 2007). In 5–10% of pregnancies, premature rupture of the membranes (PROM) occurs spontaneously before the onset of uterine contractions as the earliest sign of labour (Duff, 1996); about 60% of these are classified as term gestation. Spontaneous rupture of the membranes before 37 weeks' gestation often culminates in premature labour and delivery. Early rupture of the membranes as the first event in the course of labour is a cause for concern as it may indicate an ill-fitting presentation or high head at term in a primigravida, polyhydramnios or chorioamnionitis (a local infection which may be due to chlamydia or streptococcus).

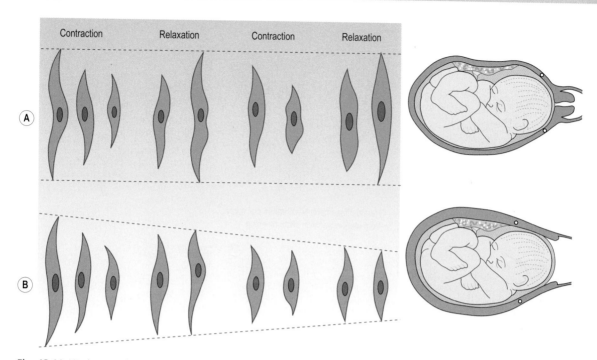

Fig. 13.11 Uterine muscle contraction. Rather than the uterine myometrial cells relaxing fully (as in A), during labour the myometrial cells in the upper segment of the uterus retract getting progressively shorter (as in B). The lower uterine segment and the cervix dilate in response to the forces of contraction generated by the shortening upper segment thus the fetus is expelled.

Rupture of the amniotic membrane is associated with collagen degradation in the membrane (Hampson et al., 1997). Usually coordinated contractions and dilatation of the cervix follow rupture of the membranes but if there is a delay the fetus is at risk from ascending infections so clinical intervention may be necessary if labour has not followed within 24 h. There is controversy about artificial rupture of membranes and the effect it has on speeding up labour; it is thought that labour may progress more abruptly and painfully (Barret et al., 1992).

Size changes in the uterus and cervix

As the size of the upper segment of the uterus gradually diminishes because of the repeated cycles of contraction and retraction, the fetus is pushed into the lower segment so its presenting part (Box 13.2) exerts pressure on the obstructing maternal tissues. This results in increased oxytocin release from the posterior pituitary gland, which increases uterine activity by positive feedback mechanisms (see Chapter 1). Later in labour, when the baby has been born and the placenta has been expelled, retraction aids the uterine walls to come together so the cavity is obliterated as the uterine walls lie in apposition. A physiological retraction ring forms at the junction between the thick retracted segment of the upper segment and the thin distended wall of the lower segment. Under normal conditions, this ring is not visibly evident or palpable by abdominal examination. A pathological visible 'Bandl's ring' is the consequence of failure to recognize and manage obstructed labour appropriately and is a sign of imminent uterine rupture.

The rate of cervical dilatation is not constant; initially the cervix dilates slowly, but early changes are reinforced by positive feedback mechanisms and the rate accelerates. The latent phase of the first stage is slower and can take up to 12 h (Box 13.3, Fig. 13.13). It is during this stage, when dilatation to 3–4 cm is achieved, that the cervix positively contracts in response to oxytocin (Olah et al., 1993). This probably facilitates effacement. After a transition stage of about 15 min when the cervix does not contract, the cervix then dilates in response to myometrial contractions during the faster active phase.

Case study 13.1 is an example of the first stage of labour.

Table 13.2 details the possible types of intervention in labour.

THE SECOND STAGE OF LABOUR

By the end of the first stage of labour, the lower uterine segment, the cervix, the pelvic floor and the vulval outlet form one continuous dilated birth canal. The forces required to expel the fetus are both from the uterine

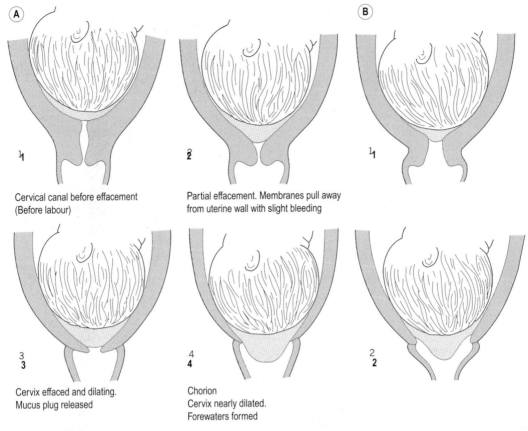

A
1 Cervical canal before effacement (Before labour)

2 Partial effacement. Membranes pull away from uterine wall with slight bleeding

B
1

3 Cervix effaced and dilating. Mucus plug released

4 Chorion Cervix nearly dilated. Forewaters formed

2

Fig. 13.12 Effacement and dilatation of the cervix: (A) in a primigravidae; (B) occurring simultaneously in a multigravidae. (Reproduced with permission from Sweet and Tiran, 1996.)

Box 13.2 Terms used for fetal presentation

- Attitude: relationship between fetal head and limbs and fetal trunk
- Lie: relationship of fetus to long axis of uterus
- Presentation: part of fetus presenting in lower aspect of uterus
- Presenting part: part of presentation immediately inside internal os
- Position: relationship of presentation, or presenting part, to maternal pelvis
- Denominator: part of presenting part marking position

Box 13.3 Progression of labour

The medical model of care in labour has defined an acceptable rate of progress in labour. Failure of labour to progress at this rate is described as abnormal and used as the rationale for medical intervention. Progress in labour is assessed through the use of a partogram. Cervical dilatation at the rate of 0.5 cm/h is accepted as normal. Intervention (such as amniotomy or use of Oxytocinon) is usually recommended if the rate of progress falls below 2 cm of the expected progress in 4 h. If in a further 4 h, following the use of Oxytocinon, if further progress is less than a further 2 cm then surgical intervention should be considered (NCCWCH, 2007).

---

muscle activity and from the secondary muscles of the abdomen and diaphragm, which augment the contractions of the uterus. The forces generated by the uterus can be described as the primary power and the complementary force from the voluntary movement of the respiratory muscles as the secondary power. By this stage, the uterus is markedly retracted and undergoing a pattern of

strong, regular and repetitive contractions. The mother is compelled involuntarily to bear down or push. As she inspires before pushing, the diaphragm is lowered and the abdominal muscles contract, augmenting the contractile forces of the uterus. Bearing down by the mother

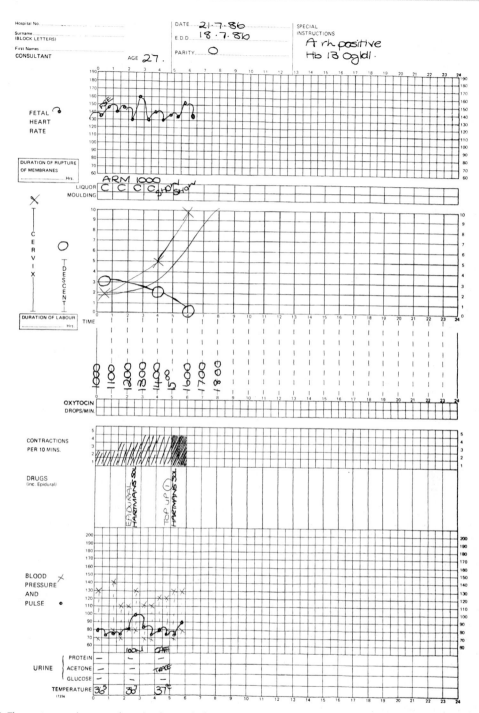

Fig. 13.13 The partogram is a complete visual record of measurements made during labour and delivery. (Reproduced with permission from Symonds and Symonds, 1997.)

Case study 13.1

Martha is a para 3; her previous pregnancies and labour were uneventful. She was admitted to the labour ward and confirmed to be in labour as her cervix was 6 cm dilated at 13:00 h. Four hours later on a repeat vaginal examination there was no further dilation, the membranes were intact, and cephalic presentation at the spines was judged to be in a direct occipito-anterior position. Martha was coping well and there were no concerns raised over the fetal condition.

- Should the midwife refer Martha for an obstetric opinion?
- Is the fact that Martha has made no progress enough to justify intervention?
- How could the midwife justify her decision to leave Martha alone, if she felt that this were appropriate?
- What physiological processes/influences may be contributing to this situation?

helps to overcome the resistance of the soft tissues of the vagina and the pelvic floor. The fetal attitude (see Box 13.2) extends as it is directed through the birth canal, which aids the efficiency of the uterine contractions. The pain experienced in the second stage of labour is often less as cervical dilatation is complete and the woman is aware that progress is more rapid.

As the fetal head passes through the pelvis, the pressure on the sacral nerves may be associated with cramp in the legs and pain from the trauma to the tissue. The fetus distends the vagina and displaces the pelvic floor. The anterior part of the pelvic floor is drawn up causing the urethra to elongate and become compressed. The bladder is therefore repositioned within the protective environs of the abdomen. Posteriorly, the pelvic floor is stretched forward in relation to the presenting part and the rectum is compressed, which may lead to defecation (which is often a sign the second stage has commenced). The perineum is flattened, lengthened and thinned by the presenting part of the fetus.

During a contraction, the presenting part (usually the fetal head) advances forward and, if not in a direct anterior position, rotates forwards facilitated by the shape and resistance of the pelvic floor. If the fetal head is completely flexed, then the top of the head (the flexion point) meets the resistance of the pelvic floor optimising rotation. In the interval between contractions, the presenting part recedes slightly and may rotate back but, as the uterine muscle retracts with each contraction, progression in the forward direction is maintained. This progression has been likened to taking two steps forward and one step back. Once the flexion point is positioned over the uretogenital hiatus, the fetal head starts to distend the perineum and vaginal opening. When the widest part of the fetal head (the biparietal diameter) distends the vulva, the stretching is at its maximum, hence pain may be severe

if not managed effectively with analgesia. This is described as 'crowning' of the head. The severity of the pain may cause a labouring woman to gasp and inhale sharply. The momentary break in the bearing-down movement has an important role in protecting the perineum from too much trauma, which can cause tearing of the tissue. Once the head is delivered, it realigns itself with the original internal position of the fetal body (so the baby's head moves from facing the maternal anus to facing one of the maternal buttocks); this is called restitution. Following restitution, the next contraction forces the anterior shoulder to contact the perineum and therefore further external rotation of the head occurs with the fetus facing at right angles with the maternal midline. The birth of the baby is usually accomplished with the next contraction following 'crowning' with the posterior shoulder leading. A gush of amniotic fluid escapes. The fetus undergoes a pattern of passive corkscrew movements as it follows the shape and curvature of the pelvis (curvature of Carus). The gutter shape of the pelvic floor facilitates the rotation of the presenting part enabling the widest diameters of the pelvis to accommodate the largest dimensions of the fetal head and shoulders (Fig. 13.14). In breach presentations, the anterior buttock of the fetus contacts with the perineum first and so rotates forward and once the anterior buttock lies over the uretogenital hiatus the breech will distend the perineum and vaginal opening as it is born.

Influences of pelvic and pelvic floor morphology and parturition

The passage of the fetus through the pelvis is described in practice as the mechanism of labour. Engagement describes the descent of the presenting part into the true pelvic cavity; the term relates to the widest transverse diameter of the fetal skull having negotiated the pelvic brim or inlet. If the baby has a cephalic (head-first) presentation, this is described in terms of number of fifths palpable (Fig. 13.15). Verification of the degree of engagement can be achieved through vaginal examination. With a cephalic presentation, the level of the biparietal prominences is judged in relation to the pelvic brim and the pelvic outlet at the level of the ischial spines. Engagement may occur long before the onset of labour, or may occur during, or even late on in, labour (more common in multiparous women). In a primigravida, engagement usually occurs at about 36 weeks' gestation in response to effacement of the cervix. Engagement does not indicate cavity and outlet measurements.

THE THIRD STAGE OF LABOUR

During the third stage, the placenta separates from the wall of the uterus and is expelled. Before separation, the placental extracellular matrix is thought to be weakened

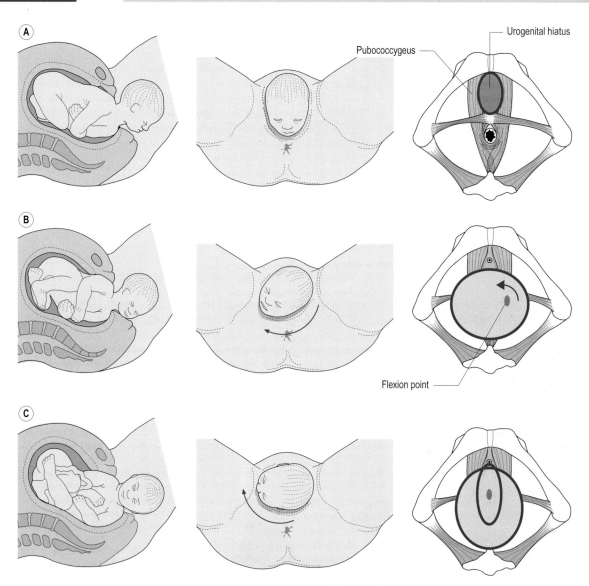

Fig. 13.14 Rotation of the presenting part: (A) delivery of the head; (B) restitution; (C) external rotation. (Adapted with permission from Bennett and Brown, 1999.)

by proteases including MMP produced by the decidua and fetal membranes (Weiss et al., 2007). The uterus retracts markedly and bleeding from the placental wound site is constrained. Following the safe delivery of a healthy baby, the third stage of labour still presents a number of potential hazards. Should part of the placenta be retained, control of bleeding is impaired and a life-threatening postpartum haemorrhage could ensue. Immediately after delivery, the uterus markedly decreases in size. The pattern of contractions is interrupted for a minute or so, until contractions resume at a slow rate. As the uterus retracts, the placental site is greatly diminished. The placenta is

not elastic, thus it tends to wrinkle and buckle and be sheared off the elastic uterine wall (like a paper label coming away from a deflating balloon). It is at this stage that some fetal blood from the placental circulation can enter the maternal circulation, potentially causing problems if there is Rhesus incompatibility (see Chapter 10). The marked retraction of the uterus impedes the venous drainage of the maternal intervillous spaces. Separation usually begins in the centre of the placenta and the extravasculated blood forms a haematoma or retroplacental clot between the placenta and decidua aiding its separation as the clot adds to the placental weight peeling the

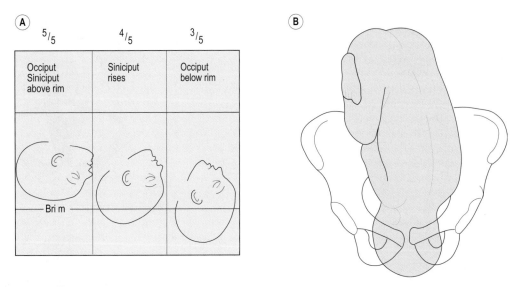

Fig. 13.15 (A) Flexion and descent of the presenting part into the pelvic cavity; (B) engagement of the head. (A, reproduced with permission from Bennett and Brown, 1999; B, reproduced with permission from Sweet and Tiran, 1996.)

membranes from the uterine wall. As the uterus retracts, its progressively shortening muscle fibres tighten around the maternal vessels, forming 'living ligatures', which impede blood flow. This restricts the flow of maternal blood to the uterus and placental wound site, preventing excessive blood loss.

It is the commencement of spontaneous or stimulated uterine contractions following the completion of the

second stage of labour that causes the placenta to separate from the uterine wall. The weight of the placenta completes the detachment of the membranes, which peel off and are expelled (Fig. 13.16). The site of placental implantation determines the speed of separation and the method of placental expulsion. The fetal membranes are expelled with the maternal or fetal surface prominent. The Schultze method of expulsion whereby the fetal side presents

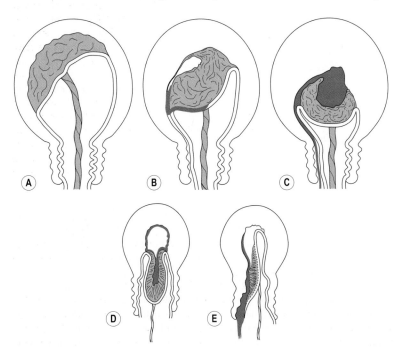

Fig. 13.16 The mechanism of placental separation and expulsion: (A) uterine wall partially retracted but not sufficiently to cause placental separation; (B) further contraction and retraction thicken uterine wall, reduce placental site and aid placental separation; (C) complete separation and formation of retroplacental clot (note: the thin lower segment has collapsed like a concertina following the birth of the baby); (D) Schultze method of expulsion; (E) Matthews-Duncan method of expulsion.

is most common and is associated with a fundal site implantation and the Matthews-Duncan expulsion (whereby the placenta slips out sideways like a button through a buttonhole) is more likely with a lateral implantation. In some cultures, the placenta has important significance and women keep it for ritual ceremonies.

Active management

The third stage of labour can be physiologically managed (passive management), taking about 20–30 min to complete, but active management is widely practised by midwives, shortening the time of placental delivery to a few minutes. Active management involves the injection of an anti-tocolytic agent such as Syntometrine (see below) at the birth of the anterior shoulder or shortly after the delivery of the baby and delivering the placenta and membranes by controlled cord traction (CCT; also known as the Brandt–Andrews manoeuvre). The sheared-off placenta is extracted rather than expelled if active management of the third stage of labour is implemented. The use of CCT is subject to some discussion and is not practised in all countries. The placenta should be separated and the uterus should be well contracted before CCT to ensure that it does not cause uterine inversion. The woman may be asked to bear down to assist expulsion of the placenta.

Syntometrine is a combination of oxytocinon (also called syntocinon; synthetic oxytocin) and ergometrine which is used to reduce the risk of postpartum haemorrhage. Oxytocinon acts within 2–3 min following intramuscular injection, by causing intermittent contractions. These effectively continue the retraction process behind the placental site, thus encouraging separation and early expulsion. Ergometrine becomes effective about 5–7 min after administration. By this time, aided by CCT (commenced as soon as the uterus contracts down), the placenta has been expelled. The midwife applies cord traction by gripping the umbilical cord with one hand and applying a downward traction (Fig. 13.17). The other hand is placed on the lower abdomen, thumb and index finger stretched out to provide a line of contact) applying pressure to avoid inversion of the uterus. Ergometrine produces a sustained uterine contraction, which promotes the haemostatic action of the living ligatures. It is essential, therefore, to deliver the placenta before ergometrine stimulates closure of the cervix as this could result in a retained placenta. The third stage of labour can also be managed using intramuscular injections of Oxytocinon only following delivery as it has fewer side effects. Oxytocinon should not be used if there is a history of hypertension as ergometrine can increase blood pressure further.

Physiological management of the third stage of labour involves no routine use of anti-tocolytic drugs, not clamping the umbilical cord until pulsations cease, no uterine manipulation or controlled cord traction, and delivery of

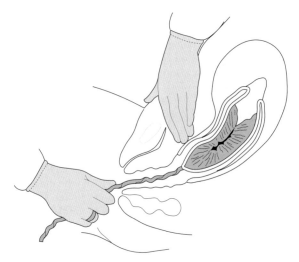

Fig. 13.17 Controlled cord traction (Brandt–Andrews method). (Reproduced with permission from Bennett and Brown, 1999.)

the placenta and membranes solely by maternal effort should be completed within 1 h of birth. Skin-to-skin contact and early breast feeding may facilitate the delivery of the placenta in the third stage by stimulating endogenous maternal oxytocin release. Women should be encouraged to empty their bladders and adopt an upright position as gravity will aid delivery of the placenta. During this time, palpation of the uterus should be avoided but careful observation is required especially of vaginal blood loss to identify haemorrhage. As placental separation occurs, there is usually an increase in blood loss but this is reduced as the uterus contracts down and the presence of the placenta in the upper part of the birth canal stimulates the mother to bear down. This may stimulate more oxytocin release due to Ferguson's reflex. Division of the umbilical cord should not be rushed unless the baby needs attention and ideally the cord should not be cut until it is pulse-less. Many practitioners advocate not clamping the maternal end of the cord to facilitate spontaneous delivery of the placenta as the free draining of the blood softens the placental body making it easier to pass through the birth canal.

THE EFFECTS OF LABOUR ON MATERNAL PHYSIOLOGY

Cardiovascular system

The stress of labour prepares the woman for the inevitable blood loss at delivery and limitation of bleeding after placental separation. Dehydration and muscle activity increase the haemoglobin concentration. Erythropoiesis and white blood cell number also increase as part of the normal response to stress. Concentrations of clotting factors increase, clotting times shorten and fibrinolytic activity is decreased on completion of the third stage of labour. The placenta and decidua are very rich sources of thromboplastin which can activate coagulation (see Chapter 1). About 5–10% of the total body fibrin is deposited as a haemostatic endometrial mesh over the placental wound site (Blackburn, 2007). This hypercoagulable state is further developed in the puerperium (see Chapter 14).

The cardiovascular system is affected by pain, anxiety, apprehension, position and anaesthesia, as well as by the muscular activity of the uterus itself and the dramatic increase in catecholamine production during labour. Uterine contractions progressively increase cardiac output as venous return and circulating volume are increased. Each contraction can contribute 300–500 mL of blood to the circulation (Sullivan and Ramanathan, 1985), which significantly increases cardiac output and blood pressure. In the supine position, stroke volume and cardiac output tend to be lower and heart rate raised.

Catecholamines affect vascular tone and increase blood pressure; this effect is reduced with anaesthetics. Pain and anxiety result in tachycardia (increased heart rate) and affect blood pressure. During a contraction, systolic blood pressure increases by at least 35 mmHg and diastolic blood pressure may increase between 25 and 65 mmHg (Blackburn, 2007). The increment in blood pressure precedes each contraction and falls to baseline between contractions. The greatest haemodynamic changes occur in women delivering their baby vaginally, which is an important consideration for women who have cardiac disease.

The respiratory system

Labour affects the respiratory system as the muscular work increases metabolic rate and oxygen consumption. Respiratory rate and depth of respiration increase. Anxiety, drugs and use of a gas mask mouthpiece can all affect respiratory rate. There is a tendency for a labouring woman to hyperventilate. Hyperventilation is a natural response to pain. Contractions occurring at high frequency can affect oxygenation causing muscular hypoxia and acidosis. Hypoxia can increase the amount of pain experienced.

The increased ventilation causes a progressive and marked decrease in partial pressure of carbon dioxide (to about 25 mmHg) particularly if the contractions are painful. In early labour, hyperventilation can cause respiratory alkalosis and increased blood pH. This can result in the woman experiencing dizziness and tingling of her fingers and toes, and possibly developing muscle spasms. At extremely low $PaCO_2$, blood flow can be affected and the oxygen–haemoglobin dissociation curve (see Chapter 1) shifts to the left so release of oxygen is impaired.

The remedy of breath counting to slow respiratory rate, especially if the woman counts them with her partner or a midwife who deliberately slows down counting, can prevent or correct hyperventilatory effects.

By the end of the first stage, maternal acidosis due to isometric muscle contractions is likely and is compensated for, to a degree, by the respiratory alkalosis. The muscle contractions reduce blood flow to the uterine muscle, which becomes hypoxic and undergoes anaerobic metabolism. Flow to the intervillous space also decreases so fetal levels of carbon dioxide increase and the fetus tends to become acidotic. During bearing down, when the mother's accessory respiratory muscles are involved, mild respiratory acidosis is likely. In the second stage of labour lactate levels increase, thus pH falls. This metabolic acidosis is not compensated for.

The renin–angiotensin system

Labour and delivery affect the renin–angiotensin system of both fetus and mother. Levels of renin and angiotensinogen increase, which are important in maintaining blood flow, but can also affect handling and excretion of drugs. Glomerular filtration rate, renal blood flow and sodium excretion are also affected by raised catecholamine levels or general anaesthetic. Oxytocin has structural similarities with ADH and has inherent antidiuretic properties; therefore fluid retention is increased in labour. Women in labour can be at risk of iatrogenic water intoxication due to loss of electrolytes, use of Oxytocinon, or intravenous fluid administration.

Metabolic rate

Maternal glucose consumption markedly increases in labour to provide energy required by the uterus and skeletal muscles. Glucose and triacylglycerides are used as energy sources. Oxytocin has some insulin-like properties. An increased body temperature during labour may indicate dehydration or infection. It is common for women to experience a transient postpartum chill about 15 min after the birth of the baby or delivery of the placenta. In the following 24 h, postpartum women frequently have a slightly raised temperature secondary to dehydration.

NUTRITION IN LABOUR

Food and drink consumption in labour is controversial. There are two conflicting arguments. The first is that a woman in labour might possibly require a general anaesthetic and therefore should be treated as a preoperative patient at risk of gastric aspiration. Pulmonary aspiration of gastric acid (Mendelson's syndrome) or particulate food matter, although rare, is a major cause of morbidity and mortality for women in labour. The risks of gastric aspiration are thought to be greatly reduced if oral intake is limited (Rowe, 1997). Pregnant women have a slower gastric emptying rate (see Chapter 11), which is further delayed by labour (Carp et al., 1992), and decreased tone of the lower oesophageal sphincter but it is not known whether this delayed gastric emptying predisposes to gastric aspiration.

The opposing view is that a more liberal policy is more beneficial and that women are being needlessly deprived of food. It is argued that general anaesthesia is relatively rare now and that techniques have improved, which make aspiration of gastric contents unlikely. It is argued that prolonged fasting could have detrimental psychological and physiological effects, including increased anxiety and stress.

Pregnant women are predisposed to ketosis, particularly in labour. Pregnancy is a ketotic state and fasting in pregnancy is invariably associated with ketonuria (Scheepers et al., 2001). It is estimated that a woman in labour has an energy requirement of 700–1100 kcal/h. When glycogen stores are exhausted, adipose tissue is mobilized. Fatty acid oxidation increases ketosis, an excess of ketone bodies in the plasma, which are excreted into the urine. Lipolysis provides fatty acid substrates for maternal energy needs and spares glucose for the fetus. The critical question is whether ketosis is detrimental to the progress of labour. Ketones can increase acidity, cause excessive renal excretion of sodium and cross the placenta to the fetus. Although the length of labour is correlated with the degree of ketosis, it is not clear whether longer labour results in increased ketosis or whether ketosis prolongs labour.

It is suggested that fasting in labour can increase the need for medical intervention. Allowing women to eat in labour reduces the plasma level of ketones, which may aid the progress of labour (Scutton et al., 1996). Ketonuria can be treated by administration of intravenous dextrose but this is associated with fluid and electrolyte imbalance. A number of women experience nausea and vomiting in labour. But, in practice, more maternity units are cautiously adopting a liberal policy offering a non-particulate diet while using antacids and H_2-antagonists to reduce gastric pH and decrease volume of gastric contents, thus minimizing the risk of aspiration and lung damage.

THE EFFECTS OF LABOUR ON THE FETUS

Labour has profound effects on the fetus and is important in aiding the adaptation to extrauterine life (see Chapter 15). Understanding the effects of labour on the fetus is important in differentiating between normal healthy responses and diagnosing fetal distress.

Behaviour of the fetus during pregnancy

The use of ultrasound led to the observation that, after 36 weeks, the fetus exhibits a number of clearly definable behavioural states, which are analogous to the neonatal states (see Chapter 15). These states have characteristic patterns of fetal heart rate (FHR), FBM, eye movements, voiding and mouthing movements (Table 13.3). The patterns of fetal behaviour change with gestational age and are assumed to reflect the activity of the fetal central nervous system and can potentially be used to recognize a compromised fetus (Nijhuis, 2003). The movements evidently demonstrate fetal ability to respond to external stimuli. Many factors such as time of day, meals, smoking, etc. affect fetal behaviour. Most of the movements that are discernible in the third trimester can be traced back to the first trimester. Both the movements and the periods of quiescence between them are important.

FBM can be detected from the end of the first trimester (Nijhuis, 2003). FBM are more regular in state 1F than in state 2F, they occur more frequently in state 2F and are present but irregular in states 3F and 4F. It has been suggested that FBM are more likely to be state-dependent when maternal glucose levels are lower (Mulder et al., 1994). There is a postprandial increase in FBM and smoking diminishes them. Fetal voiding movements are inhibited in state 1F but occur at the transition to state 2F. Sucking and swallowing can be seen from the end of the first trimester. Regular or rhythmic mouthing movements

Table 13.3 Fetal behavioural states	
State 1F (1 fetal); quiet sleep	Fetal quiescence with brief gross startles; high-voltage electrocortical activity; no eye movement; FHR accelerations; minimal heart rate variability; isolated fetal heart rate
State 2F (2 fetal); active sleep	Paradoxical/irregular sleep; frequent and periodic stretches; retroflexion and movements of extremities; low-voltage electrocortical activity; continuous eye movements; increased FHR variability with frequent accelerations
State 3F (3 fetal); quiet awake	Absence of gross movements; continuous rapid eye movements; stable, but widely oscillating FHR, no accelerations
State 4F (4 fetal); active awake	Vigorous and continual movements; rapid eye movement; unstable heart rate – large, long accelerations and tachycardia

are most often observed in state 1F, when they occur in bursts of 10–20 min, whereas powerful sucking movements can be seen in state 3F. Both regular mouthing and sucking can entrain FHR patterns which can bewilder clinical interpretation.

States 1F and 2F account for about 90% of fetal life in late gestation. FHR patterns during these four behavioural states may mimic fetal distress. The fetal behavioural states and the transitions between them can be observed throughout labour. States 1F and 2F predominate as they do before labour. It is thought that diminished FHR variability and absent accelerations in a healthy term fetus probably represent fetal sleep rather than fetal distress. In the deep sleep state 1F, FHR pattern is usually unaffected even by strong uterine contractions. A period of low fetal heart variability (FHV) or tachycardia may indicate that fetal oxygenation is being compromised. In the second stage of labour, the length of the behavioural cycles decreases; this is related to the gamut of sensory stimuli and head compression incurred during this stage of labour.

FBM increase in frequency and in length of episode as gestation progresses. By the third trimester, FBM occur for 30% of the time and are closely associated with behavioural state, especially active sleep (2F). A few days before the onset of labour, FBM are depressed, probably because increased levels of prostaglandin, especially PGE_2, inhibit the fetal respiratory centre. During the latent stage of labour, FBM occur for about 10% of the time but almost cease in the active stage. In preterm labour, the decrease in FBM is less acute. FBM may be affected by changes in oxygenation and pH. FBM require energy so the fetus decreases FBM in response to hypoxia as an adaptive response to conserve oxygen. The hypoxia-induced decrease in FBM is more marked near term possibly because the responses to hypoxia have become more sensitive as the respiratory centre becomes more mature.

Although hypoxia normally decreases FBM, deeper, sustained inspiration or gasping is stimulated synergistically by raised carbon dioxide levels in the presence of hypoxia. In perinatal aspiration, this gasping can cause meconium inspiration. Paradoxically, maternal hyperventilation decreases FBM. Hypoglycaemia and central nervous system depressants, such as ethanol, barbiturates and diazepam, decrease FBM. Theophylline increases FBM and is used to treat postnatal apnoea in premature infants. Prostaglandin inhibitors, such as indomethacin, stimulate FBM but have to be used with caution because of their effects on fetal vascular function.

Changes in fetal behaviour over the course of pregnancy are summarized in Box 13.4.

Changes during labour

The stress of labour causes a reflex increase in maternal catecholamine levels well above those seen in non-pregnant women or pregnant women before labour.

Box 13.4 Changes in fetal behaviour during pregnancy

First trimester
- Specific sequence of movements
- Continual activity
- Coordinated and graceful quality

Second trimester
- Body movements diminish
- Breathing movements increase
- Quiescence increases
- Rest–activity cycles develop

Third trimester
- Clear fetal behavioural states
- Specific combination of variables
- Stable with state transitions
- Breathing is state-dependent

The physiological stress and hypoxia associated with the pain and anxiety increase adrenaline secretion. The physiological work of labour, which is highest in the second stage of labour, increases noradrenaline release. Placental metabolism of maternal catecholamines reduces the transfer to the fetus. However, maternal catecholamines can affect placental blood flow and affect the fetus in labour. Animal studies show that adrenaline is associated with vasoconstriction and a reduction in uterine blood flow. As the rise in adrenaline level is associated with maternal stress in labour, there is a clear advantage to limiting maternal psychological distress and pain.

Normal labour and delivery are associated with increased physiological stress resulting in raised cord levels of catecholamines in the neonate (Gluckman et al., 1999). This increase in fetal catecholamines may be a response to fetal compression, mild acidosis and other stimuli experienced during the birth. It is suggested that this is an adaptive response that facilitates extrauterine adaptation. The increased catecholamines stimulate breathing, increase fluid absorption from the lungs, stimulate surfactant release, enhance irritability, and play a role in metabolism by mobilizing glucose and fatty acids (Gluckman et al., 1999).

Fetal tissues are metabolically active; heat dissipation is via the placenta to the mother. Cord exclusion in animals results in an increase in fetal temperature. It seems likely that uterine contractions affecting uterine blood flow will impair heat transfer, particularly in active labour. At delivery, there is a transition from a heat-producing fetus to a neonate dependent on heat generation. In utero, PGE_2 and adenosine derived from the placenta may have a role in suppressing the activity of brown adipose tissue and therefore minimizing heat production by the fetus. Occlusion of the umbilical cord is the signal to increase heat generation. Non-shivering thermogenesis by brown adipose tissue is under the control of noradrenaline (see Chapter 1) released during labour.

A healthy term fetus has good energy stores and a normal base excess so it can tolerate temporary reductions in uterine perfusion in labour. There is a marked increase in fetal glycogen storage in the last month of gestation. The fetus also has the enzymes required for glycogenolysis. However, under normal uterine conditions, placental transfer of maternal glucose means that the fetal glucose pool is of maternal origin. Until labour, the fetus still depends on maternal sources of glucose. The changes in catecholamine secretion boost neonatal metabolism.

The placenta also provides the route of oxygen transfer and carbon dioxide removal. Maternal hyperventilation in labour increases carbon dioxide diffusion across the placenta, therefore increasing respiratory alkalosis (increasing pH). However, respiratory depression caused by oversedation or magnesium sulphate could have the opposite effect. In the presence of a reduced oxygen supply, anaerobic metabolism will cause metabolic acidosis. Lactate diffusion across the placenta is slow and the fetal kidney is not efficient at clearing organic acids. It seems likely that the respiratory alkalosis related to maternal hyperventilation compensates for at least some of the metabolic acidosis, owing to anaerobic glycolysis, thus restoring fetal pH to a normal range. Normal labour nevertheless will cause a gradual decrease in fetal pH, oxygen and bicarbonate ions and a corresponding rise in partial pressure of carbon dioxide.

Uterine blood flow is largely determined by maternal blood pressure, cardiac output and uterine muscular tone. Labour compromises uterine blood flow. The maternal spiral arteries, which perfuse the intervillous spaces, are occluded and venous drainage of the spaces is obstructed during uterine contractions. Doppler measurements show that blood flow through the uterine arteries is gradually reduced during a contraction and gradually returns when the uterus relaxes. Most animal models demonstrate that the placenta has an anatomical redundancy; over 70% of the placental capillary bed must be occluded before impedance to gas exchange rises significantly. If placental reserve is reduced, uterine contractions may have a significant effect on fetal hypoxia and acidosis. Even with a healthy placenta and normal uterine blood flow, contractions with excessive strength of frequency can cause fetal hypoxia and bradycardia. Maternal conditions may exacerbate this by reducing uterine perfusion; supine posture can reduce venous return, therefore cardiac output and regional anaesthesia can cause vasodilation so decreasing maternal cardiac output.

Labour promotes the clearance of fetal lung fluid. Transient tachypnoea, caused by residual lung fluid, is more common in babies born by elective caesarean section than in those experiencing a vaginal delivery. Chest compression mechanically expels a small volume of fluid. Late in gestation, the pulmonary epithelial cells actively secrete chloride ions, which create a gradient maintaining adequate lung volume *in utero*. Before birth the lung epithelial cells change from being predominantly chloride-secreting to being sodium-absorbing, which draws fluid into the interstitial spaces. The sodium-pumping activity is increased in spontaneous labour; this may be related to the catecholamine surge.

A mature sucking pattern is evident from 36 weeks of gestation. Although fetal swallowing can be observed as early as 11 weeks' gestation, near-term discrete episodes of swallowing occur, probably triggered by 'thirst', gastric emptying or changed composition of amniotic fluid (Boyle, 1992). This swallowing may be important for gut development and maturation. In labour there is some evidence that swallowing increases. Meconium passage is rare until about 38 weeks when the control of intestinal peristalsis is more mature. Early meconium passage is associated with listeriosis. Meconium-stained amniotic fluid occurs in about a third of pregnancies beyond 42 weeks. Hypoxia induces vasoconstriction of the fetal gut, hyperperistalsis and anal sphincter relaxation, so passage of meconium has been associated with fetal distress (Houlihan and Knuppel, 1994). However, it has been argued that meconium-stained fluid could reflect normal maturity of the fetal gut function (Katz and Bowes, 1992). Less than 2% of babies born with meconium-stained fluid go on to develop severe meconium aspiration syndrome. It has been suggested that the primary cause of this syndrome is pulmonary epithelial damage or airway obstruction, which results in ineffectual clearance of meconium. The residual meconium can interfere with surfactant dispersal and increase the severity of the respiratory problems.

THE FETAL SKULL AND FETAL PRESENTATION

The dimensions of the fetal head correlate well with those of the maternal pelvis. Examination of the shape of the baby's head soon after delivery shows how it passed through the pelvis (Fig. 13.18). The bones of the fetal skull are relatively mobile and mould under compression during labour. The sutures and fontanelles (Fig. 13.19) allow the skull bones to overlap partially so the dimensions of the presenting part can be reduced by about 0.5–1 cm. Diameters that are not compressed elongate to compensate for those that are reduced. If the pressure generated against the cervix impedes the circulation in the scalp then oedema may occur forming a caput or swelling. The area of the caput and the degree of moulding indicate the degree of head compression endured in

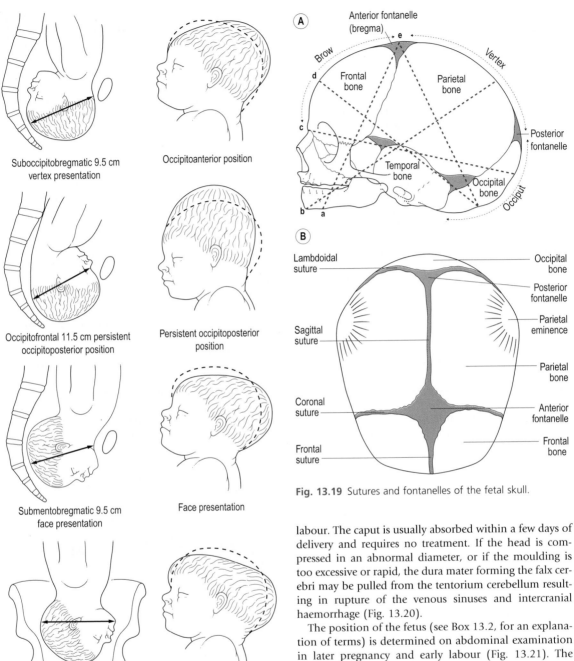

Suboccipitobregmatic 9.5 cm vertex presentation

Occipitoanterior position

Occipitofrontal 11.5 cm persistent occipitoposterior position

Persistent occipitoposterior position

Submentobregmatic 9.5 cm face presentation

Face presentation

Mentovertical 13.5 cm brow presentation

Brow presentation

Fig. 13.18 The relationship between the shape of the baby's head and the moulding of the fetal skull.

A

Anterior fontanelle (bregma)

Brow

Vertex

e

d

Frontal bone

Parietal bone

c

Posterior fontanelle

Temporal bone

Occipital bone

b a

Occiput

B

Lambdoidal suture

Occipital bone

Posterior fontanelle

Parietal eminence

Sagittal suture

Parietal bone

Coronal suture

Anterior fontanelle

Frontal suture

Frontal bone

Fig. 13.19 Sutures and fontanelles of the fetal skull.

labour. The caput is usually absorbed within a few days of delivery and requires no treatment. If the head is compressed in an abnormal diameter, or if the moulding is too excessive or rapid, the dura mater forming the falx cerebri may be pulled from the tentorium cerebellum resulting in rupture of the venous sinuses and intercranial haemorrhage (Fig. 13.20).

The position of the fetus (see Box 13.2, for an explanation of terms) is determined on abdominal examination in later pregnancy and early labour (Fig. 13.21). The midwife can gently palpate the pregnant woman's abdomen to determine how the fetus is lying and how the presenting part of the fetus relates to the pelvis. The degree of engagement of the fetal head into the brim of the pelvis can also be ascertained. Auscultation of the fetal heart confirms the initial findings. The lie of the fetus describes the relative position of the long axis of the fetus to the long axis of the uterus. Usually the lie is longitudinal, rather than oblique or transverse,

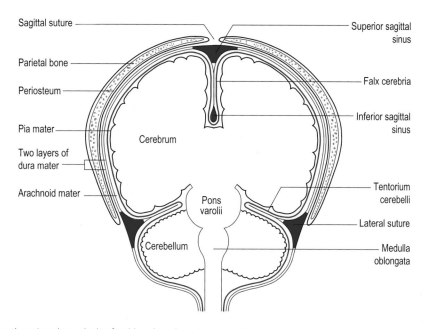

Fig. 13.20 Coronal section through the fetal head to show intracranial membranes and venous sinuses. (Reproduced with permission from Bennett and Brown, 1999.)

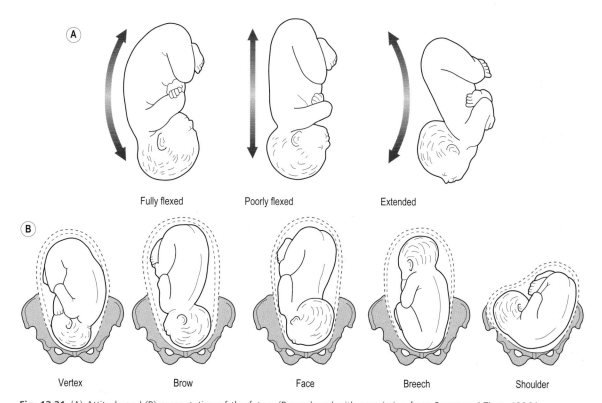

Fig. 13.21 (A) Attitude and (B) presentation of the fetus. (Reproduced with permission from Sweet and Tiran, 1996.)

particularly in the last weeks of pregnancy. The attitude is the degree of flexion of the fetus. In the fully flexed attitude, the fit of the fetus in the uterus is comfortable. The presentation describes the presenting part of the fetus. Cephalic presentation occurs in most pregnancies. The fetal position is described by the relationship of the denominator (the presenting part) to areas of the maternal pelvis. The pelvic areas are: left and right, anterior, lateral or posterior areas. The occiput (the bone at the back of the fetal skull) is the denominator of a cephalic position so the fetus could, for instance, be described to be in a right occipitoanterior position. Anterior positions are more common because the fetal spine is against the mother's abdominal wall. Occipitoposterior positions tend to result in the fetus assuming a deflexed attitude, which can result in less-effective contraction, prolonged labour, uneven cervical dilatation, increased risk of trauma to the perineum and unfavourable compression of the fetal head.

PAIN IN LABOUR

Many women experience severe pain in labour. Pain is a complex and personal phenomenon. Although it is easier to understand the neurophysiological aspects of tissue damage, the experience of pain is always subjective and is related to psychological state and past experience. Pain can be defined as a sensation (sensory and emotional experience) usually evoked by tissue damage or inflammation that stimulates the activity of specific receptors transmitting information to pain centres in the brain. Although pain can often be considered to be part of a protective mechanism (a rapid warning system) against tissue damage, there are some exceptions. For instance, pain associated with radiation (as in sunburn) or tumour growth tends to occur well after the tissue damage has occurred so it does not function as a warning. Chronic pain associated with degenerative diseases, such as arthritis, also cannot be regarded as a protective reflex. In labour, some aspects of pain experienced can be protective, such as the pain due to stretching of the soft tissue as the baby's head is crowned, which causes the woman to gasp.

The perception of pain depends on a number of physiological factors. The location and intensity of the stimuli affect the quality and severity of the perceived pain; generally, the higher the intensity of the stimuli, the greater is the pain experienced. However, psychological and cultural factors are important in the perception of pain (Box 13.5). Mood and personality type are important; generally, anxious or tired people are less able to tolerate pain but emotional arousal limits pain perception. In certain primitive cultures, the father has the 'labour pains' and the mother quietly gives birth.

Box 13.5 **Factors affecting pain perception**

- Anatomy
- Physiology
- Psychology
- Sociology
- Culture
- Cognition
- Learning

Pain receptors

Pain or nociceptive receptors respond to stimuli that cause tissue damage. They are specific, responding to chemical mediators of tissue damage, such as plasmakinins, acetylcholine, histamine and substance P. Pain receptors are distributed unevenly with a higher density in skin, dental pulp, some internal organs, periosteum, meninges, arterial walls and joint surfaces. Pain receptors are free nerve endings that form part of small afferent myelinated $A\delta$ fibres and larger (but unmyelinated) C fibres (Table 13.4). There is controversy over the pain being caused by overstimulation of other receptor types such as those that respond to temperature and pressure (Box 13.6).

Pain transmission

Transmission of pain depends on the type of fibre in which the nerve ending triggers the impulse. In general the speed of transmission is faster in larger fibres and those that are myelinated (see Chapter 1). Sharp stabbing sensations are thought to be conducted by $A\delta$ fibres and dull aching or burning pain by the slower unmyelinated

Table 13.4 Fast and slow pain receptors

FAST PAIN	SLOW PAIN
Bright, sharp, localized sensation	Dull, intense, diffuse unpleasant feeling
$A\delta$	C fibres
2–5 μm diameter	0.4–1.2 μm diameter
Myelinated	Non-myelinated
Conduct at 12–30 m/s	Conduct at 0.5–2 m/s
Terminate on neurons laminars I and II	Terminate on neurons in laminars I and V
Spinothalamic tract	Spinorecticular tract
Somatic pain	Visceral pain

Box 13.6 Pain receptors

Large

- Aα (Ia and Ib) (myelinated): position proprioception, touch, pressure, vibration
- Aβ (II) (myelinated): fine discriminative touch, pressure, vibration
- Aγ (myelinated): burning sensation

Small

- Aδ (III) (myelinated): well-localizable sharp pain, temperature
- C (IV) (unmyelinated): dull aching pain, temperature

C fibres. Myelinated fibres are more sensitive to ischaemia. Small unmyelinated fibres are more susceptible to local anaesthetics such as procaine, which is effective at blocking aching pain.

The nerve fibres enter the spinal cord and terminate in the grey matter of the dorsal horn (Fig. 13.22). Aδ fibres have a relatively direct route of transmission, synapsing with neurons in the dorsal horn to the brain stem and via the spinothalamic tract to the thalamus and cerebral cortex. Therefore the pain is perceived as sharp and is easy to localize. The unmyelinated C fibres synapse in the grey matter of the spinal cord as well but are routed through the spinoreticular tract and reticular formation to the thalamus and cortex. Within the reticular formation, a number of physiological processes take place, stimulating the nervous system and affecting electrical activity in the brain, wakefulness and attention. The state of excitement that is generated means the pain is difficult to localize and produces unpleasant symptoms. The limbic system (which includes the hypothalamus and the amygdala) at the base of the brain is stimulated, which affects emotional responses such as fear, anger, pleasure and satisfaction. The thalamus integrates the sensation of pain and relays the information that tissue damage has occurred.

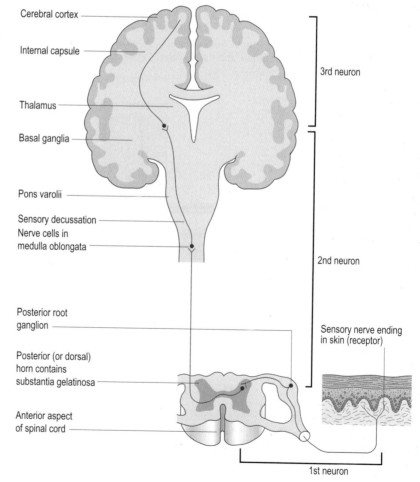

Fig. 13.22 Pathways of pain transmission. (Reproduced with permission from Bennett and Brown, 1999.)

Cerebral cortex

Internal capsule

3rd neuron

Thalamus

Basal ganglia

Pons varolii

Sensory decussation
Nerve cells in medulla oblongata

2nd neuron

Posterior root ganglion

Sensory nerve ending in skin (receptor)

Posterior (or dorsal) horn contains substantia gelatinosa

Anterior aspect of spinal cord

1st neuron

The somatosensory cortex discriminates and identifies the precise position of the tissue damage and the parietal cortex is involved in interpreting the information and relating the learned meaningfulness to past experience. The main excitatory neurotransmitter in pain perception is glutamate.

The gate control theory

There is a relationship between the pain receptors and the touch receptors at the level of the spinal cord. The pain gate control theory, proposed by Melzack and Wall (1965), suggests that interneurons in the substantia gelatinosa of the dorsal horn of the spinal cord can regulate the conduction of the ascending afferent nerve (Fig. 13.23). So input from the large-diameter myelinated fibres from the touch receptors can inhibit the impulses on the smaller-diameter fibres from the pain receptors, acting as a gate. This means that touch, like massage, can inhibit transmission from the pain receptor unless activity along the smaller fibres markedly increases. Descending fibres from the brain can also modify transmission of pain signals, thus 'opening' or 'closing' the gate. This explains the relationship between psychological factors and pain perception. If a labouring woman is feeling relaxed and confident, the descending

inhibition is high so less pain is perceived. If she becomes tired or anxious, the descending inhibition is reduced. Transcutaneous electrical nerve stimulation (TENS) acts both to stimulate the large-diameter touch afferent nerves and possibly to stimulate powerful descending inhibitory pathways.

Pain from muscle contractions

Both visceral pain from the uterus and somatic pain from trauma to the soft tissues of the birth canal are experienced in labour. Visceral pain tends to predominate in the first stage of labour when the uterus is contracting and the cervix is stretching and dilating. Rhythmic muscle contraction in the presence of an adequate blood flow does not usually cause pain. In labour, uterine contractions compress blood vessels and reduce flow; the ischaemic pain persists until the flow is restored. It is hypothesized that a chemical mediator reaches critical levels when flow is limited and stimulates the pain receptors. When flow is restored, the chemical mediator is diluted or metabolized. This is similar to exertion causing myocardial ischaemia and angina pain, which is relieved by rest and decreased myocardial oxygen requirements. Initially, pain is transmitted by the afferent fibres entering the spinal cord at T11 and T12, spreading to T10 and L1.

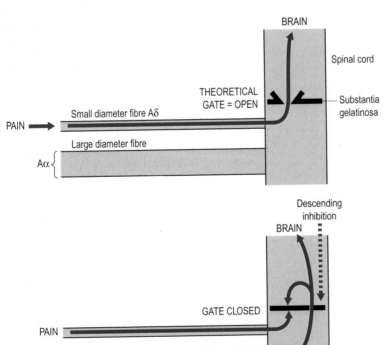

Fig. 13.23 The gate control theory of pain.

Referred pain

In referred pain, damage from one part of the body is experienced as though it had occurred in another part of the body. The pain fibres from the damaged area enter the spinal cord at the same level as the afferent nerves from the referred area. Usually the pain is referred to another tissue or structure that developed from the same embryonic structure or dermatome in which the pain originates. So, for instance, development of the diaphragm begins in the neck but, as the lungs develop, the diaphragm and the phrenic nerve migrate towards the abdomen. The afferent fibres in the phrenic nerve enter the spinal cord with the afferent fibres from the tip of the shoulder. Irritation of the diaphragm is therefore referred as a pain in the shoulder. However, previous experience is important in referred pain. Pain from the abdominal viscera including the uterus is usually referred to the midline. But in patients who have experienced abdominal surgery, such as a caesarean section, the pain is referred to the scar site. Pain during this stage arising from the uterus and cervix may be referred. A labouring woman may experience pain over her abdominal wall, between the naval and pubic bone, radiating down her thighs and in the lumbar and sacral regions.

Somatic pain

Somatic pain caused by the presenting part impinging on the birth canal, vulva and perineum tends to occur in the transition and in second stage of labour. Pain is transmitted by the pudendal nerves S2, S3 and S4. The conscious sensation of pain is accompanied by a number of physiological responses including increased ventilation and cardiac output, inhibition of gastrointestinal function, increased oxygen demand and metabolic rate and increased catecholamine release. The increased catecholamine release may detrimentally affect placental perfusion and uterine contractions. Non-pharmacological methods of pain relief, such as imagery, relaxation techniques and provision of information about the progress of labour, probably decrease anxiety and stress and responses mediated by the sympathetic nervous system.

Women with epidurals in situ may experience pain during the second stage of labour even if the epidural has been effective earlier. This is because epidurals are more effective at blocking visceral pathways that the somatic pathways. Following delivery with an epidural still in situ, if perineal repair is required, it is good practice to ensure the women remains pain free and this often requires local anaesthetic even if the epidural is topped up.

Endogenous opiates

The endogenous opiates are of particular interest in pain perceived in labour. These include β-endorphin, enkephalins and dynorphin, which are analgesic peptides. They bind to the presynaptic receptors on the neuron membrane and block pain transmission. Enkephalins comprise two short peptide chains (consisting of five amino acids) that are very unstable and have a half-life of less than a minute. Enkephalins are fragments of β-endorphin, which is more stable and also binds to opiate receptors; β-endorphin is a fragment of the pituitary hormone β-lipotrophin. β-Lipotrophin and ACTH are both derived from the same precursor.

Endogenous opiates inhibit prostaglandin synthesis. Prostaglandins are possible chemical mediators of pain. They also inhibit actions of a number of other pain transmitters. β-Endorphin levels increase throughout pregnancy, peaking at delivery, and may be further stimulated by the stress of labour. It is suggested that it is this high level of endogenous opiates that allows women to tolerate surprisingly high levels of pain during delivery; this phenomenon is known as 'pregnancy-induced analgesia'. Acupuncture may increase enkephalin activity. Placebo responses where pain relief occurs as a result of expectation of pain relief rather than because of being given an analgesic may be due to release of endogenous opiates and genuine analgesia.

Pain relief

Pain relief in labour needs to work rapidly and effectively relieve the pain without slowing down the course of labour. It needs to be safe for the mother and fetus and not adversely affect the neonate. There is no ideal analgesic (Table 13.5);

Table 13.5 Types of analgesics

PAIN RELIEF	EXAMPLE	MECHANISM	DISADVANTAGES/ADVANTAGES
Opioids	Pethidine	Depression of CNS	Nausea, vomiting, sedation; potentiate effect of epidural
Paracervical block	Spinal	Action potentials blocked from nerves	Risk of fetal injection; could provide surgical anaesthesia
Epidural	Bolus, intermittent or continuous infusion	Inhibition of neurotransmission across synapses	Maternal hypotension, motor blockade

all have some side-effects but pain also can adversely affect the fetus. Maternal analgesia can alter the balance of factors promoting uterine contraction and can potentially result in increased effects of oxytocin, promoting tetanic uterine contractions, decreasing oxygen delivery and causing transient fetal bradycardia (Eberle and Norris, 1996). There are three main mechanisms of pain relief blocking the pain receptors, the propagation of the action potential or the perception of pain within the central nervous system (CNS). Mild analgesics block at the pain receptor level. The sensitivity of the pain receptors is increased by prostaglandins. Drugs which inhibit prostaglandin synthesis, such as aspirin, decrease levels of prostaglandins both at the receptor and where prostaglandins are involved in pain transmission higher in the pathway.

Local anaesthetics

Local anaesthetics prevent the propagation of action potentials by blocking the sodium channels. They are particularly effective in blocking pain carried by the C fibres, possibly because unmyelinated fibres allow easier penetration. For instance, lignocaine (lidocaine) injected into the perineum is effective at blocking the pain of episiotomy.

Centrally acting opiates

Centrally acting opiates or narcotics, such as morphine and pethidine, block nerve transmission in the brain and spinal cord and decrease pain perception. There are also opiate-binding sites in the substantia gelatinosa of the dorsal horn of the spinal cord, which affect the release of neurotransmitters. Opiates increase the activity of the descending inhibitory pathways from the brain stem and act on the limbic system to elevate mood. Opiates have other physiological effects such as depressing the medullary respiratory centre, causing nausea and vomiting, sedating and affecting the heart rate.

POSITION IN LABOUR

Certain positions have advantages in optimizing uterine efficiency or increasing maternal comfort (Blackburn, 2007) (see Box 13.7). The lithotomy position and lying supine are probably advantageous only to those assisting at the delivery, unless medical intervention/delivery is required. Fetal monitoring and a number of procedures can usually be adapted to a variety of maternal positions. There seems to be no physiological advantage in lying supine. Fetal alignment, pelvic diameter and efficiency of contractions are not optimal. Contractions are more frequent but less intense so labour is prolonged and drug use seems to be increased. Many women appear to choose a supine position because they are presented with a bed and have no alternative option.

Box 13.7 Waterbirth

Over the last 20 years delivering babies in water has, increasingly, become popular and is available in many hospitals, birth centres and within the home environment (Cluett and Burns, 2009). Many women perceive waterbirth as a natural process without the need for analgesia. There have been concerns raised over the safety of waterbirth such as water inhalation and other complications such as hyponatremia, infection, haemorrhage associated with cord rupture, hypoxia and death (although these complications are rare). Research studies that show there is no significant difference in infant outcomes comparing waterbirth with conventional deliveries (Bodner et al., 2002; Geissbuehler et al., 2004). These studies show that there is a reduction in episiotomies and a reduction in the use of analgesia in women who choose waterbirth. Evidence that the new born baby is no more at risk from infection following a waterbirth compared to a conventional delivery has been presented (Thoeni et al., 2004). The intensity of pain does not seem to be reduced by waterbirth but waterbirth does appear to reduce the use of conventional anaesthesia in the advanced stages of labour (Eberhard et al., 2005).

It is important that guidelines are referred and followed so that safety of both mother and baby is optimised (Geissbuehler et al., 2004). There is also some evidence to suggest that waterbirth is effective in lowering maternal blood pressure and so may be a useful intervention in mild preeclampsia. This may be a combination of relaxation and peripheral dilatation of the blood vessels due to the warming of the skin by the water. It is important to ensure the pool water temperature does not exceed 37.5 °C as prolonged immersion in hot water will eventually raise the maternal core temperature and as a consequence the fetal heart rate will be affected. The buoyancy of the water provides support and reduces the stress of weight bearing so enabling the mother move freely and change positions easily.

A lateral recumbent position reduces obstructive pressure on maternal blood vessels so venous return and cardiac output are optimal for uterine perfusion and fetal oxygenation. Uterine contractions are more intense but less frequent and have increased efficiency. In an upright position, the abdominal wall relaxes and the effect of gravity will augment the effect of the fetal head pressing on the cervix and the subsequent feedback to the myometrial activity. Both frequency and intensity of contractions are increased so uterine activity is enhanced and labour tends to be shorter. Squatting increases maternal pelvic diameter, enhances engagement and the descent of the fetal head.

During bearing down, in the second stage of labour, directed pushing with a Valsalva manoeuvre against a closed glottis increases sympathetic discharge and catecholamine release. Minimal straining with an open glottis has fewer negative effects on maternal blood pressure, maternal and fetal oxygenation levels and is associated with reduced need for episiotomy.

Key points

- Parturition in humans is poorly understood; animal studies offer limited insight into the process owing to the evolution of species-specific differences.
- Parturition is a continuous process: the defining of the various stages of labour enables clinical judgement of progress and thus intervention under the biomedical model of care.
- The fundal region of the uterus has the highest density of smooth muscle so it is responsible for the strong expelling contractions of the uterus during labour.
- Human cervical structure is complex owing to the upright stance causing an increased gravitational force as the contents of the uterus increase in mass. Structural changes within the cervix have to occur before dilatation can be achieved by uterine contractions.
- Coordinated effective contractions are facilitated by the development of gap junctions between the myometrial cells.
- The first stage of labour is measured from the onset of strong and regular effective contractions to full effacement and dilation of the cervix.
- The second stage of labour is characterized by strong expulsive contractions, aided by respiratory muscle involvement, until the fetus is delivered.
- The passage of the fetus through the pelvis is described as the mechanism of labour and is achieved through the contractions forcing the presenting part to rotate against the muscle tone, structural resistance and shape of the pelvic floor.
- The third stage of labour covers the delivery of the placenta and fetal membranes and staunching of maternal blood loss.
- Maternal blood loss immediately following separation of the placenta is limited by the myometrial fibres contracting, thus occluding the uterine vessels.

- The onset of labour is poorly understood; a fetal signal probably alters the ratio of progesterone and oestrogen and other factors, such as prostaglandin secretion and oxytocin receptor expression, are involved in the amplification of the signal.
- The evolution of bipedal locomotion and increasing cephalization have influenced parturition in humans so the presenting part has to negotiate, by rotational manoeuvres, rather than just pass through the pelvic girdle.
- The process of labour induces many changes within the fetus in preparation for extrauterine existence, which are mediated by increasing hypoxia and catecholamine production.
- Pain in labour has a complex aetiology; there are visceral and somatic components further complicated by psychological and social factors.

Application to practice

Midwives need to understand the physiological interactions and external factors that can affect human labour in order to underpin intrapartum care.

The development of observational skills allows the midwife not only to interpret how a woman may be coping with labour, but also to determine how the labour is progressing from observing behaviour and physical responses of the labouring woman. By ignoring, not noticing or misunderstanding certain physical cues, the midwife may inadvertently provide suboptimal support.

Intervention in labour must be justified and decisions surrounding this must be underpinned to maximize maternal and fetal well-being. Knowledge of the effects of intervention upon fetal and maternal physiology is essential so that the midwife can judge the effectiveness and quickly identify possible adverse outcomes of such interventions.

ANNOTATED FURTHER READING

Abitbol MM: *Birth and human evolution: anatomical and obstetric mechanics in primates*, 1996, Greenwood Press.
This book describes the evolutionary development of the mechanisms of birth in monkeys and primates including humans.
Baston H, Hall J: *Midwifery Essentials: Labour*, (ed 1), 2009, Churchill Livingstone (Vol. 3).

This book provides a comprehensive guide but easy to follow guide to care in labour including waterbirth and caesarean section.
Blackburn ST: *Maternal, fetal and neonatal physiology: a clinical perspective*, (ed 3), Philadelphia, 2007, Saunders.
An excellent in-depth description of physiological adaptation to pregnancy and consequent development of the fetus and

neonate that draws from physiological research studies. The chapters are clearly organized by physiological systems and link physiological concepts to clinical applications including the assessment and management of low- and high-risk pregnancies.
Challis JR, Lockwood CJ, Myatt L, et al: Inflammation and pregnancy, *Reprod Sci* 16:206–215, 2009.

A brief review of the inflammatory changes in pregnancy which considers how inflammation is involved in preterm delivery.

Chapman V Charles C, editors: *The Midwife's Labour and Birth Handbook,* (ed 2), 2008, Wiley Blackwell Location.

This book focuses on the promotion of normality through a women centred approach to care in labour. It includes chapters on waterbirth, homebirth, breech, Caesarean section and vaginal birth after Caesarean section.

Dick-Read G Odent M *Childbirth without Fear: The Principles and Practice of Natural Childbirth,* (ed 4), 2007, Pinter & Martin Ltd (Revised).

This Classic book was first published in 1942 and remains in print today. It challenges modern medical obstetric practice and essential reading for those interested in the development of modern intrapartum care.

Gary *Cunningham FG: Williams Obstetrics,* (ed 23), 2009, McGraw-Hill Medical.

This book, is a comprehensive book for obstetrics and is a useful reference book for midwives interested in reproductive pathophysiology.

Iams JD, Romero R, Culhane JF, et al: Primary, secondary, and tertiary interventions to reduce the morbidity and mortality of preterm birth, *Lancet* 371:164–175, 2008.

A balanced discussion of the medical and therapeutic approaches to reduce the morbidity and mortality of preterm birth classified as primary (directed to all women), secondary (aimed at eliminating or reducing existing risk), or tertiary (intended to improve outcomes for preterm infants).

Liu D: *Labour Ward Manual,* (ed 4), Edinburgh, 2007, Churchill Livingstone Elsevier.

This book provides guidance on the clinical management of complications associated with labour.

López Bernal A: The regulation of uterine relaxation, *Semin Cell Dev Biol* 18:340–347, 2007.

A review of the mechanisms controlling myometrial contraction which describes how uterine quiescence changes during pregnancy and tocolytic therapy in preterm labour.

National Collaborating Centre for Women's and Children's Health: *Intrapartum care – care of healthy women and their babies during childbirth,* 2007, National Institute of Clinical Excellence (Clinical guideline 55).

This guideline presents clinical based labour care from an evidenced based care perspective.

Quigley EM: Impact of pregnancy and parturition on the anal sphincters

and pelvic floor, *Best Pract Res Clin Gastroenterol* 21:879–891, 2007.

A thorough discussion of the underlying pathophysiology of anal sphincter and pelvic floor damage in childbirth which can lead to incontinence and defaecation difficulties.

Reuwer P: *Proactive Support of Labor: The Challenge of Normal Childbirth,* (ed 1), Cambridge, 2009, Cambridge University Press.

Written by obstetricians, this book challenges current obstetric practice within the United States of America by focusing on the promotion of normality.

Walsh D: *Evidence-based Care for Normal Labour and Birth, A Guide for Midwives,* (Paperback), (ed 1), London, 2007, Routledge.

This is essential reading for practitioners wanting to extend their knowledge and skills in intrapartum care outside current medical models of care.

Walsh D, Downe S, editors: *Intrapartum Care, Essential Midwifery Practice,* (ed 1), 2010, Wiley-Blackwell.

This book describes how intrapartum care has evolved and developed in relation with the development of midwifery practice. It has chapters that explore issues such as psychology, sexuality, spirituality, feminism and complimentary therapies in relation to intrapartum care.

REFERENCES

Aitken MA, Rice GE, Brennecke SP: Gestational tissue phospholipase A2 messenger RNA content and the onset of spontaneous labour in the human, *Reprod Fertil Dev* 2:575–580, 1990.

Apostolakis EM, Rice KE, Longo LD, et al: Time of day of birth and absence of endocrine and uterine contractile activity rhythms in sheep, *Am J Physiol* 264:E534–E540, 1993.

Bani D: Relaxin: a pleiotropic hormone, *Gen Pharmacol* 28:13–22, 1997.

Barret JFR, Savage J, Phillips K, et al: Randomised trial of amniotomy in labour versus the intention to leave membranes intact until the second stage, *Br J Obstet Gynaecol* 99:5, 1992.

Beck S, Wojdyla D, Say L, et al: The worldwide incidence of preterm birth: a systematic review of maternal

mortality and morbidity, *Bull World Health Organ* 88:31–38, 2010.

Bennett VR, Brown LK: *Myles' textbook for midwives,* (ed 13), Edinburgh, 1999, Churchill Livingstone, pp 393, 396 431, 451, 468, 473, 509, 993.

Berkman ND, Thorp JM Jr., Lohr KN, et al: Tocolytic treatment for the management of preterm labor: a review of the evidence, *Am J Obstet Gynecol* 188:1648–1659, 2003.

Bernal AL, Europe-Finner GN, Phaneuf S, et al: Preterm labour: a pharmacological challenge, *Trends Pharmacol Sci* 16:129–133, 1995.

Blackburn ST: *Maternal, fetal, and neonatal physiology: a clinical perspective,* (ed 3), Philadelphia, 2007, Saunders.

Blumenfeld YJ, Lyell DJ: Prematurity prevention: the role of acute

tocolysis, *Curr Opin Obstet Gynecol* 21:136–141, 2009.

Bodner K, Bodner-Adler B, Wierrani F, et al: Effects of water birth on maternal and neonatal outcomes, *Wien Klin Wochenschr* 114(10–11):391–395, 2002.

Bowen JM, Chamley L, Keelan JA, et al: Cytokines of the placenta and extra-placental membranes: roles and regulation during human pregnancy and parturition, *Placenta* 23(4):257–273, 2002.

Boyle JT: Motility of the upper gastrointestinal tract in the fetus and neonate. In Polin RA, Fox WW,, editors: *Fetal and neonatal physiology* (Vol. 2). Philadelphia, 1992, Saunders, pp 1028–1032.

Carp H, Jayaram A, Stoll M: Ultrasound examination of the stomach contents of parturients, *Anesth Analg* 74:683–687, 1992.

Challis JRG, Matthews SG, Gibb W, et al: Endocrine and paracrine regulation of birth at term and preterm, *Endocr Rev* 21:514–550, 2000.

Clifton VL, Read MA, Leitch IM, et al: Corticotropin-releasing hormone-induced vasodilatation in the human fetal placental circulation, *J Clin Endocrinol Metab* 79(2):666–669, 1994.

Cluett ER, Burns E: Immersion in water in labour and birth, *Cochrane Database Syst Rev* CD000111, 2009.

De Ziegler D, Bulletti C, Fanchin R, et al: Contractility of the nonpregnant uterus: the follicular phase, *Ann N Y Acad Sci* 943:172–184, 2001.

Duff P: Premature rupture of the membranes in term patients, *Semin Perinatol* 20:401–408, 1996.

Eberhard J, Stein S, Geissbuehler V, et al: Experience of pain and analgesia with water and land births, *J Psychosom Obstet Gynecol* 26(2):127–133, 2005.

Eberle RL, Norris MC: Labor analgesia: a risk-benefit analysis, *Drug Saf* 14:239–251, 1996.

Field DJ, Dorling JS, Manktelow BN, et al: Survival of extremely premature babies in a geographically defined population: prospective cohort study of 1994–9 compared with 2000–5, *BMJ* 336:1221–1223, 2008.

Fuchs AR, Fuchs F, Husslein P, et al: Oxytocin receptors in the human uterus during pregnancy and parturition, *Am J Obstet Gynecol* 150:734–741, 1984.

Fuchs AR, Romero R, Keefe D, et al: Oxytocin secretion and human parturition: pulse frequency and duration increase during spontaneous labour in women, *Am J Obstet Gynecol* 165:1515–1522, 1991.

Garfield RE, Blennerhassett MG, Miller SM: Control of myometrial contractility: role and regulation of gap junctions, *Oxf Rev Reprod Biol* 10:436–490, 1988.

Gee H, Olah KS: Failure to progress in labour, *Prog Obstet Gynaecol* 10:159–181, 1993.

Geissbuehler V, Stein S, Eberhard J, et al: Waterbirths compared with landbirths: an observational study of nine years, *J Perinat Med* 32 (4):308–314, 2004.

Germain AM, Valenzuela GJ, Ivankovic M, et al: Relationship of circadian rhythms of uterine activity with term and preterm delivery, *Am J Obstet Gynecol* 168:1271–1277, 1993.

Gluckman PD, Sizonenko SV, Bassett NS: The transition from fetus to neonate: an endocrine perspective, *Acta Paediatr Suppl* 88(428):7–11, 1999.

Goldenberg RL, Culhane JF, Iams JD, et al: Epidemiology and causes of preterm birth, *Lancet* 371:75–84, 2008.

Goldman S, Shalev E: Progesterone receptor profile in the decidua and fetal membrane, *Front Biosci* 12:634–648, 2007.

Goodwin TM: A role for estriol in human labor, term and preterm, *Am J Obstet Gynecol* 180(1 Pt 3): S208–S213, 1999.

Grummer R, Winterhager E: Regulation of gap junction connexins in the endometrium during early pregnancy, *Cell Tissue Res* 293 (2):189–194, 1998.

Hampson V, Lui D, Billett E, et al: Amniotic membrane collagen content and type distribution in women with preterm premature rupture of the membranes in pregnancy, *Br J Obstet Gynaecol* 104:1087–1091, 1997.

Hertelendy F, Zakar T: Prostaglandins and the myometrium and cervix, *Prostaglandins Leukot Essent Fatty Acids* 70(2):207–222, 2004.

Hillhouse EW, Grammatopoulos DK: Role of stress peptides during human pregnancy and labour, *Reproduction* 124(3):323–329, 2002.

Honnebier MBOM, Nathanielsz PW: Primate parturition and the role of the maternal circadian system. European Journal of Obstetrics, *Gynecol Reprod Biol* 55:193–203, 1994.

Honnebier WJ, Jobsis AC, Swaab DF: The effect of hypophysial hormones and human chorionic gonadotrophin (HCG) on the anencephalic fetal adrenal cortex and on parturition in the human, *J Obstet Gynaecol Br Commonw* 81(6):423–438, 1974.

Houlihan CM, Knuppel RA: Meconium-stained amniotic fluid: current controversies, *J Reprod Med* 39 (11):888–898, 1994.

Husslein P: Pregnancy and plasma oxytocin levels, *J Perinat Med* 13:314–315, 1985.

Jenkin G, Young IR: Mechanisms responsible for parturition; the use of experimental models, *Anim Reprod Sci* 82–83:567–581, 2004.

Karalis K, Goodwin G, Majzoub JA: Cortisol blockade of progesterone: a possible mechanism involved in the initiation of labour, *Nat Med* 2:556–560, 1996.

Karteris E, Grammatopoulos D, Dai Y, et al: The human placenta and fetal membranes express the corticotropin-releasing hormone receptor 1alpha (CRH-1alpha) and the CRH-C variant receptor, *J Clin Endocrinol Metab* 83 (4):1376–1379, 1998.

Katz V, Bowes WA: Meconium aspiration syndrome: reflections on a murky subject, *Am J Obstet Gynecol* 166(1 Pt 1): 171–183, 1992.

Lawn JE, Lee AC, Kinney M, et al: Two million intrapartum-related stillbirths and neonatal deaths: where, why, and what can be done? *Int J Gynaecol Obstet* 107(Suppl. 1):S5–S18, S19 2009.

Leppert PC: Anatomy and physiology of cervical ripening, *Clin Obstet Gynaecol* 38(2):267–279, 1995.

López Bernal A: Mechanisms of labour: biochemical aspects, *Br J Obstet Gynaecol* 110(Suppl. 20):39–45, 2003.

MacLaughlin SM, McMillen IC: Impact of periconceptional undernutrition on the development of the hypothalamo-pituitary-adrenal axis: does the timing of parturition start at conception? *Curr Drug Targets* 8:880–887, 2007.

Melzack R, Wall PD: Pain mechanisms: a new theory, *Science* 150 (699):971–979, 1965.

Mesiano S: Myometrial progesterone responsiveness and the control of human parturition, *J Soc Gynecol Investig* 11(4):193–202, 2004.

Miller FD, Chibbar R, Mitchell BF: Synthesis of oxytocin in amnion, chorion and decidua: a potential paracrine role for oxytocin in the onset of human parturition, *Regul Pept* 45:247, 1993.

Mitchell BF, Taggart MJ: Are animal models relevant to key aspects of human parturition? *Am J Physiol Regul Integr Comp Physiol* 297:R525–R545, 2009.

Mitchell BF, Wong S: Changes in 17 beta,20 alpha-hydroxysteroid dehydrogenase activity supporting an increase in the estrogen/progesterone ratio of human fetal membranes at parturition, *Am J Obstet Gynecol* 168:1377–1385, 1993.

Mulder EJH, Boersma M, Meeuse M, et al: Patterns of breathing movements in the near-term fetus: relationship to behavioural states, *Early Hum Dev* 36:127–135, 1994.

Nakamura K, Sheps S, Arck PC: Stress and reproductive failure: past notions, present insights and future directions, *J Assist Reprod Genet* 25:47–62, 2008.

NCCWCH: *Intrapartum care – care of healthy women and their babies during childbirth*, 2007, National Institute of Clinical Excellence (Clinical guideline 55).

Neulen J, Breckwoldt M: Placental progesterone, prostaglandins and mechanisms leading to initiation of parturition in the human, *Exp Clin Endocrinol* 102(3):195–202, 1994.

Nijhuis JG: Fetal behavior, *Neurobiol Aging* 24(Suppl. 1):S41–S46, 2003.

Odent M: New reasons and new ways to study birth physiology, *Int J Gynecol Obstet* 75:S39–S45, 2001.

Olah KS: Changes in cervical electromyographic activity and their correlation with cervical response to myometrial activity during labour, *Eur J Obstet Gynecol Reprod Biol* 3:157–159, 1994.

Olah KS, Gee H, Brown JS: Cervical contractions: the response of the cervix to oxytocic stimulation in the latent phase of labour, *Br J Obstet Gynaecol* 100:635–640, 1993.

Olson DM, Zaragoza DB, Shallow MC, et al: Myometrial activation and preterm labour: evidence supporting a role for the prostaglandin F receptor: a review, *Placenta* 24(Suppl. A):S47–S54, 2003.

Petersen LK, Oxlund H, Uldberg N, et al: In vitro analysis of muscular contractile ability and passive biomechanical properties of uterine cervical samples from non-pregnant women, *Obstet Gynaecol* 77:772–776, 1991.

Petraglia F, Benedetto C, Florio P, et al: Effect of corticotropin-releasing factor-binding protein on prostaglandin release from cultured maternal decidua and on contractile activity of human myometrium in-vitro, , *J Clin Endocrinol Metab* 80:3073–3076, 1995.

Romero R, Chaiworapongsa T, Espinoza J: Micronutrients and intrauterine infection, preterm birth and the fetal inflammatory response syndrome, *J Nutr* 133 (5 Suppl. 2):1668S–1673S, 2003.

Rosenberg K, Trevathan W: Birth, obstetrics and human evolution, *Br J Obstet Gynaecol* 109(11):1199–1206, 2002.

Rowe TF: Acute gastric aspiration: prevention and treatment, *Semin Perinatol* 21:313–319, 1997.

Saigal S, Doyle LW: An overview of mortality and sequelae of preterm birth from infancy to adulthood, *Lancet* 371:261–269, 2008.

Scheepers HC, de Jong PA, Essed GG, et al: Fetal and maternal energy metabolism during labor in relation to the available caloric sustrate, *J Perinat Med* 29 (6):457–464, 2001.

Scutton M, Lowy C, O'Sullivan G: Eating in labour: an assessment of the risks and benefits, *Int J Obstet Anesth* 5:214–215, 1996.

Shynlova O, Tsui P, Jaffer S, et al: Integration of endocrine and mechanical signals in the regulation of myometrial functions during pregnancy and labour, *Eur J Obstet Gynecol Reprod Biol* 144(Suppl. 1): S2–110, 2009.

Slattery MM, Brennan C, O'Leary MJ, et al: Human chorionic gonadotrophin inhibition of pregnant human myometrial contractility, *Br J Obstet Gynaecol* 108 (7):704–708, 2001.

Smith R: Parturition, *N Engl J Med* 356:271–283, 2007.

Smith R, Nicholson RC: Corticotrophin releasing hormone and the timing of birth, *Front Biosci* 12:912–918, 2007.

Smith R, Van Helden D, Hirst J, et al: Pathological interactions with the timing of birth and uterine activation, *Aust N Z J Obstet Gynaecol* 47:430–437, 2007.

Steer PJ, Johnson MR: The genital system. In Chamberlain G, Broughton Pipkin F, editors: *Clinical physiology in obstetrics*, (ed 3), Oxford, 1998, Blackwell, pp 308–355.

Stephens BE, Vohr BR: Neurodevelopmental outcome of the premature infant, *Pediatr Clin North Am* 56:631–646, 2009.

Stewart DB: The pelvis as a passageway I. Evolution and adaptations, *Br J Obstet Gynaecol* 91:611–617, 1984.

Stjernholm Y, Sahlin L, Akerberg S, et al: Cervical ripening in humans: potential roles of estrogen, progesterone and insulin-like growth factor-I, *Am J Obstet Gynecol* 174:1065–1071, 1996.

Sullivan JM, Ramanathan KB: Management of medical problems in pregnancy: severe cardiac disease, *N Engl J Med* 313:304–309, 1985.

Sweet B, Tiran D: *Mayes' midwifery*, (ed 12), London, 1996, Baillière Tindall, pp 31, 224 225, 340, 358, 993.

Symonds EM, Symonds IM: *Essential obstetrics and gynaecology*, (ed 3), Edinburgh, 1997, Churchill Livingstone, p 134.

Terzidou V: Preterm labour. Biochemical and endocrinological preparation for parturition, *Best Pract Res Clin Obstet Gynaecol* 21:729–756, 2007.

Thoeni A, Zech N, Moroder L, et al: Water birth and the risk of infection. Experience after 1500 water births, *Pol J Gyn Invest* 7(1/4):21–26, 2004.

Thong KJ, Baird DT: Induction of abortion with mifepristone and misoprostol in early pregnancy, *Br J Obstet Gynaecol* 99:1004–1007, 1992.

Thorburn GD: The placenta, PGE_2 and parturition, *Early Hum Dev* 29:63–73, 1992.

Uldbjerg N, Malstrom A: The role of proteoglycans in cervical dilatation, *Semin Perinatol* 15:127–132, 1991.

Warnes KE, Morris MJ, Symonds ME, et al: Effects of increasing gestation, cortisol and maternal undernutrition on hypothalamic neuropeptide Y expression in the sheep fetus, *J Neuroendocrinol* 10:51–57, 1998.

Weiss A, Goldman S, Shalev E: The matrix metalloproteinases MMPS in the decidua and fetal membranes, *Front Biosci* 12:649–659, 2007.

Wilmsatt J, Myers DA, Myers TR, et al: Prostaglandin synthase activity of fetal sheep cotyledons at 122 days of gestation and term-expression of prostaglandin synthetic capacity in fetal cotyledonary tissue near labor is location-dependent, *Biol Reprod* 52:737–744, 1995.

Wolfe CDA, Petruckevitch A, Quartero R, et al: The rate of rise of corticotropin releasing-factor and endogenous digoxin-like immunoreactivity in normal and abnormal pregnancy, *Br J Obstet Gynaecol* 97:832–837, 1990.

Wray S: Uterine contraction and physiological mechanisms of modulation, *Am J Physiol* 264: C1–C18, 1993.

Wray S, Jones K, Kupittayanant S, et al: Calcium signaling and uterine contractility, *J Soc Gynecol Investig* 10(5):252–264, 2003.

Yuan W, López Bernal A: Cyclic AMP signalling pathways in the regulation of uterine relaxation, *BMC Pregnancy Childbirth* 7 (Suppl. 1):S10, 2007.

Chapter | **14** |

The puerperium

INTRODUCTION

The puerperium has been traditionally defined as the 6-week period immediately following the birth of a baby and represents the period of time in which maternal physiology, particularly the reproductive system, returns to a near pre-pregnant state. It probably originates from the tradition of 'churching' or the 'lying-in period', which was a religious ceremony where women were accepted back into the church after a period of 40 days during which they were considered unclean. The time after childbirth is imbued with social, cultural and religious significance and, in many cultures, the puerperal woman is given special treatment. Two important landmarks are often observed: the cessation of lochial discharge (women often being considered 'unclean' when lochia is present) and the shrivelling and loss of the remnants of the umbilical cord from the infant. With the rise of medical dominance, the end of the puerperium was marked by the postnatal examination of the woman by a doctor. This has structured the traditional descriptions of the puerperium as a period of maternal recovery, underpinned by the medicalization of pregnancy. It is the midwife's responsibility to maintain a careful watch on the physiological changes in the puerperium and to recognize early signs of pathological conditions.

Chapter case study

Zak was born 2 days after his expected date of delivery and was the first son born to his proud parents, Zara and James. Zak was delivered at around 04:30 hours and Zara had laboured in a birthing pool attended by her named midwife. As labour had progressed quickly without complications, the midwife followed Zara's request for no active management in the third stage of labour. The midwife was unable to accurately estimate Zara's blood loss due to the waterbirth. Once out of the bath, the midwife assessed Zara's perineal trauma, which appeared to be a first-degree tear that was not bleeding and did not require suturing.
- How can the midwife effectively assess Zara's well-being following the delivery, given that she has been unable to estimate Zara's total blood loss?
- What factors that have occurred during Zak's delivery will optimize Zara's transition to parenthood?

The puerperium is sometimes considered to be the 'Cinderella' of midwifery and obstetrics as the excitement of the birth is over and after delivery the effects of pregnancy on maternal physiology receive little emphasis. There is not very much research into the timing or mechanisms of the changes in the puerperium. However, the puerperal woman can be very vulnerable to physiological stress, which can become pathological. The midwife's role is to observe and monitor the early changes and to be able to differentiate between those which are normal and abnormal.

A woman adapts to pregnancy progressively over a period of months, but after childbirth she suddenly no longer needs the physiological changes. During the puerperium, there is a marked decrease in the levels of oestrogen and progesterone within the maternal system. Although the placenta is the main source of progesterone in pregnancy, the corpus luteum continues to produce progesterone for several days into the puerperal period. The fall in concentrations of steroid hormones facilitates the initiation of lactation (see Chapter 16) and allows the physiological systems to return to their pre-pregnant state. In reality, the puerperium should be described as a transitional phase. It begins at the birth of a child and it ends with the return of fertility. Women do not return to the same physiological and anatomical state, however. The puerperium also, within a social context, represents many transitions for the parents, child and other members of the family. Many of the physiological changes within the puerperium, such as the establishment of parenting skills, lactation and feeding, are modified by the past and present social interactions of the individuals within the new family situation.

PHYSIOLOGICAL AND STRUCTURAL CHANGES

Involution of the uterus

Clinical observation and management of the puerperium is essentially based on the return of the uterus to its 'normal' size. The puerperium begins as soon as the placenta and

membranes are expelled from the uterus together with a substantial proportion of the endometrium. Oxytocin released from the posterior pituitary gland induces strong intermittent myometrial contractions, and as the uterine cavity is empty the whole uterus contracts down fully and the uterine walls become realigned in apposition to each other. The myometrial spiral fibres that occlude the uterine blood vessels (see Chapter 13) constrict the blood supply to the placental site (Fig. 14.1). Uterine vascular resistance increases soon after delivery (Tekay and Jouppila, 1993).

About an hour after delivery, the myometrium relaxes slightly but further active bleeding is prevented by the activation of the blood-clotting mechanisms, which are altered greatly during pregnancy to facilitate a swift clotting response. Haemostasis is achieved in three ways:

- Ischaemia
- Pressure: apposition of the uterine walls forming the T-shaped cavity
- Clotting mechanisms.

The midwife has the responsibility to inspect the placenta and membranes to assess that they are complete and that no tissue remains within the uterine cavity. Retained products impede the contraction of the uterus and may be the source of abnormal bleeding and cause secondary postpartum haemorrhage (secondary PPH) as they become the focus of infection. Retained products are often spontaneously voided usually associated with the passing of a blood clot, which facilitates the cleansing of the uterine cavity. Blood clots should always be checked for the presence of placental and membranous tissue.

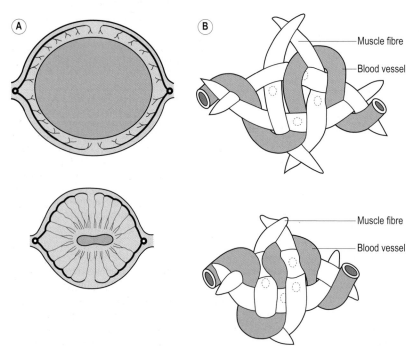

Fig. 14.1 (A) Myometrial spiral fibres around uterine blood vessels; (B) occlusion of blood supply to the placental site. (Reproduced with permission from Sweet and Tiran, 1996.)

Muscle fibre

Blood vessel

Muscle fibre

Blood vessel

Immediately after delivery, the uterus weighs about 900–1000 g and the fundus is palpable about 11–12 cm above the symphysis pubis (Howie, 1995) at around the level of the umbilicus. The placental site is raw and exposed. Initially, the uterus is continuous with the vagina with the cervix draping from the body of the uterus. Uterine involution is rapid so 50% of the total mass of the tissue is lost within a week (Howie, 1995). This physiological destruction of most of the uterine tissue is unique in adult life and the mechanisms are not clearly understood. It is suggested that 90% of uterine protein is degraded in the first 10 days of the puerperium (Hytten, 1995). There are rapid and marked changes in collagen and elastin content (Stone and Franzblau, 1995), and water and protein are lost. Involution results from a withdrawal of placental hormones and is thought to be mediated by hydrolytic and proteolytic enzymes released from myometrial cells, endothelial cells of blood vessels and macrophages. Cytoplasmic organelles are autodigested, and intracellular cytoplasm and extracellular collagen are reduced (Howie, 1995). The breakdown of protein from the myometrial cells releases the amino acid components into the circulation and thence into the urine; thus, a puerperal woman is in a state of negative nitrogen balance (see Chapter 12). The myometrial cells are thought to reduce in size (Fig. 14.2) rather than being destroyed and replaced, although there may be an 'overshoot' in uterine involution with rebuilding to the resting non-pregnant state. The uterus ultimately returns almost to its prepregnant size (Fig. 14.3), although the proportion of fibrous tissue present in the uterus is progressively increased with successive pregnancies.

Initially, the cervix is soft, bruised and lacerated following a vaginal delivery (particularly so in primiparae and with premature labour). The cervix rapidly reforms and closes; by the end of the first puerperal week it will admit one finger. However, the cervix never returns to its original state and always shows evidence of parturition. The external os reforms with a slit rather than the nulliparous dimple (Fig. 14.4).

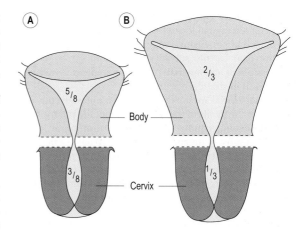

Fig. 14.3 Return of uterus to a size close to the prepregnant dimensions: A nulliparous uterus; B parous uterus. (Reproduced with permission from Miller and Hanretty, 1998.)

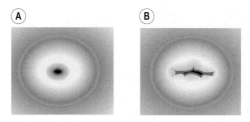

Fig. 14.4 Reformation of the external os: (A) nulliparous cervix; (B) parous cervix. (Reproduced with permission from Miller and Hanretty, 1998.)

The uterus involutes quite quickly, initially at about 1 cm/day; thus by the tenth day it should no longer be palpable above the symphysis pubis. Involution is slower in women who have undergone lower-segment caesarean section (LSCS), but it can be judged by a detectable decrease in fundal height. Subinvolution (a slow rate of uterine involution) may indicate retained products of conception (ERPC) and/or a secondary infection, which is usually found in conjunction with continued lochia rubra that may have an offensive odour. The uterus should be well contracted, hard and central; if it is higher than the umbilicus and soft on palpation (often described as 'boggy') then this may also indicate the presence of infection. The endometrial cavity is a potential space in non-pregnant women but gas is commonly detected in the endometrial cavity puerperally (Hytten, 1995).

The initiation of breastfeeding and the infant suckling in the early puerperium augments stimulation of oxytocin release. The oxytocin stimulates further contraction of the myometrium and so uterine evacuation. Involution of the uterus in breastfeeding mothers is more efficient. 'Afterpains' associated with lactation are often experienced,

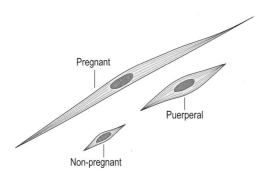

Fig. 14.2 Reduction in size of myometrial cells. (Reproduced with permission from Miller and Hanretty, 1998.)

particularly, by multiparous women who often complain of increased vaginal loss while feeding. Initially, oral analgesia such as paracetamol may be offered but the intensity of the pain usually subsides after about 24 h because expression of myometrial oxytocin receptors is reduced as a result of oestrogen withdrawal.

The superficial layer of the decidua becomes necrotic and is shed in the lochia in the first few days of the puerperium. The epithelium rapidly regenerates, re-forming an intact layer over most of the surface within 7–10 days of delivery. The placental site takes 3 weeks or longer to recover. The endometrium regenerates from the basal layers and grows in from the margins of the placental wound site and from glandular remnants within it (Howie, 1995).

Soft tissue damage and repair

It is not uncommon for soft tissue damage to occur during the delivery of a baby. Trauma to the female genital tract is described as follows:

- Superficial—this usually describes grazes to the skin where the epidermis has split owing to pressure of distension. These require no treatment; however, they often cause discomfort through stinging because of the disruption of the many nerve endings found within the superficial layer of the tissue. Voiding of urine can also be uncomfortable as the urine comes in contact with the grazes.
- First degree—this describes a tear in the skin and underlying superficial tissues (not including the muscle). Often the wound will heal spontaneously as the skin edges are usually in apposition. Ragged tears may result in the formation of excess scar tissue which can cause dyspareunia (pain during intercourse). Tears on the labia minora, a well-innervated area, can cause a lot of discomfort. If bilateral tears are present, suturing needs to be considered as the labia may fuse together if the tears are in close apposition forming a band of tissue over the vaginal opening.
- Second degree—when a tear involves perineal muscle damage it is described as being second degree. Usually these wounds are sutured to aid healing. Simple second degree tears are usually in the midline and involve one line of tearing. Some second degree tears can be complex with more than one tear line radiating in both lateral and downward directions involving larger amounts of muscle trauma.
- Episiotomy—this is a surgical incision to enlarge the introitus to facilitate the delivery of the baby which used to be thought to be beneficial and so done routinely. It falls into the same category as the second-degree tear. Although episiotomies can be performed in the midline, because of the increased risk of extension to a third degree tear and anal sphincter rupture they are usually performed to the side (mediolateral).

- Third degree—here the muscle of the anal sphincter is involved. Obstetric repair is essential so that the sphincter activity of the muscle is restored thus avoiding complications of faecal incontinence at a later time.
- Fourth degree—when the tear is extensive, the anal sphincter may become completely divided and the tear continues through the rectal mucosa. Specialist surgical repair is required to ensure the resumption of normal anal function.

Repair to the perineum involves the clinician suturing the perineum. There is a wide variety of suture materials and techniques for repair; however, suturing aims to achieve the following:

- Haemostasis—this is to ensure that any active bleeding points are ligated to minimize blood loss and the postnatal complication of a haematoma (formation of a blood clot within the wound) which can be extremely painful.
- Alignment—this is to bring the tissues back into alignment to optimize healing and to achieve a near pre-tear condition. If wounds are left gaping, alignment may not occur and as healing is by granulation this can result in the formation of scar tissue. This can result in a rigid misshapen perineum, which can cause dyspareunia (pain on intercourse).

The majority of perineal traumas can be described as being deep wounds as the tissue trauma involves layers below the epidermis and the dermis. Wound healing occurs in three phases: inflammation, tissue formation and tissue remodelling (see also Box 14.1). Some features of wound healing are common to all tissues; others are specific to the tissue involved. For instance, granulation tissue does not develop in the endometrium and the wounds do not heal with scarring. In this respect, there are similarities with fetal wounds which also heal without scarring suggesting that the process of endometrial remodelling is more a developmental mechanism than merely repair.

1. First is the inflammatory response; inflammation is a normal reaction to tissue trauma. Perineal inflammation can initially cause great discomfort for women in the very early postnatal period. An analgesic such as diclofenac sodium is useful as it acts as an anti-inflammatory agent (though it should be used with caution if the woman is asthmatic). Paracetamol and codeine-based products can also be used but codeine can cause or exacerbate bowel constipation so appropriate advice is required. However, a degree of inflammation is vital to ensure tissue healing, so analgesics should be used only when the response is severe and perineal pain restricts normal activity. The inflammation acts to isolate the damaged tissues, reducing the spread of infection. White blood cells, such as neutrophils and

Box 14.1 **The stages of wound healing**

0–3 days

- Blood clot forms, reinforced with fibrin fibres.
- Acute inflammatory response occurs: polymorphs and macrophages migrate to site; high-protein exudate leads to local oedema.

1 week later

- Eschar dries out, hardens and eventually becomes detached.
- Wound contracts.
- Mitotic activity occurs in epidermal cells, which migrate over living tissue.
- New blood capillaries form from endothelial buds, bringing nutrients to healing tissue.
- New connective tissue, formed by fibroblasts, supports capillary loops.

6 months later

- Surface depression may still be visible at wound site; scar tissue becomes paler.
- Epithelialization is complete.
- Connective tissue is reorganized, less vascular and stronger.

Box 14.2 **Lochia**

- **Lochia rubra (red)**
  - decidua and frank blood loss from placental site
  - initially sterile then uterus begins to be colonized by vaginal flora
  - red colour persists for about 3 days
- **Lochia serosa (pink/brown)**
  - contains leukocytes, mucus, vaginal epithelial cells, necrotic decidua, non-pathological bacteria
  - may be blood stained for 3–4 weeks
  - characteristic sweetish odour
- **Lochia alba (yellow–white)**
  - mostly serous fluid and leukocytes
  - plus some cervical mucus and microorganisms

macrophages, invade the tissue owing to the increased vasodilatation in the surrounding blood vessels. These cells ingest any invading bacteria and break down any necrotic tissue within the wound.

2. The migratory phase involves the infiltration of the wound by mesenchymal cells that form fibroblasts, initially creating a scab over the open wound site. Following this, blood vessels grow into the wound and the wound is gradually filled from the bottom up by new tissue growth called granulation tissue.

3. There then follows a proliferative phase where epithelial cells grow under the scab. It concludes with the maturation of the new cells and the shedding of the scab.

LOCHIA

The initial vaginal loss is termed the lochia rubra and consists of blood that has collected within the reproductive tract together with autolytic products of degenerated necrotic decidua from the placental site and any trophoblastic remains. The outward flow of blood lost at delivery and the subsequent discharge of lochia are important in removal of potential sources of ascending infection and, thus, protection of the placental wound site. The alkalinity of the lochia is also important in protecting the vulnerable site. Lochia is the normal discharge in the puerperium; it has a characteristic sweetish smell unless there is an infection.

Lochia may be described by its visual appearance (Box 14.2); normally, the lochia lightens progressively in both volume and colour. However, at about day 7 after delivery, the fibrinous mesh deposited over the placental site may be shed as part of the normal healing process so the vaginal loss may be transiently heavier and flushed with fresh blood. By day 10, the lochia is normally scant and pink in colour although discharge of lochia may persist for up to 6 weeks. Prolonged duration of lochia discharge suggests the placental wound site is not completely epithelialized or that the woman has some retained debris which is still disintegrating (Hytten, 1995). The duration of lochia discharge tends to be longer with the first pregnancy and is also related to birth weight.

Heavy discharge of lochia with an offensive odour, maternal pyrexia and/or a feeling of general malaise can all indicate possible intrauterine infection. If the lochia remains abnormally heavy and further bleeding occurs, dilatation and curettage (D&C) to empty the uterine cavity may be necessary. The procedure is also termed evacuation of ERPC. The cervix is dilated and the retained products are scraped from the decidua. This procedure is not without complications, however. Excessive scraping can damage or remove the entire endometrium. If the basal layer of the endometrium is removed (see Chapter 2) then proliferation during the menstrual cycle fails to occur, affecting fertility; this is termed Asherman's syndrome.

Blood loss

Excessive blood loss, that is, more than 500 mL or any amount that jeopardizes the well-being of the mother, at and within 24 h of delivery is termed a primary postpartum haemorrhage (primary PPH). It is usually caused by failure of the myometrium to contract completely, or failure of the blood-clotting mechanisms, or both (see Chapter 13); PPH may be very serious (Box 14.3, Case study 14.1). Women may also loose significant amounts of blood from trauma to the genital tract and perineum. If there is excessive bleeding but the uterus is well contracted, examination of the genital tract and perineum should not be delayed to identify bleeding points and any trauma repaired as quickly as possible to minimize blood loss.

Occasionally, there may be concealed bleeding, either into the peritoneum from ruptured blood vessels in the broad ligament or into the tissues forming large collections of blood clots called haematomas. Therefore, even in the absence of visible blood loss, women can still be physically in shock if concealed bleeding is present.

The risk of primary PPH is lower 24–72 h following delivery, but until involution of the uterus is complete there is a risk of a secondary PPH if there is an infection within the uterine cavity. The bleeding is usually due to the fibrinolytic action of bacteria such as haemolytic streptococcus. These bacteria are usually anaerobes (able to thrive in the absence of oxygen) and so specific antibiotic treatment with antibiotics such as metronidazole may be required.

Hormonal changes

In late pregnancy, most of the steroid hormones are derived from the placenta, although the corpus luteum and ovary continue to contribute some progesterone. Levels of progesterone and oestrogen fall to non-pregnant levels within 72 h of delivery. The placental protein hormones have a longer half-life so plasma levels fall more slowly. During pregnancy, production of the gonadotrophins is suppressed. Follicle-stimulating hormone (FSH) levels are restored to prepregnant concentrations within 3 weeks of delivery, but restoration of luteinizing hormone (LH) secretion takes longer, depending on the duration of lactation. Levels of oxytocin and prolactin also depend on lactational performance.

The haematological system and cardiovascular changes

The blood lost at delivery, accepted to be about 300–500 mL normally and about 1000 mL in caesarean sections, is adequately compensated for by the increase in blood volume acquired during pregnancy (see Chapter 11). Women can lose about 1000 mL of their predelivery blood volume before postnatal haemoglobin concentration is compromised (Letsky, 1998; Case study 14.2). Erythropoiesis is

Case study 14.1

Lucy is a 35-year-old primigravida who is delivered by emergency LSCS at 30 weeks' gestation owing to fulminating pre-eclampsia. Following delivery, the blood loss per vaginum is noted to be quite brisk and a Syntocinon (oxytocin) infusion is commenced in an attempt to control the bleeding. On investigation, it is discovered that Lucy's platelet count is extremely low and that the clotting time for her blood is greatly prolonged. A provisional diagnosis of DIC secondary to HELLP syndrome is made.
- What predisposing factors may have contributed to Lucy's condition?
- What intervention would Lucy require and what care would she need following this diagnosis?

Case study 14.2

Prior to delivery, Megan had a haemoglobin (Hb) concentration of 10.1 g/dL. At delivery, her blood loss is estimated at around 1000 mL. The midwife is quite concerned over this although Megan was asymptomatic. Prior to discharge on day 3, Megan's Hb concentration is rechecked and is estimated at being 9.8 g/dL.
- How can you account for the Megan's Hb concentration being relatively stable despite her suffering a postpartum haemorrhage?
- What advice/treatment would you give to Megan following her discharge?

stimulated before and after delivery (Richter et al., 1995). Diuresis further decreases plasma volume in the first days, although as interstitial fluid is mobilized subsequently the plasma volume tends to increase transiently causing haemodilution of both haemoglobin and plasma proteins, such as clotting factors. It is this variability in blood lost at delivery and restoration of normal water balance that may result in raised concentrations of clotting factor and hypercoagulability. The tendency to coagulate is also affected by the loss of placental and fetal factors affecting clotting and water regulation (Blackburn, 2007).

Haemoglobin levels return to normal prepregnant levels within 4–6 weeks and white blood cell numbers fall to normal within a week of delivery (Blackburn, 2007). Platelet number increases in the first few days following delivery, thereafter falling gradually to prepregnant levels. Fibrinolytic activity is maximal for about 48 h after delivery in response to the removal of the placenta, which produces fibrinolytic inhibitors (Lanir et al., 2003). Clotting factors, which peaked in labour, gradually decrease. The net result is that the hypercoagulable state of pregnancy is increased in the early puerperium and then slowly returns to a prepregnant state over a few weeks. This period of prolonged hypercoagulability is why women are at significantly increased risk of thromboembolic episodes in the postnatal period.

In previous eras, wealthy women were advised to rest in bed after childbirth and received indulgent cosseting (Hytten, 1995). However, trials of early ambulation led to early mobility being highly recommended as it facilitates improved vena caval blood flow and rapid disposal of oedema and thus optimizes cardiovascular health. Mobilization is essential to optimize venous return and avoid stasis within the vascular bed, in order to minimize the risk of deep vein thrombosis (DVT) formation (see p. 373). Women who are unable to mobilize owing to obstetric complications, such as an LSCS, are given prophylactic treatment as the risks of DVT and complications are much increased. Women are advised to report any discomfort or swelling in the lower legs as this may indicate DVT formation (especially if one leg appears more swollen than the other although bilateral DVTs are possible); the risks of DVT progressively diminish.

The cardiovascular system is rendered transiently unstable by delivery owing to the blood loss and the ensuing compensatory mechanisms. During the brief period of instability of fluid balance in the first week after delivery, many women experience headaches. Initially, there is a marked increase in cardiac output as the uteroplacental flow is returned to the venous system and the gravid uterus no longer impedes the vena cava blood flow. This is augmented by the mobilization of extracellular fluid. Although pregnant women are normally able to tolerate normal blood lost at delivery, those women who had decreased vascular expansion during pregnancy, such as those with pre-eclampsia (see Chapter 11), may be less able to tolerate blood loss. Vaginal delivery is associated with a higher haemoglobin concentration than operative deliveries because vaginal delivery tends to have less blood loss and to promote diuresis more markedly (Blackburn, 2007).

Parameters of the cardiovascular system return towards prepregnant values but remain significantly different. Resolution of ventricular hypertrophy is slow. Vascular remodelling of pregnancy persists for at least a year after delivery and is enhanced by second and subsequent pregnancies (Clapp and Capeless, 1997). Because circulating blood volume and cardiac output fall early in the puerperium and the hypertrophied ventricle is slowly remodelled over a period of 4–6 months, the stroke volume remains relatively high for up to 12 weeks or longer (Blackburn, 2007). This means that heart rate falls in the puerperium, as the stroke volume contributes proportionately more to the decreased cardiac output. Thus, it is normal for puerperal women to exhibit bradycardia (a reduced pulse rate of about 60–70 beats per minute). A raised (or normal) pulse may indicate severe anaemia, venous thrombosis or infection (see below).

Respiratory system

The decreased progesterone concentration following delivery of the placenta restores prepregnant sensitivity to carbon dioxide concentration promptly so partial pressures of carbon dioxide return to prepregnant levels. The diaphragm can increase its excursion distance once the gravid uterus no longer impedes it so full ventilation of the basal lobes of the lung is possible. Chest wall compliance, tidal volume and respiratory rate return to normal within 1–3 weeks. Changes in the elasticity of the rib cage may persist for months (Blackburn, 2007).

Urinary system

It is important that bladder function is assessed in the early postnatal period. The trauma experienced by the bladder during delivery usually results in oedema and hyperaemia of the bladder, which has reduced muscle tone in pregnancy. Effects on the bladder are increased by prolonged labour, use of forceps, analgesia and anaesthetic procedures and pressure of the descending presenting part during delivery. The resulting transient loss of bladder sensation, which may result in overdistension and incomplete emptying, can last from days to weeks. Bladder changes are associated with increased risk of urinary tract infections (UTI) in the puerperium. Trauma to the sphincter of the bladder increases the frequency of stress incontinence, which is marked by urine leakage occurring with coughing, laughing, sudden movement or exercise.

If bladder function is impaired, an indwelling catheter may be inserted to enable the damaged tissue to recover;

however, catheterization itself increases the risk of a UTI. If the uterus can be palpated high up or is displaced over to one side following the woman voiding urine, this indicates that there is retention of urine as the full bladder displaces the uterus. This is compounded by the increased diuresis that occurs in the postnatal period due to the reduction of the increased plasma volume acquired during pregnancy. It is normal for women to have frequency of micturition as long as they are voiding large amounts of urine each time. Frequency involving just small amounts of urine being voided may indicate a degree of urinary retention. Further assessment of bladder function by ultrasound scanning will confirm if an abnormal amount of residual urine is present following micturition.

Pain associated with micturition may indicate a UTI. Dilation of the ureters, overdistension of the bladder and instrumental or operative deliveries all increase the risk of infection. By day 10, full bladder function should be observed and assessed; there should be no evidence of unprovoked urinary incontinence.

Parameters of the renal system, such as renal plasma flow, glomerular filtration rate and plasma creatinine, are usually back to normal non-pregnant levels by the 6-week check. Urinary excretion of mineral and vitamins is normal within the first week after delivery. Plasma renin and angiotensin levels adjust to the loss of fetal hormones affecting their control so levels fall and then increase before returning back to normal (Blackburn, 2007). This fluctuation in hormone levels affecting water retention, together with the redistribution of body fluid, results in rapid and sustained natriuresis and diuresis, which is particularly marked between the second and fifth day after delivery. Fluid and electrolyte balance is normal with 21 days after delivery. Oxytocin, which has antidiuretic hormone (ADH)-like activity, falls after delivery, augmenting diuresis. The voiding volume increases and many women experience night sweats in the puerperium, which also increase fluid loss. Pregnancy-induced changes in the urinary system may persist for several months. Although the dilated smooth muscle of the urinary tract appears normal within a week of delivery, it remains potentially distensible. The kidneys return to their prepregnant size within 6 months of pregnancy.

Gastrointestinal system and defaecation

During labour, gastric motility is reduced, particularly in association with pain, fear and narcotic drugs. The reduced tone of the lower oesophageal sphincter, reduced gastric motility and increased gastric acidity result in delayed gastric emptying. The tone and pressure of the lower oesophageal sphincter are normal by 6 weeks after delivery. However, in the early puerperium, the reduced gastrointestinal muscle tone and motility and the relaxed abdomen can increase gas distension and constipation

immediately after delivery. Gallbladder muscle tone and contractility is enhanced after delivery so the gallbladder may expel small gallstones that developed during pregnancy (Blackburn, 2007).

The first bowel movements usually occur within 2 or 3 days following delivery. This may become complicated by the presence of haemorrhoids, which are associated with evacuation problems. Haemorrhoids are common during late pregnancy because of the effects of progesterone on vascular smooth muscle tone. Usually haemorrhoids resolve quickly after birth and cause only minor discomfort in the postnatal period. Sometimes, particularly if they are severe, owing to displacement by the passage of the presenting part through the birth canal, they can become traumatized and localized thrombosis can occur. This can be further complicated if constipation develops and the woman, because of perineal trauma, resists opening her bowels. Problems with constipation are increased by intestinal atony, lax abdominal musculature, irregular food intake and dehydration in labour. By day 10, the woman should have achieved normal bowel function. Faecal incontinence may indicate anal sphincter damage or inadequate repair.

Weight change

Although weight is lost at delivery of the products of conception, many women experience a weight gain in the first couple of days following delivery. This is due to a combination of increased adrenocorticotrophin (ACTH), ADH and stress, all of which increase sodium and water retention. Women who have a higher blood loss at delivery tend to gain slightly more weight during the early days of the puerperium as water is retained for compensatory expansion of their blood volume. Weight usually starts to fall from the fourth day after delivery as diuresis increases. Weight is lost steadily, usually over a period of several months. Postpartum weight retention is affected by changes in lifestyle during and after pregnancy rather than by pregnancy itself (Ohlin and Rossner, 1994). Weight loss tends to be greater with lower parity, maternal age and lower prepregnant weight. Lactation and maternal nutrition also affect the rate of weight loss (see Chapter 16).

Other structural changes

Immediately after delivery, the vagina is smooth, soft and oedematous. The elasticity of the tissue returns within a few days. As the vagina is extremely well vascularized, episiotomies and tears usually heal well. The rugae of the vagina re-form in the third week but are less prominent than prior to pregnancy. The labia regress to a less prominent and fleshy state than in nulliparous women. The fall in oestrogen at delivery results in the vaginal epithelium becoming thinner and many women experience problems

Fig. 14.5 Carunculae myrtiformes. (Reproduced with permission from Miller and Hanretty, 1998.)

with vaginal lubrication immediately after delivery. Tags of the hymen remain and are renamed carunculae myrtiformes (Fig. 14.5).

Pelvic floor muscle strength and neuromuscular control are impaired to a greater extent in women who deliver vaginally and experience more mechanical trauma, particularly in the first week of the puerperium (Peschers et al., 1997); however, for most women, muscular tone and strength are normal within 2 months. Weakened circumvaginal muscles are associated with perineal outcome, episiotomy, length of second stage of labour, the weight of the baby and pushing techniques (Cosner et al., 1991). Problems associated with a lax ineffective pelvic floor such as uterine prolapse, urinary incontinence and prolapse of the rectum are more likely as parity increases. Pelvic floor exercises help to restore the muscle tone and function of the pelvic floor; specialist advice from an obstetric physiotherapist may be required for persistent problems with incontinence.

The abdominal wall may remain soft and flabby for several weeks. Severe stretching, for instance in a multiple pregnancy or with polyhydramnios, can result in permanently lax muscles. The softened pelvic joints and ligaments slowly return to normal over a period of a few months. Relaxation of pelvic joints may cause backache in the puerperium. The striae gravidarum become paler over a period of several months but fade rather than completely disappear.

Pregnancy-induced changes in the skin spontaneously regress or fade, though hyperpigmentation and melasma may persist in women with darker skin and hair. Hair loss may be marked following delivery and initial regrowth may be initially less abundant. Corneal sensitivity and pressure return to normal within 2 months of delivery. Nasal congestion and effects on the ear and larynx are restored to prepregnant status within a few days of delivery.

Body temperature

In the first 24 h following delivery, body temperature may increase slightly (to 38°C) in response to the stress of labour, particularly dehydration. This temperature fluctuation is normally transient; a persistent raised temperature may indicate infection (see below).

SLEEP

The puerperium is associated with disrupted sleep patterns, particularly immediately after delivery (Swain et al., 1997). The first 3 days can be extremely difficult for the mother compounded by fatigue accumulated during labour and being unable to rest comfortably due to perineal pain (see Case study 14.3). Postpartum perineal pain correlates well with the duration of the second stage of labour (Thranov et al., 1990). Euphoria, urinary, breast and perineal discomfort and infant disturbances can all lead to reduced sleep, which may affect memory and psychomotor tasks. Theoretically, sleep patterns are close to normal within 2 or 3 weeks of delivery but breastfeeding mothers obviously have more disrupted sleep (Quillin, 1997).

PSYCHOLOGICAL STATE

Usually by day 10 the mother and baby have established a feeding cycle. Although fatigue is common and normal, the mother should be developing strategies to cope with this, such as daytime sleeps. The mother should be independently caring for herself and the baby and interacting fully with members of her family and other people. Offspring provide their mothers with stimuli that elicit behavioural responses and emotional reactions; comparative studies suggest that these nurturing responses are evolutionarily conserved (Stern, 1997).

Case study 14.3

Sandra is a first-time mother who delivered a healthy male infant 3 days ago. She went home on the day of the birth as she appeared to be coping well with breastfeeding and caring for her infant. The community midwife visits at lunchtime on the third day to find a very distressed mother, partner and infant. They have had no sleep and the baby has been very fractious and wakeful.

- What are the possible physiological causes that have contributed to this situation?
- What would reassure the midwife that everything was normal and what support, help and advice could the midwife give to the family during this difficult period?

Many women experience a lack of libido (sex drive) during the first few months following delivery. This may be complicated by trauma to the reproductive tract during delivery. Sexual desire, expression and satisfaction may be reduced after delivery. Sexual activity may be affected by fatigue, altered body image, marital adjustment, dyspareunia, lactation, traditional taboos, vaginal bleeding or discharge, insufficient lubrication or fear of waking the baby.

Return to fertility

In pregnancy, ovarian function is suppressed by the high level of placental steroids. Women who do not breastfeed begin to menstruate, on average, about 55–60 days after delivery and to ovulate at about 40–50 days after delivery (Wang and Fraser, 1994), whereas lactation can delay ovulation to 30–40 weeks after delivery and menstruation to 8–15 months, depending on the duration and extent of breastfeeding. Although ovarian activity is almost invariably suspended, there have been reported cases of women who conceive within 2 weeks of giving birth (Hytten, 1995). The return to fertility exhibits similar hormonal profiles as puberty with a circadian pattern of LH secretion. A proportion of women become pregnant during lactational amenorrhoea but the degree of suppression of fertility depends on infant-feeding patterns and perhaps on maternal nutrition. Lactational effects on fertility are reduced as the spaces between the feeds increase and as the baby receives supplementary feeding. Where the number of sucking episodes is 10–20 per day, as is normal in many developing countries, resumption of ovarian activity is unlikely. With 5–6 feeds per day, the duration of feeds is important in suppressing ovulation. However, lactational amenorrhoea appears to reduce the likelihood of conception for a few months (Lewis et al., 1991), although it is probably more successful in achieving birth spacing.

Many women purposely choose to limit the number of children they wish to have. There are many economical and social issues that impinge on this; however, it is important to recognize that there are some women for whom certain (or all) methods of contraception are not acceptable on cultural and religious grounds. The return of fertility is very difficult to assess as factors such as breastfeeding, cultural and religious practice, genetic variation and disease may all compound the identification of return of the fertility cycle. It is important to emphasize that ovulation precedes menstruation so amenorrhoea does not guarantee the absence of fertility.

THE ROLE OF THE MIDWIFE

In the UK, most women are discharged from midwifery care by day 10; however, the midwife may visit up to day 28 in the postnatal period if required. Once the midwife is satisfied that the physiological transition is progressing normally then the discharge can be completed. The health visitor and general practitioner (GP) continue care of the mother and baby. The responsibilities of the midwife in the puerperium and at discharge include giving advice to women on a number of issues including infant feeding, parent craft, pelvic floor exercises, contraception and sources of psychological support.

COMPLICATIONS OF THE PUERPERIUM

Thromboembolic disorders

Hypercoagulability of pregnancy probably evolved to protect women from excessive bleeding associated with miscarriage and delivery (James, 2009). However, the increase in potential clot formation can have a physiological disadvantage both in pregnancy and following delivery because thrombi (blood clots) can form within the venous system. During the third trimester, the pregnant woman develops a pronounced state of hypercoagulation, such that her blood is more likely to clot than it would in the non-pregnant state and the effects of progesterone on venous muscle tone increase stasis of flow and decrease venous capacitance. In addition, mechanical obstruction by the uterus can decrease venous outflow and women may become less mobile. The risk of thromboembolic disorders in pregnancy is about six times higher than previously, and increases further in the puerperium. This is enhanced by a decrease in fibrinolytic activity (the breakdown of fibrin forming a blood clot) and raised concentration of clotting factors. Vascular trauma during delivery and haemoconcentration of the blood from physiological diuresis following delivery augments the increase in clotting factors. Some women may suffer from protein C and protein S deficiencies, these proteins are anticoagulants and so in pregnancy and the postnatal period these women are at greater risk of developing DVT (Mahmoodi et al., 2010). The risk of thrombosis persists for at least 8 weeks following deliver (James, 2009).

Thrombophlebitis

Thrombophlebitis is inflammation due to the formation of a thrombus (clot) in a superficial vein. The commonest site of thrombus formation is in the saphenous vein supplying the calf of the leg. Symptoms include a tender reddened area over the thrombosed vein and possibly a small increase in pulse and temperature. Motility and elevating the legs at rest reduce the risk of thrombus formation; compression stockings may be helpful. Thrombophlebitis is unlikely to progress to pulmonary embolism (PE).

Deep vein thrombosis

DVT is less common but carries the risk of a clot dislodging, which can cause PE. Hypercoagulability is increased with increased maternal age, parity, dehydration following delivery and delivery by caesarean section. Risk factors include immobility, pelvic or leg trauma, obesity, pre-eclampsia, caesarean section, instrument-assisted delivery, haemorrhage, multiparity, varicose veins, a previous history of a thromboembolic event and hereditary or acquired thrombophilias (Colman-Brochu, 2004). It has been observed clinically that there is an increased risk of DVT in the left leg, especially after a caesarean section, because blood flow velocity is reduced to a greater extent (Macklon and Greer, 1997). DVT may cause no symptoms or the woman may experience pain and swelling over the affected area and occasionally pyrexia. There may be marked differences in calf size or, in extreme cases, circulation to the leg below the thrombosis may be affected so the leg appears cold and white and possibly oedematous. DVT is confirmed by Doppler ultrasound or impedance plethysmography.

Pulmonary embolism

PE is an obstetric emergency that may follow DVT or occur without warning. PE is a condition that contributes towards maternal mortality associated with pregnancy (Bourjeily et al., 2010). If a thrombus (a fragment of the blood clot) breaks away and enters the venous system, it is then carried in the venous system to the right side of the heart and the pulmonary circulation. As the pulmonary arteries reduce in size, the thrombus may occlude arterial vessels within the lungs, causing major damage. Symptoms are sudden collapse, acute severe chest pain, dyspnoea, cyanosis, haemoptysis and shock. A woman with a PE will require intensive treatment and care.

A PE is more common in the postnatal period compared to the antepartum period. This may be due to the physiological reversal of haemodilution happening much faster (usually by day 3) than the physiological reversal of increased clotting factors which may take up to 6 weeks to return to prepregnancy values.

Women assessed to be at increased risk of thrombus formation are treated with prophylactic anticoagulants, such as heparin and synthetic analogues such as enoxaparin. DVT is usually treated with heparin and, if required, long-term anticoagulation therapy with drugs such as warfarin is commenced. Warfarin use in pregnancy is contraindicated as it is transported across the placenta; but postnatal women who choose to breastfeed can have warfarin treatment as it not secreted in significant levels in the breast milk.

Postpartum thyroid disorders

Transient thyroid disorders are fairly common during the postpartum period (Okosieme et al., 2008). Postpartum women, especially if older than 35, are at increased risk of developing Graves' disease and postpartum thyroid disorder (PPTD) transiently affects 6–9% of postpartum women. It is thought that PPTD is probably due to changes in the immune system as it switches back to being Th1 dominated (see Chapter 10). The syndrome is biphasic (Weetman, 2010). The initial effects are thyrotoxicosis with thyroid cell destruction and excessive release of stored thyroid hormone from the damaged thyroid tissue causing mild hyperthyroidism for 2–4 weeks. This is followed by a period of hypothyroidism as the damage to the thyroid progresses, which usually lasts 2–4 months. Typical symptoms are mild and include fatigue, cold intolerance, hair damage and weight gain with high TSH and low free T4 levels. Normal thyroid function is established in most women with PPTD within a year but a proportion of women remain hypothyroidic (Stuckey et al., 2010). The condition may recur in subsequent pregnancies (Weetman, 2010) and the risk of developing permanent hypothyroidism is increased.

Risk of infection

In the puerperium, the woman is at increased risk of infection, particularly that associated with the genital tract, urinary system, breast and any site of thrombophlebitis. The placental wound site, lacerations and incisions of the perineum and the lax urinary system are especially vulnerable. The lochia provides ideal culture conditions for microorganisms. Other predisposing factors include anaemia, fatigue, malnutrition, traumatic delivery and the presence of retained tissue in the uterus. Both maternal and neonatal infection (see Chapter 15) may be caused by endogenous or exogenous organisms (Box 14.4).

Common symptoms of infection include:

- pyrexia (up to 40 °C)
- tachycardia (up to 140 beats per minute)
- subinvolution of the uterus
- headache

Box 14.4 **Examples of microorganisms causing puerperal infection**

Endogenous
- *Escherichia coli*
- *Clostridium perfringens*
- *Streptococcus faecalis*
- *Pseudomonas aeruginosa*

Exogenous
- β-Haemolytic streptococci
- *Staphylococcus aureus*

- malaise, lower abdominal pain and back pain
- heavy offensive-smelling lochia.

Less common symptoms usually associated with severe sepsis (Dellinger et al., 2008) are:

- hypothermia
- tachypnoea
- altered mental status
- marked oedema and positive fluid balance with acute oliguria
- hyperglycaemia in the absence of diabetes
  - markers of inflammation such as high WBC count, high plasma C-reactive protein or procalcitonin levels
  - haemodynamic variables such as arterial hypotension or hypoxia, signs of organ dysfunction, coagulation abnormalities and/or thrombocytopenia, high creatinine, ileus (absent bowel sounds)
  - markers of impaired tissue perfusion such as hyperlactataemia or decreased capillary refill (or mottling).

Infection in the acute phase can inhibit lactation. When choosing antibiotics to treat infection in the puerperium, one needs to take into consideration whether the woman is breastfeeding and the potential effect of the transfer of the drug into breast milk.

Breast discomfort and after-pains

The establishment of lactation is covered in detail in Chapter 16; however, it is worth mentioning here two common problems that can occur during this period in relation to breastfeeding.

- If the baby has been incorrectly positioned, often because it is fractious or hungry and wanting to feed constantly, the nipple may become sore, cracked and bleed as a consequence. A break in the integrity of the nipple skin increases the risk of mastitis (localized and ascending infection usually caused by Staphylococcus aureus). Women experiencing early feeding problems need a lot of help and support. The baby needs to 'fix' or 'latch on' properly in order to provide adequate nipple stimulation to establish the feeding cycle.
- Sometimes the breasts become engorged or extended. Initially, this may be a venous cause due to the increased vascularization of the breast. However, when milk production increases (described as the milk 'coming in'), the breast may initially be overproductive. The breasts may overfill with milk causing them to become distended and hardened, which may be uncomfortable or painful. The baby may need help achieving an appropriate position; however, once the feeding cycle is established the demand/supply balance is achieved and the breast engorgement problems will resolve.

Pharmacological effects

The majority of deliveries within the UK have the third stage actively managed as opposed to passive or physiological management where the women deliver the placenta naturally (see Chapter 13). However, the administration of an anti-tocolytic (or 'uterotonic') drug such as Syntometrine (which contains ergometrine and oxytocin) may cause side effects following completion of the third stage; for example:

- nausea and vomiting
- transient rise in blood pressure
- palpitations and tachycardia
- chest pain
- headache.

Most of these side effects are strongly associated with ergometrine so it is recommended that administration of intramuscular injection of syntocinon is used instead (NCCWCH, 2008). Also during the early puerperium, women may suffer side effects from pharmacological methods of pain relief administered during labour. Pethidine may induce drowsiness, fatigue and nausea within the mother and reduce the suckling instinct of the infant, thus interfering with feeding. The effects of an epidural anaesthetic may take several hours to wear off, which affects maternal mobility and the ability to void urine.

Psychological problems

Women in the postpartum period have increased vulnerability to affective disorders which are classified on the basis of severity, such as postpartum 'blues', postpartum depression and postpartum psychosis. It is estimated that as many as 80% of women may experience some fluctuations in mood, mostly transient emotional disorders at about day 3 described as 'the blues' (Steiner, 1998). Ten to twenty percent of puerperal women develop true depressive illness, which may have a later onset (or referral) and delayed recovery. A few women (0.1–0.2%) develop severe prolonged psychotic illness following childbirth. Although many of these cases may be recognized in the early postnatal period, some become evident much later and depression is frequently under-reported and not always recognized. Certain symptoms are recognized to be important in the diagnosis of postnatal depression (Box 14.5). Overall, these figures mean that postnatal depression is the most common disorder of the puerperium.

The aetiology of these depressive disorders is not fully understood. Immediately after delivery, the infant may feed often and this may be increased at night adding to maternal fatigue. Initially, the mother's fatigue is overcome by intense feelings of relief and excitement at the birth of her baby. By day 3, however, the woman may become emotional, tearful and tired and need a lot of

Box 14.5 Classic signs of postnatal depression

- Depressed mood
- Sleep disturbance not related to discomfort and infant wakening
- Unable to cope—guilt
- Thoughts of harming self or baby
- Rejection of baby
- Altered libido
- Anxiety

Case study 14.4

At delivery, Sarah suffered a large haemorrhage that was difficult to control; she finally underwent a hysterectomy following a total blood loss of over 4 L. Her recovery was uneventful but within 6 months she was diagnosed as suffering from Sheehan's syndrome—necrosis of the pituitary gland.

- What would her symptoms be?
- What endocrine function would be disrupted as a result of this condition?

support and comfort during this period. This low ebb of hormonal withdrawal is physiologically marked by the commencement of full lactogenesis following the initial production of small volumes of colostrum (see Chapter 16). The 'blues' coincide with lactation, breast engorgement, perineal pain and wound discomfort.

As the withdrawal of steroid hormones has been postulated to have a role in the aetiology of postnatal depression, clinical trials have investigated whether either progesterone or oestrogen supplementation might be of prophylactic or therapeutic value in postnatal depression. Some uncontrolled studies (e.g. Dalton, 1980) reported the benefit of progesterone in preventing postnatal depression. However, use of synthetic progesterone is positively associated with depression in the postnatal period and should be used with caution (Karuppaswamy and Vlies, 2003).

Oestrogen has also been associated with psychological well-being (Brace and McCauley, 1997); sudden changes in oestrogen levels such as those experienced in the puerperium may result in effects on neurotransmitter release. Oestrogen therapy may be of modest value in severe postnatal depression but more research is needed.

Other authors suggest that levels of cortisol or β-endorphin have a stronger association with postnatal depression (Harris et al., 1996). The hypothalamic–pituitary–adrenal (HPA) axis is very active in the third trimester as placental corticotrophin-releasing hormone (CRH) production increases and CRH-binding protein (CRH-BP) levels fall. Suppression of hypothalamic CRH secretion is implicated in the aetiology of postnatal depression (Magiakou et al., 1996). The relationship between breastfeeding and postnatal depression is controversial. However, hormones involved in lactation affect cortisol levels (Amico et al., 1994). Lactation may also predispose the breastfeeding mother to depression by isolating her and increasing levels of fatigue. Women who develop postnatal depression make a good recovery with the right treatment and support. Exercise programmes have been found to decrease anxiety and depression in the puerperium significantly (Koltyn and Schultes, 1997). The recurrence of postnatal depression is high, which allows identification of women at increased risk. It has been suggested that women who have a low intake of fish (and omega-3 fatty acids) are more likely to suffer from postnatal depression (Hibbeln, 2002). Certainly, the high docosahexaenoic acid (DHA) requirements of the fetus and for breast milk may deplete women. Although a number of studies have investigated possible relationships between dietary factors, including omega-3 fatty acids and various micronutrients, and the aetiology and treatment of postnatal depression, the results are generally inconsistent and inconclusive (Derbyshire and Costarelli, 2008).

Case study 14.4 describes an example of a hormonal complication of the puerperium.

Key points

- Maternal physiology and anatomy adapt rapidly to the withdrawal of steroid hormones, following the delivery of the placenta. These dramatic physiological changes increase the risk of infection, haemorrhage and psychological and emotional changes.
- The uterus rapidly involutes after delivery; normal involution can be monitored by assessment of fundal height and characteristics of the lochia.
- After delivery, there is a dramatic and rapid decrease in circulating blood volume followed by a return to normal cardiovascular parameters. As stroke volume initially remains high, bradycardia is usual, particularly in the first 2 weeks.
- The postpartum physiological changes allow the woman to tolerate considerable blood loss at delivery, but alteration in clotting factor concentration and venous stasis predispose the woman to thromboembolic disorders; the risk is enhanced by immobility and sepsis.
- Marked diuresis is normal in the puerperium but overdistension, or decreased sensitivity, of the bladder can predispose the woman to urinary problems.
- Ovulation occurs before menstruation and is delayed by breastfeeding; lactational amenorrhoea is useful in birth spacing rather than being a reliable method of contraception.

Application to practice

In comparison to pregnancy, when the changes induced by endocrine effects are at a relatively slow pace, the reversal of this in the puerperium is much more dramatic. These rapid changes occur at the same time as another endocrine-induced change resulting in the initiation of lactation.

Fatigue from labour, perineal pain from trauma and the demands of a newborn infant can also complicate the situation.

The midwife needs to use her knowledge of the puerperium to support women through this often difficult period of adaptation.

Knowledge of mental health issues in the postnatal period is essential in differentiating between mild depressive states and recognizing severe psychotic disorders.

ANNOTATED FURTHER READING

Lynch C, Keith LG, Loonde A, et al: *A textbook of postpartum haemorrhage: a comprehensive guide to evaluation, management and surgical intervention,* 2006, Sapiens Publishing.

This book provides an in-depth guide to the management of postpartum haemorrhage in relation to the possible causes and factors that contribute to excess bleeding post delivery. Midwives will find the detail of this obstetric text very useful in developing their understanding and ability to deal with this often complex situation.

Barlow J, Svanberg PO: *Keeping the baby in mind,* London, 2009, Routledge.

An interesting book which covers the transition to parenthood from the infant's mental health and development perspective.

Baston H, Hall J: *Midwifery essentials: postnatal,* vol. 4, 2009, Churchill Livingstone.

The fourth title in the Midwifery Essentials series which includes the postnatal examination of the woman and neonate, hospital postnatal care and caesarean section, emotional wellbeing, postnatal fertility issues and lactational support.

Byrom S, Edwards G, Bick D: *Essential midwifery practice: postnatal care,* 2009, Wiley-Blackwell.

An edited textbook written by midwifery experts which covers postnatal clinical care in hospital and community settings, transition into parenthood, empowering parents and supporting vulnerable women and their families.

Hanley V: *Perinatal mental health: a guide for health professionals and users,* 2009, Wiley-Blackwell.

A comprehensive reference book health professionals which focuses on perinatal mood and mental health disorders and includes topics on the antenatal period, postnatal depression, bipolar disorder, psychosis, personality disorders, eating disorders, sexual issues, self harm and suicide.

Hughes H: Postpartum contraception, *J Fam Health Care* 19, 9–10, 12, 2009.

A review covering the advantages and disadvantages of commonly used methods of postpartum contraception including lactational amenorrhoea, combined oral contraception, the progesterone-only pill, injectable methods, implants, intrauterine devices and systems, barrier methods and sterilization, and emergency contraception.

Moore LJ, Jones SL, Kreiner LA, et al: Validation of a screening tool for the early identification of sepsis, *J Trauma* 66:1539–1546, 2009.

Practitioners may find this tool and guidelines useful in assessing women for signs of sepsis throughout the pregnancy continuum.

National Collaborating Centre for Mental Health: *Antenatal and postnatal mental health: the NICE guideline on clinical management and service guidance,* (NICE guideline), 2007, British Psychological Society/ RCPsych Publications.

This is a very comprehensive guide to a wide range of mental health issues in relation to pregnancy, childbirth and the postnatal period.

Royal College of Obstetricians and Gynaecologists: *Thromboembolic disease in pregnancy and the puerperium: acute management green top guideline 28,* London, 2007, RCOG.

Clinical guidance and management for the treatment of venous thromboembolism.

Royal College of Obstetricians and Gynaecologists: *Reducing the risk of thrombosis and embolism during pregnancy and the puerperium Green-top Guideline NO. 37,* London, 2009, RCOG.

Clinical guidance and management for the prevention of venous thromboembolism.

van Dillen J, Zwart J, Schutte J, et al: Maternal sepsis: epidemiology, etiology and outcome, *Curr Opin Infect Dis* 23:249–254, 2010.

This review focuses on focus on new findings concerning epidemiology, etiology and outcome of maternal sepsis in low-income as well as high-income countries.

REFERENCES

Amico JA, Johnston JM, Vagnucci AH: Suckling-induced attenuation of plasma cortisol concentrations in postpartum lactating women, *Endocrinol Res* 20:79–87, 1994.

Blackburn ST: *Maternal, fetal, and neonatal physiology: a clinical perspective,* ed 3, Philadelphia, 2007, Saunders.

Bourjeily G, Paidas M, Khalil H, et al: Pulmonary embolism in pregnancy, *Lancet* 375:500–512, 2010.

Brace M, McCauley E: Oestrogens and psychological well-being, *Ann Med* 29:283–290, 1997.

Clapp JF, Capeless E: Cardiovascular function before, during, and after the first and subsequent pregnancies, *Am J Cardio.* 80:1469–1473, 1997.

Colman-Brochu S: Deep vein thrombosis in pregnancy, *MCN Am J Matern Child Nurs* 29(3):186–192, 2004.

Cosner KR, Dougherty MC, Bishop KR: Dynamic characteristics of the circumvaginal muscles during pregnancy and the postpartum, *J Nurse Midwifery* 36:221–225, 1991.

Dalton K: *Depression after childbirth*, Oxford, 1980, OUP.

Dellinger RP, Levy MM, Carlet JM, et al: Surviving Sepsis Campaign: international guidelines for management of severe sepsis and septic shock: 2008, *Crit Care Med* 36:296–327, 2008.

Derbyshire E and Costarelli V: Dietary factors in the aetiology of postnatal depression, *Nutr Bull* 33:162–168, 2008.

Harris B, Lovett L, Smith J, et al: Cardiff puerperal mood and hormone study III: postnatal depression at 5 to 6 weeks postpartum, and its hormonal correlates across the peripartum period, *Br J Psychol* 168:739–744, 1996.

Hibbeln JR: Seafood consumption, the DHA content of mothers' milk and prevalence rates of postpartum depression: a cross-national, ecological analysis, *J Affect Disord* 69 (1–3):15–29, 2002.

Howie PW: The physiology of the puerperium and lactation. In Chamberlain G, editor: *Turnbull's obstetrics*, ed 2, New York, 1995, pp 756–771, Churchill Livingstone.

Hytten F: *The clinical physiology of the puerperium*, London, 1995, Farand Press.

James AH: Venous thromboembolism in pregnancy, *Arterioscler Thromb Vasc Biol* 29:326–331, 2009.

Karuppaswamy J, Vlies R: The benefit of oestrogens and progestogens in postnatal depression, *J Obstet Gynaecol* 23(4):341–346, 2003.

Koltyn KF, Schultes SS: Psychological effects of an aerobic exercise session and rest session following pregnancy, *J Sports Med Phys Fitness* 37:287–291, 1997.

Lanir N, Aharon A, Brenner B: Haemostatic mechanisms in human placenta, *Best Pract Res Clin Haematol* 16(2):183–195, 2003.

Letsky E: The haematological system. In Chamberlain G, Broughton Pipkin F, editors: *Clinical physiology in obstetrics*, ed 3, Oxford, pp 71–110, 1998, Blackwell.

Lewis PR, Brown JB, Renfree MB, et al: The resumption of ovulation and menstruation in a well-nourished population of women breastfeeding for an extended period of time, *Fertil Steril* 55:529–536, 1991.

Macklon NS, Greer IA: The deep venous system in the puerperium: an ultrasound study, *Br J Obstet Gynaecol* 104:198–200, 1997.

Magiakou MA, Mastorakos G, Rabin D, et al: Hypothalamic corticotrophin-releasing hormone suppression during the postpartum period: implications for the increase in psychiatric manifestations at this time, *J Clin Endocrinol Metab* 81 (5):1912–1917, 1996.

Mahmoodi BK, Brouwer JL, Ten Kate MK, et al: A prospective cohort study on the absolute risks of venous thromboembolism and predictive value of screening asymptomatic relatives of patients with hereditary deficiencies of protein S, protein C or antithrombin, *J Thromb Haemost*, 8(6):1193–1200, 2010.

Miller AWF, Hanretty KP: *Obstetrics illustrated*, ed 5, New York, 1998, Churchill Livingstone, p 336.

NCCWCH National Collaborating Centre for Women and Children's Health: *Intrapartum care clinical (NICE guideline 55)*, London, 2008, NICE.

Ohlin A, Rossner S: Trends in eating patterns, physical activity and socio-demographic factors in relation to postpartum body weight development, *Br J Nutr* 71:457–470, 1994.

Okosieme OE, Marx H, Lazarus JH: Medical management of thyroid dysfunction in pregnancy and the postpartum, *Expert Opin Pharmacother* 9:2281–2293, 2008.

Peschers UM, Schaer GN, DeLancey JO, et al: Levator ani function before and after childbirth, *Br J Obstet Gynaecol* 104:1004–1008, 1997.

Quillin SL: Infant and mother sleep patterns during the 4th postpartum week, *Issues Compr Pediatr Nurs* 20:115–123, 1997.

Richter C, Huch A, Huch R: Erythropoiesis in the postpartum period, *J Perinat Med* 23:51–59, 1995.

Steiner M: Perinatal mood disorders: position paper, *Psychopharmacol Bull* 34(3):301–306, 1998.

Stern JM: Offspring-induced nuturance: animal–human parallels, *Dev Psychobiol* 31:19–37, 1997.

Stone PJ, Franzblau C: Increase in urinary desmoline and pyridoline during postpartum involution of the uterus in humans, *Proc Soc Exp Biol Med* 210:39–42, 1995.

Stuckey B, Kent G, Ward L, et al: Postpartum thyroid dysfunction and the long-term risk of hypothyroidism: results from a 12 year follow-up study of women with and without postpartum thyroid dysfunction, *Clin Endocrinol (Oxf)* 73:389–395, 2010.

Swain AM, O'Hara MW, Starr KR, et al: A prospective study of sleep, mood, and cognitive function in postpartum and nonpostpartum women, *Obstet Gynecol* 90:381–386, 1997.

Sweet B, Tiran D: *Mayes' midwifery*, ed 12, London, 1996, Baillière Tindall, pp 405, 406.

Tekay A, Jouppila P: A longitudinal Doppler ultrasonographic assessment of the alterations in peripheral vascular resistance of uterine arteries and ultrasonographic findings of the involuting uterus during the puerperium, *Am J Obstet Gynecol* 168:190–198, 1993.

Thranov I, Kringelbachh AM, Melchior E, et al: Postpartum symptoms: episiotomy or tear at vaginal delivery, *Acta Obstet Gynecol Scand* 69:11–15, 1990.

Wang IY, Fraser IS: Reproductive function and contraception in the postpartum period, *Obstet Gynecol Surv* 49:56–63, 1994.

Weetman AP: Immunity, thyroid function and pregnancy: molecular mechanisms, *Nat Rev Endocrinol* 6:311–318, 2010.

Chapter | 15 |

The transition to neonatal life

LEARNING OBJECTIVES

- To identify the key steps in the transition to successful neonatal life.
- To describe the vulnerability of the neonate, with particular reference to the potential risk of respiratory problems, hypoglycaemia and jaundice.
- To outline the principles of thermoregulation in the newborn.
- To compare the fetal and neonatal circulatory and respiratory systems, describing the transition stages.
- To describe factors relating to the neonatal gastrointestinal, renal and nervous systems that make breast milk the ideal food.
- To describe normal physiological fetal to neonatal transition and to recognise signs of a neonate experiencing compromised transition.

INTRODUCTION

During fetal life, the placenta carries out the crucial physiological roles of gas exchange, nutrition, elimination of waste products and additional aspects of circulation. Within minutes of birth, the placental support ceases so the baby's own cardiovascular, respiratory, gastrointestinal, renal and metabolic systems must function independently. The transition from fetal to neonatal life needs to be smooth, swift and successful; the majority of infant deaths occur within the neonatal period (first 28 days) and these are linked to inadequate progression to neonatal physiological functions. Millennium Development Goal 4, set by UNICEF in 2000, is to reduce child mortality (deaths under 5 years of age) by two-thirds between 1990 and 2015. Although under-5 mortality rates have improved, neonatal rates have increased (Lawn et al., 2010). The leading cause of neonatal mortality is complications of preterm birth and compromised transition to neonatal life.

The transition to extrauterine life depends on the degree of maturation in late gestation, the process of delivery itself and establishment of independent physiological processes for regulating homeostasis after placental separation. These physiological processes include establishing continuous respiration, changing from a parallel to a serial circulatory organization and ceasing the right-to-left shunting across the heart so oxygenated blood can be delivered to the tissues, establishing oral intermittent feeding and independent thermoregulation and glucose homeostasis. These complex physiological changes must occur within a relatively short time frame. Monitoring and assessing neonatal transition are important in order to recognise delayed or compromised adaptation or the warning signs of more serious conditions such as birth injury, congenital abnormality or disease (Askin, 2009a).

	Chapter case study

The midwife officially recorded Zak as having an Apgar score of 9 at approximately 1 min of age. Following the delivery James was surprised how alert his son Zak was, that he seemed to be aware of his surroundings and appeared to be actively looking around.
- What factors could have contributed to Zak's behaviour and what are the possible explanations for Zak being so alert following his delivery?
  Zara asks the midwife if she can attempt to breastfeed.
- What could the midwife do to encourage Zak to suckle?

The process of birth is physiologically stressful with fluctuations in placental blood flow resulting in a degree of hypoxia and respiratory acidosis. Increased secretion of adrenal catecholamines, stimulation of the sympathetic nervous system and the subsequent mobilization of glycogen and lipid stores are fundamental in the activation of essential physiological mechanisms that result in an alert and active baby at birth. However, a prolonged or difficult delivery and marked hypoxia/anoxia and acidosis can result in an overstressed or seriously asphyxiated baby (Box 15.1).

Both the fetus and the neonate can tolerate degrees of hypoxia and anoxia that would result in serious morbidity or mortality in an adult. The neonate retains the capability to divert a considerable proportion of its cardiac output to the brain thus protecting it. Although the brain is vulnerable to hypoxia, the compensatory mechanisms can increase tolerance to hypoxic states (Parer, 1998). However, severe asphyxia can cause cerebral microhaemorrhages resulting in a spectrum of damage from impaired intellectual development to spasticity and irreversible brain damage (Box 15.2). Neonates are also vulnerable to infection.

Although there is usually a good correlation between gestational length and degree of maturity, infants affected by intrauterine growth retardation (IUGR) may have precocious organ development because undernutrition and the resulting fetal stress promote increased fetal cortisol secretion thus enhancing fetal organ maturation. In humans, fetal cortisol appears not to have a role in inducing labour as has been demonstrated in other species (see Chapter 13). The major problems of premature

Box 15.1 **Fetal asphyxia**

Fetal asphyxia is due to a significant reduction in the amount of oxygen available via the placenta and the maternal circulation. There are many possible causes for example placental abruption, rapid deterioration in the maternal condition, such as eclampsia, uterine hyperstimulation in response to syntocinon augmentation. Whatever the reason, prolonged fetal hypoxia will result in asphyxia (low oxygen levels and raised carbon dioxide levels). Fetal hypoxia, if suspected during labour, can be assessed by obtaining a small sample of blood from the fetal scalp, from which the pH and base excess can be measured. Acidaemia is diagnosed if the pH of the fetal blood is below 7.2, however many babies can tolerate moderate acidaemia without long term problems. A base excess above 12 mmol indicates chronic or prolonged acidaemia. The risk of asphyxia rises with lower pH and higher base excess. Babies born with asphyxia require active resuscitation to restore pH and base excess. In extreme cases, severe asphyxia results in irreversible brain damage.

Box 15.2 **Neonatal head cooling**

In extreme cases of neonatal asphyxia, brain cell distruction triggers apotosis in surrounding cells. The number of apoptotic neural cells can be reduced by neonatal head cooling thus potentially reducing the severity of brain damage (Wyatt et al, 2007; Polderman, 2008).

infants can be attributed to a shorter duration of glucocorticoid exposure (even though fetal stress results in actual levels being higher); this results in an increased risk of persistent fetal circulation, increased likelihood of lung immaturity and respiratory diseases syndrome and immaturity of thermoregulatory responses, the gastrointestinal system and enzymes involved in maintaining glucose homeostasis.

Fetal preparation for birth includes storing glycogen, producing catecholamines and laying brown and white fat. The glucocorticoid system is pivotal in the fetal preparation for birth. Fetal cortisol levels rise from about 35 weeks. Glucocorticoids cause the natural decrease in growth that occurs towards term and are also thought to be responsible for the growth retardation associated with physiological stress in utero such as that due to hypoxia and undernutrition. Glucocorticoids bring about functional and morphological changes in many biochemical pathways and fetal tissues including lungs, liver, gut, adipose tissue and skeletal muscle (Fowden and Forhead, 2009). Glucocorticoids influence surfactant production and maturation of the alveoli and other respiratory tissues thus promoting lung maturation. They stimulate glycogen deposition in the fetal liver and skeletal muscle and also induce hepatic gluconeogenesis enzymes by promoting adrenaline synthesis (and potential effective response to stress), inducing hormone receptors and affecting thyroid hormone synthesis. They also enhance proteolysis so fetal protein accretion is reduced. Fetal corticotrophin-releasing factor (CRF) and antidiuretic hormone (ADH) and placental CRF orchestrate the increase in fetal cortisol production, which influence adrenocorticotrophin (ACTH) production by the maturing fetal pituitary gland; increased ACTH stimulates cortisol production.

At birth, there are also changes in the regulation of growth. Fetal growth is substrate-limited and actively constrained to optimize successful delivery (see Chapter 9). The rise in glucocorticoids towards term suppresses growth and is responsible for the natural decrease in growth that occurs at this time (Fowden and Forhead, 2009); the increase in glucocorticoids also induces growth hormone receptors and changes in expression of insulin-like growth factor I (IGF-I).

THE CARDIOVASCULAR SYSTEM

Blood

Before birth

Fetal blood (Table 15.1) is structurally and functionally different to adult blood; it contains larger and more numerous erythrocytes (red blood cells) with a higher haemoglobin content which maximizes their uptake of oxygen (Palis and Segel, 1998). Fetal haemoglobin with its two α-chains and two γ-chains has a higher affinity for oxygen in the slightly more acid fetal environment. Less-effective binding of 2,3-bisphosphoglycerate (or 2,3-diphosphoglycerate) to the γ-chains means that the oxygen–haemoglobin dissociation curve of the fetus and neonate is shifted to the left (Fig. 15.1). Shifts of pH in the placenta further increase both dissociation of oxygen from maternal haemoglobin and its uptake by fetal hae-moglobin. This means that, although fetal haemoglobin has an increased oxygen uptake, it is less efficient at releas-ing oxygen to the tissues.

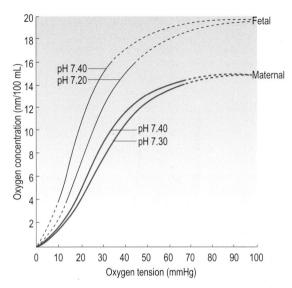

Fig. 15.1 The maternal and fetal oxyhaemoglobin dissociation curves.

At term, the ratio of fetal haemoglobin to adult haemo-globin (HbF:HbA) is 80:20; by 6 months production of the β-chain replaces the γ-chain so the ratio is 1:99 (Fig. 15.2). Preterm infants tend to have an even higher HbF level and a decreased 2,3-bisphosphoglycerate concen-tration therefore oxygen unloading at the tissue level is even less efficient. The raised levels of HbF in the neonate mean that haemoglobinopathies caused by altered synthe-sis of β-chains (such as β-thalassaemia) or altered structure of β-chains (such as sickle-cell anaemia) are not evident immediately at birth but become evident when the infant is at least 2 months old. It is possible to detect fetal blood cells in the maternal circulation, an observation that is utilized in the management of Rhesus incompatibility (see Chapter 10) (Lamvu and Kuller, 1997).

After birth

At birth, fetal blood has an increased population of nucle-ated erythrocytes (even more so if the baby has been sub-jected to increased stress, is immature or has Down's syndrome). For the first 3 months of life, the erythrocytes are more fragile, have an increased metabolism and a shorter half-life and erythropoietin production is sup-pressed (Box 15.3). Once respiration in the neonate is established, the excess red blood cells compensating for the lower oxygen saturation within the uterine environ-ment are no longer needed. These red blood cells are bro-ken down and physiological jaundice may result, usually around day 3 of life as the neonatal liver is immature and initially cannot keep up with the rate of bilirubin pro-duction from red blood cell breakdown.

Table 15.1 Fetal and adult blood

	FETAL/NEONATAL	ADULT
Blood volume	80–100 mL/kg 90–105 mL/kg (preterm)	75 mL/kg
Red blood cell number	6–7 ∞ 10^6/mL	Female: 4.8 ∞ 10^6/mL Male: 5.4 ∞ 10^6/mL
Haemoglobin content	20.7 g/dL	Female: 14 g/dL Male: 16 g/dL
Oxygen content of 100 mL saturated blood	21 mL (theory) 13 mL (practice)	16 mL (theory) 15.7 mL (practice)
Red blood cell lifespan	80–100 days 60–80 days (preterm)	120 days
Haemoglobin type	HbF: $\alpha_2\gamma_2$	HbA: $\alpha_2\beta_2$

Note: the theoretical value is the amount of oxygen the blood can be saturated with whereas, in practice, the blood is saturated to a lesser degree because the transfer of oxygen across the placenta is less efficient than the transfer of oxygen across the alveoli.

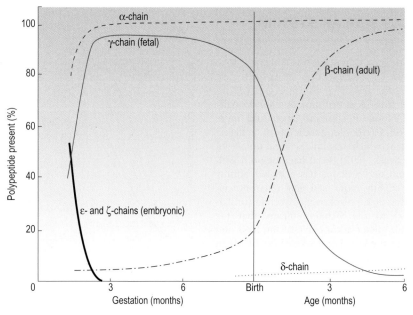

Fig. 15.2 Changes in fetal:adult haemoglobin (HbF:HbA) ratios in fetal and infant blood. (Reproduced with permission from Begley et al., 1978.)

Box 15.3 **Physiological anaemia of infancy**

Haemopoiesis (red blood cell production) is controlled by the hormone erythropoietin, which increases when oxygen delivery to the kidney is reduced; it stimulates red blood cell production by the bone marrow. The increased oxygen levels inhibit erythropoietin levels in the neonate postnatally (Strauss, 1994). Levels remain low for 2–3 months (longer in preterm infants) and then increase, resulting in increased bone marrow activity and red blood cell production. As the neonate appears to tolerate the fall in haemoglobin concentration without ill-effects, it is deemed to be physiological. The haemodilution effects are increased by rapid growth being matched by total blood volume, which precedes any change in red blood cell number.

Haemostasis

Neonates, particularly those born prematurely but those who are healthy as well, have an increased risk of haemostatic problems because they are born with a deficiency of plasma coagulation factors, inhibitors of haemostasis and other components of the fibrinolytic system (Aronis-Vournas, 2006). However, despite this, because the deficiencies in components of the coagulation and fibrinolytic system tend to be balanced, the healthy term neonate does not usually have thrombotic or haemorrhagic problems. The most common example of neonatal haemostatic problem is (Kuehl, 1997) disseminated intravascular coagulation (DIC) due to accelerated and inappropriate coagulation, which depletes the body's supply of platelets and clotting factors and paradoxically increases the risk of haemorrhage. Susceptibility is increased because, first, the immature neonatal reticuloendothelial system has a decreased capacity to remove intermediary products of coagulation so they can further stimulate coagulation and consumption of clotting factors, and, second, synthesis of clotting factors by the immature liver is inefficient. Vitamin K levels in the neonate are about 50% of adult values, which affect the efficiency of the clotting cascade. Vitamin K levels are low because placental transport of the vitamin is poor and colonization of the gut by bacteria that synthesize vitamin K is not immediate. The consequent reduced level of all vitamin K-dependent clotting factors is associated with an increased bleeding tendency, which can predispose to haemorrhagic disease of the newborn (HDNB) (Box 15.4). Neonatal platelets exhibit decreased aggregation and adhesiveness because their production of thromboxane A_2 (TxA_2) is impaired. This appears to protect the term neonate against thrombosis but to increase the vulnerability to bleeding of the preterm or sick baby. Placental transfer of maternal drugs such as aspirin can affect coagulation in the neonate.

Box 15.4 **Haemorrhagic disease of the newborn (HDNB)**

- Bleeding from the gut, umbilicus, circumcision wounds and oozing from puncture sites
- Evident 2–3 days after birth
- Associated with antibiotics, which affect colonization of the gut with vitamin K-synthesizing bacteria
- Associated with anticonvulsant drugs (e.g. phenobarbital, diphenylhydantoin), which concentrate in the fetal liver and antagonize the effect of vitamin K
- Associated with maternal warfarin treatment, which decreases levels of vitamin K-dependent clotting factors and prolongs prolonged clotting times
- Prophylactic vitamin K is routinely administered to all babies born in the UK (Paediatric Formulary Committee, 2010)
- Term babies respond well to vitamin K therapy but synthesis of clotting factors is further limited in preterm babies by inadequate hepatic synthesis of precursor proteins

The circulation

Before birth

As the fetal oxygen source is the placenta rather than the lungs, blood in the fetal circulation flows in a circuit that perfuses the placenta and largely bypasses the lungs (Fig. 15.3). In order to do this, the fetal circulation has several additional structures: the umbilical vein, which carries blood rich in oxygen and nutrients to the underside of the liver, the ductus venosus (a venosus is a shunt that connects a vein to a vein), which bypasses the liver taking blood from the umbilical vein to the inferior umbilical vein en route to the right side of the heart. With increasing gestational age, more blood goes to the liver rather than bypassing it (Askin, 2009a). The hypogastric arteries, which branch off the internal iliac arteries, are contiguous with the umbilical arteries of the umbilical cord, returning blood to the placenta. The lungs are bypassed by two structures: the foramen ovale, which allows blood to move directly from the right atrium to the left atrium, and the ductus arteriosus, which connects the pulmonary arterial trunk to the descending aorta (an arteriosus is a vascular shunt that connects an artery to an artery).

The oxygenated and nutrient-enriched blood is taken from the placenta in the umbilical vein that goes through the abdominal wall to the underside of the liver. This is the only unmixed blood and is about 80% saturated with oxygen; the blood goes through the ductus venosus to the inferior vena cava where it mixes with oxygen-depleted blood returning to the heart from the lower body

(Fig. 15.4A). The inflows of blood from the inferior and superior venae cavae do not mix thoroughly because of their angle of entry and the shape of the right atrium. Because the entry of the inferior vena cava is aligned with the foramen ovale, most (about 60%) of the blood from the inferior vena cava travels from the right atrium through the foramen ovale into the left atrium and thence to the left ventricle and the ascending aorta. The foramen ovale is kept open because the high pulmonary vascular resistance (PVR) means that the pressure in the right atrium is also high.

Most blood entering the right atrium from the superior vena cava passes through the tricuspid valve into the right ventricle and to the pulmonary arterial trunk. The ductus arteriosus is inserted into the vessel at the bifurcation of the right and left pulmonary artery (taking blood to the right and left lung, respectively); it shunts blood from the pulmonary arterial route into the descending aorta. The pulmonary circulation is vasoconstricted and has a high PVR, because the pulmonary environment is relatively hypoxic. Systemic vascular resistance (SVR) is low. Only about 10% of the output of the right ventricle continues into the pulmonary circulation for the growth and metabolic needs of the lungs; the rest is diverted through the ductus arteriosus which has a low resistance; its patency is maintained by the low fetal PO_2 and by high levels of prostaglandins produced by the placenta. Towards the end of gestation, the proportion of blood perfusing the lungs tends to increase. From the descending aorta, the blood supplies the remaining organs and the lower body. The hypogastric arteries branch off the internal iliac arteries and return to the placenta via the umbilical arteries.

The upper body and head are fed from arteries which branch off from the aortic arch before the insertion of the ductus arteriosus and the subsequent mixing of slightly less-well-oxygenated blood. The early branching of the coronary and carotid arteries means the heart and brain receive slightly better oxygenated blood. The advantages conferred by the early branching of the subclavian arteries which supply the upper limbs can be illustrated by the enhanced development of arms compared to the legs.

After birth

One of the most important transitional stages in the adaptation to extrauterine life is the establishment of the neonatal circulation. In fetal life, the source of oxygen is the placenta so most of the blood flow bypasses the fetal lungs. At birth, blood fully perfuses the lungs and flow through the fetal vascular structures ceases. At birth, these changes that mark the transfer of the fetal into adult-type circulation (see Fig. 15.4B) are not rapid or immediate. They are initiated within 60 s of delivery but may not be fully completed for a few weeks. The two determining

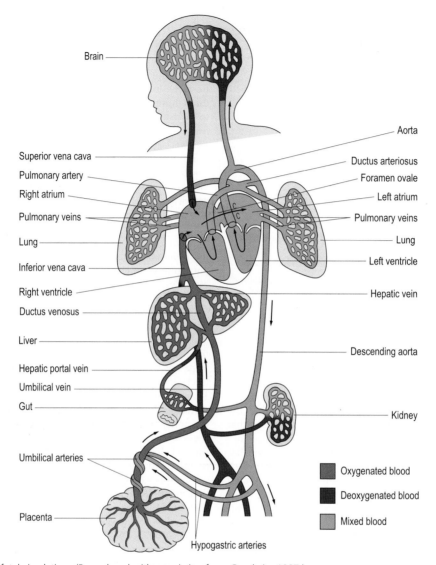

Fig. 15.3 The fetal circulation. (Reproduced with permission from Goodwin, 1997.)

events that initiate the closure of the fetal shunts are the arrest of the umbilical circulation, and therefore placental perfusion, and lung inflation and expansion, which results in increased pulmonary blood flow. The first breath results in lung expansion and vasodilatation of the pulmonary vessels in response to increased partial pressure of oxygen so blood flow to the lungs increases. The tortuosity of the capillaries is reduced and the pulmonary circulation changes from a high-resistance to a low-resistance pathway so 90% of the blood flows through the pulmonary vascular bed. There is a brief reversal of flow through the ductus arteriosus, which vasoconstricts in response to the change in oxygen level, mediated by prostaglandins, especially decreased prostaglandin PGE$_2$

(Thorburn, 1992). The placenta no longer contributes to prostaglandin production and prostaglandin breakdown is increased because more blood flows to the lungs where significant prostaglandin metabolism and breakdown occur.

The smooth muscle of the umbilical artery walls is not innervated but is irritable. Vasoconstriction is stimulated by stretching and handling the cord, by cooling and in response to stress-related catecholamine release. The thicker walls of the umbilical arteries are able to generate high intraluminal pressure, which arrests the placental circulation, preventing flow from the infant to the placenta. This is augmented by the increased synthesis of prostaglandins and thromboxanes in response to the raised

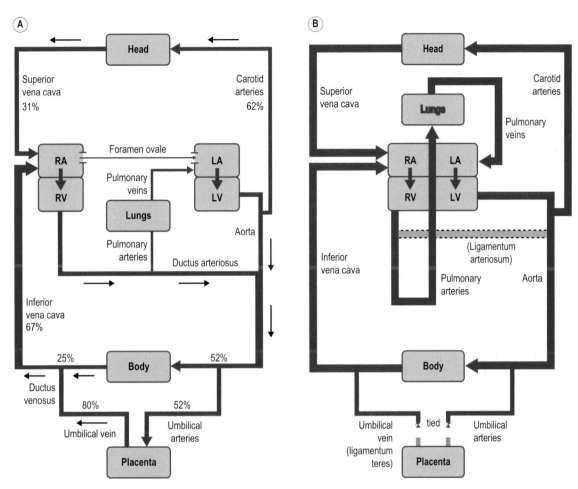

Fig. 15.4 Changes in circulation at birth: (A) fetal circulation showing oxygen saturation of blood; (B) neonatal circulation. (Reproduced with permission from Chamberlain et al., 1991.)

oxygen level due to breathing, which increases vessel irritability and vasoconstriction. The umbilical vein remains dilated; blood flow from the placenta to the infant can continue via gravity. Thus, initial neonatal blood volume is affected by the timing of clamping of the umbilical cord and by the relative positions of the infant and placenta at the time of clamping. The usual practice is to clamp the umbilical cord earlier if the baby is subject to fluid overload (hydropic), or if the baby is polycythaemic (e.g. infants of diabetic mothers or growth retarded), to limit the transfer of maternal analgesic agents or antibodies or to avoid possible baby-to-baby transfusions in the cases of multiple births (Kinmond et al., 1993).

The flap of the foramen ovale (Fig. 15.5) is pushed closed because the decreased umbilical flow results in a decreased venous return from the inferior vena cava so the pressure in the right atrium and PVR falls in response to changes in oxygenation. The increased pulmonary blood flow results

in an increased return to the left atrium and consequent increase in pressure. Thus, the pressure gradient across the foramen ovale is reversed. So at birth, PVR falls and SVR increases. The relatively thick layer of smooth muscle in the pulmonary blood vessels begins to thin from birth.

The closure of the fetal structures may not be immediate or permanent and may never be completed. The closure of the foramen ovale is reversible at first; interruption of ventilation or a drop in alveolar oxygenation results in constriction of the pulmonary capillaries and consequent reversal of pressure across the atria and reversion to fetal circulation. The incomplete closure can result in intermittent and reversible cyanotic episodes. After a few days of functional closure, the tissue associated with the foramen ovale fuses and closure becomes permanent. In many adults, a patent foramen ovale can be demonstrated (a probe can be passed through) although the pressure gradient maintains effective functional closure.

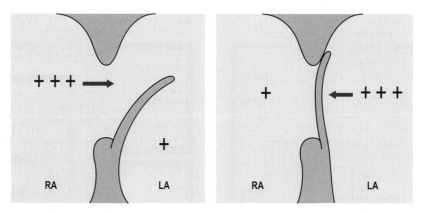

Fig. 15.5 Initiation of neonatal circulation and closure of the foramen ovale between the right atrium (RA) and left atrium (LA).

Intermittent flow through the ductus arteriosus may initially occur during each cardiac cycle when aortic pressure is maximal following ventricular contraction. Bradykinin released from the newly inflated lungs mediates the constriction of the ductus arteriosus. Production of prostaglandins, which had maintained the open ductus arteriosus in the fetus, is decreased as oxygenation increases. Most neonates have some degree of patency of the ductus arteriosus in the first 8 h of life but it becomes functionally closed within the first or second day (Askin, 2009a). Fibrolysis and obliteration of the lumen of the ductus arteriosus are usually complete within 3 weeks; continued patency is very serious and can result in left ventricular failure. The ductus venosus constricts when umbilical flow is halted. The obliterated vessels remain as anatomical ligaments; the slow closure of the umbilical vein and its degeneration into ligamentum teres are utilized as a route for neonatal blood transfusions if required.

The nervous control of the cardiovascular system is well developed in the neonate with mature physiological control of blood pressure and cardiac output demonstrable. The systemic arterial blood pressure is relatively low in the first few weeks as vascular tone develops which increases vascular resistance. Pulmonary arterial blood pressure is initially high but falls to mature values as pulmonary resistance falls. The neonate's heart rate is fast, as in the fetus. As in the fetus, control of cardiac output is largely achieved by changing heart rate because the heart is small and non-compliant and has a relatively thick wall. At birth, the wall of the right ventricle is thicker than the left, which hypertrophies in response to the changed postnatal circulation.

THE RESPIRATORY SYSTEM

The primitive air sacs are developed by the 20th week of gestation, and by 26 weeks respiratory bronchioles with a rich capillary supply are evident. Although the enzymes for synthesis of phospholipid/lipoprotein components of surfactant are present from week 18, the type II pneumocytes secrete surfactant only from week 26 with a surge in production after week 30. Surfactant, a detergent-like wetting agent, allows increased compliance, so the force required to inflate the alveoli is reduced thus increasing compliance. A lack of surfactant causes respiratory distress syndrome (RDS) (see below). The lecithin:sphingomyelin (L:S) ratio of the surfactant can be determined by amniocentesis indicating the maturity of the respiratory system (Fig. 15.6). By week 35, the L:S ratio in a healthily developing fetus is 2:1. This ratio is decreased in pre-eclampsia, prematurity, narcotic addiction, maternal diabetes and other problems in pregnancy. Administration of cortisol (dexamethasone) to the mother prior to delivery of a baby born from 24 to 34 weeks' gestation increases fetal surfactant production within 24 h and can be used to decrease the risk of RDS (Hutchison, 1994).Variations (polymorphisms) in the genes for components of surfactant are associated with a range of inherited neonatal respiratory problems including bronchopulmonary dysplasia (BPD), (RDS) and respiratory syncytial virus (RSV) bronchiolitis and may influence susceptibility to influenza virus (Hallman and Haataja, 2006). Premature infants, particularly those born before 28 weeks, have immature alveoli with fewer type II cells and may require instillation of exogenous surfactant down endotracheal tubes to alleviate respiratory distress. Poor ventilation suppresses surfactant secretion so the severity of hypoxia, hypercapnia and acidosis is worsened and respiratory muscle activity is compromised which further compromises surfactant production.

The lungs

Before birth

In fetal life, the lungs are filled by fluid secreted by the lung epithelium; the lung fluid is essential for growth and development of the lungs and this fluid exchanges

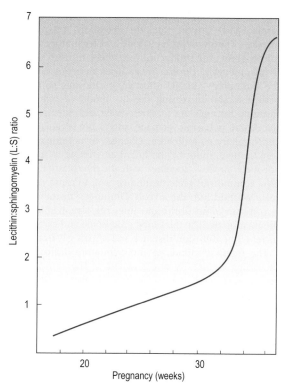

Fig. 15.6 Lecithin:sphingomyelin (L:S) concentration in the amniotic fluid; the concentration rises very sharply after 30 weeks' gestation. (Reproduced with permission from Chamberlain et al., 1991.)

with amniotic fluid. At birth, the neonate has to rapidly clear fluid from its air-spaces; 10–25 mL/kg fluid will be expelled or resorbed. Fetal breathing movements (FBM) are observed on ultrasound from the first trimester. Initially, they are intermittent, rapid and irregular. As gestation progresses, FBM increase in strength and frequency, occurring up to 80% of the time in an organized episodic pattern (Nijhuis, 2003). The lung fluid is 'breathed' out by the fetus into the amniotic fluid. Patterns of FBM dominate during the daytime and are correlated with fetal behavioural states. Fetal wakefulness and arousal are associated with sustained vigorous respiratory patterns. Quiet sleep is associated with an absence of FBM. Adrenergic and cholinergic compounds, prostaglandin synthesis inhibitors and raised maternal carbon dioxide levels stimulate FBM. They are inhibited by hypoglycaemia, cigarette smoking, alcohol consumption and accelerated labour. Despite the relatively low partial pressure of oxygen and high partial pressure of carbon dioxide, the fetus makes only shallow respiratory movements although severe hypoxia and acidosis may stimulate gasping. Mild hypoxia leads to quiet sleep and reduced energy expenditure and oxygen consumption, which may be protective.

The movement of the diaphragm generates about 25 mmHg pressure for between 1 and 4 h per day in a pattern that coincides with rapid eye movement (REM) sleep but not during slow-wave sleep or fetal 'wakefulness'. FBM are important in lung development (Harding and Hooper, 1996), promoting growth and allowing rehearsal of the respiratory actions. Lung development is retarded in conditions where FBM are limited such as congenital disorders of the diaphragm or nervous system. The fluid volume in the fetal airways correlates with the functional residual capacity in postnatal life (Strang, 1991).

After birth

The most urgent need after delivery is the initiation of ventilation; the neonate has to clear its lungs of fluid, establish regular breathing and increase pulmonary blood flow to match pulmonary perfusion to ventilation. Many factors interact to stimulate the first breath, including changes in temperature and state. The mild asphyxia (decreased oxygen concentration, raised carbon dioxide concentration) and acidosis (decreased pH) due to flow in the cord ceasing sensitize the fetal aortic, carotid and central (medullary) chemoreceptors that increase ventilatory drive. Tactile stimulation, such as that which occurs during delivery, also promotes respiration. In additional, it is thought that the placental prostaglandins may inhibit breathing (decreased oxygen concentration, raised carbon dioxide concentration). The surge of endogenous steroids and catecholamines associated with labour also contributes; infants who do not experience labour are more likely to retain residual fluid in their lungs and have less efficient respiratory performance.

The fluid-filled lung with collapsed alveoli and undispersed surfactant proffers a high resistance to inflation and the first breath requires considerable effort. The diaphragm contracts strongly and the complaint flexible ribs and sternum of the newborn baby are pulled concave in the effort of the first breath. Once the lungs are inflated, the lung fluid is forced into the alveoli where it aids dispersal of surfactant and is rapidly resorbed into the pulmonary lymphatic vessels. Subsequent breaths require fewer changes in pressure and less mechanical work. The thoracic compression of a vaginal delivery contributes to fluid loss from the upper respiratory tract; the compression of the chest (known as the 'vaginal squeeze') creates negative pressure which draws air into the lungs and they re-expand. Most of the fluid clearance is due to a change in the lung epithelium from being a predominantly chloride-secreting membrane at birth to being predominantly a sodium absorbing membrane after birth (Jain and Eaton, 2006).

Most babies gasp within 6 s and have patterns of normal breathing and gas exchange within 15 min. Initially the newborn infant has metabolic and respiratory acidosis due to decreased oxygen concentrations (resulting in increased lactic acid) and increased carbon dioxide levels, respectively; this acid–base imbalance is corrected as ventilation improves. The risk of transient tachypnoea of the newborn (TTN) is increased in babies who are delivered by caesarean section or those who experience perinatal hypoxia. It is thought that TTN is due to immaturity of the sodium transport mechanisms of the lung epithelium (Jain and Eaton, 2006).

The rate of ventilation of the newborn is high compared with an adult but is similar when relative size is taken into account. Ventilation is often irregular with the baby exhibiting periods of fetal-like shallow breathing. The reflexes associated with lung inflation also appear to be different. As well as the Hering–Breuer Reflex (where filling of the lungs increases expiratory centre activity), the newborn infant demonstrates Paradoxical Reflex of Head (where filling the lungs excites the inspiratory centre thus stimulating further inspiration) (Givan, 2003). For the first few weeks, babies breathe via the nose and suck via the mouth. Control of ventilation by chemoreceptors is functional but qualitatively different in that hypoxia tends to increase depth of respiration (rather than respiratory rate) and that the response is temperature-dependent and is abolished in cold temperatures. The chemoreceptors seem to be more sensitive to raised carbon dioxide levels.

Babies have a relatively large oxygen consumption, which reflects their heat generation and that their more metabolically active tissues (e.g. liver and brain) are proportionately larger. The high airway resistance means that the energy cost of respiration is higher. PVR drops 6–8 weeks after birth when the diameter of the small arterioles increases. The relatively high requirement for oxygen means that neonates are more susceptible to asphyxia than other age groups. Neonatal resuscitation aims to prevent mortality and morbidity. Hypothermic neonates are predisposed to hypoglycaemia and acidosis. Acidosis compromises respiration because it increases PVR and suppresses both respiratory drive and surfactant production. The aims of neonatal resuscitation are to promote and maintain adequate ventilation and oxygenation, to initiate and maintain adequate cardiac output and perfusion and to maintain body temperature and adequate blood glucose levels.

Respiratory distress syndrome

RDS is caused by a deficiency in surfactant, which results in alveolar collapse and increased airway resistance. Surfactant deficiency is usually inversely related to gestational age and lung maturity. Abnormal pH, stress and inadequate pulmonary perfusion also inhibit surfactant synthesis and recycling. RDS is worsened by asphyxia and is the most common cause of respiratory failure in the preterm infant. The reduced surface tension affects alveoli expansion. Small alveoli tend to collapse and normal alveoli are overdistended. Segments of the lung close and hypoxaemia and carbon dioxide retention progressively increase. The resulting metabolic and respiratory acidosis further limits the production of surfactant from the type II pneumocytes. Hypoxaemia causes vasoconstriction of the pulmonary arteries thus compromising pulmonary perfusion and increasing the likelihood of right-to-left shunting through the foramen ovale and ductus arteriosus. Local ischaemic damage affects the alveolar tissue and capillary endothelium. Changes in pulmonary pressure brought about by the infant attempting to maintain adequate air flow, together with the low plasma protein level common in preterm infants, tend to cause displacement of fluid into the alveoli. Fibrinogen in the exudate is converted into fibrin and lines the alveoli thickening the membrane. The thickened membrane and excess fluid increase the diffusion distance and impair gas transfer.

The infant responds to the respiratory difficulties by increasing respiratory rate and effort. The clinical signs appear early and increase in severity over 2 or 3 days. The infant may grunt and exhibit oedema and cyanosis. Cyanosis tends to be progressive and is due to high levels of deoxygenated haemoglobin in the capillaries. It is enhanced by right-to-left shunting, alveolar hypoventilation and impaired gas diffusion across the alveolar membranes. The baby grunts because expiration is against a partially closed glottis, which increases pressure and retards expiratory flow, therefore increasing gas exchange. RDS risk is increased in prematurity, babies of diabetic mothers (because insulin is antagonistic to cortisol), antepartum haemorrhage and second-born twins. Male babies are twice as susceptible to RDS. Chronic hypertension, maternal heroin addiction, pre-eclampsia and growth retardation appear to protect against RDS.

TEMPERATURE REGULATION

Before birth

In utero, the fetus depends on its mother for temperature regulation. It loses heat via the placenta and via conduction (from skin to amniotic fluid to uterus). The fetus is a net heat producer although raised maternal temperature may compromise it (Edwards et al., 1997). Brown fat is actively inhibited and fetal oxygen consumption is about 30% of postnatal levels. Fetal temperature is maintained at about 0.5°C above maternal temperature and the fetus does not expend energy in keeping warm. Research has focused on raised maternal temperature due to fever, exercise and external raised temperature (such as hot baths and saunas). The results are inconclusive. However, maternal fever has effects not only on temperature gradients but also on oxygen consumption and haemodynamics and may be associated with teratogenesis and preterm labour.

After birth

The infant is usually born into a wet and relatively cold environment. As environmental temperature is usually lower than maternal temperature, the baby will experience a temperature loss at birth. Heat transfer is affected by two gradients: the internal gradient involving transfer from the core to the surface of the baby and the external gradient involving heat transfer from the body surface to the environment. Cooling is usually rapid at a rate of 0.2–1.0°C per minute depending on the environmental factors and the gestational age of the infant (which affects body composition). Transfer of heat through the internal gradient depends on insulation and blood flow. Neonates are predisposed to heat loss; they have less subcutaneous fat than adults do (about 16% body fat compared with 30%), a higher surface area:mass ratio (about three times the relative surface area of an adult) and a lower ability to shiver. Should the baby be born small, it will not only have an even larger surface area:mass ratio but also the insulation provided by its subcutaneous fat will also be further compromised and skin permeability will be increased. Small-for-dates babies have proportionately bigger heads and higher metabolism and are disadvantaged in that their heat losses are higher. Changes in peripheral circulation affect heat loss via conduction.

Heat loss across the external gradient depends on the temperature difference between the body and the environment. Conduction, convection, evaporation and radiation transfer heat from the baby. Warming objects that will come into contact with the neonate, and increasing insulation by wrapping, limit heat loss by conduction. Evaporation offers the greatest route for heat loss immediately after delivery but drying the baby, especially the head, immediately after delivery is effective at reducing the loss. Skin keratinization is inadequate in immature infants so evaporative heat losses are higher. Evaporative insensible heat loss increases with respiratory problems, activity, the use of radiant heaters or phototherapy and low relative humidity. Convective losses are related to draughts and are affected by ambient temperature and humidity. Higher air temperatures, minimal air circulation, swaddling and baby hats reduce heat loss by convection. Radiation is the major form of heat loss from babies in incubators. It involves the transfer of radiant energy to surrounding objects not directly in contact with the baby. Consideration therefore has to be given to the temperature of objects in the local environment including the incubator, walls and windows. Skin-to-skin contact with the mother immediately following birth is a very efficient way of reducing heat loss from the neonate. The large skin area and the softness of the breasts enable a large amount of maternal skin to come into direct contact with the baby's skin surface.

The mechanisms of heat conservation and generation mediated by the peripheral nervous system are insufficient in the neonate (Okken, 1991). Infants can produce heat from metabolic processes and by increasing activity. Postural changes are also important in conserving heat. Shivering is not so important in infants but heat generation by non-shivering thermogenesis (NST) is important. NST takes place in brown adipose tissue (BAT), a specialized type of adipose tissue that is well vascularized, particularly by sympathetic nerves, and has cells densely packed with mitochondria (Fig. 15.7).

Fig. 15.7 Structures and development of white and brown adipose tissue. (Reproduced with permission from Hull, 1966.)

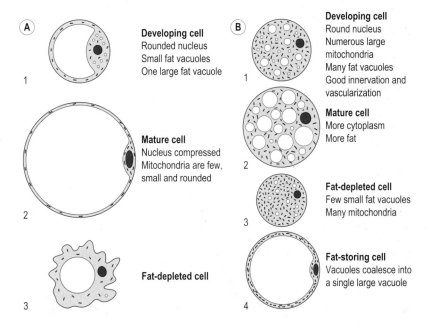

(A)

1 Developing cell
Rounded nucleus
Small fat vacuoles
One large fat vacuole

2 Mature cell
Nucleus compressed
Mitochondria are few, small and rounded

3 Fat-depleted cell

(B)

1 Developing cell
Round nucleus
Numerous large mitochondria
Many fat vacuoles
Good innervation and vascularization

2 Mature cell
More cytoplasm
More fat

3 Fat-depleted cell
Few small fat vacuoles
Many mitochondria

4 Fat-storing cell
Vacuoles coalesce into a single large vacuole

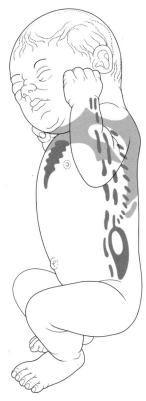

Fig. 15.8 Location of brown adipose tissue in the human infant.

In humans, BAT is mostly replaced by white adipose tissue (WAT); adults have very few BAT cells which are interspersed with WAT (Wolf, 2009). However, BAT has a major role in heat production in the neonate. BAT is formed from about 30 weeks' gestation until about 4 weeks' postbirth. Fat mass is significantly altered by maternal nutrition and gestational length; stores of BAT (and white fat) are lower in preterm infants. BAT comprises about 2–7% of birth weight and is predominantly located around the core organs (Fig. 15.8). It generates heat by uncoupling electron transport from oxidative phosphorylation in the mitochondria so the energy released by electron transport will not be used to synthesize ATP but will be liberated as heat instead (Fig. 15.9). Fifty percentage of cellular respiration is uncoupled from ATP formation in BAT (Wolf, 2009). The unique uncoupling protein (UCP1) is a proton transporter located in the inner mitochondrial membrane. UCP1 causes protons to leak across the inner mitochondrial membrane so the electrochemical gradient, that usually drives ATP production, is lost and heat is produced. When UCP1 is maximally activated, it allows the production of at least 100 times as much heat from BAT compared to other tissue. UCP1 is synthesized during the maturation of fetal fat (Symonds et al., 2003). At birth, the activation of BAT is accompanied by mobilization of fat and a marked increase in lipolysis. Thermogenesis by BAT is inhibited in the fetus by PGE_2 and prostacyclin (PGI_2) produced by the placenta. The placenta also suppresses formation of active T_3 (tri-iodothyronine) from T_4 (thyroxine) (see below).

Heat production per unit mass of the neonate is higher than that of an adult; thermogenesis begins when a critical temperature difference of 12 °C between the environment and the skin is exceeded. The drop in temperature stimulates release of noradrenaline from sympathetic nerve endings that stimulate the brown adipose cells (Gunn et al., 1991). At birth, catecholamines from the adrenal medulla and rise in T_3 production by the thyroid gland augment the effect of noradrenaline. Inhibition of BAT by the placenta ceases. Oxygen consumption and metabolic rate increase markedly in response to a drop in temperature. Heat generation involves lipolysis of BAT, which depends on the availability of oxygen, ATP and glucose. There is a strong interrelationship between ventilation, feeding and temperature regulation, which means that hypoglycaemia, hypoxia or acidosis can affect the ability of the neonate to produce heat (Fig. 15.10). Persistent hypothermia can therefore result in metabolic acidosis (due to increased lactic acid production), decreased surfactant production and, if it is chronic, compromised growth. Cold stress or hypothermia will increase metabolic rate and peripheral and pulmonary vasoconstriction. The increased metabolic rate will increase oxygen demand. Peripheral and pulmonary vasoconstriction can compromise oxygenation and perfusion efficiency. Tissue hypoxia may increase acidosis because anaerobic metabolism increases lactic acid production. Hypoxia inhibits metabolic rate and compromises the thermal response; it also affects surfactant production.

Mechanisms for losing heat are not well developed in the neonate (Power, 1992). The neonate can lose some heat by sweating (which increases evaporation) but peripheral vasodilatation is the main source of heat loss. Although the density of neonatal sweat glands is high in some areas, they are less responsive and less efficient at sweat production. Phototherapy increases water loss. Sweating is more inefficient in preterm babies and those with central nervous system dysfunction. As the baby gets older and can rely on physical methods of generating heat, NST becomes less important. BAT gradually diminishes in the first year.

WAT provides both insulation and an energy reserve. Development of body fat in the fetus is under nutritional constraint whereas postnatal growth is controlled by genetic potential. Compared to other mammals,

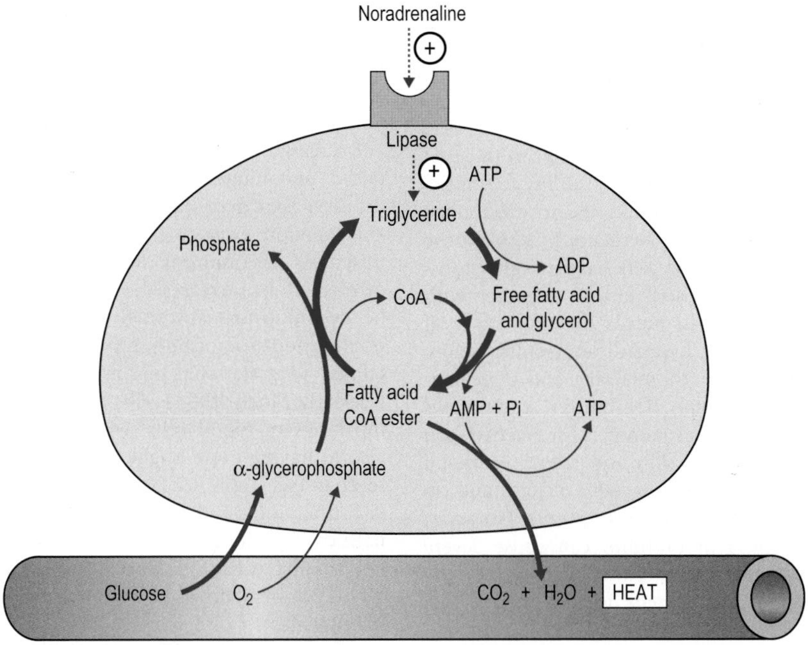

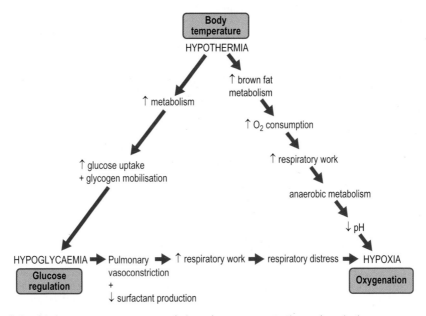

Fig. 15.9 Metabolic pathways in brown adipose tissue: triglycerides break down to yield useful heat (about 160 kcal/mol are produced during each turn of the cycle). (Reproduced with permission from Begley et al., 1978.)

Fig. 15.10 Interrelationship between temperature regulation, glucose concentration and respiration.

human infants are not only extremely fat at birth but also they continue to increase in adiposity during early postnatal life. Although it has been suggested that the role of the fat is insulation required as compensation for human hairlessness, evidence to support this is weak. A more likely explanation is that the adipose tissue acts as an energy reserve both to support the demands of a large brain and to protect the infant from nutritional disruption at birth and weaning or during infection (Kuzawa, 1998).

THE NEONATAL LIVER

Bilirubin

The functions of the neonatal liver are similar to those of an adult but are relatively immature. The ability to synthesize plasma proteins such as albumin and to metabolize foreign substances is inefficient. Neonates produce more bilirubin because the red blood cells have a higher turnover and shorter lifespan. These factors, together with immature intestinal processes, means the neonate is at increased risk of developing hyperbilirubinaemia. Before birth, bilirubin is cleared by the placenta and then handled by maternal metabolism. If bilirubin accumulates in the serum of the neonate, jaundice (or icterus) can occur; yellow staining of the skin and sclera. Neonatal jaundice is common affecting up to 60% of term and up to 80% of preterm infants (Juretschke, 2005). However, markedly elevated levels of bilirubin can cause severe jaundice and potentially cause brain damage. As the blood–brain barrier of the neonate is more permeable, free bilirubin can access the brain easily and in sufficient concentrations can deposit in the basal ganglia causing kernicterus (brain tissue is heavily stained with bilirubin). Bilirubin encephalopathy, damage to the brain by bilirubin deposits, results in a range of symptoms from convulsions and abnormal behaviour such as lethargy, hypotonia and poor suck to cerebral palsy, deafness or death.

Physiological jaundice is due to normal breakdown of red blood cells and neonatal immaturity; it is usually mild and resolves relatively quickly. Severe jaundice may result from increased production of bilirubin and/or decreased excretion. Risk factors include sepsis (which compromises the liver's ability to breakdown excess haemoglobin), excessive trauma and interstitial bleeding (e.g. haematomas, excess bruising, etc), polycythaemia, AB rhesus incompatibility (neonatal blood cells are destroyed by maternal antibodies) and liver abnormalities. In such cases, kernicterus is more likely to occur and so careful monitoring of serum bilirubin levels is required.

Bilirubin is a breakdown product of haemoglobin from red blood cells (Fig. 15.11). Iron from red blood cells is recycled. Haem, the pigment, is degraded by macrophages of the reticuloendothelial system to biliverdin and then to bilirubin. Unconjugated (indirect) bilirubin is insoluble and cannot be excreted. It is transported bound to plasma albumin to the liver to be metabolized into conjugated (direct) bilirubin, which is soluble. Conjugation involves binding of glucuronide sugars to bilirubin forming bilirubin diglucuronide. Conjugated bilirubin is excreted into bile and so into the duodenum. It is a major component of bile and faeces. In the intestine, conjugated bilirubin is further metabolized by bacterial flora to produce urobilin and stercobilin (which give the characteristic colour of faeces). Some of the breakdown products of bacterial metabolism of bilirubin are deconjugated and absorbed across the gut wall to be recirculated. Small amounts of bilirubin are also excreted via the kidneys.

Decreased production of plasma proteins can result in raised unconjugated bilirubin levels. The pathways in the liver that deconjugate bilirubin to its water soluble, and therefore excretable, metabolite may also be compromised. As meconium is rich in bilirubin, delayed passage of meconium increases the possibility that bilirubin will be deconjugated, absorbed and re-enter the circulating pool. Production of bilirubin in neonates is inversely correlated to gestational age and remains high for a few weeks (Lockitch, 1994). This is partly due to high circulating levels of blood cells, which are then removed, and also to having more fragile red blood cells with a shorter lifespan (see Table 15.1). The risk of hyperbilirubinaemia is further increased by other conditions that stress this pathway such as excess blood cell breakdown (as in excessive trauma at birth or due to infection) or increased red blood cell breakdown (as in polycythaemia due to maternal diabetes).

Infants are vulnerable to a number of diseases which are associated with oxidative injury including retinopathy of prematurity, necrotising enterocolitis, intraventricular haemorrhage and BPD. It has been suggested that as bilirubin has antioxidant properties, there may be a potential benefit of raised levels of bilirubin in early infancy to help protect infants from oxidative damage (Juretschke, 2005).

Fuel storage

Fetal metabolism is dominated by anabolic pathways, whereas the neonate has to catabolize fuel stores to provide nutrients between periodic neonatal feeds (Hay, 1994). The last weeks of gestation are an important time for laying down lipids and glycogen. During fetal life, glycogen is stored in the liver and skeletal muscle. Hepatic glycogen provides the substrate for energy metabolism during delivery and the first few hours of postnatal life (Nelson, 1994). Fat stores serve as an alternative energy source; the neonate markedly increases fatty acid oxidation and uses ketone bodies for energy production. In the first few days of life, the respiratory quotient falls from 1.0 (as glucose sources are exhausted) to about 0.7 (a value similar to that seen in adult diabetics) as fat and protein are mobilized until adequate milk is consumed.

Glucose regulation

Thyroxine (T_4) is relatively inactive and is usually converted to active tri-iodothyronine (T_3). Fetal T_3 levels are low because fetal liver levels of outer-ring deiodinase are low and placental levels of inner-ring deiodinase are high,

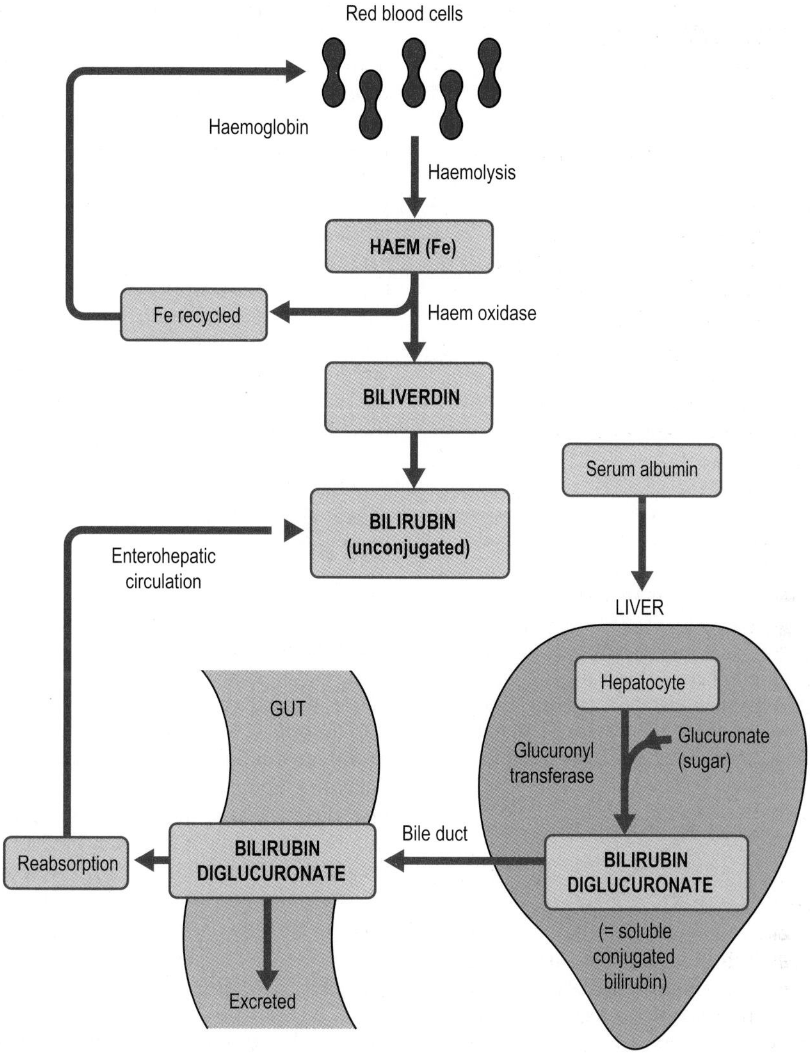

Fig. 15.11 Breakdown of haemoglobin to form bilirubin.

both of which drive preferential production of inactive reverse T_3. The resulting low level of the active thyroid hormone T_3 can support brain development but suppresses oxygen consumption by non-neural tissues and inhibits thermogenesis. In late gestation, the rise in glucocorticoids induces expression of outer-ring deiodinase in the fetal liver so production of fetal T_3 increases markedly. The rise in T_3 plays a role not only in hepatic enzyme activity but also in tissue maturation and lung and bone development. At birth, the T_3 levels increase further as the inner-ring deiodinase is reduced on placental separation, and evaporative cooling induces a rise in thyroid-stimulating hormone (TSH, thyrotrophin), which further stimulates hormone production by the thyroid gland.

Adipose tissue significantly contributes to the conversion of T_4 to T_3 after delivery; smaller fat depots result in less thyroid hormone production, potentially further compromising thermogenesis in premature infants.

Blood glucose levels in the neonate tend to fall after delivery because the immature liver is better at promoting glycogen synthesis than glycogenolysis, and because the baby has increased activity and metabolism at birth. At birth, neonatal glucose concentrations are about 70% of maternal levels (Aylott, 2006) and falls to its lowest point 1–2 h later. The neonate has a high requirement for glucose because it has a relatively large brain and more and larger red blood cells. The stress of delivery and cooling at birth stimulate the release of catecholamines, which stimulate glucagon release and suppress insulin release and are important in activating the metabolic pathways in the liver. The neonate is unable to regulate blood glucose efficiently (Smith, 1995) and is usually hypoglycaemic (glucose levels are about 2 mmol/L) (Box 15.5). The enzymes involving glucose metabolism do not reach optimal levels in the liver for 2–3 weeks, so glycogenolysis (mobilization of glycogen stores) and gluconeogenesis (hepatic synthesis of glucose from substrates) are relatively slow in correcting falls in blood glucose. Lipolysis generates ketones which are used as alternative sources of energy for brain metabolism. If the delivery is protracted, the neonate may deplete its glycogen stores. Also the response to raised levels of glucose is slow; although adequate concentrations of insulin are present in the pancreas, the β-cells initially lack sensitivity to glucose, responding better to amino acids. Thus, neonatal blood glucose levels fluctuate and hypoglycaemia may occur because hepatic glucose production is inadequate or there is excess insulin secretion (common in the infants of mothers with gestational diabetes). Hypoxia and hypothermia can exacerbate hypoglycaemia because of the

energetic costs of respiration and heat production, respectively. Blood glucose values as low as 1.0 mmol/L have been recorded. In an adult, such a level of hypoglycaemia would cause convulsions, hypoglycaemic coma and probable neurological damage, whereas in the newborn they might cause an apnoeic attack. The central nervous system of the neonate exhibits a degree of plasticity and is partially protected as it can utilize fatty acids and ketones efficiently. Physiological responses to hypoglycaemia activate the sympathetic nervous system and cause neuroglycopenia. Clinical signs of hypoglycaemia can include changes in level of consciousness (such as lethargy and drowsiness), changes in behaviour (such as irritability and jitteriness, hypotonia and poor feeding) and changes in vital signs (such as apnoea, hypothermia, bradycardia, bounding pulse and sweating).

THE GASTROINTESTINAL SYSTEM AT BIRTH

The gut completes anatomical development by week 24 and the term neonate is able to digest and absorb milk from birth. The fetus swallows amniotic fluid which passes through the gut. Water, electrolytes and glucose are absorbed in the small intestine. Species-specific growth factors in milk are important in promoting postnatal development of the gut. The neonatal gut has immature digestive and absorptive capacities but there are a number of compensatory mechanisms, particularly for babies who are breastfed who receive both digestive enzymes and growth factors that stimulate gut development in the milk (Lonnerdal, 2003).

Feeding reflexes

From birth, a normal infant can suck from the breast, convey milk to the back of the mouth and swallow it for a period of 5–10 min while breathing normally. There is an innate programme of reflexes and behaviour, which become evident within an hour or so following delivery, including the ability to move from the mother's abdomen to her breast, coordinated hand–mouth activity, rooting for the nipple, attaching to the breast and feeding vigorously before falling asleep. Touching the palate triggers the sucking reflex. The neonate exhibits rhythmic jaw action, which creates a negative pressure, and the peristaltic action of the tongue and jaw strips milk from the breast and moves it to the throat thus triggering the swallowing reflex. These breastfeeding reflexes are strong at birth in the normal neonate and are evident in preterm babies from about 32 weeks (about 1200 g). Extremely preterm babies and those that are sick or have a very low birth weight have markedly decreased or absent reflexes. Other babies who experience feeding problems include those with physical problems such as cleft lip or palate and those subjected to obstetric sedation, analgesia or extreme stress at birth.

The sucking and swallowing reflexes are aided by the particular morphological configuration of the neonate's mouth, which has a proportionately longer soft palate. The neonate also has an extrusion reflex in response to the presence of solid or semisolid material in the mouth. This reflex is lost at 4–6 months and is replaced by a pattern of rhythmic biting movements coinciding with the development of the first teeth at 7–9 months.

Hormone and enzyme production

Gastric secretion is developed but low; responses to gut regulatory hormones appear also to be low. The effect is that the gastric juice has a pH close to neutral (compared with a pH of 2 in an adult's stomach). The high gastric pH means that salivary amylase is not inactivated in the stomach so starch digestion can continue. Reflux of gastric contents is common, as the lower oesophageal sphincter is immature in both musculature and neurological control. Less-acidic gastric juice does not cause painful tissue damage to the oesophageal mucosa but also it is less effective at denaturing proteins including microorganisms. It has been suggested that a reflux of human milk is advantageous as very small amounts of milk may reach the upper part of the respiratory tract conferring an immunological benefit there. Breastfed babies have a lower incidence of respiratory problems. Decreased acid production in the stomach means that the activation of pepsinogen to pepsin is restricted, limiting protein digestion in the stomach. The decreased acidity and protein digestion may enhance the defence mechanism promoting the activity of immunoglobulins and antigen recognition in the gastrointestinal tract as these proteins survive the gentler gastric environment.

Pancreatic amylase levels are low in the newborn but breast milk contains mammary amylase, which can augment starch digestion. Colostrum is particularly rich in mammary amylase. Lactase activity is relatively late in developing, reaching adequate levels after 36 weeks' gestation. However, many preterm babies can digest lactose satisfactorily as unabsorbed lactose can be metabolized by colonic bacteria to short-chain fatty acids, which can then be absorbed thus salvaging the energy. The low pancreatic lipase levels are compensated for by lingual and gastric lipase produced by the neonate (stimulated by suckling) and by bile salt-stimulated lipase in human milk. Bile acid formation is low but human milk is rich in taurine, which is used for neonatal conjugation of bile salts.

Bowel movements

Passage of meconium, a mix of mucus, epithelial and gut cells, larger molecules and skin cell debris from the amniotic fluid, fatty acids and bile pigments (which gives it the characteristic greenish-black colour) confirms that the lower bowel is patent. (Usually defaecation does not occur in utero unless the fetus is stressed.) Passage of a changing stool (meconium and food residue), usually within 24 h, indicates the whole gut is patent. Slow (more than 48 h after birth) or absent passage of meconium can indicate Hirschsprung's disease, impaired motility of the colon due to the absence of ganglion cells; diagnosis is usually made following biopsy of the bowel wall. At birth, the stomach capacity is 10–20 mL, which rapidly increases to 200 mL by 1 year.

THE KIDNEYS

Before birth

In utero, from 9 to 10 weeks' gestation, the fetus produces large volumes of hypotonic (dilute) urine, which is an important contributor to amniotic fluid (Box 15.6). However, the regulatory and excretory functions of the kidneys are minimal before birth (Guillery, 1997). The placenta corrects any osmotic imbalance. Mature kidney function is not developed until about 1 month; until then the urine is fetal-like. The neonatal kidneys, weighing about 12.5 g each, have a low glomerular filtration rate (GFR) and relatively low surface area. The ability to reabsorb or excrete sodium (Na^+) is poor so the urine produced is of low specific gravity and hypotonic, reaching 1.5 times plasma concentration (700–800 mOsm) compared to adult values of three to five times plasma concentration (1200–1400 mOsm).

After birth

At birth, the normal obligatory water loss means the baby loses 5–10% of its birth weight in the first 4 days as a

---

Box 15.6 **Clinical symptoms of Potter's syndrome**

- Bilateral renal agenesis (absence of kidneys)
- Urine is not excreted into amniotic fluid
- Results in oligohydramnios (defined as less than 500 mL of amniotic fluid at term)
- Incidence: about one in 3000 live births
- Incompatible with postnatal life; most affected babies die within a few hours of birth
- Causes: pulmonary hypoplasia because of restricted space for thoracic expansion and an imbalance of fluid for filling the lungs; musculoskeletal abnormalities because fetal movement is constrained; abnormal facies because face is moulded by compression; cord compression in labour and fetal distress (Scott and Goodburn, 1995)

result of the loss of water and Na^+. Neonatal renal function can efficiently prevent dehydration and eliminate the lower level of metabolic waste products of the breastfed infant. Because the newborn infant does not retain Na^+ efficiently, it is vulnerable to dehydration. Changing fluid intake (or increasing the solute load) can result in osmotic imbalance, acidosis or dehydration. The risks are lower if the baby is feeding on demand; however, the very immature renal function of preterm babies requires careful calculation of fluid and electrolyte balance as Na^+-rich urine may be produced despite low plasma Na^+ levels. This can be crucial if there is high extrarenal water loss, for instance in the presence of fever or high ambient temperature.

The ability to excrete protons or hydrogen ions (H^+) is also limited, thus increasing the neonate's susceptibility to acidosis. Elimination of drugs such as antibiotics cleared by the renal system is decreased so the half-life of the drug in the circulation is increased necessitating a requirement for decreased frequency of dose. The neonate should urinate within 24 h of delivery. Initially, 15–30 mL/kg of urine is produced per day increasing to 100–200 mL/kg by day 7 as the fluid intake increases. Mature renal function is not achieved until 12 months to 2 years.

THE NERVOUS SYSTEM

Before birth

The fetus responds to noises, intense light, noxious stimulation of the skin and decreased temperature by changing autonomic responses such as heart rate and by moving. Fetal movements can be felt from about week 14; the 'exercise' is thought to aid muscle growth and limb development. By term, the nervous system is prepared to process and receive information. Human cortical function is relatively immature compared with that of some other mammalian species. Complete myelination of the long motor pathways occurs after birth, therefore fine movements of the fingers, for instance, are not evident until several months after birth.

After birth

After birth, the nervous system undergoes accelerated development in response to increased sensory input. Reflexes may be slightly depressed for the first 24 h, particularly if there has been transplacental transfer of narcotic analgesia, after which several reflexes can be elicited. In cases of severe asphyxia, low Apgar scores (see p. 399) or neurological damage, reflexes are depressed, abnormal and may take longer to appear. The grasping reflex and the Moro embrace are used to assess the reflex ability of the newborn. Babies also demonstrate a strong palmar grasp and a rhythmic stepping movement. Many reflexes common to the neonate disappear unless there is pathological interference, in which case they may be exhibited in the adult, for example Babinski's reflex. The baby exhibits general awareness to its surroundings and reacts to sound and light.

Babies are born with active sensory pathways. Studies have demonstrated that neonates can recognize the smell of their mother's milk. They can differentiate between tastes and appear to have a preference for sweet tastes. Although babies can see at birth, there are big postnatal developments in visual capability, particularly in the first 6 months. The neonate has limited visual acuity but appears to focus at a distance of 20 cm. From birth, babies can discriminate between contrast and contours and can follow movement. The neonate is able to hear and discriminate between sounds particularly those of low- to middle-range frequency. Studies have demonstrated a neonate's ability to recognize the characteristics of their mother's voice and to demonstrate a preference for rhythmic sing-song intonation. Neonates are reassured by the rhythmic sounds of breathing, heartbeat and gut peristalsis, which they hear, for instance, while being held. Newborn infants can be trained to activate a tape recorder by sucking non-nutritively on a modified nipple; they demonstrate that they recognize not only their mother's voice but also particular passages of a book that they were read in utero (Lipsitt and Rovee-Collier, 2001). The development of motor function is described by the 'Jacksonian principle', a hierarchical model whereby the last reflexes to develop are the first to be lost when the organism degenerates and dies. This pattern occurs because the first reflexes to develop are well rehearsed and require less oxygen to be initiated than more recent reflexes. The order of sensory development (tactile, vestibular, thermal, chemical, auditory and visual) is also reversed during injury, disease or ageing.

SLEEP AND BEHAVIOURAL STATES

The fetus exhibits slow-wave and REM sleep between patterns of wakefulness. The neonate sleeps about 16 h per day, 40% in REM sleep, compared with a total of 12 h asleep at 2 years of age (20% in REM sleep). Sleep patterns are not diurnal and do not follow a light–dark cycle. Six sleep–wake states are recognized: quiet (deep) sleep, active (light) sleep, drowsy state, awake (quiet) alert, active alert and crying (Wolff, 1966). The proportion of time in each state varies with postconceptual age. Quiet deep sleep is restful and the baby is in an anabolic state when growth hormone secretion is high, mitotic rate is high, oxygen consumption is low and there is little movement. In active sleep, the eyes are closed but the baby moves its face and extremities. Respiration and heart rate are irregular. The baby exhibits 'paradoxical' REM sleep, in which the brain activity is similar to awake states. This state is associated with learning and synapse development. The drowsy state is transitional between being awake and asleep. The eyes are open and the baby is alert but has little movement. The baby appears to focus on visual stimuli and appears to be processing sensory information. In the active alert state, respiration rate is increased and is irregular. There are skin colour changes, much activity and the baby has increased sensitivity to stimuli. Crying is the method of communication usually in response to unpleasant stimuli. Characteristically, neonates close their eyes, grimace and make sounds. However, preterm infants may not be capable of making a noise.

At one time, it was believed that the immature degree of myelination and lack of experience meant that neonates were unable to perceive pain. In fact, not only do the anatomical and functional requirements for pain perception develop early and the fetus, preterm and term infant demonstrate similar physiological responses to the adult, but there is also evidence that pain perception is more intense and that early experience of pain has long-term developmental and behavioural consequences (Taddio and Katz, 2004). Abundant sensory fibres, a functional spinal reflex, connections to the thalamus and connections to subplate neurons are evident by 20 weeks of fetal development but mature thalamocortical projections are not present until about 30 weeks (Lowery et al., 2007). It is obviously difficult to measure and interpret pain in the fetus during gestation but many countries are introducing legislation to require consideration of possible fetal pain during intentional termination of pregnancy. In the neonate, procedures likely to cause pain cause catecholamine and cortisol release to increase, heart rate and respiration rates to change, metabolic rate and oxygen consumption to increase and blood glucose levels to rise. The rate of transmission may be slower but a probable shorter distance between the pain receptor and brain compensates for this. Assessment of pain can be difficult as pain may be expressed differently in neonates; facial expressions may be used but some babies tend to withdraw and increase passivity and sleep more in response to pain.

THE SKIN AND IMMUNE SYSTEM

The skin of a neonate appears relatively transparent and soft and velvety. It is important in temperature regulation, as a barrier and as a sensory organ. Part of the appearance is due to the lack of large skin folds and localized oedema. Melanin production and pigmentation are low in the newborn so the skin is vulnerable to damage by ultraviolet rays. However, residual levels of maternal and placental hormones can produce transient pigmentation of certain skin areas. During delivery, the skin is subject to

changes in blood flow and mechanical stress from the pressure of contractions and from maternal structures which can result in abrasions and ischaemia. Obstetric interventions, for example, fetal monitoring, scalp sampling and use of amnio-hooks, forceps and vacuum extraction, also compromise the integrity of the skin. Immediately after birth, most fair-skinned babies have characteristic pink coloration with blue but warm extremities.

Vernix caseosa is a superficial fatty substance that coats the fetal skin from the middle of gestation and subsequently decreases as gestation progresses. Lanugo is the first generation of downy body hair that is fine and unpigmented; it appears from the 12th week and is mostly shed before birth. Vernix caseosa tends to accumulate at the sites of dense lanugo growth and is evident on the preterm baby on the face, ears and shoulders and in folds. At term, traces of vernix are present on the brow, ears and in the skin creases. Vernix caseosa is composed of sebaceous gland secretion and skin cells and is rich in triacylglycerides, cholesterol and fats. Its role is to protect the fetus from the amniotic fluid and to prevent loss of water and electrolytes. It provides insulation for the skin and helps to reduce friction at delivery; it may also have antibacterial properties.

The barrier properties of the stratum corneum of the skin increase with increased gestational age, especially after 24 weeks (Rutter, 1996). The epidermis of a preterm baby might be only five layers thick compared with about 15 layers in a term infant. A thinner epidermal layer results in increased transepidermal water loss, decreased ability to cope with friction, thermal instability because of the increased blood supply to the surface and increased permeability to microorganisms and chemicals (such as topically applied substances and reagents on clothes). Premature babies have translucent shiny red skin that becomes pinker through to the white thick skin of term infants. Drying out of the skin is a normal maturation process. Substances that interfere with the keratinization process, such as emollients, can delay the development of the skin becoming effective as a barrier. The transepidermal water loss can be limited by use of a thermal blanket, altering the air flow and maintaining an insulating layer of saturated air in contact with the skin.

The neonate is a compromised host, vulnerable to nocosomial (cross) infection. Host defence mechanisms are immature, partly because of lack of previous exposure to common organisms and partly because the neonate has limited cellular responses (see Chapter 10). Breaks in the delicate mucosa and skin from delivery and invasive obstetric procedures provide opportunities for the entry of pathogenic bacteria. In relation to artificial feeding, neonates are at increased risk of developing gastrointestinal infections, which may be associated with later development of allergies. Preterm infants, especially those of less than 34 weeks' gestation, are very vulnerable as they have less maternal IgG transfer. At birth, the neonate leaves the sterile fetal environment for one loaded with microorganisms (Jarvis, 1996). Ingestion and inhalation provide routes for bacterial colonization after birth, initially with organisms derived from the maternal genital tract. The neonate's skin, umbilical cord and genitalia are colonized first, followed by the face, respiratory system and gut. Skin flora is increased in infants with little vernix caseosa and is limited by antiseptic agents and alkaline soaps. The use of detergents may affect the integrity of the skin and cause dermatitis by interfering with the pH mantle; therefore, the use of only water to clean neonatal skin is advocated. If heavy soiling is present, then the use of pH neutral products may minimize skin irritation (Cork et al., 2009). There seems to be no differences to the effects on the skin whether the infant is bathed or washed using a cloth (Blume-Peytavi et al., 2009).

Initially, gut colonization is with organisms that the infant comes into contact with at and immediately after delivery. The profile of organisms is affected by the diet; breastfed babies have optimal conditions for the growth of the protective lactobacilli and bifidobacterium. Different patterns are seen in babies of very low birth weight and those who require feeding or ventilatory assistance. Meconium *in vivo* is usually sterile but when excreted provides rich culture conditions for microorganisms. The use of antibiotics changes the pattern of bacterial colonization of the neonate and can encourage the growth of resistant bacteria.

Case study 15.1 gives an example of neonatal infection.

 Case study 15.1

During a routine visit, the midwife examines Tracy, a 3-day-old baby, who was delivered in hospital and discharged the day before. Her umbilicus appears moist and sticky so the midwife takes a swab for culture and sensitivity. Two days later it is revealed that Tracy's umbilicus has been colonized with methicillin-resistant Staphylococcus aureus (MRSA). The infant appears well, has been exclusively breastfed and has regained her birth weight.

- What treatment, if any, would Tracy require and what reasons could be applied to argue against the use of antibiotic therapy?
- Do you think it is necessary to try to identify the source of the infection?
- What should the midwife do to ensure that further cross-infections do not occur?
- What factors may put other individuals at risk?

NORMAL NEONATAL TRANSITION

Much of the physiological adaptation to extrauterine life takes place during the first few hours following birth but final cardiovascular changes may not take up to 6 weeks. During the first few hours, most of the fetal lung fluid is absorbed, normal lung function is established and the normal neonatal blood flow to the lungs and tissues is initiated. This results in a pattern of predictable changes which can be monitored as changes in heart rate, respiratory pattern, gastrointestinal function and body temperature. Three discrete phases of neonatal transition were identified (Askin, 2009a). The first phase (0–30 min) is a period of reactivity; heart rate increases, respiration is irregular and fine crackles in the chest are accompanied by nasal flaring and grunting. This is followed by a phase of decreased responsiveness (30 min to 3 h) in which respiration is more shallow, heart rate decreases and muscle activity is decreased but jerks, twitches and sleep may occur. The third phase is another phase of reactivity (3–8 h after birth) in which tachycardia and a labile heart rate are common, tone and colour may change and aging and vomiting are not uncommon. Healthy infants may continue to exhibit normal signs of transition in the first 24 h of life; these may include lung crackles, a soft heart murmur (due to turbulent blood flow following the closure of fetal vascular shunts), tachypnoea, tachycardia and acrocyanosis. Some infants may also exhibit mild-to-moderate respiratory distress, slight temperature instability and slightly low blood sugar levels. Immediately following delivery, it is considered normal for infants to exhibit transient acrocyanosis during episodes of crying.

Delayed or complicated adaptation or increased signs of distress are important to identify quickly to ensure appropriate interventions. Risk factors for abnormal transition include maternal factors such as diabetes, hypertension, anaemia and shock, prenatal factors such as growth restriction, placental problems, multiple gestation, malpresentation and drug exposure, intrapartum factors such as infection, instrumental delivery, meconium-stained amniotic fluid and fetal distress or factors affecting the neonate directly such as prematurity or postmaturity, birth trauma and congenital malformations. Moderate to severe respiratory distress is indicated by intermittent grunting, nasal flaring, marked retractions, tachypnoea (respiratory rates of 100–120 breaths per minute) and prolonged need for supplemental oxygen. Persistent pulmonary hypertension of the newborn (PPHN) is due to the normal drop in PVR not occurring so there is continued shunting of blood away from the lungs in a fetal circulatory pattern. The resulting hypoxia causes further constriction of the pulmonary vessels and on-going shunting. Mild respiratory problems such as TTN may result in acrocyanosis whereas more severe problems can be evident as central cyanosis, pallor or greyness. Cyanosis is due to the presence of desaturated (unoxygenated) haemoglobin so hypoxia can be masked by anaemia and polycythaemic babies can look cyanotic at higher oxygen saturation levels because they have more haemoglobin. Pallor might indicate anaemia. Although a soft heart murmur is common in the first 24 h after birth, a cardiac murmur accompanied by respiratory distress, cyanosis or signs of congestive heart failure needs further investigation. Abnormal heart rate and rhythm might indicate compromised cardiovascular function. Persistent bradycardia (heart rate less than 80 bpm) can be due to heart block associated with maternal SLE and bradycardia during rest and sleep can indicate hypoxia and sepsis.

INITIAL EXAMINATION OF THE NEWBORN

After delivery, the baby is always examined by a midwife who, in accordance with professional legislative requirements, must refer any deviation from the normal to a medical practitioner. There is a statutory requirement to document findings.

The Apgar score

The baby's condition, including mental and physical development and level of alertness, is assessed using the Apgar score (Table 15.2). Although 'Apgar' is named after Virginia Apgar, the doctor who developed the scoring system, the mnemonic **A**ppearance, **P**ulse, **G**rimace, **A**ctivity and **R**espiration can be useful.

Table 15.2 Apgar score			
	0	**1**	**2**
Heart rate	Absent	Slow (<100 beats per minute)	Fast (>100 beats per minute)
Respiratory effort	Absent	Irregular, slow	Regular, cry
Muscle tone	Limp	Some flexion in limbs	Well-flexed limbs
Reflex irritability	Nil	Grimace	Cough, cry
Colour	White, blue	Body pink, extremities blue	Completely pink

Although the interpretative value of the Apgar score has been questioned, it is a means of assessing a baby for the absence or presence and degree of birth asphyxia. It is quick and simple and no other test has been routinely adopted. The Apgar test scores the baby's heart rate, respiratory effort, colour (of the skin in pale-skinned infants and of the mucous membrane in dark-skinned babies), muscle tone and reflex responses at 1 and 5 min following birth. It is repeated at 5-min intervals when active resuscitation measures are undertaken. The 1-min score may be low as the baby has been subjected to physical stress including a drop in temperature. Measurement of heart rate can be done by listening to the heart with a stethoscope or palpating the heart via the anterior chest wall. A heart rate of 110–150 beats per minute is considered normal. A heart rate persistently above 160 may be due to respiratory problems or sepsis. A heart rate of 90 or less may be indicative of congenital heart block, for example, associated with antiphospholipid syndrome or maternal SLE. A baby who is crying is obviously breathing in order to produce sound. Breathing can be seen easily, even on quiet babies. The respiratory rate of a healthy newborn baby is about 40–60 breaths per minute and should not be punctuated by grunting. A high-pitched or irritable cry may indicate brain damage or cerebral irritation due to oedema or haemorrhage. Rapid respirations in conjunction with chest retractions should be observed closely – early resolution is common in TTN but if prolonged may indicate sepsis.

The colour of the mucous membranes inside the mouth and the eyelids is assessed. If the blood flow is good, as in a healthy baby, these areas will be pink. If the tissues are being deprived of oxygen, they appear purplish or navy blue if the deprivation is severe. Healthy babies often appear bluish at the extremities but this may be due to cold rather than poor circulation. The face may appear congested if the cord was around the neck or if pressure from the delivery was prolonged. Pale babies may be anaemic, and polycythaemic babies (with an excess of red blood cells) tend to look very red.

The rooting reflex, turning of the head towards a touch on the cheek, is noted. Alternative reflexes include the baby curling the toes if the sole of the foot is stroked or responding with a grabbing movement if the palm of the hand is stroked (palmar grasp reflex). Abnormal responses such as the toes curling upwards (Babinski's sign) are often associated with abnormalities. The Moro reflex is looked for by startling the baby. If the head is allowed to drop back a few centimetres, the baby responds by flinging the arms outwards, usually accompanied by crying.

Muscle tone is more difficult to assess. All newborn babies have poorly developed musculature and seem fairly floppy, but babies who are especially floppy because they have immature coordination do not resist limb movement. Healthy babies have flexed limbs and respond to handling; the normal procedure is to lay the baby on the midwife's hand resting on its stomach and to observe position of the limbs.

A baby that needs urgent resuscitation is pale and floppy has a sluggish pulse and makes no respiratory effort. This is apparent and needs immediate response without having to calculate the Apgar score first. The Apgar score indicates the baby's capability to survive without intervention. If the Apgar score is above 7, little intervention is required, but a baby with an Apgar score of 5–7 will often need cutaneous stimulation and oxygen via a face mask. A score of 3–5 usually requires administration of oxygen via an 'Ambu' bag or equipment that allows facial oxygen to be delivered under cycles of positive pressure to inflate the lungs. A lower score requires immediate active treatment usually requiring ventilation via an endotracheal tube.

Case study 15.2 is an example of a baby possibly in need of resuscitation.

Body measurements and inspection

Once these tests are completed, further examination of the newborn can take place. An initial development check is followed by a fuller examination about 24 h later. It is becoming more common for midwives to undertake this more detailed examination of the newborn which traditionally was always undertaken by a paediatrician or general practitioner. This examination includes screening for common conditions such as congenital cataracts, cardiac and circulatory abnormalities, congenital hip dysplasia (CHD). Minor physical anomalies and variations can be found in 15–20% of newborns but most are not significant; some specific anomalies may indicate an underlying medical condition or genetic syndrome (Askin, 2009b). Major congenital anomalies are structural defects, such as cleft palate, gastroschisis and spina bifida, present at

birth that significantly affect function or social acceptability. Minor congenital anomalies, such as birth marks and skin tags, have minimal effect on function but have social significance; they predominantly occur on the face or hands because there are the areas which are complex. Developmental or normal variations are found in about 4% of the population and have no functional or social significance. Chromosomal investigation is recommended if three or more congenital anomalies are present (Askin, 2009b).

The baby's weight, length and head circumference are measured and recorded, however, it is important to note that head circumference and length may change as moulding of the fetal skull and oedema in the scalp resolves. Babies with birth weights above the 90th centile or below the 10th centile have an increased risk of becoming hypoglycaemic.

Examination of the genitalia allows assignation of the sex of the baby. Small genetalia may indicate underlying endocrine disorders or genetic syndromes. In male infants, the scrotum is felt for the presence of both testes and the position of the urethral exit on the penis is checked. In female babies, the vaginal and urethral orifices are inspected. Presence of meconium demonstrates patency of the anus; this may become evident on rectal temperature measurement although rectal temperature recording should be avoided unless the baby is very cold and the core temperature needs assessing due to the increased risk of developing necrotizing enterocolitis.

Moulding of the head, oedema of the scalp and distortion of the face are common at birth because of intrauterine pressure, the pressure imposed by the birth canal (see Chapter 13) and birth trauma. Microcephaly or macrocephaly feature in a number of syndromes and may indicate intrauterine infection. The normal term infant is well endowed with subcutaneous fat and usually has vernix caseosa in the skin folds. Postmature babies may have dry and peeling skin. The fontanelles and suture lines are observed. Bulging fontanelles may indicate an increased pressure and sunken fontanelles that the baby is dehydrated. An abnormal-shaped head indicates abnormal moulding (see Chapter 13). Eyes and ears are checked for abnormalities; the eyes should be clear and free from discharge. Low-set, absent or deformed ears may be associated with chromosomal abnormalities. The baby's mouth is inspected for the presence of teeth, which can be removed, or other extraneous material. Both the soft and hard palate are checked; the baby should demonstrate a sucking reflex. Minor skin blemishes are common. Hypertrophic sebaceous glands or milia present as white spots on about 40% babies. Both these spots and 'stork marks' – minor capillary haemangiomas – usually on the nose or eyelids, disappear within a few months of delivery.

The overall morphology of the baby should be symmetrical. The insertion of the umbilicus should be central, and is checked for swellings. The nipples, of either male

Case study 15.2

Paul is only 10 s old. He appears blue, not moving and limp and does not respond to touch. The midwife summons help and a paediatrician is called. The paediatrician arrives 4 min later to find a healthy, well-perfused infant, crying while being held by his mother.

- Was the midwife justified in being cautious by summoning a paediatrician early?
- How many midwives in practice wait a full minute before their initial assessment of the newborn?
- What actions do you think the midwife took prior to the arrival of the paediatrician?
- What care will Paul require in the first few hours of his life and are there any specific observations that the midwives should be carrying out during this period?

or female babies, may be swollen and producing milk in response to circulating maternal hormones. Respiratory movement of the chest of a healthy baby is symmetrical and the abdomen is rounded. The limbs are checked for equal length and free movement; short limbs can indicate achondroplasia. A single crease across the hand (Simian crease) is a common variant but occurs with higher incidence in Down's syndrome. The digits are counted; extra digits (polydactyly), a curved fifth finger (clinodactyly), fused fingers (syndactyly) and webbing between the digits are relatively common. The feet and ankles are examined for talipes and other abnormalities.

Visible signs of congenital dislocation of the hips (CDH) also known as CHD are asymmetry of the pelvis, asymmetrical creases in the groin and apparent differences in leg length. Midwives may be discouraged from undertaking manipulative tests of the hips as there is a danger of malpositioning the head of the femur into the acetabular cup, which can trap the femoral blood flow resulting in necrosis of the head of the femur. Midwifery units usually have local policies and protocols for the screening of hips for congenital dislocation.

The neck is observed for shortness, webbing or folds of skin on the back of the neck; these characteristics are associated with chromosomal abnormalities, such as Turner's syndrome. The spine is checked for swellings or defects and for pilonidal dimples or hairy patches, which may indicate occult spina bifida. Before the baby is discharged from the postnatal ward, there should be confirmation that the baby is feeding normally; excretion of urine and meconium normally occurs within 24 and 48 h of delivery, respectively. Early screening is important both to reassure the parents and to detect any abnormality or problem requiring further investigation.

Key points

- Many changes must occur at birth for successful transition to neonatal life, including initiation of breathing, conversion from fetal to neonatal circulation and physiological homeostatic control of thermoregulation and metabolism.

- The transition to neonatal circulation requires closure of the fetal shunts and vasodilatation of the pulmonary circulation; oxygen is a major stimulant.
- Successful breathing requires adequate maturation of the lungs, particularly the presence of adequate surfactant and neuromuscular control, and clearance of lung fluid.
- The relatively large surface area of neonates means they are vulnerable to excessive heat loss; body temperature is maintained by non-shivering thermogenesis. Efforts to reduce heat loss at birth are essential.
- Normal newborn infants are able to maintain adequate blood glucose levels be compromised by a stressful labour, abnormal maternal metabolism, restricted fetal growth and prematurity.
- Human milk and early physiological conditions compensate for the immature development of the neonatal gut.

Application to practice

An understanding of the transition to neonatal life is important for the following reasons. Many infants require some degree of intervention to support establishment of respiration after birth. An infant who does not appear to adapt fully at birth (i.e. is cyanotic) may for example have an underlying cardiac defect or be suffering from sepsis.

The midwife should use her or his assessment of adaptation as part of the neonatal check and not check solely for visible abnormalities therefore assessment of factors such as alertness, movement, muscle tone and vital signs, in the context of maternal, family and antenatal/perinatal history, is an important component of the initial and 24-h detailed examinations.

Many parents are distressed at the appearance of a baby that has just been born and need reassurance that the transition is not always completely spontaneous and that this is quite normal. An understanding of the effects of hypoxia and anoxia during labour are important in the planning the subsequent care of an affected neonate following delivery.

ANNOTATED FURTHER READING

Askin DF: Physical assessment of the newborn: part 1 of 2: preparation through auscultation, *Nurs Womens Health* 11:292–301, 2007.

Askin DF: Physical assessment of the newborn: part 2 of 2: inspection

through palpation, *Nurs Womens Health* 11:304–313, 2007.

A comprehensive description, published in two parts, of a thorough and structured approach to undertaking a head-to-toe physical inspection of the newborn using

palpation and auscultation. These guides provide a practical and structured approach for practitioners undertaking examination of the newborn.

Askin DF: Fetal-to-neonatal transition – what is normal and what is not? Part 2:

red Flags, *Neonatal Netw* 28:e37–e40, 2009.

A clear summary of the signs and symptoms of the common complications of neonatal physiological transition to extrauterine life which warrant further investigation in order to identify infants with underlying disease or abnormalities.

Baston H, Durward H: *Examination of the newborn*, ed 2, London, Routledge, 2010.

For practitioners wanting to develop their skills in undertaking examination of the newborn this book is a comprehensive text covering all aspects of the physical examination.

Blackburn S: *Maternal, fetal, & neonatal physiology: a clinical perspective*, ed 3, 2007, Saunders.

An in-depth and well-illustrated description of physiological adaptation to pregnancy and development of the fetus and neonate that draws from physiological research studies. The chapters are clearly organized by physiological systems and link physiological concepts to clinical applications, including the assessment and management of low- and high-risk pregnancies.

Burke C: Perinatal sepsis, *J Perinatal Neonatal Nurs* 23:42–51, 2009.

A guide to the risk factors, symptoms, diagnosis, management and physiological effects of sepsis in the neonate. Recognition of sepsis in the neonate is often difficult and this guide is useful in enabling practitioners recognise the early subtle signs of sepsis.

Christensen RD, Henry E, Jopling J, et al: The CBC: reference ranges for neonates, *Semin Perinatol* 33:3–11, 2009.

A review, based on recent research reports, which proposes references ranges for parameters of the complete blood count for neonates of various gestational and postnatal ages and discusses the physiological reasons for the different normal values.

Davies L, McDonald S: *Examination of the newborn and neonatal health: a multidimensional approach*, 2008, Churchill Livingstone.

This book has chapters that focus on pre-birth influences that should be considered when undertaking the examination of the newborn. It also focuses on the screening elements of the newborn examination.

Di Renzo GC, Simeoni U: An atlas of the prenate and neonate: the transition to extrauteine life informa, 2006..

Practitioners undertaking the examination of the newborn will find the diagrams and illustrations in this book useful in developing knowledge to underpin the examination process.

Hansmann G: *Neonatal emergencies*, ed 1, Cambridge, 2009, Cambridge University Press.

This book provides a useful and easy to use reference guide to neonatal emergencies common in the first 72 h of life. It provides a multidisciplinary approach in such emergency situations including the role of the midwife.

Johnson MH: *Essential reproduction*, ed 6, Oxford, 2007, Blackwell.

An excellent, well-organized research-based textbook that explores comparative reproductive physiology of mammals including a chapter on the fetus and its preparations for birth.

In Meeks M, Hallsworth M, Yeo H, editors: *Nursing the neonate*, 2009, Wiley-Blackwell.

This book is a useful reference guide for midwives with little or no experience in caring for the sick neonate. It focuses on body systems in a systematic and comprehensive way.

Rennie JM: *Roberton's textbook of neonatology*, ed 4, 2005, Churchill Livingstone.

This book is invaluable for practitioners who require information on congenital disorders and pathological conditions in the neonate. It covers a wide range of conditions but it is especially useful for the rarer conditions not commonly observed in clinical practice.

Williamson A, Crozier K: *Neonatal care: a textbook for student midwives and nurses*, 2008, Reflect Press Ltd.

This book provides a basic and simple guide which may be useful not only for midwifery and nursing students but for maternity care assistants who require to develop skills in caring for neonates within the maternity services.

REFERENCES

Aronis-Vournas S: The bleeding neonate, *Haematol Rep* 12:66–70, 2006.

Askin DF: Fetal-to-neonatal transition – what is normal and what is not? *Neonatal Netw* 28:e33–e40, 2009a.

Askin DF: Physical assessment of the newborn: minor congenital anomalies, *Nurs Womens Health* 13:140–148, 2009b.

Aylott M: The neonatal energy triangle. Part 1: metabolic adaptation, *Paediatr Nurs* 18:38–42, 2006.

Begley DJ, Firth JA, Hoult JRS: *Human reproduction and developmental biology*, New York, 1978, Macmillan pp 160, 199.

Blume-Peytavi U, Cork MJ, Faergemann J, et al: Bathing and cleansing in newborns from day 1 to first year of life: recommendations

from a European round table meeting, *J Eur Acad Dermatol Venereol* 23:751–759, 2009.

Chamberlain G, Dewhurst J, Harvey D: *Illustrated textbook of obstetrics*, London, 1991, Gower Medical (Mosby), pp 14–16.

Cork MJ, Danby SG, Vasilopoulos Y, et al: Epidermal barrier dysfunction in atopic dermatitis, *J Invest Dermatol* 129:1892–1908, 2009.

Edwards MJ, Walsh DA, Li Z: Hyperthermia, teratogenesis and the heat shock response in mammalian embryos in culture, *Int J Dev Biol* 41:345–358, 1997.

Fowden AL, Forhead AJ: Endocrine regulation of feto-placental growth, *Horm Res* 72:257–265, 2009.

Givan DC: Physiology of breathing and related pathological processes in infants, *Semin Pediatr Neurol* 10(4):271–280, 2003.

Goodwin B: *Health and development: conceptions to birth*, Milton Keynes, 1997, Open University, p 259.

Guillery EN: Fetal and neonatal nephrology, *Curr Opin Pediatr* 9:148–153, 1997.

Gunn TR, Ball KT, Power GG, et al: Factors influencing the initiation of nonshivering thermogenesis, *Am J Obstet Gynecol* 164(1 Pt 1):210–217, 1991.

Hallman M, Haataja R: Surfactant protein polymorphisms and neonatal lung disease, *Semin Perinatol* 30:350–361, 2006.

Harding R, Hooper SB: Regulation of lung expansion and lung growth before birth, *J Appl Physiol* 81:209–224, 1996.

Hay W Jr: Placental supply of energy and protein substrates to the fetus, *Acta Paediatr Suppl* 405:13–19, 1994.

Hull D: The structure and function of brown adipose tissue, *British Medical Bulletin* 22:92–93, 1966.

Hutchison AA: Respiratory disorders of the neonate, *Curr Opin Pediatr* 6:142–153, 1994.

Jain L, Eaton DC: Physiology of fetal lung fluid clearance and the effect of labor, *Semin Perinatol* 30:34–43, 2006.

Jarvis WR: The epidemiology of colonisation, *Infect Control Hosp Epidemiol* 17:47–52, 1996.

Juretschke LJ: Kernicterus: still a concern, *Neonatal Netw* 24:7–19, 2005.

Kinmond S, Aitchison TC, Holland BM, et al: Umbilical cord clamping and preterm infants: a randomised trial, *Br Med J* 306:172–175, 1993.

Kuehl J: Neonatal disseminated intravascular coagulation, *J Perinat Neonatal Nursing* 11:69–77, 1997.

Kuzawa CW: Adipose tissue in human infancy and childhood: an evolutionary perspective, *Am J Phys Anthropol* Suppl 27:177–209, 1998.

Lamvu G, Kuller JA: Prenatal diagnosis using fetal cells from the maternal circulation, *Obstet Gynecol Surv* 52:433–437, 1997.

Lawn JE, Gravett MG, Nunes TM, et al: Global report on preterm birth and stillbirth 1 of 7: definitions, description of the burden and opportunities to improve data, *BMC Pregnancy Childbirth* 1(10 Suppl):S1, 2010.

Lipsitt LP, Rovee-Collier C: Prenatal and infant development. In Smelser NJ, Baltes PB, editors: *International encyclopedia of the social and behavioral sciences* London, 2001, Elsevier, pp 11994–11997.

Lockitch G: Beyond the umbilical cord: interpreting laboratory tests in the neonate, *Clin Biochem* 27:1–6, 1994.

Lonnerdal B: Nutritional and physiologic significance of human milk proteins, *Am J Clin Nutr* 77(6):1537S–1543S, 2003.

Lowery CL, Hardman MP, Manning N, et al: Neurodevelopmental changes of fetal pain, *Semin Perinatol* 31:275–282, 2007.

Nelson N: Physiology of transition. In Avery GB, Fletcher MA, MacDonald MG, editors: *Neonatology, pathophysiology and management of the newborn*, ed 4, Philadelphia, 1994, Lippincott, pp 223–247.

Nijhuis JG: Fetal behavior, *Neurobiol Aging* 24(Suppl 1):S41–S46, 2003.

Okken A: Postnatal adaptation in thermoregulation, *J Perinat Med* 19(Suppl 1):67–73, 1991.

Paediatric Formulary Committee: *British National Formulary for Children 2008, vitamin K*, London, 2010, Pharmaceutical Press, pp 570–572.

Palis J, Segel GB: Developmental biology of erythropoiesis, *Blood Rev* 12(2):106–114, 1998.

Parer JT: Effects of fetal asphyxia on brain cell structure and function: limits of tolerance, *Comp Biochem Physiol A: Mol Integr Physiol* 119:711–716, 1998.

Polderman KH: Induced hypothermia and fever control for prevention and treatment of neurological injuries. *Lancet* 371:1955–1969, 2008.

Power GG: Fetal thermoregulation: animal and human. In Polin RA, Fox WW, editors: *Fetal and neonatal physiology*, Philadelphia, 1992, Saunders, p 447.

Rutter N: The immature skin, *Eur J Pediatr* 155(Suppl 2):S18–S20, 1996.

Scott RJ, Goodburn SF: Potter's syndrome in the second trimester: prenatal screening and pathological findings in 60 cases of oligohydramnios sequence, *Prenat Diagn* 15:519–525, 1995.

Smith SL: Hypoglycaemia in the neonate. In Alexander J, Levy V, Roch S, editors: *Aspects of midwifery practice: a research-based approach*, Basingstoke, 1995, Macmillan, pp 154–176.

Strang LB: Fetal lung liquid: secretion and reabsorption, *Physiol Rev* 71:991–1016, 1991.

Strauss RG: Erythropoietin and neonatal anemia, *N Engl J Med* 330:1227–1228, 1994.

Symonds ME, Mostyn A, Pearce S, et al: Endocrine and nutritional regulation of fetal adipose tissue development, *J Endocrinol* 179:293–299, 2003.

Taddio A, Katz J: Pain, opioid tolerance and sensitisation to nociception in the neonate, *Best Pract Res Clin Anaesthesiol* 18(2):291–302, 2004.

Thorburn GD: The placenta, PGE$_2$ and parturition, *Early Hum Dev* 29:63–73, 1992.

Wolf G: Brown adipose tissue: the molecular mechanism of its formation, *Nutr Rev* 67:167–171, 2009.

Wolff PH: The causes, controls and organization of behaviour in the neonate, *Psychol Issues* 5(Monogram 1), 1966.

Wyatt JS, Gluckman PD, Liu PY, et al: Determinants of outcomes after head cooling for neonatal encephalopathy, *Pediatrics* 119:912–921, 2007.

Chapter | **16** |

Lactation and infant nutrition

LEARNING OBJECTIVES

- To describe the anatomical structure of the breast.
- To outline the hormonal control of lactation.
- To describe how the physiology of lactation can be applied clinically.
- To describe the mechanisms of milk secretion.
- To discuss maternal adaptations during lactation: the effects on fertility, maternal behaviour and nutritional requirements.
- To explain why breastfeeding provides optimal nutrition of the neonate.
- To describe the non-nutritional advantages of breast milk.

INTRODUCTION

Infant feeding is the result of multifaceted interactions between infant nutritional demand and maternal physiology. The physiological basis of lactation is important in understanding and facilitating successful breastfeeding. Despite increased awareness of the health benefits of human milk, many women discontinue breastfeeding because they perceive that they have insufficient milk supply. Most breastfeeding problems have identifiable physiological, rather than pathological, causes and are best addressed by considering the interactions between the mother and the baby. Successful breastfeeding has nutritional, emotional, developmental and economic benefits. It can be argued that the nutrient requirement of the infant is one of the best understood areas of

nutrition. Human milk, however, does not just provide the optimal balance of nutrients in a form appropriate to the developmental needs of the infant, it also compensates for the immature digestive capability and vulnerable immune status of the neonate. Breast milk is the most appropriate food for growth, development, and protection of the neonate. Short-term benefits are a result of the immunological properties of breast milk and protection against infectious diseases. Medium-term benefits are associated with the lower prevalence of inflammatory bowel diseases, type-1 diabetes and childhood cancers. In addition, there are long-term benefits; health in later life appears to be optimized for those individuals who were breastfed as infants. Breastfeeding is universally agreed to be one of the most effective preventative measures of reducing the death rate of children under 5 years old. There are also health benefits associated with breastfeeding; lactation contributes to birth spacing and women who have breastfed seem to have reduced incidence of breast and ovarian cancer.

Chapter case study

Almost immediately following his birth, Zara placed Zak in her arms and he instinctively latched onto the breast and started feeding before the cord was cut. Zak fed on the breast for over 45 min before detaching himself.
- What are the advantages of offering the baby the breast as soon as possible after delivery for both mother and baby?
- What factors could have a negative influence on the early establishment of breastfeeding and how can the midwife optimize breastfeeding?

ANATOMY OF THE BREAST

The tissue of the breast extends from about the second to the sixth rib (depending on posture). The extension of the tail of the tissue into the axilla (Fig. 16.1) can result in discomfort in the early puerperium when it may become swollen. The mammary gland is made up of a branching network of ducts ending in lobular–alveolar clusters which are the sites of milk secretion. The breast also has a variable amount of adipose tissue and connective tissue. The breast is divided into sections or lobes by fibrous septae, which run from behind the nipple towards the pectoralis muscle. These septae are important in localizing infections, which are often visually evident as a wedge of red inflamed skin on the surface of the breast. Each of the 8–12 lobes, separated by connective tissue, contains glandular tissue composed of clusters of alveoli and small ducts (Fig. 16.2). The alveolar secretory cells are grouped in grape-like lobules around an extensive branching system of small ducts, which lead to the nipple. Fat is interspersed throughout the lobules. Ultrasound studies of

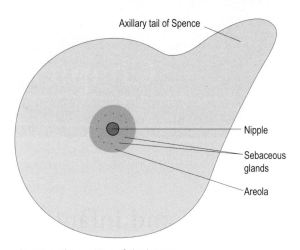

Fig. 16.1 The position of the breast.

babies feeding at the breast show that there are no discernible lactiferous sinuses in the human breast and that the ducts, even close to the nipple, can branch and be very small and compressible (Ramsay et al., 2005).

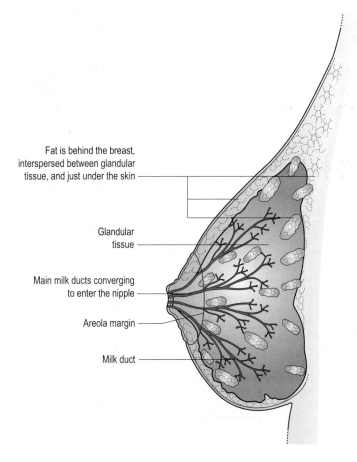

Fig. 16.2 Anatomy of the human breast. (Reproduced with permission from Ramsay et al., 2005.)

The nipple is surrounded by the areola, a pigmented area of varying size, which darkens during pregnancy and has a rich vascular supply and sensory nerve inputs. Surrounding the nipple are Montgomery's tubercles which are sebaceous glands that hypertrophy and become prominent during pregnancy, providing lubrication and protection. Heavy use of soap can increase the risk of nipple damage, particularly drying and cracking. The sensitivity of the nipple and surrounding area increases markedly immediately after delivery. Suckling results in an influx of afferent nerve impulses to the hypothalamus controlling lactation and maternal behaviour.

Each lobe consists of 20–40 lobules, each containing 10–100 alveoli, the glandular physiological units. Alveolar cells are cuboidal in the resting non-pregnant breast and change remarkably to develop full secretory features during lactation. The alveolar cells secrete milk into the lumen of the small ducts. These secretory cells are surrounded by oxytocin-sensitive myoepithelial (contractile) cells, which are important in milk ejection. The ducts are also lined by contractile cells that open the ducts widely during the milk ejection reflex to assist flow.

BREAST GROWTH AND DEVELOPMENT

Mammary growth and development can be divided into four phases: resting, development (pregnancy), milk secreting (lactation) and involution. At birth, the structure is simply the nipple and a few rudimentary ducts, with few or no alveoli, reflecting their evolutionary origin of modified apocrine sweat glands. Until puberty, the only degree of development may be a little branching of the ducts. There is a decreased incidence of breast cancer in populations with a high consumption of phytoestrogens (oestrogen-like compounds derived from plants). It is suggested that the phytoestrogens stimulate development of the mammary cells in childhood and puberty before pregnancy; these well-differentiated cells may be more resistant to tumour formation (Adlercreutz, 1995).

The human is unusual, even compared with other primates, having extensive breast development at puberty, rather than at pregnancy, resulting in an erotic significance. During puberty, the proliferation of the milk ducts, which elongate, sprout and branch, is primarily dependent on secretion of oestrogen with further contributions from growth hormone (GH) and adrenal hormones. The modest alveolar development at this stage is stimulated by progesterone, providing the tissue has been primed by oestrogen. Prolactin may also play a role although the interaction between the adrenal and pituitary glands and the ovaries is not fully understood. The hormonal fluctuations of the menstrual cycle give repeated exposure of the tissue to oestrogen and progesterone, which allow additional but limited growth. Many non-pregnant women experience cyclical changes, especially premenstrually, in breast volume, which is associated with water retention. Occasionally, some secretory activity may occur within the alveoli and a mammary secretion may be expressed premenstrually.

Once an adult woman has developed breasts, minimal stimulation is required to begin milk secretion (Box 16.1). Growth in breast size is most marked in early pregnancy (Hytten, 1995). The hormones required for breast development during pregnancy are less than those required for other species. In humans, neither human placental lactogen (hPL) nor GH is essential.

In early pregnancy, breast size and areolar pigmentation increase. The tubercles of Montgomery enlarge and the nipples become more erect. Blood flow to the breast doubles so blood vessels become more prominent and the skin may appear to have a translucent marbled appearance. There is a sharp increase in ductal and glandular elements so the breasts tend to feel slightly lumpy in early pregnancy. This initial hyperplasia is followed by alveolar cell hypertrophy and initiation of secretory activity in later pregnancy.

Oestrogen plays the dominant role in development of the ducts and progesterone in the development of glandular tissue, although insulin and other growth factors, such as epidermal growth factor (EGF) and transforming growth factor (TGFα), have a role in regulation. Changes in pregnancy depend on the lactogenic hormones, prolactin and hPL, with placental oestrogen and progesterone playing important modulatory roles. Under these hormonal influences, prominent lobules, resembling bunches of grapes,

Box 16.1 Relactation

Relactation, or induced lactation, is the process whereby lactation is initiated at a time not associated with delivery. For instance, an adoptive mother who has not borne a child may wish to breastfeed her adopted baby or a mother may want to resume feeding her own child. Relactation is easier if the woman has previously lactated or been pregnant and if the infant is young. Hormonal support such as oxytocin nasal sprays may be used. The woman is advised to eat well and rest, and to stimulate the nipple and breast often, either by hand or with a breast pump. Supplementary formula milk is given to the baby by spoon or dropper; bottle teats and dummies are avoided. Use of a 'Lact-Aid' supplementer is often found helpful. This device allows the baby to feed on formula milk from a tube attached to the mother's nipple. As the baby feeds, it stimulates the nipple and increases endogenous prolactin secretion. The formula milk is in a bag maintained at body temperature because it is in contact with the mother's body. As breast milk production increases, the amount of formula milk can be reduced.

- Increased vascularization – may cause tingling
- Dilatation of superficial veins – fair skin appears 'marbled'
- Hypertrophy – full development of lobules
- Dilatation of alveoli and ducts – may feel nodular
- Thickening of nipple skin
- Pigmentation of nipple and areolar – persists after pregnancy
- Secondary areola may appear in dark-skinned women
- Montgomery's tubercles become prominent
- Small quantity of clear colostrum can be expressed in latter half of pregnancy

form in the breast so the alveolar lumen becomes dilated by mid-pregnancy and the secretory cells fully differentiated (Box 16.2). The areola becomes pigmented and a secondary patchily pigmented areola may develop. The nipple enlarges and becomes more mobile and protractile, as the connective tissue anchorages soften and become more stretchable with the oestrogen-driven increase in hydration (see Chapter 11). By the 4th month of pregnancy, the epithelial cells accumulate substantial amounts of secretory material and the mammary glands are fully developed. Prolactin levels progressively increase throughout the pregnancy and are maximal at term. Although it is possible to expel a breast secretion in pregnancy, this is not true colostrum. Full colostrum and milk production is inhibited by high progesterone levels so copious milk production is not established until after parturition. Placental hPL may also contribute to blocking of prolactin responses in pregnancy. Even if very small amounts of the placenta or fetal membranes are retained after delivery, lactation is inhibited (Neifert et al., 1981) (see Chapters 13 and 14).

The increase in glucocorticoids that occurs in association with the raised levels of free placental corticotrophin releasing hormone prior to the onset of labour (see Chapter 13) is also important for the breast secretory activity and milk synthesis and secretion (Casey and Plaut, 2007). Glucocorticoids play a significant role in the formation of cellular components such as rough endoplasmic reticulum and tight junctions which are required for milk synthesis and secretion. They are also involved in the regulation of milk protein gene expression and the maintenance of secretory cell differentiation and lactation by preventing the second phase of involution.

PHYSIOLOGY OF LACTATION

Mammary differentiation and milk secretion are co-ordinated by the endocrine system and involve three categories of hormones: reproductive hormones which change during reproductive development and affect mammary gland development and coordinate milk delivery; metabolic hormones which regulate metabolic responses to nutrient intake or stress; and mammary hormones produced by the lactating mammary gland (Neville et al., 2002). Lactation can be considered as two phases: lactogenesis, the initiation of lactation; and galactopoiesis (sometimes referred to as lactogenesis stage 3), the maintenance of milk secretion. Lactogenesis itself has two stages. Stage 1 is the enzymatic and cellular differentiation of the alveolar cells, which result in colostrum formation, and uptake of immunoglobulins prior to parturition but very little milk synthesis and secretion. Lactogenesis stage 2 is the onset of copious secretion of all milk components about 2–4 days after parturition following the progesterone withdrawal at parturition and concurrent stimulation by prolactin and cortisol. Lactogenesis is normally robust but may be delayed with stressful deliveries and in poorly controlled diabetes (Neville and Morton, 2001) and in obese women, probably because adipose tissue abrogates the decrease in progesterone concentration (Rasmussen et al., 2001). Maternal obesity is associated with a lower breastfeeding rate but not solely related to physiological issues; obesity affects breastfeeding intention, initiation and duration (Amir and Donath, 2007). Other factors that may delay lactogenesis are increasing maternal age, infant birthweight (over 3.6 kg), use of formula milk (especially more than 60 mL in the first 48 h of life), lower maternal educational status, low Apgar scores and caesarean section (Nommsen-Rivers et al., 2009). Once lactation is commenced, it is maintained by the removal of milk which is orchestrated by prolactin, which stimulates production of milk, and oxytocin, which is involved in milk ejection (Table 16.1, Fig. 16.4). Maternal perception of inadequate milk supply may influence mothers to augment breast feeding with formula milk and thus interfere with the establishment of lactogenesis and galactopoiesis (Huang et al., 2009). Women at risk of lactational failure will need careful support and encouragement in the initiation of breast feeding. Augmentation with formula milk should be discouraged unless there are medical indications and women whose babies suckle frequently must be reassured that this does not mean their milk supply is inadequate but is an important component in establishing lactation.

Prolactin

Suckling results in the firing of afferent impulses via the anterolateral columns of the spinal cord to the brain stem and hypothalamus. The hypothalamus subsequently decreases release of dopamine (formerly described as prolactin inhibitory factor) into the portal circulation to the pituitary gland. It was postulated that a dopamine-stimulating factor existed but, although several hormones

Table 16.1 Prolactin and oxytocin

SOURCE	ANTERIOR PITUITARY GLAND	POSTERIOR PITUITARY GLAND (BUT SYNTHESIZED IN HYPOTHALAMUS)
Primary control	Lifting of dopamine inhibition	Neural pathway
Modulating factors	Positively stimulated by oestrogen, TSH, VIP	Neurotransmitters
Peak response	30 min	30 s
Stimulus	Suckling	Suckling, sound, sight and thought of baby
Target cell	Alveolar cell	Myoepithelial cell
Effect	Milk synthesis	Milk ejection

positively modulate prolactin secretion, control is largely by the lifting of the tonic inhibition from dopamine. The abrogation of thedopamine inhibition stimulates the release of prolactin from the cells of the anterior pituitary. Secretion of prolactin is modified by oestrogen and thyroid-stimulating hormone (TSH). Studies in rats have demonstrated that vasoactive intestinal peptide (VIP), released from the pituitary gland, is an extremely potent prolactin-releasing factor and affects mammary blood flow. The number of signals affecting prolactin release indicates a complex neuroendocrine axis (Ben-Jonathan et al., 1991). β-Endorphin and melanocyte-stimulating hormone (MSH), which are co-released from the intermediate lobe of the pituitary gland, also seem to have a role. β-Endorphin blocks dopamine inhibition of prolactin and MSH stimulates the release of prolactin by lowering the threshold of the lactotrophs (Porter et al., 1994).

Levels of prolactin begin to rise within 10 min of suckling, peak about 30 min after initial stimulation and then progressively fall back to basal levels within a further 3 h. This delay in prolactin secretion following suckling led to the concept that the rise in prolactin was the 'order for the next meal'. Areolar stimulation is essential for prolactin release; negative pressure alone is not adequate and denervation of the nipple prevents prolactin release in response to nipple stimulation.

Prolactin levels fall abruptly about 2 h before delivery then dramatically rebound. These fluctuations in prolactin level probably relate to changing oestrogen concentrations. The level of prolactin seems to be important in establishing lactation but levels are much diminished after 6 weeks at a rate dependent on suckling frequency and duration (Johnston and Amico, 1986). The peak prolactin levels in response to suckling also fall progressively.

Prolactin has a pulsatile release. A diurnal rhythm of prolactin secretion is apparent, with higher circulating levels during sleep. The exact quantitative relationship between prolactin levels and milk production is not clear. In the early puerperium bromocriptine, a dopamine D_2 receptor agonist causes a fall in prolactin levels and abolishes milk secretion. Dopamine-receptor blockers (such as metoclopramide, haloperidol, domperidone and sulpiride) increase prolactin levels and milk production. The use of drugs which stimulate prolactin should be the last resort after excluding all the other factors which might negatively affect milk supply such as checking the positioning of the infant. All the drugs are a risk of side effects. Domperidone is usually preferred because it has a lower risk of toxicity as it crosses into the breast milk and brain to a lesser extent (it has a large molecular weight, is less soluble and is usually bound to proteins). Dopamine binds to receptors on the pituitary and is internalized resulting in the increased breakdown of prolactin within the secretory granules. However, women who have had pituitary surgery and have prolactin levels just above non-pregnant level can breastfeed. The evidence seems to suggest that a threshold prolactin level is required but then there is no correlation between prolactin level and milk production (Howie et al., 1980).

Prolactin binds to receptors on the secretory alveolar (acinar) cells acting at several sites to increase synthesis of several components of the milk including casein, lactalbumin and fatty acids. During pregnancy, secretory alveolar cells proliferate and acquire the characteristics of highly active secretory cells including numerous mitochondria, an extensive endoplasmic reticulum, well-developed Golgi apparatus and many secretory vesicles. Early suckling is important to stimulate prolactin to ensure that milk production is optimal and sustained. Infrequent and/or poor suckling in the early postnatal period may significantly reduce the optimal long term milk production as less prolactin receptor complexes are formed so stimulation of the acinar cells is sub-optimal and the potential for milk production is reduced (Manuel et al., 2007). It is important to support and reassure mothers whose infants frequently suckle in the early postnatal period to promote prolactin release and establish long term breast feeding (Case Study 16.1). Introduction of formula feeds in the belief that the infant is hungry will interfere with the establishment of lactation. In the first few hours of birth, spontaneous suckling may be facilitated by maternal–neonatal skin-to-skin contact (Bramson et al., 2010).

As well as the dopamine-antagonist drugs, there are a number of herbal galactogogues which have been traditionally used to promote milk production; these include

Case study 16.1

Almost immediately following his birth, Zara held Zak in her arms; he was naked and in direct contact with Zara's skin and he instinctively latched onto the breast and started feeding before the cord was cut. Zak fed on the breast for over 45 min before falling asleep.

- What are the advantages of offering the baby the breast as soon as possible after delivery for both mother and baby?
- What can the midwife do to encourage Zak to spontaneously suckle at the breast with future feeding?
- What factors could have a negative influence on the early establishment of breastfeeding and how can the midwife optimize breastfeeding?

fenugreek seeds, fennel, brewer's yeast, alfalfa, asparagus, rescue remedy and ignatia 6x (Gabay, 2002). There is a lack of scientific evidence for the effectiveness of these herbal galactogogues. Smoking has been shown to reduce prolactin production (Andersen et al., 1984); in addition, psychosocial factors tend to result in lower rates of breast-feeding in women who smoke (Amir and Donath, 2003).

Biosynthesis of milk

The secretory cells of the alveoli (Fig. 16.3) synthesize or extract the components of milk, which are secreted into the alveolar lumen. The cells are joined near their apical surface by adherins and tight junctions. The apical plasma membrane has a smooth surface with few microvilli, in contrast to the tightly folded basal membrane, which facilitates uptake of substrates such as amino acids,

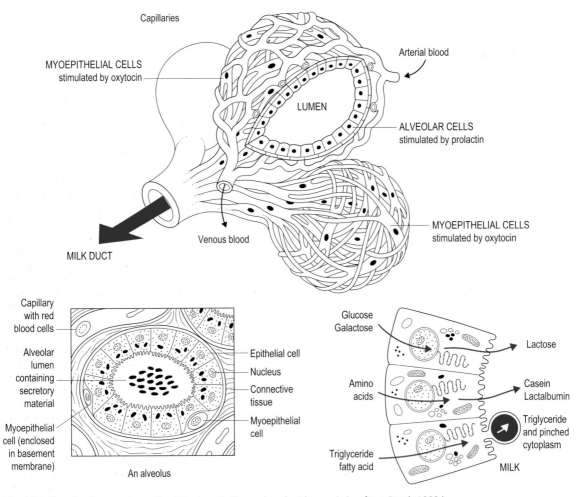

Fig. 16.3 The alveolar secretory cells of the breast. (Reproduced with permission from Pond, 1992.)

glucose, acetate and fats from the extracellular space. Proteins, fats and lactose are synthesized in the cell and packaged into vesicles. The vesicles move to the apex of the cell where exocytosis takes place.

The composition of the maternal diet can influence the components of breast milk, especially those passing from blood to milk with little modification by the alveolar cell, such as lipids. The alveolar cells have a unique mechanism for lipid secretion whereby microlipid droplets coalesce forming progressively larger lipid droplets that are eventually enclosed by a specialized milk fat droplet membrane prior to secretion (McManaman and Neville, 2003). Aqueous solutes including the proteins, oligosaccharides, lactose, citrate, phosphate and calcium are secreted into the milk by exocytosis after being packaged into secretory vesicles by the Golgi apparatus. Macromolecular substances derived from maternal serum, such as serum proteins (IgA, albumin and transferrin), endocrine hormones (insulin, prolactin and oestrogen), cytokines and lipoprotein lipase, are transported by a transcytosis pathway. Various membrane transport pathways transfer small molecules and ions such as glucose, amino acids and water. Large blood cells and serum follow a paracellular route, squeezing between the alveolar cells.

Oxytocin

Oxytocin levels control the milk ejection reflex, which is responsible for the transfer of the milk from the breast to the baby. Oxytocin stimulates the myoepithelial cells so the alveolar sacs are compressed, increasing the pressure, and the ducts shorten and widen. Although secretion of oxytocin is under a similar neuroendocrine reflex to prolactin, it is physiologically independent. Oxytocin synthesis in the hypothalamus, and its release from the posterior lobe of the pituitary gland, is increased in response to handling the baby, hearing cries or thinking about feeding as well as by tactile stimulation at the nipple. Oxytocin is released in short-lived bursts of less than a minute immediately in response to stimuli. Frequently, the largest response is to the baby crying before feeding so maximum release of oxytocin may occur before suckling even starts. Between feeds, isolated pulses of oxytocin are released (McNeilly, 2001) possibly in response to other babies' cries or fleeting images of the baby. Unlike prolactin secretion, the milk ejection reflex can be conditioned, as demonstrated by dairy farmers who clang their buckets to stimulate oxytocin and a good milk yield. Similarly, a baby's cry can often trigger oxytocin secretion, which is why the practice of babies 'rooming-in' with their mothers (sleeping close to their mother's bed) is often associated with successful breastfeeding.

The milk ejection reflex is very sensitive to inhibition by physical and psychological stresses such as pain and discomfort, anxiety, emotional swings, tiredness, embarrassment, worry and alcohol. Women who have had long labours, high levels of intervention and traumatic deliveries may be particularly at risk of impaired oxytocin production. In addition, the use of oxytocin to augment labour may reduce endogenous oxytocin levels in the early postnatal period and also affect the milk ejection reflex (Jonas et al., 2009). The limbic system, which coordinates the body's responses to emotions, is involved in oxytocin release. The likely mechanism is catecholamine inhibition of oxytocin release and adrenergic vasoconstriction of mammary blood vessels limiting access of the oxytocin to the myoepithelial cells. Women experiencing problems in establishing milk flow are often helped by covering their breasts with warm flannels which appears to aid blood flow and oxytocin access. Women may be embarrassed by exposing their breasts or being touched by practitioners helping them to establish breastfeeding and so a 'hands-off' approach is best adopted whilst focusing on maintaining privacy and dignity and minimizing inhibition. Stress reducing interventions such as relaxation therapies and skin-to-skin contact have been shown to improve lactation performance (Lau, 2001).

Surprisingly, denervation of mammary glands in experimental animals appears to have little effect on milk production (Williams et al., 1993). This suggests that the afferent nerve pathway may not be as important as the interactions of neurotransmitters. Transmitters that have been implicated in the control of the milk ejection reflex include noradrenaline, β-endorphin, serotonin and dopamine. As with control of prolactin secretion, the number of factors influencing oxytocin secretion suggests that the pathway is much more complicated than originally thought. Stimulation of the female reproductive tract, especially the vagina and cervix, increases oxytocin release so milk may be ejected from the breasts during coitus.

Oxytocin binds to specific receptors on the myoepithelial cells around the milk-secreting cells and to longitudinal cells in the duct walls. Contraction of the myoepithelial cells results in milk being expelled into the ducts, which shorten as the longitudinal cells contract. Oxytocin-induced contraction generates pressure waves within the breasts and is responsible for prickly sensations associated with breastfeeding. When the milk ejection reflex is well established, milk may be spontaneously ejected from both breasts.

Oxytocin pulses increase in amplitude during labour and are involved in the positive-feedback amplification in labour (see Chapter 1). Oxytocin is associated with changes in maternal behaviour and increased alertness at delivery. The pulses of oxytocin induced by feeding have an effect on the uterus, stimulating uterine contractions and involution. Multiparous women tend to feel these contractions or 'after-pains' with increased intensity. Women who do not want to breastfeed may find the physiological changes in the breasts at delivery uncomfortable; various techniques are recommended to inhibit lactation (Box 16.3).

Box 16.3 **Methods for suppression of lactation**

- Bromocriptine (dopamine agonist) (use with great caution)
- Treatment with sex steroids to antagonize prolactin effects
- Breast-binding
- Application of ice-packs

SUCKLING AND MILK TRANSFER

In feeding from the breast, the baby takes the whole nipple into its mouth and places its tongue under the adjacent areola. When the baby's tongue moves down, ducts in the nipple fill with milk which is expelled when the tongue moves upwards. The milk is expressed from the nipple and sucking aids the process.

Babies exhibit two distinct patterns of suckling (Turgeon-O'Brien et al., 1996). Nutritive suckling is a continuous stream of strong slow sucks, which efficiently allows milk transfer. This occurs predominantly in the early part of the feed. Non-nutritive suckling increasingly replaces nutritive suckling during the progression of the feed. It is characterized by alternation of rapid shallow bursts of suckling and rests. It is thought that patterns of thumb sucking may reflect these two conducts. Breastfed babies have two distinct rhythms of thumb sucking and tend to put more of the root of the thumb into their mouths. Although non-nutritive suckling is associated with a decreased transfer of milk, it is still very effective in stimulating prolactin release and so may be important in successful lactation. It has been suggested that odours from volatile compounds in the secretions from the Montgomery's tubercles may promote positive feeding behaviour such as rooting and contribute to the establishment of effective milk production and transfer (Doucet et al., 2009).

The amount of milk produced is extremely variable; that mothers can feed multiple babies and produce additional milk for banking or storage suggests that the mammary synthetic capacity exceeds the normal requirement of single infants. A demand-fed baby consumes irregular quantities of milk at irregular times. The suggestion that the baby determines milk yield by local control is supported by the strong correlation between degree of breast emptying and rate of milk synthesis. Some women feed exclusively from one breast (and not at all from the other). The autocrine factor capable of overriding the central hormone control, feedback inhibitor of lactation (FIL), was first identified in goats (Wilde et al., 1995). This protein inhibitory factor has also been found in the whey fraction of human milk.

It is secreted from the alveolar cells and accumulates in milk. The factor inhibits secretion of lactose, probably by blocking the action of prolactin, and therefore provides the mechanism to adjust supply to demand. When milk is not removed from the breast, the concentration of the factor increases and blocks the action of prolactin thus reducing the rate of milk synthesis. It helps to explain why maternal dietary intake has relatively little influence on the amount of milk produced. Women in traditional societies have a much greater frequency of breastfeeding so their production of FIL is probably not enough to have an autocrine effect on lactation; milk synthesis is most likely to be influenced solely by metabolic and endocrine mechanisms (Hartmann et al., 1998). Ankyloglossia or tongue tie may interfere with the suckling reflex and the division of the tie (frenulotomy) may be effective in improving breastfeeding (Miranda et al., 2010).

INVOLUTION

After cessation of lactation, involution takes about 3 months. Milk accumulates in the alveoli and small lactiferous ducts, which causes distension and mechanical atrophy of the epithelial cells and rupture of the alveolar walls, creating large spaces. Milk secretion is therefore suppressed by local mechanical factors rather than by diminishing prolactin levels. Phagocytosis of the cells and glandular debris results in fewer and smaller lobular–acinar structures. The alveolar lumens decrease in size and may disappear. The alveolar lining changes from a single secretory layer to a non-secretory double layer. If breastfeeding is stopped suddenly, the process is more intense and painful. The breasts remain larger after lactation as the deposits of fat and connective tissue are increased. Involution after lactation is different to the structural atrophy and loss of adipose tissue occurring in postmenopausal mammary cells deprived of oestrogen.

PROBLEMS ASSOCIATED WITH LACTATION

Milk insufficiency

Most problems have an identifiable physiological basis; breast milk insufficiency is frequently over-diagnosed and is usually simply resolved (Woolridge, 1996). The majority of women with apparently insufficient milk supply have unsubstantiated worries and require confidence, improved technique (especially positioning), encouragement or advice. This can be supported by physiological strategies such as electric breast pumps and pharmacological (anti-dopamine) agents. Avoiding pressure on the breasts (such as that due to wearing a tight bra or other tight clothing or sleeping prone) is important as it can negatively affect milk supply. Iatrogenic low milk supply may be attributed to excessive down-regulation of supply probably during the calibration period. It is possible that baby milk manufacturers inadvertently exploit the importance of the calibration period by offering free milk samples early in lactation. If the initial calibrated volume cannot be increased, the mother will then be unable to increase her milk supply later and will be forced to provide alternative inferior sources of milk, which are expensive and can be harmful if water supplies are contaminated, as happens in a number of developing countries.

Behavioural problems that are acquired by the baby as coping strategies to avoid aversive events may also induce a low milk supply. These problems include discomfort during positioning at the breast and problems with breathing. Self-limitation of intake and lack of persistence may account for the condition described as 'contented underfed babies' (Woolridge, 1996). Pathophysiological failure is rare and probably affects less than 2% of women with apparent milk insufficiency. Rare causes include mammary hypoplasia, or absence of normal breast development at puberty or in pregnancy. Retained placental products affect lactation reversibly but Sheehan's syndrome, necrosis of the anterior pituitary due to acute hypovolaemic shock, as in antepartum haemorrhage (e.g. due to placental abruption) or postpartum haemorrhage, is more serious.

Drugs

Many drugs are secreted into breast milk, but the data on the effects of specific drugs on the breastfed infant is often not available. Of particular concern are those drugs with central nervous system (CNS) activity as the postnatal development of the infant's nervous system is vulnerable. The benefits of maternal treatment and the advantages of breastfeeding have to be balanced against the risk of exposure of the neonate to the medication. Passive diffusion of the unbound, unionized form of the drug into the breast milk is the major mechanism of transfer. Therefore, it is affected by maternal compartmentalization and molecular properties and the composition of the breast milk (McManaman and Neville, 2003). Assessment of adverse drug reactions in infants is difficult. Drugs that are minimally excreted into the breast milk, are metabolized quickly by the neonate and are not associated with adverse effects are obviously the preferred choice.

Socially used drugs such as alcohol (Mennella and Beauchamp, 1991), nicotine and illicit drugs (heroin and cocaine) (Golding, 1997) also cross into the milk. How much these affect the baby is not clear. Women who smoke are less likely to want to breastfeed, or initiate breastfeeding, and more likely to breastfeed for a shorter duration (Amir and Donath, 2003). Drug metabolism and elimination by the neonate is often limited, so exposure to apparently low doses of the drug in milk can have a cumulative effect, particularly in premature babies and those who have prolonged exposure. Drugs tend not to accumulate in the milk but have a bidirectional transfer. Therefore, the amount of drug received by the infant will be reduced if the mother takes the drug immediately after a feed so the baby does not feed when the drug is at peak concentration in the maternal plasma and milk. Production of breast milk is also a method of excretion and contains drugs, viruses, food additives, chemical contamination (such as lead), volatile solvents, pesticides and radioactivity. Chemical residues of pollutants are detected in most human milk throughout the world. Heavy metals are of concern because of the susceptibility of the infant's nervous system. Mammals do not have a mechanism to excrete pesticide residues such as polychlorinated biphenyls and 1,1,1-trichloro-2,2-bis(p-chlorophenyl)ethane (DDT). However, the residues do cross the blood–breast barrier so lactation is the only way to reduce the body load. The burden of persistent organic pollutants is then transferred to the breastfed infant (Nickerson, 2006). Usually, breastfeeding is not contraindicated but a slow and steady rate of maternal weight loss during lactation is important to limit the mobilization of maternal fat and release of the environmental contaminants which can then partition in the breast milk.

Psychological stress and breast diseases

Women often cease breastfeeding prematurely in the first 6 months after birth because they experience breastfeeding related problems such as pain, cracked nipples, milk stasis and mastitis (Abou-Dakn et al., 2009). These conditions may occur in isolation or may be compounded by anxiety about milk sufficiency. It is estimated that a significant proportion of breastfeeding women will experience some problem in the first few days of feeding. Women experiencing breastfeeding problems are likely to have a higher level of psychological stress. Although lactation may be protective against stress in the short-term, longer lasting psychological stress may negatively affect the endocrine, immune and nervous systems (Wöckel et al., 2010).

Viruses

Maternal viruses may enter the milk. Vertical transmission and subsequent infection of the infant via breast milk have been confirmed for human immunodeficiency virus (HIV), tuberculosis (TB), cytomegalovirus (CMV) and hepatitis B. It is probably inadvisable for mothers with TB to breastfeed as the infection tends to be reactivated by maternal tiredness and stress (Box 16.4). However, advice for HIV-positive mothers is unclear. The immunological

---

Box 16.4 **Contraindications to breastfeeding**

- Maternal illness
- Maternal drug consumption
- Congenital abnormalities, for example, cleft palate
- HIV-positive – controversial
- TB infection (depending on strain and treatment)

Case study 16.2

Elma expressed concerns about breastfeeding throughout her pregnancy. She complained that the midwives running the antenatal classes were biased towards breastfeeding and that bottle-feeding was just as good. Elma described her own family as an example; she is the oldest of five children all of whom were bottle-fed by her mother and were well and healthy. Two days after delivery, Elma experienced breast discomfort and tentatively asked a midwife whether it was too late to try breastfeeding.

- How would you as the midwife explain and encourage Elma to breastfeed throughout the antenatal period?
- What are the health advantages for mothers and their babies who choose to breast feed? Do you think women should be informed of the higher risks of infection for the baby if the mother chooses to feed with formula milk? If so, remember it is not just because of the need to ensure sterilization of feeding equipment but formula milk lacks many of the components of breast milk that actively reduce infection in the newborn.
- What factors would increase her chances of being successful in breastfeeding?
- What support would she require from the midwives?
- Would breastfeeding or anything else help to relieve the breast discomfort?

---

properties of breast milk are probably important in protecting against illnesses that accelerate the development of AIDS (acquired immune deficiency syndrome), particularly in areas of the world where it is endemic (Van de Perre, 1995). The likelihood of HIV transmission is affected by maternal viral load, the volume of the milk consumed, the duration of breastfeeding, inflammation of the breast (e.g. caused by cracked nipples), the presence of oral thrush and the introduction of formula milk (Warner and Sapsford, 2004). (Note that several medications used in HIV prophylaxis can transfer to the breast milk and have potentially serious side effects, including anaemia, seizures, hepatitis and feeding difficulties.) The WHO recommends exclusive breastfeeding for the first 6 months of life (and breastfeeding with complementary feeding for the first 2 years of life). The rationale for this is the protective effect of breastfeeding on infection rate. However, in developed countries where the water supply is clean and good quality, alternatives to breast milk are feasible and affordable, it may be preferable for mothers with serious infections not to breastfeed to prevent vertical transmission. However, it should be noted that whatever method is chosen, it should be exclusive as mixed feeding is thought to increase the risk of transmission of HIV.

Case study 16.2 is an example of concerns about breastfeeding.

INHIBITION OF FERTILITY

Breast milk is also important to the infant because suppression of fertility is an advantage. An adequate birth interval is important for both maternal and child health. Lactational amenorrhoea may last from 2 months to 4 years. It is particularly important in developing countries where breastfeeding prevents more pregnancies than all the other methods of contraception put together. The variability in duration of suppressed fertility seems to be related to a number of factors; the most important seems to be frequency of suckling. At the end of pregnancy, levels of gonadotrophins are very low because high levels of oestrogen continue to impose negative feedback. At delivery, the placental hormones begin to disappear, at different rates depending on their half-life. hPL disappears from the plasma within hours. Oestrogen and progesterone levels fall to pre-pregnant levels within a week of the placental loss (Hytten, 1995). Levels of human chorionic gonadotrophin (hCG) are negligible about 3 weeks after delivery. There is a gradual recovery in the ovarian–pituitary axis over the first 4 months after delivery; this recovery is delayed by regular suckling.

In non-lactating women, body temperature measurements and the first menstrual bleeding suggest that the earliest ovulation may occur at 4 weeks after delivery but is usually delayed until 8–10 weeks (McNeilly, 2001); most women have resumed normal menstrual patterns by 15 weeks. The first menstrual cycle is often anovulatory or associated with an inadequate luteal phase. Most women ovulate by the third cycle. Fifty percent of non-lactating women who do not use contraception conceive within 6–7 months.

Menstruation and ovulation return more slowly in a lactating woman. Ovarian activity usually returns before the end of lactational amenorrhoea. Therefore, menstruation is a poor indicator of fertility; conception can occur before the resumption of menstrual cycles. Neither ovulation nor menstruation normally occurs within 6 weeks, but about half of all contraceptive-unprotected breastfeeding mothers conceive within 9 months of lactation, 1–10% during lactational amenorrhoea. Between 30% and 70% of first cycles are ovulatory; the longer the period of lactational amenorrhoea, the more likely the woman is to ovulate prior to the first menstruation.

The precise mechanisms involved in lactational amenorrhoea are not clear. High prolactin levels abolish the pulsatile luteinizing hormone (LH) secretion and decrease the pituitary response to gonadotrophin-releasing hormone. The mid-cycle positive feedback in response to oestrogen is absent. The sensitivity to negative feedback is enhanced and that to positive feedback is decreased. So, even if enough LH and follicle-stimulating hormone (FSH) are present to stimulate follicular development, the inhibitory effect of oestrogen results in an inadequate luteal phase. Prolactin is inhibitory at the level of the ovary, blocking the effects of LH and FSH. It also has a direct effect on the brain, possibly affecting libido.

As prolactin secretion has a pulsatile rhythm with larger amounts being released at night, the frequency of stimulation by suckling and the night-time feeds are particularly important in maintaining prolactin levels high enough to suppress fertility (McNeilly, 2001). The duration and number of feeds are important because the prolactin levels are augmented before they return completely to the basal secretory level. Prolonged amenorrhoea is associated with maternal malnutrition (Rogers, 1997). Poor nutrition is associated with suppression of fertility in non-lactating women. The extra nutrient requirement for milk production can increase the degree of maternal malnutrition. Also, although women receiving less than optimal nutrition can breastfeed their babies adequately, they secrete milk more slowly so the infants feed more often and for longer which raises their circulating prolactin levels.

MATERNAL BEHAVIOUR

Maternal commitment to reproduction is more than pregnancy; it involves the establishment of lactation and appropriate maternal behaviour (Grattan, 2002). The demands of the parents and offspring during lactation may conflict. It is suggested that parents will tend to maximize the survival of their young but not to the extent that would limit investment in other offspring, including those as yet unborn (Peaker, 1989). This theory means that, although mothers will try to recoup the investment of pregnancy by favouring the offspring's survival, should this cost compromise their future reproductive ability there are definite advantages in discontinuing this investment in favour of a more favourable future offspring. There may be genetic components affecting the time course of lactation or the upper limit of milk production. The rate of milk secretion and duration of lactation vary with nutritional state. Some mammals respond to decreased food supply in ways that favour the succeeding pregnancies, such as killing some or all of the litter. Species with long gestation and long-term commitment to the offspring, such as humans, tend to favour the well being of live offspring.

Behavioural changes include preparatory behaviour such as nest building and increased aggression. Care and protection are associated with lactation, particularly the maternal level of oxytocin (Gordon et al., 2010). These behavioural patterns are associated with the progressive independence of the young. In humans, this behaviour is more difficult to observe than in other species.

The nutritional status of the mother may affect feeding and interaction with her infant (Britton, 1993). The effect of maternal malnutrition can affect infant development, depending on its duration and the timing. Infants malnourished in utero may have decreased capacity to respond to appropriate cues and therefore an increased likelihood of social and further nutritional deprivation. Malnourished infants have poorer muscle tone, increased lethargy, irritability and frequency of illness, decreased attention and responsiveness and altered sleep–wake states. Malnourished mothers experience more fatigue, which can affect their own sensitivity to cues from the baby, such as responses to stress and attention–behavioural patterns.

NUTRITION OF THE LACTATING MOTHER

Human growth rate is much slower than that of other animals. Neurological development is relatively late and the duration of human lactation is longer. During lactation, daily nutrient input and reserves laid down in pregnancy are juggled. Milk output is largely independent of the mother's ethnic origin and nutritional status. A balanced diet in lactation appears to favour the health of the mother. However, it should be noted that substrates required for milk synthesis are not flexible. Mammary glands are not able to synthesize essential amino acids or long-chain polyunsaturated fatty acids (LC-PUFAs); they also require non-essential amino acids for protein synthesis and glucose or glucose precursors for lactose and oligosaccharide synthesis. These have to be provided from the maternal diet or from maternal body reserves. Indeed, it has been suggested that the maternal brain may act as a reservoir of PUFAs for both fetal and neonatal brain requirements (Dewar and Psych, 2004) and that increased transfer of nutrients to the developing brain during pregnancy and lactation might contribute to postnatal depression.

Energy requirements for milk production

The energy output of milk is a significant proportion of the total energy output of the lactating woman; it is suggested that peak lactation requires an increase of energy intake of about 25%. In dairy animals, the level of food intake strongly correlates with milk yield. In a number of species, lactation results in a significant increase in size and complexity (such as villus size) of the maternal intestine (Hammond, 1997), but it is obviously not possible to study any such adaptive changes in lactating women. It may not be valid to apply knowledge of nutrition and physiology of dairy animals, which are completely milked twice a day, to mammals that suckle their young according to natural patterns of behaviour. Anthropological studies on human hunter–gatherer communities suggest that babies feed every half hour at 2 weeks and every 4 h at 4 months. The characteristics of mammalian milk relate directly to the interaction between the mother and child. Marsupials and animals that bear their young during hibernation are always present and produce milk that is dilute and has a low fat content. In contrast, in animals where the mother nurses her young at widely spaced intervals, for instance a hunting lioness, the milk is very concentrated and high in fat. Human milk has most resemblance to the former; it is dilute with a low fat content suggesting that humans have evolved as a species where the young have unlimited access to milk and there is high attentiveness shown by a constantly present mother (Prentice and Prentice, 1995). The stress of human lactation is relatively low compared with species with faster growing or multiple young, but this is countered by the high cost of maintaining a dependent infant for a prolonged period. The high level of maternal investment in pregnancy and slow reproductive cycle mean that humans are committed to sustain a conception.

There is a discrepancy between the theoretical calculated energy requirement for milk production and the actual intake of lactating women, even taking into account the fat reserves laid down in pregnancy. Current recommendations are that an exclusively breastfeeding woman requires an additional 2700 kJ (650 kcal) per day and an increase of 20 g of protein per day (Dewey, 1997). However, it is thought that about 600 kJ (150 kcal) per day will be provided by the maternal fat stores for the first 6 months so the net increment needed is 2100 kJ (500 kcal) per day. In practice, these requirements are much higher than the observed intakes in successfully lactating women even when offered unlimited access to food. Lactational performance is particularly resilient in humans as demonstrated by the efficiency of lactation in undernourished and impoverished communities. In animals, a decrease in non-shivering thermogenesis (inhibition of brown-fat heat generation) (NST) and therefore the provision of extra energy for milk production are suggested to account for this difference. The mechanism in humans is not thought to be mediated by changes in NST but the lactating woman has increased sensitivity to insulin (Illingworth et al., 1986). This energy-sparing effect and efficient energy utilization of lactating women have a particularly big implication in developing countries.

Increased incidence of obesity in Western societies is of concern with about a third of women having a body mass index (BMI) greater than 25 kg/m^2. Pregnancy is a risk factor for the development of obesity; it is suggested that postpartum weight loss may not be inevitable and gestational weight gain may not be lost postpartum (Chin et al., 2010). Possibly, the changes in energy metabolism associated with pregnancy and lactation may remain after weaning. If so, lactation could contribute to the problem. Different species of mammal lay down body fat during pregnancy to different degrees. In lactation, mammals rely on the deposited fat to different extents. Whales and seals, for instance, rely entirely on body fat and protein reserves to sustain lactation whereas dairy cows and laboratory rats are very dependent on increased intake to provide energy for milk yield. Pregnant women deposit fat and have a changed hormonal environment. The reported studies tend to conflict and do not show significant differences in weight loss with different patterns of infant feeding. However, interpretation of the studies is confused by confounding factors such as different duration and extent of feeding and the increased tendency of women who are not breastfeeding to reduce their weight deliberately. There is also a large variation in the energy content of the milk produced (see below). Lactating women produce adequate-to-abundant quantities of milk of sufficient quality to promote growth of healthy infants, even when maternal nutrition is not adequate. Whereas the health of the breastfeeding infant is apparently protected should maternal nutrition be compromised, it is probably at the cost of depletion of maternal nutrient stores and potential effects on subsequent pregnancies. Deliberate weight loss in well-nourished healthy breastfeeding woman has no effect on the yield or composition of breast milk. However, it is recommended that weight loss should not be more than 1–2 kg per month (Institute of Medicine, 2002). Although reduction in energy intake does not affect milk synthesis, lower intakes of food mean that micronutrient intake, particularly calcium and vitamin D, might be compromised (Lovelady et al., 2006). As energy intake falls, the likelihood of a number of nutrients failing to reach the recommended intake progressively increases. In order of vulnerability, the nutrients most likely to be affected are calcium, zinc, magnesium, thiamin, vitamin B$_6$, vitamin E, riboflavin, folate, phosphorus and iron (Lawrence, 2010). Overweight lactating women are advised to restrict their energy intake by decreasing consumption of foods high in simple sugars and fat and by increasing their intake of calcium-rich foods, vegetables and fruit.

Minerals

Both pregnancy and lactation present a tremendous challenge to maternal calcium status (Prentice, 2000). The fetal skeleton requires 5 mmol of calcium per day. The lactational drain of calcium is greater; average daily production of 800 mL milk contains 6.25 mmol of calcium. It is estimated that about 10% of total maternal calcium stores (about 105 g) is transferred to the fetus/neonate, predominantly duration lactation (Wysolmerski, 2002). One or more of the following can meet demand for calcium: increased dietary calcium, increased absorption, decreased excretion or increased bone demineralization (net loss of bone). In the third trimester, absorption of calcium increases together with a modest increase in bone resorption. This increase in calcium absorption appears to be independent of vitamin D status (Fudge and Kovacs, 2010). Calcium demands of lactation are met by an increase in the rate of bone resorption and a decrease in renal calcium excretion which are speculated to have evolved from the adaptations in bone and mineral metabolism that supply calcium for egg production in lower vertebrates (Wysolmerski, 2002). The oestrogen level during lactation is relatively low so the bone mass is not protected to the same extent.

Lactation is the period of most rapid bone loss in a woman's life; there is a net drain of calcium from the body, with a selective decrease in trabecular bone. This reduction is independent of parathyroid hormone and vitamin D levels. So lactation may appear to increase future risk of osteoporosis, but risk factors shown to be associated with fractures do not necessarily include breastfeeding (Sowers, 1996). During weaning, an imbalance between bone resorption and bone formation results in a rapid and complete recovery of bone mass. The implications for birth spacing and prolonged breastfeeding are not clear. Modern practices of delaying childbearing resulting in decreased time for recovery before menopause are probably countered by the cumulative effect of having fewer children. Prolonged lactational amenorrhoea may help to restore maternal iron status.

The mammary gland homeostatically controls milk concentration of essential nutrients; levels of major minerals including calcium, sodium, potassium, phosphorus and magnesium are not affected by the diet. The mammary gland can adapt to maternal deficiency (or excess) of iron, zinc and copper (Lönnerdal, 2007) suggesting there are active transport mechanisms for these nutrients in the mammary gland. When milk production falls during weaning, milk iron levels decrease and milk zinc levels increase. However, maternal intakes of iodine and selenium do affect levels in milk. As iodine is so important for fetal and neonatal brain and nervous system development and many women do not have an optimal intake of iodine (partly because salt use is decreasing and fewer iodine-containing cleaning agents are used in the dairy industry), iodine supplements are widely recommended for pregnant and lactating women and for women considering pregnancy (Zimmermann, 2009).

Water and fluids

The volume of milk produced is robust; only very severe dehydration and extreme malnutrition affect the volume of milk produced. There is no evidence that increasing fluid intake increases the volume of milk produced or that reducing fluid intake prevents engorgement. When fluids are restricted, urine output decreases and the woman is at risk of dehydration. Breastfeeding women should be advised to drink when they are thirsty and to be aware that they will need more fluid than normal.

INFANT NUTRITION AND THE COMPOSITION OF HUMAN MILK

Human milk optimally fulfils the nutritional requirements of the human neonate. It has a unique composition that is particularly suitable for the rapid growth and development of the infant born with immature digestive, renal and hepatic systems. Unique features of human milk are able to compensate for the underdeveloped neonatal capabilities. Human milk contains not only the macronutrients, vitamins and minerals but also non-nutrient growth factors, hormones and protective factors.

There are at least 100 components of human milk, including substances yet to be identified and their roles elucidated. In the Koran, breast milk is described as 'white blood'. This is a particularly apt description, because the early milk has more white blood cells than blood itself. Milk is a solution in which other substances are dissolved, emulsified or colloidally dispersed. The value of breast milk is undisputed; rarely should breastfeeding be discouraged.

Both the volume and composition of human milk are extremely variable. Some of this variability is genetic (any genetic mutation leading to inadequate mammary development in humans would no longer be eliminated as alternatives to human milk are available). Postponing childbearing until long after sexual maturity has an effect on breast development as advancing age causes some atrophy of the mammary tissue (Hytten, 1995). However, there is little relationship between the size of the breast and milk output.

The unique characteristic of humans is the large complex brain, which undergoes much development in the first 2 years of life. Human milk provides levels of lactose, cysteine, cholesterol and thromboplastin, which are required for CNS tissue synthesis. However, as breast milk provides a model of optimum nutrition, analysis of its composition has allowed good substitutes to be produced as formula feeds. Infant formula milk will never completely mimic human milk, however, as the quality of the nutrients is not reproducible and the immunological aspects of the milk make it superior.

Although breast milk may be considered perfect nutrition, its composition is variable. It varies from woman to woman, from one period of lactation to another, and hourly through the day. Its composition is related to the timing of the feed, how much is produced and parameters relating to the last feed (Emmett and Rogers, 1997); it has also been suggested that maternal age, parity, health and social class affect the composition of the milk. Mothers of premature infants produce milk that has a higher concentration of some nutrients, but this probably reflects the small volumes produced for small infants. Except for vitamin and fat content, the composition is largely independent of maternal nutrition unless the mother experiences severe malnutrition. Supplementation may improve maternal health rather than affect milk composition and volume.

There are many difficulties encountered in the estimation of the volume of milk produced. Weighing either the mother or baby before and after the feed is fraught with problems. Although double-labelled water measurements have allowed more accurate estimations (Lucas et al., 1987), the variability within a feed and from feed to feed makes it very difficult to ascertain precisely the nutrient consumption of a healthy growing baby. These estimates of about 60 kcal per 100 mL are lower than UK food composition tables (69 kcal per 100 mL). The volume of daily milk intake by healthy infants has a wide range. Factors that influence frequency, intensity or duration of feeds will affect volume consumed. Breastfed infants appear to self-regulate their energy intake and consume more milk if it has a lower energy level. This is thought to be related to the lower incidence of obesity in individuals who were breastfed as infants (Dewey, 2003). Breastfeeding allows infants to learn self-regulation of energy intake whereas bottle-fed infants may be encouraged to finish the bottle which suppresses their autoregulatory mechanism. Breast milk may also contain appetite inhibitors and stimulators. It is suggested that different modes of infant feeding have different metabolic programming effects. Formula-fed infants tend to receive more protein which results in an increased insulin response. Insulin stimulates adipose tissue deposition (increased number and fat content of adipocytes) which is associated with weight gain and obesity. Alternatively, breastfeeding may affect leptin metabolism; the higher level of fatness in formula-fed infants may programme reduced sensitivity to leptin in later life. However, it should be noted that there is confounding by parental attributes and the family environment. Parents who choose to breastfeed tend to have a healthier lifestyle with more optimal dietary habits and higher levels of physical activity; they also exert less parental control over child-feeding practices (Dewey, 2003).

The low levels of gastric secretion and other immature digestive characteristics of the neonatal gut confer a number of immunological advantages which were described in Chapter 15 (p. 397).

Colostrum

In the first 3 days postdelivery, the mother produces about 2–10 mL of colostrum per day. More colostrum is produced sooner if the woman has had previous pregnancies, particularly if she has lactated before. In some cultures, colostrum is thought to be old milk or 'pus' and is discarded rather than fed to infants.

Colostrum is transparent and is yellow from the high β-carotene content. Mature milk in contrast looks less viscous and slightly blue. Colostrum has more protein and vitamins A and K and less carbohydrate and fat than mature milk. It is easily digested and well absorbed. It has a lower energy content of 58 kcal per 100 mL compared with 70 kcal per 100 mL in mature milk. Levels of sodium, potassium, chloride and zinc are high in colostrum but these reflect the low volume produced rather than the infant's requirements for a bolus dose of certain nutrients. The composition is extremely variable, which reflects its unstable secretory pattern.

Colostrum facilitates the colonization of the gut with *Lactobacillus bifidus* (Wharton et al., 1994). Meconium also contains growth factors for *L. bifidus*. Colostrum seems to have a laxative effect, stimulating the passage of meconium. The high protein content is largely due to the abundant antibodies, which protect against gastrointestinal tract infection. IgA forms 50% of the protein content of colostrum, falling to 10% by 6 months. In the first few days of life, priming and maturation of the mucosal immune system is maximal and the gut is permeable and able to absorb macromolecules; colostrum contains many immunomodulatory molecules particularly anti-inflammatory agents which help to protect the vulnerable immature gut from mucosal damage.

During the first 30 h or so, the secretion (colostrum) has a high protein:lactose ratio. In the following days, as the baby suckles more and stimulates milk production, the resulting increase in prolactin secretion stimulates production of the major whey protein α-lactalbumin, which is a specific component of the enzyme lactose synthetase and so regulates lactose production. The effect of increasing lactose production is that water is drawn into the secretion to maintain osmotic equilibrium so the volume increases thus diluting the protein content. The absolute amounts of protein secreted into the milk are maintained or increased even though the concentration falls.

The composition of the milk becomes relatively stable from about day 5 but is variable in volume. The amount of breast milk produced is related to the weight and requirement of the infant; there is a steady increase in volume in the first few weeks. Milk production appears to get under way regardless of the size and requirements of the baby, although hPL levels may play a role in the increased production of milk in mothers of twins. The early weeks of lactation can be considered to be a time of calibration between maternal production and the infant's demand. The volume of milk produced is usually increased to match demand. Down-regulation may be irreversible. It is suggested that mothers of small or preterm babies should express as much milk as they can (i.e. peak yield rather than only enough for the baby's transiently limited requirement).

Milk secretion in women who do not suckle their baby may persist scantily for 3 or 4 weeks while prolactin levels are still high. The effect of suckling is to stimulate the release of prolactin and oxytocin, which are essential for the maintenance of lactation (Fig. 16.4). Provided breastfeeding is regular, lactation can last for several years. Most studies suggest that the average daily volume of milk produced is about 800 mL. Measurement of the milk produced is notoriously difficult but it is clear that there is much variation depending on demand: mothers of twins produce about twice as much milk (Saint et al., 1986) (see Box 16.5).

Energy

The energy requirements of infants can be estimated from total energy expenditure and the energetic cost of tissue deposition during growth (Butte, 2005). Energy

Box 16.5 Breastfeeding twins and multiples

Human milk is nutritionally and immunologically superior to formula milks which is particularly important for twins as multiple pregnancies have a relatively high incidence of prematurity and low birthweight infants. There is no physiological reason for not breastfeeding multiple infants; milk supply will be increased in response to increased demand. Mothers feeding multiple infants are advised to increase their nutrient intake and to rest more. Advice about simultaneous feeding or feeding the infants individually will need to be given (Flidel-Rimon and Shinwell, 2006). Simultaneous feeding saves time and can mean that a more vigorous infant on one breast can stimulate the let-down reflex for the other infant. There are three commonly used positions for feeding twins: 'double cradle' (where the two infants' bodies cross on the mother's abdomen), 'double football' (where the infants' bodies are tucked under the mother's arms) and a cradle-football combination. Mother feeding triplets or quadruplets choose between the various combinations; these mothers often intend to provide their infants with some exposure to human milk rather than feeding them exclusively.

Fig. 16.4 Suckling stimulates the release of prolactin and oxytocin.

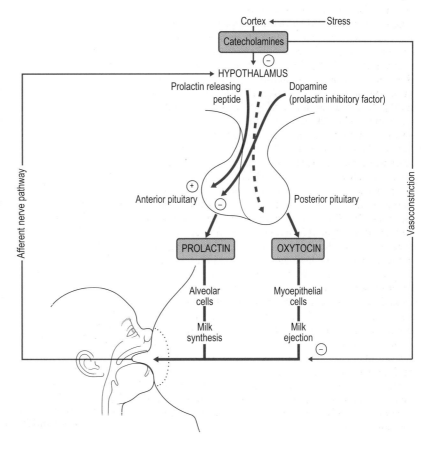

expenditure includes basal metabolism, thermic effect of feeding, thermoregulation and physical activity. The energy requirement to maintain the tissue takes precedence over the energy requirements to synthesize new tissue. So satisfactory growth is a sensitive indicator of whether energy needs are met. Infectious diseases increase energy requirement because there is an increased protein turnover, production of cytokines and phagocytotic cells and repairing tissue are costly and lipids are metabolized less efficiently. Originally, infant energy requirements and recommendations were based on a compilation of energy intakes of well-nourished infants. Measurement of infant energy expenditure using doubly labelled water was subsequently used as the basis for revised energy requirements which were lower than the original recommendations.

Total energy requirements increase with age. Energy requirements are higher in male infants because male infants are heavier. This has an influence on lactation; increased energy content of milk is associated with a male infant. It is proposed that this increased nutritional investment may account for the often observed greater growth rates in male infants (Powe et al., 2010).

Protein

Protein is the limiting nutrient for growth and development. It also provides nitrogen and amino acids required for membrane and transport proteins, hormones, enzymes, growth factors, neurotransmitters and immunoglobulins. Human neonates have a slow growth rate compared with other species which is reflected in the low protein concentrations (0.7–0.9 g protein per 100 mL compared with 3.5 g per 100 mL in cow's milk). (Note that early estimates of protein neglected the high concentration of non-protein nitrogen (NPN) thus significantly overestimating protein level; see below.) Excess protein intake can present an excessive solute load to the immature kidneys, which results in acid–base imbalance and metabolic acidosis. The faster growth rates of formula-fed infants is probably related to the higher level of protein and different ratio of amino acids in formula milks compared to breast milk; as appropriate infant growth has short- and long-term health implications, reducing the protein content and improving the protein quality of formula milks may be desirable. The growth rate of infants fed formula milk or breast milk is different from the first days of life and diverges markedly after 2–3 months. Breastfed infants have lower weight-for-length (Nommsen-Rivers and Dewey, 2009) but it is evident that this is not related to insufficient breast milk. Breastfed infants are also taller as adults (Schack-Nielsen and Michaelsen, 2007).

Chronic maternal protein undernutrition or prolonged lactation may result in changes in the protein composition of milk. Protein supplementation of the mother's diet tends to increase milk volume rather than affecting protein concentration but has an important role in supplementing maternal health.

When milk proteins are exposed to the relatively acidic environment of the neonatal stomach they separate into casein (proteins that precipitate, forming curds) and whey (those proteins that remain soluble). This means that there is a continuous flow of nutrients, initially as soluble lactose and whey proteins, and later from digested curd. Whey proteins include serum albumin, α-lactalbumin, lactoferrin, secretory IgA and some enzymes and protein hormones transported from the maternal circulation. Whey proteins are easy to digest by a human neonatal gut, which has particularly low levels of trypsin and pepsin. The whey-dominant content of milk reduces the risk of lactobezoars (obstructive milk curd balls) forming in the stomach. Human α-lactalbumin is easier to digest than bovine β-lactalbumin.

The ratio of whey to casein in human milk is 60:40 (1.5). The β-casein in human milk forms curds that are soft and flocculent with a low curd tension, which are easily digested. Bioactive peptides formed from partial hydrolysis of human milk casein may be important in stimulating the neonatal immune system (Ebrahim, 1990). In contrast, cow's milk has a whey:casein ratio of 20:80 (0.25). Bovine casein is predominantly α-casein, which forms a tough rubbery precipitate unless heat treated, which is more difficult for human infants to digest and decreases the bioavailability of calcium and other cations. Human β-casein tends to form smaller micelles incorporating minerals that are easier for the neonate to digest. κ-Casein in cow's milk has a marked effect on the development of the bovine gastrointestinal physiology, stimulating the secretion of chymosin, which is the dominant protease of the fourth stomach. Casein associates with calcium, phosphate and magnesium in the micelles.

Colonization of the neonatal gut

The infant at birth has a sterile gut and lacks a fully functional immune system. The neonate is quickly colonized; in a vaginal delivery, the neonate comes into close proximity to its mother's vagina, skin and faeces. Infants born by caesarean section have a reduced number of bacteria. Breast milk also provides a source of bacteria; there are up to 10^9 microbial cells per litre of human milk. Initially, the gut is colonized with aerobic species of bacteria such as Enterobacteriaceae, streptococci and staphylococci (Morelli, 2008). Although these are potentially pathogenic species, their metabolism optimizes subsequent colonization by beneficial enteric bacteria within a couple of days.

The intestinal microbiota or microflora of breastfed and formula fed infants are distinctively different. Breastfed infants have a high preponderance of lactobacilli (especially *Bifidobacterium bifidum* formerly known as *L. bifidus*) which generates a lower pH and inhibits enteric pathogens. Human milk contains large amounts and numbers of complex carbohydrates such as glycans and oligosaccharides. Some glycans inhibit pathogens binding to the gut; there is structural homology between the milk glycan and the gut cell so the pathogen binds to the glycan which effectively acts as a decoy binding site. The glycans are indigestible and so arrive in the colon in an undigested state where they have a prebiotic effect and influence the composition of the intestinal microbiota. This may be particularly important as modern day hygiene practices limit exposure of the neonatal gut to environmental microbiota. Optimizing gut colonization is thought to be important in developing a stable microbial ecosystem which promotes the growth of symbiotic microorganisms and inhibits the colonization by enteric pathogens. The intestinal bacteria also appear to have a role in reducing the risk of developing allergy (Kalliomäki and Isolauri, 2003).

The immune response to cow's milk

A high proportion of dietary casein of bovine origin is associated with an increased incidence of intestinal allergy and inflammation and is implicated as one of the possible triggers of necrotizing enterocolitis (NEC). As the neonatal gut is permeable, large proteins can be absorbed intact across the gut. Some of these proteins stimulate maturation of the gut and immune system. However, others may present an immunological challenge that produces a response which can cause problems later in life. It has been controversially hypothesized that proteins in cow's milk formula are associated with an increased incidence of diabetes (Karjalainen et al., 1992). The hypothesis suggests that a large bovine protein crosses the infant's gut and stimulates the immune system (Monte et al., 1994). Because of similarities between this protein and proteins of the endocrine pancreas, the immune system may direct an autoimmune response against the cells of the pancreas destroying the insulin-producing β-cells. For whatever reason, the incidence of insulin-dependent diabetes mellitus is lower in children who have been breastfed.

Protein

Proteins are formed of chains of 20 amino acids. Some of the amino acids cannot be made in the body; these are essential or indispensable amino acids (see Table 12.1). Non-essential amino acids can be synthesized from glucose and ammonia via the Krebs cycle or from free amino acids by transamination. Some amino acids are conditionally essential for the neonate because the neonate has limited synthetic capability. The amounts and proportions of essential amino acids determine the quality of a protein. A protein that is rich in all essential amino acids has a high biological value or net protein utilization which means all the amino acids supplied are converted into proteins. A food with a deficiency of an amino acid has a low biological value. Human milk has a very high biological value because it is fully utilized by the neonate as its amino acids are exactly in proportion to requirement. Few other foods have such a high value. By the end of the second week of life, 90% of the ingested nitrogen-containing substances in milk are absorbed, suggesting that milk contains the optimal pattern of amino acids.

The amino acid content of human milk, especially whey proteins, is ideal for the growth requirements of the human infant. Neonatal metabolism of certain amino acids (e.g. phenylalanine, tyrosine and methionine) is initially limited because the enzymes involved in their metabolism are expressed late in development. If these amino acids reach high concentrations, they can cause damaging effects. Human milk is relatively low in tyrosine, phenylalanine and methionine but high in amino acids that the infant cannot synthesize in adequate amounts. The inability to synthesis adequate quantities of histidine, cysteine and taurine means that these amino acids become conditionally essential for infants and need to be provided in the diet. The enzyme that converts methionine to cysteine, cystathionase, is low or undetectable in the neonate. Cysteine is required for growth and development. Infants, especially preterm infants, fed unmodified cow's milk may develop hyperphenylalaninaemia and hypertyrosinaemia, which can increase the net acid load and adversely affect development of the CNS.

Taurine is the second most abundant free amino acid in human milk. Infants use taurine for bile acid conjugation (in contrast to adult conjugation by glycine) so this amino acid is important in the digestion and metabolism of cholesterol and fats. There are also high levels of taurine in fetal brain tissue where it may act as a neurotransmitter or neuromodulator, and be involved in myelinization of nerves and the optimal maintenance of retinal integrity (Chesney et al., 1998). The absolute requirement for taurine is unknown but it is added to formula milk at the levels found in human milk.

Aspartame is a sweetener composed of aspartic acid and phenylalanine. If maternal consumption of foods containing aspartame is increased, there is an increase in plasma levels of phenylalanine but levels in milk only increase marginally suggesting that the mammary gland regulates the transfer of amino acids into the milk.

Non-protein nitrogen

More than 25% of the nitrogen found in human milk comes from sources other than protein. This is the NPN fraction (Box 16.6). Methods for protein determination

Box 16.6 **Non-protein nitrogen**

The protein content of human milk was initially overestimated because it was based on the assumption that the nitrogen fractions within the milk would all be components of protein. In fact, about 25% of the nitrogen-containing components in the milk are not within proteins. This is high compared with other species; for instance, cow's milk contains only 5% of the total nitrogen as NPN.

NPN includes:

- Amino sugars: which promote the growth of *Lactobacillus bifidus* and are also incorporated into neural tissue and gut epithelial membrane
- Taurine: a free amino acid that is a component of bile salts and therefore contributes to fat digestion
- Peptides: these have roles as growth factors and hormones
- Cysteine: a free amino acid that is conditionally essential in the infant because the conversion of methionine to cysteine is limited
- Binding factors: these facilitate absorption of other nutrients
- Urea
- Creatine: the role of these factors is not clear
- Creatinine
- Uric acid

usually rely on measuring the total nitrogen in a foodstuff and calculating the average amount of protein that would contain that much nitrogen. Therefore, the protein content of human milk was overestimated before it was clear how large the proportion of NPN was. Each mammalian species has a characteristic amount and profile of NPN, which is of nutritional significance. The NPN of human milk includes a variety of compounds such as peptides and free amino acids (such as those that are conditionally essential), nucleotides, traces of inorganic compounds, urea, creatinine, *N*-acetyl sugars and glycosylated amines. Some of the NPN compounds are of developmental importance but the biological significance of others is uncertain. Urea is high in early milk, reflecting high plasma levels due to uterine involution (see Chapter 14).

Fat

Fat is the main source of energy in the milk. The nutritional status of the mother can affect the fat concentration of the milk and therefore the energy content, fatty acid composition and immunological properties. Of all the macronutrients in milk, fat is the most variable component; it is influenced by the maternal diet, parity, the season of the year and amount of milk removed at the last and current feed, the length of the time between feeds and the fat content of the last feed (Mitoulas et al., 2002). The sampling method used to measure fat is important as hindmilk has three to five times the fat content of foremilk. Averaging foremilk and hindmilk is unlikely to produce a good estimate of the overall composition. The fat content of milk is lowest in the early morning (about 6 a.m.) and then rises to a peak mid-morning (about 10 a.m.) before falling during the day (Hytten, 1995). There is also a progressive decline in the average fat content with increasing maternal age but with much individual variability. The diurnal rhythm of milk composition is related to GH secretion. The fatty acid pattern is variable, reflecting maternal energy intake and dietary fat consumption (Innis, 2007). It is possible to discriminate between the milk of vegetarian and non-vegetarian mothers. The concentration of the LC-PUFAs (such as docosahexaenoic acid (DHA), a component of membrane phospholipids of the brain and retina) in human milk is related to maternal intake and status (Jensen and Lapillonne, 2009). DHA supplementation of lactating women to optimize their status may confer neurodevelopmental and immunological benefits to the breastfed infants and, in addition, may possibly affect postnatal depression and cognitive function of the mothers. If maternal energy and fat intake fall, the fat composition of the milk resembles maternal adipose fat composition as fat stores are mobilized. If the maternal diet is high in energy but low in fat, milk triglycerides are higher in medium-length fatty acids (lauric acid, C_{12}, and myristic acid, C_{14}) indicating synthesis of fatty acids from carbohydrates is increased (Lawrence, 2010). Women of high parity (greater than 10) may have decreased capacity for milk synthesis and therefore produce milk of lower fat (and energy) level.

As fat concentration affects the energy content of the milk, these variations in fat content make it particularly difficult to arrive at the average energy content of human milk. Previous overestimation of energy levels in breast milk resulted in formula milk providing too high an energy level which may have led to overfeeding and potential obesity problems of previous generations.

Ninety percent of fat is present as triacylglycerides. The remaining 10% is made up of free fatty acids, phospholipids, cholesterol, diglycerides and monoglycerides, glycolipids and sterol esters. Fat provides the vehicle for fat-soluble vitamins and essential fatty acids required for brain development. Phospholipids are critical components of cell membranes and are a component of surfactant. The fatty acid composition of human milk is very different to that of cow's milk. Human milk has more essential fatty acids (linoleic and α-linolenic acids), has a higher proportion of unsaturated fatty acids and is rich in long-chain fatty acids. Cow's milk has more short-chain fatty acids (C_4–C_8) and a higher content of saturated fatty acids. The products of lipase digestion are predominantly 2-monoglycerides and free fatty acids, which can be absorbed. Free fatty acids, such as linoleic and lauric acid, and monoglycerides at the concentrations found in the stomachs of breastfed babies are toxic to many pathogens including viruses and some parasites. Monoglycerides act as detergents damaging the membranes of pathogens. Free oleic acid converts the α-lactalbumin in human milk to an altered complex known as HAMLET which induces apoptosis specifically in tumour and virus cells and promotes their regression (Svensson et al., 2002). Most of the triacylglycerides in human milk have palmitic acid (16:0) or oleic acid (18:0) at position 2 of the molecule. Bovine triacylglycerides usually have palmitic acid at position 1 or 3 so digestion of cow's milk fat can release free palmitic acid, which is precipitated by calcium as soap. This can result in the loss of absorption of both fat and calcium.

Human milk and vegetable oil fats are better absorbed than is the saturated fat of cow's milk. Long-chain fatty acids require bile salt micelle formation and lipase activity. Short- and medium-chain fatty acids can be absorbed intact.

Human milk has a high content of cholesterol, which is required for myelin synthesis (important for the CNS development). The cholesterol content of breast milk is not affected by maternal diet. There may be a connection between cholesterol exposure early in life and the development of enzymes for cholesterol degradation and amounts of endogenous cholesterol synthesized (Bayley et al., 1998), which results in lower cholesterol levels in individuals who were breastfed as infants.

As lactation progresses, triacylglyceride levels increase and cholesterol levels fall but phospholipid content remains stable. Usually, 20% of the milk in a feed remains in the breast; this contains about half of the fat. This effect may be due to absorption of fat globules on the surface of the alveolar cells in the secretory and ductal surfaces of the breast. It has been observed that babies suck in longer bursts and decrease the rest intervals when they are feeding on hindmilk (Woolridge and Fisher, 1988).

Essential fatty acids

Human milk provides all the dietary essential fatty acids (see Chapter 12) (Table 16.2) which are required for cell proliferation, retinal development and myelinization of the CNS. The LC-PUFAs DHA and arachidonic acid (AA) are essential constituents of cell membranes, particularly of the nervous system, occurring at notably high concentrations in the brain and retina. The brain undergoes a brain growth spurt in late gestation and early neonatal life when the brain weight increases about 60-fold from 20 g in the second trimester to about 1200 g by the age of 2 years (Dobbing and Sands, 1979). The neonate has a limited ability to desaturate and elongate fatty acid chains thus limiting the conversion of linoleic acid

Table 16.2 Long-chain polyunsaturated fatty acids

	OMEGA-6 (N − 6)	OMEGA-3 (N − 3)
Predominant source	Vegetable oils	Marine oils
Essential fatty acid	Linoleic	α-Linolenic
Converted to	Arachidonic acid	Docosahexaenoic acid

into AA and α-linolenic acid into DHA, so these PUFAs may be conditionally essential in the neonatal diet. Infants acquire PUFAs prenatally via the placenta and postnatally in milk. Human milk is particularly rich in DHA which is suggested to be associated with the raised IQ levels and better visual perception of breastfed infants (Lucas et al., 1992). Maternal PUFA status, and therefore milk levels, varies with fish and fatty acid intake but there is a lack of specific dietary fat recommendations for pregnancy and lactation. As the raised levels of oestrogen in pregnancy would increase the conversion of dietary essential acids to long chain fatty acids, the most vulnerable time seems to be lactation when oestrogen levels are low. It is suggested that lactating women who do not consume the currently recommended intakes of oily fish (two portions per week) should use a supplement (1 g fish oil per day) to achieve the equivalent breast milk levels of DHA (Innis, 2007).

LC-PUFAs are important for synaptogenesis in the visual system which is assessed by measuring visual acuity and speed of processing in infants. Breastfed infants appear to have a slight neurodevelopment advantage which is attributed to the high PUFA level of human milk. However, it should be noted that there are a number of selection biases, as women who choose to breastfeed tend to have higher IQ, educational level and socioeconomic status. Patterns of parent–child interactions may also be different.

The variation in milk fat reflects the variation in maternal diet. A low-fat maternal diet may maximize *de novo* synthesis of fatty acids for milk triacylglycerols but should contain adequate quantities of LC-PUFAs. As a species, humans have a uniquely large brain, which is composed of about 60% lipid. The essential dietary requirement for LC-PUFAs required for the development of the human cerebral cortex has some interesting evolutionary aspects. It has been proposed that the freshwater lakes of the Rift Valley in East Africa provided the optimal environment to promote development of Homo sapiens (Broadhurst et al., 1998). Freshwater fish and shellfish are particularly rich in LC-PUFAs and have an AA:DHA ratio similar to that of the human brain.

The importance of the long-chain fatty acid ratios may explain some of the observed benefits of breast milk such as the decreased incidence of multiple sclerosis (Pisacane et al., 1994). Animal fats, including human milk, tend to be rich in omega-6 fatty acids (Crawford, 1993). Formula milks are supplemented with fat derived from vegetable sources so tend to be far richer in linoleic acid than the omega-3 family of long-chain polyunsaturated fats. Milk intended for preterm babies is now supplemented with AA and DHA because premature babies have a very limited capability in elongating and desaturating fatty acids and have not experienced as much transfer of fatty acids in the third trimester. As premature infants have a high requirement, optimal levels of these LC-PUFAs in breast milk of mothers of preterm infants can be achieved by giving the mothers a supplement or by adding DHA directly to expressed milk (Lapillonne and Jensen, 2009).

Lipases

Human milk contains lipases, which are supplemented by unique production of neonatal lipases; these together compensate for limited pancreatic lipase activity. Lipoprotein lipase (serum-stimulated lipase) may appear in milk because of leakage from mammary tissue. Refrigerated and frozen milk undergo lipolysis. The enzyme responsible for this appears to have activity similar to that of pancreatic lipase; it is present in the fat fraction of the milk and is inhibited by bile salts. The most important lipase is the bile salt-stimulated lipase, which occurs in milk of humans and other primates. This enzyme, which is stable and active in the gut, has a significant effect on hydrolysis of milk triacylglycerides and is activated by concentrations of bile salts even lower than those required for micelle formation.

Lipase activity occurs in the saliva (and there may be additional gastric lipase activity). This lingual lipase is stimulated by the presence of milk in the mouth and by suckling, even non-nutritive suckling. Human milk fat digestion is 85–90% efficient compared with less than 70% efficiency of the fat digestion in cow's milk-derived formulas. Human milk fat globules are enclosed in maternal alveolar cell membranes, which aid in maintaining optimal surface area for emulsification and absorption and also protect the fat from lipolysis and oxidation. These factors mean that human milk stores well.

Carnitine

Human milk contains carnitine, which has an important role in facilitating the entry of long-chain fatty acids into mitochondria where they are oxidized. Carnitine is synthesized from the essential amino acids, lysine and methionine, but neonates may have limited synthetic capacity. Carnitine also is involved in the initiation of ketogenesis and in the regulation of heat generation from brown adipose tissue. As infants use fat as a major source of energy and have limited ability to synthesize carnitine, they have an increased need for carnitine.

Carbohydrate

Lactose, which is unique to mammalian milk (and probably therefore important in the development of the mammalian order), is the principal carbohydrate of milk, present at about 7 g per 100 mL. The lactose concentration of mature human milk is thought to be related to the size of the adult brain. Levels of lactose are stable as lactose drives the volume of milk produced. There is no evidence that maternal nutrition affects lactose concentration. As well as lactose, there is also a significant amount of 130 other sugars, the most prevalent of which are glucose, galactose, glucosamine and other oligosaccharides (see below). Some of the non-lactose sugars may contribute to favourable gut colonization. Nitrogen-containing oligosaccharides, including the complex sugar l-fucose, promote the growth of *L. bifidus* resulting in increased gut acidity, which suppresses the growth of pathogenic bacteria and may facilitate calcium absorption.

Lactose is a disaccharide that is digested by the enzyme lactase into its component monosaccharides, glucose and galactose. Lactase activity develops rapidly in late gestation and is adequate from 36 weeks; its activity cannot be prematurely induced by exposure. Most mammals and many humans do not produce lactase after infancy. The ability to produce lactase throughout life seems to be related to continual exposure to lactose in communities that have a strong economic dependence on dairy farming.

Lactose is relatively insoluble and is slowly digested and absorbed in the small intestine. It promotes the growth of microorganisms that produce organic acids and synthesize many B vitamins. The acidic environment is inhospitable to many pathogenic bacteria. Lactose forms soluble salts so the absorption of calcium, phosphorus, magnesium and other metals is increased in the presence of lactose.

Clinical application: nutritional problems of preterm infants

Human milk is nutritionally inadequate for preterm infants, leading to poor growth rates and osteopaenia. However, it does have clear advantages. It has valuable immunological properties, protecting against NEC; 90% of infants affected by NEC have not been exposed to any human milk. Human milk is associated with improved cognition and it stimulates gut maturity and immunomodulation. The ideal food for a preterm infant able to tolerate lactose is the baby's own mother's milk fortified with additional calories, protein and minerals. Babies requiring parenteral feeding benefit from receiving some milk in the gut. One of the problems of tube feeding is the loss of energy, as the fat tends to stick to the tubes. If the mother has a good supply of milk, fractionating the milk and feeding the baby the fat-rich hindmilk can increase the energy content. Skin-to-skin contact has also been found to be important for premature babies and it helps to stimulate the mother's lactational capabilities. It also increases the maternal IgA in the milk, which will be specific to the nocosomial flora of the hospital environs or other environment that the mother and infant have been exposed to.

In preterm babies, with low lactase activity, a large proportion of lactose reaches the large intestine in an undigested form. Here, it is metabolized by colonic bacteria to produce organic acids, hydrogen and carbon dioxide. The organic acids are absorbed across the intestinal mucosa and a proportion of the energy is recovered. This means that preterm babies are able to utilize a large proportion of the energy contributed from lactose. The extent of colonic salvage can be determined by measuring the amount of hydrogen in the baby's breath and can be severely compromised by antibiotics or surgery disrupting the colonic flora. It is suggested that over-accumulation of organic acids in the lower gut may be a factor in the initiation of NEC (Lucas and Cole, 1990) (Box 16.7).

Although the evolution of mammalian species has obviously depended on the unique properties of lactose, intolerance to lactose may occur. Although galactose is directly involved in the synthesis of glycoproteins and glycolipids of the CNS, it is not essential in the diet. Galactose can be synthesized from glucose in the liver so glucose can substitute for lactose in a lactose-free diet. Alternatively, lactase can be added directly to bottles or milk can be fermented prior to ingestion.

Table 16.3 compares the composition of human colostrum, mature human milk and cow's milk.

Box 16.7 Necrotizing enterocolitis

- Seen predominantly in premature infants
- Associated with infection, hypertonic feeds, hypovolaemia and perinatal asphyxia
- Most prominent in jejunum, ileum and colon
- Clinical signs usually appear at 3–10 days old
- Symptoms may include abdominal distension, blood in stools, vomiting, lethargy, respiratory distress and poor thermoregulation
- Human milk fed enterally is protective, possibly by stimulating gut maturity and integrity, providing substrates for enzymes and increasing perfusion

---

Starch

Starch digestion in young babies is possible. Infant saliva contains some amylase activity but levels rapidly increase from 3 to 6 months. Pancreatic amylase activity is minimal in the first 3 months and remains low until about 6 months. Mammary amylase in human milk has a high activity in colostrum, which is retained for about 6 weeks. Intestinal mucosa has both disaccharidases and glucoamylase, which hydrolyse oligosaccharides and disaccharides. Glucoamylase is a brush-border enzyme that can hydrolyse glucose polymers in formula milk. Formula feeds derived from cow's milk often contain maltodextrin, a polymer of maltose and glucose. This has the advantages of being easily digested and increasing the viscosity and mineral content of the formula. Babies are born with relatively high levels of glucoamylase activity, which further increases after birth. Glucoamylase is less susceptible to being affected by intestinal mucosal damage and is distributed along the length of the small intestine, which increases the efficiency of hydrolysis and uptake of its products.

There is evidence that the ability to digest starch can be induced if starch is present in the diet. Adaptation is not quick and may take days to weeks. Undigested starch causes gastrointestinal disturbances, such as diarrhoea, interfering with the absorption of other nutrients, so affected infants may exhibit symptoms of failure to thrive. Hypoxia and ischaemia result in decreased intestinal perfusion, which alters the structure of the epithelial cells affecting uptake of monosaccharides.

Oligosaccharides

Milk contains about 130 different oligosaccharides. Human milk seems to have a particular diverse profile of oligosaccharides, which vary genetically and with the duration of lactation and the time of day. The concentration of unbound human milk oligosaccharides (HMO) is about 5–10 g per litre (similar to the amount of protein in human milk and more than the amount of lipid; Bode, 2006). The role of oligosaccharides in milk is protective. They are not absorbed and appear to act as substrates for beneficial bacteria in the colon and to bind pathogens, so the pathogens do not bind to the cells lining the gut (Bode, 2006). HMO thus promote a particular bacterial flora in the gut of breastfed babies, which results in a characteristic pH; they also serve as receptor analogues for urinary pathogens and thus protect against urinary infections. In the infant's circulation, HMO participate in interactions in the immune system, protecting breastfed infants against NEC and other inflammatory diseases. Breast milk has high concentrations of gangliosides, sialic acid-containing glycosphingolipids (McJarrow et al., 2009). Gangliosides are found in high concentrations in the brain; they are deposited in the developing brain in fetal and early neonatal life and play a role in the

Table 16.3 Compares the composition of human colostrum, mature human milk and cow's milk

	COLOSTRUM (100 ML)	MATURE HUMAN MILK (100 ML)	COW'S MILK	COMMENTS
Energy water		70 (kcal)	66 (kcal)	Colostrum is produced in small but easier digest amounts – produced during first 3 days of life; neonate may feed frequently as metabolic process adapts from the constant feed environment of the uterus to an extrauterine fast/feed cycle
Protein	Immunoglobulins account for increased protein content	1.3 g (mostly whey); lactalbumin; immunoglobulins; lactoferrin; lysozyme; enzymes; hormones	3.5 g (high casein content)	Colostrum rich in passive immunity factors to provide initial protection to infant; cow's milk harder to digest owing to increased casein, also contains lactoglobulin not found in breast milk (may be responsible for cow's milk allergy); protein ratios differ owing to the calf having a faster growth trajectory than the human infant
Lactose	Less lactose	7.0 g provides 37% of energy requirement	4.9 g	Breast milk tastes sweeter than cow's milk
Fat	Less fat	4.2 g (98% triglycerides) provides approx. 50% of energy requirements	3.7 g	All mammalian milks are rich in fats owing to the high-yielding energy from fat metabolism
Sodium		15 mg	22 mg	Higher concentrations of organic ions in cow's milk; the neonatal kidney may be unable to regulate higher ion concentrations owing to immaturity
Potassium		60 mg	35 mg	
Chloride		43 mg	29 mg	
Calcium		35 mg	117 mg	
Phosphorus		15 mg	92 mg	
Magnesium		2.8 mg		
Vitamin A	Increased level	60 μm	less	
Vitamin D		0.01 μm		
Vitamin E	Increased level	0.35 μm		
Vitamin K	Increased level	0.21 μm	6 μm	
Thiamin	16 μm	44		
Riboflavin	30 μm	175 μm		
Nicotinic acid	230 μm			
B_{12}	0.01 μm	0.4 μm		
B_6	6 μm			
Folate	5.2 μm	5.5 μm		

Table 16.3 Compares the composition of human colostrum, mature human milk and cow's milk—cont'd

	COLOSTRUM (100 ML)	MATURE HUMAN MILK (100 ML)	COW'S MILK	COMMENTS
Pantothenic acid	260 µm			
Biotin	3.8 µm			
Vitamin C	3.8 mg	1.1 mg		
Iron	76 µm	5 mg		Breast milk has low levels of iron; however, it is absorbed approx. 20 times more efficiently than iron supplements
Copper	76 µm			
Zinc	295 µm			
Iodine	7 µm			

development and maturation of the brain such as neuronal growth and myelination. They may influence cognitive function and development of the gut.

Vitamins

A plentiful supply of breast milk from a well-nourished woman contains all the vitamins required by a term neonate, with the possible exceptions of vitamins D and K. Dietary taboos practised during lactation in some cultures may affect the vitamin content of breast milk. As fat is the most variable constituent of the milk, the level of fat-soluble vitamins is relatively unstable. There is a seasonal variation in the vitamin A content of cow's milk. Water-soluble vitamins in breast milk fluctuate with maternal intake as they move readily from maternal serum to milk. Human milk has a high level of vitamin C; there may be a seasonal variation in vitamin C content and both infant and maternal requirements for vitamin C increase with stress (including lactation). B vitamin levels in milk are acutely affected by maternal diet. Vitamin B_{12}, which is found in animal protein, is likely to be deficient in the milk from strict vegetarian or vegan women who should take vitamin B_{12} supplements during pregnancy and lactation. Transfer of folate from maternal plasma into milk occurs against a steep concentration gradient so the nursing infant is well protected against maternal folate deficiency. However, maternal folate reserves may be depleted during lactation which would have important consequences for the mother and her own folate status, especially if the interpregnancy interval is short.

Vitamin D

Breastfed babies rarely develop rickets although the level of vitamin D in breast milk is low. The vitamin D content of foods is measured by assessing the vitamin D content of the fat fraction. However, breast milk may contain an aqueous vitamin D sulphate, which is not included in the fat fraction, so the vitamin D content of breast milk may be underestimated. Although the vitamin D level in breast milk has been reported to be low, it is not low if the mothers have had optimal vitamin D status themselves throughout pregnancy and lactation. Neonates have stores of all fat-soluble vitamins, including vitamin D, and they are able to synthesize vitamin D on exposure to sunlight from an early age. Vitamin D-deficient milk is associated with low exposure to sun, long winters, Northern climes, use of sun screen, dark skins and cultural practices such as covering the skin, all factors which compromise maternal vitamin D status. Increased levels of pollution may also affect vitamin D synthesis in the skin. Certain ethnic groups, such as Rastafarians in the UK, have an increased risk of vitamin D deficiency.

Vitamin E

Vitamin E, mostly in the form of α-tocopherol, is an antioxidant. Deficiency compromises the integrity of the red blood cell membrane and can lead to microhaemorrhages if severe. In formula feeds, the α-tocopherol:polyunsaturated fat ratio is held constant (1 IU vitamin E per gram of linoleic acid).

Vitamin K

Vitamin K deficiency is associated with haemorrhagic disease of the newborn (see Chapter 15) and is usually due to low stores of vitamin K rather than low levels in the milk. There is a critical need for vitamin K during birth and in the first days of life when the risk of bleeding, particularly intracranially, is high. Vitamin K is not efficiently transferred across the placenta. The major source of vitamin K in postnatal life is from the by-products of bacterial metabolism, but the baby is born with a sterile gut, and gut colonization capable of producing vitamin K is not adequate until the baby is at least 6 weeks old as lactobacilli do not synthesis menaquinones. Concentrations of vitamin K are higher in colostrum and early milk, particularly the hindmilk as the vitamin is fat-soluble. Breast milk stimulates colonization of the gut by vitamin K-producing bacteria. A prophylactic dose of vitamin K is routinely given at birth to protect against haemorrhagic disease of the newborn.

Vitamin A

Vitamin A requirement is increased if stores are inadequate or there are problems with fat absorption. A deficiency of vitamin A in infancy is associated with bronchopulmonary dysplasia. This may result from a low intake or increased requirement for the vitamin in healing the damaged lung epithelium. Breastfeeding women are advised to select plenty of vegetables and fruit rich in provitamin A.

Minerals

The mineral content of milk is slightly affected by maternal diet but milk provides all the major minerals and trace elements required by the normal term infant. Usually the mother's dietary deficiency or excess intake of mineral does not affect the composition of her milk very much as maternal homeostasis protects the infant against fluctuations of most minerals in the maternal diet. Parenteral feeding of infants, rather than frank deficiencies, has elicited most information about mineral requirements. Deficiencies are usually associated with short gestation or severe placental insufficiency.

The concentration of most minerals remains generally low but the bioavailability is high. Human milk has a number of binding proteins, notably for iron, calcium and zinc. Although the level of iron in breast milk is low, absorption of iron from human milk is particularly efficient, aided by the lactoferrin and transferrin content of milk and its low pH. Iron requirement in infants are relatively low for the first few months of life because there is recycling of the senescent red blood cells from the higher number circulating in the fetus.

The sodium content of human milk is inversely related to the volume of milk produced so it is higher initially and at weaning. Cow's milk has four times the sodium content of human milk. Hypernatraemia, caused for instance by hot weather, mild infection or over-concentrated formula reconstitution, can result in dehydration.

Calcium absorption is affected by vitamin D, calcium and phosphorus concentrations, fatty acids and lactose. It is particularly enhanced by the acid environment and low phosphorus content of human milk. The concentration of calcium in the blood is tightly regulated; there seems to be similar homeostatic mechanisms ensuring a relatively constant concentration of calcium in breast milk (Kent et al., 2009). The calcium:phosphorus ratio of human milk is 2:4 (compared with 1:3 in cow's milk). If phosphorus levels are high, there is increased phosphorus absorption at the expense of calcium absorption as they compete for the same mechanism of transfer across the gut wall. The resulting fall in plasma calcium concentration can cause hypocalcaemia with symptoms of jitteriness, tetany and convulsions.

Milk-borne trophic factors

As well as nutritive and immunological factors, human milk contains a group of biologically active factors that affect nutritional status and somatic growth. The immature neonatal mucosa can allow potentially immunogenic molecules to cross the gut; human milk accelerates maturation of the gut barrier function. Human milk contains products of the maternal adaptive immune system such as antibodies and components of the innate immune system; in addition components in human milk attenuate early inappropriate inflammatory responses. The biologically active factors in human milk can be classified into four groups: hormones and peptide growth factors, nucleotides and nucleosides, polyamines and digestive enzymes. The hormone group includes insulin, GH, insulin-like growth factors (IGF-I and IGF-II), somatostatin, EGF, prolactin, erythropoietin and GH-releasing factor. Some of these hormones and growth factors are absorbed across the permeable neonatal gut into the body where they affect metabolism and promote growth and differentiation of organs and tissues. Other hormones, such as somatostatin, appear not to be absorbed but resist proteolysis, having an effect directly on the wall of the gut. The growth factors in human milk may modulate the development of the infant gut (Goldman, 2000), protecting gastrointestinal cells and therefore reducing the risk of NEC.

Both human and bovine colostrum are rich in nucleotides, which are precursors of nucleic acids. Nucleotides appear to have a role in enhancing growth and differentiation. They are particularly involved in liver cell function, lipid metabolism and lipoprotein synthesis. They also affect the development of the gut-associated lymphoid tissue (GALT). Unlike cow's milk, mature human milk maintains high levels of nucleotides. Up to a fifth of the breastfed neonate's requirement for nucleotides is derived from milk. Dietary nucleotides may facilitate iron absorption and promote development of the immune response.

The polyamines, spermine and spermidine, are present in all cells but human milk has about 10 times as much polyamine content as cow's milk. Levels of polyamines are particularly high in the first days of lactation. They may have mitogenic, metabolic and immunological effects promoting gut development of the newborn. Enzymes include amylase, lipase and proteases which aid digestion.

Case study 16.3 is an example of concerns about newborn nutrition.

Special considerations

Breast milk can vary in taste and colour and can affect the infant's digestive system. Some components of the mother's diet such as artichokes, asparagus, peppers, legumes, brassica (vegetables from the cabbage family) and alliums (vegetables from the onion family) may occasionally result in a reaction from the infant though the evidence that maternal diet is the cause of infant colic is inconsistent. The taste and flavour of breast milk can be altered by components of maternal diet such as garlic (Mennella et al., 2001). When the breastfeeding mother consumes garlic, the infant consumes more milk. These early flavour and odour experiences may programme later food preferences including those at weaning. Rarely, breast milk colour has been reported to be affected by excessive maternal consumption of food colouring (usually in soft and sports drinks) and drug therapy (Lawrence, 2010).

Case study 16.3

Isla is 11 days old and has just regained her birth weight. She has been breastfed since birth and appears to be very healthy and alert. Julia, her mother, contacts the midwife because she is concerned about Isla who is sleeping 12 h at night and feeds only four times a day. Julia's elder sister also gave birth recently and her 21-day-old baby feeds every 2 h, day and night, and has been progressively gaining weight. Julia's sister reported that her midwife told her that this is how a newborn baby normally behaves and advises Julia to stop breastfeeding because her baby is not growing properly.

- How can the midwife reassure Julia that Isla is well, feeding normally and gaining adequate nutrition?
- What concerns, if any, would you have for Julia's niece or how would you reassure Julia that all was normal?
- Why do some babies have different patterns of feeding and weight gain?

It has been suggested that susceptible infants might be exposed to environmental allergens and dietary antigens via their mother's breast milk. In some cases, where there is a history of allergy, mothers may be advised to avoid potential allergens whilst breastfeeding such as nuts, eggs, cow's milk, berries and tropical foods. However, responses vary widely and foods should not be eliminated without medical supervision.

Caffeine and alcohol both pass into breast milk. With all substances including caffeine, nicotine, alcohol and drugs, the levels are reduced in the milk if maternal consumption is timed immediately after a feed with the longest possible time before the next feed.

Breastfeeding women are encouraged to exercise, time providing. Exercise increases blood lactic acid levels and there may be some transfer of lactic acid into breast milk. Human milk is sweet and lactic acid has a sour bitter taste which may result in infants displaying puckering facial expressions and even rejecting milk if they are offered it close to exercise. However, not all infants are sensitive to the taste of lactic acid and discarding the first few millilitres of milk by manual expression often remedies the situation (Lawrence, 2010). Physical activity and energy intake must be balanced.

IMMUNOLOGICAL PROPERTIES OF HUMAN MILK

Neonates are particularly susceptible to infection (see Chapter 15). Milk has an important non-nutritive protective role. In addition, some of the nutrient components of human milk can be multifunctional in that either in their native or partially digested state, they are immunologically active. Human milk discourages bacterial growth whereas cow's milk promotes bacterial growth in the upper small bowel, which is optimal for ruminants (Jackson and Golden, 1978). Breastfed infants have fewer infections (Box 16.8), but some of this effect may be due to a decreased exposure to other foods bearing microorganisms (Golding et al., 1997). Breast feeding appears to be protective for Sudden Infant Death Syndrome (SIDS) possibly because as well as the immunological advantages of human milk, breast fed infants have different sleeping practices and are more easily aroused from active sleep (Horne et al., 2004). (Note that there are several significant risk factors for SIDS including not being breastfed, sleeping in a prone position, overheating and exposure to smoke.) The protective properties of milk are also important in protecting the breasts themselves from infection. Many cultures use breast milk topically, for instance to treat eye infections. Immunological properties of human milk are increased with better maternal nutrition (Chang, 1990). Human milk has a high antioxidant capacity because it is rich

Box 16.8 **Advantages of breastfeeding**

- Optimal infant nutrition
- Convenience, cost and lack of contamination
- Reduced risk of mortality from necrotizing enterocolitis and sudden infant death syndrome
- Reduced infection: gastrointestinal, respiratory, urinary tract, ear, meningitis, intractable diarrhoea
- Reduced atopic disease and allergy: eczema, asthma
- Increased intelligence
- Reduced overweight and obesity in childhood and adulthood
- Reduced risk of autoimmune disease
- Enhanced immunity
- Reduced risk of maternal cancer: breast, ovarian
- Increased maternal oxytocin levels: promote expulsion of placenta, minimize postpartum blood loss, and facilitates rapid uterine involution (see Chapter 14)
- The promotion of exclusive breastfeeding for at least the first six months of life –
  - may significantly reduce the health care costs within the population both short and long term (Bartick and Reinhold, 2010)
  - may reduce the incidence and severity of mental health for the neonate in later life (Oddy et al., 2010)
  - may reduce the risk of maternal late onset diabetes (Gunderson et al., 2010)

in ascorbic acid, uric acid, α-tocopherol and β-carotene (Labbok et al., 2004); this may be particularly important for preterm infants who have an immature antioxidant defence system and so are more prone to oxidative stress (Ledo et al., 2009).

Immunoglobulins

The immunoglobulins (antibodies) in milk are distinct from those found in maternal serum. The major immunoglobulin is secretory IgA which is produced from plasma cells in the breast; milk also contains minor amounts of monomeric IgA, IgG and IgM. Secretory IgA is at very high concentrations in the colostrum but declines to lower levels by day 14 as milk volume increases. The mother will produce specific immunoglobulins to every pathogen she encounters. The transfer of IgA into the milk is a form of passive immunity (see Chapter 10), augmenting the placental transfer of IgG to the fetus. The baby's own immune system is further stimulated by factors in the milk. Breastfed babies have superior responses to vaccination programmes and have higher IgA in their saliva, nasal secretions and urine (Prentice, 1987; Prentice et al., 1987).

IgA is stable at low pH and resistant to proteolytic enzymes (because its structure has an additional secretory component that confers resistance to digestion by trypsin and chymotrypsin) so it survives in the gastrointestinal tract. IgA has an important role in the defence against infection, slowing bacterial and viral invasion of the mucosa by neutralising toxins. It adheres to the gastric mucosa and binds to antigens on the pathogen so preventing adhesion of microorganisms to the gut wall. IgA promotes closure of the gut and so decreases its permeability to allergens such as cow's milk β-lactoglobulin and serum bovine albumin.

Binding proteins

Lactoferrin is an iron-binding protein that facilitates the absorption of iron from milk. In binding iron, it reduces the amount of free iron available for microorganisms in the gut, thus inhibiting the growth of certain pathogenic bacteria and having a broad bacteriostatic effect. It is suggested that lactoferrin in breast milk helps to reduce the incidence of gastrointestinal tract infections. Excess free iron is associated with increased bacterial pathogens in the gut. These bacteria have a high iron requirement and can cause gut damage and microhaemorrhages, which themselves can lead to iron-deficiency anaemia. Lactoferrin also inhibits the pathological activity of several bacteria, stimulates macrophage phagocytotic activity and inhibits viruses such as HIV, CMV and herpes virus (Newburg and Walker, 2007). Partial digestion of lactoferrin produces lactoferricin B, a peptide which has antibacterial activity against gram-positive and gram-negative bacteria. Some lactoferrin and lactoferricin are absorbed and excreted in the urine where they probably also protect against urinary tract infections (Labbok et al., 2004). Haptocorrin, the binding protein for vitamin B12, is similarly resistant to digestion; haptocorrin inhibits the enterotoxigenic *Escherichia coli*.

Other protective properties

Breast milk contains high levels of lysozyme, an enzyme which is protective against Gram-positive bacteria and viruses because it breaks down the complex polysaccharides in bacterial cell walls. It is produced in the secretions protecting the mucosal surfaces of the gut and respiratory tract in later life but levels are very low in infancy. Lysozyme has a bacteriostatic effect against *E. coli* and can also inhibit growth of fungus such as *Candida albicans*. Breast milk contains prebiotic substances, called bifidogenic or bifidus factors, which together with lactose stimulate the growth of lactobacilli which produce organic acids thus promoting an acidic and protective environment. Bifidus factors are human milk glycans (glycopeptides and glycoproteins). Fibronectin, which is present in high concentrations in human milk, is a non-specific opsonin (see

Chapter 10) that increases phagocytosis of bacteria. Milk also contains other protective factors (Table 16.4).

Milk is not sterile but contains about $4 \infty 10^9$ cells per litre including lymphocytes from maternal Peyer's patches and scavenger macrophages and neutrophils. Levels of cells are particularly high in the colostrum. Proteins and mucins of the milk lipid globule membrane itself may also confer immunological advantages (Keenan, 2001). Other factors in human milk with anti-infective or immunological properties include anti-proteases, which inhibit the breakdown of anti-infective immunoglobulins and enzymes, free fatty acids which have antiviral properties and cytokines which stimulate an inflammatory response from the immune cells.

FORMULA FEEDING

Human milk substitutes existed before the modern age of infant formulas. There were two approaches, either using a surrogate mother or wet nurse, or feeding milk from another mammal. In Western countries, where dairy farming is established, cow's milk is modified and processed into the formula feeds, which are the basis of bottle feeding. Human children in other cultures are reared on buffalo, goat, horse, camel and yak milk. Mammalian milks may be quantitatively similar but the quality is variable, being species-specific.

Cow's milk is supplemented with carbohydrate, either lactose or maltodextrin, which dilutes the higher mineral and protein content. Cow's milk fat (which has a high commercial value as butter and cream) is substituted with vegetable oil-fat blends. This increases the absorption efficiency; unabsorbed fat decreases the energy content, lowers calcium absorption and produces steatorrhoea.

For whey-dominant formulas, demineralized whey (which is expensive) is blended with skimmed milk to increase the whey:casein ratio and decrease the electrolyte content. The profit margin of whey-dominant formulas is lower than that of casein-dominant formulas. Casein-dominant formulas are marketed for the 'hungrier baby' and, although the energy content is constant, are considered to be a progressive step in feeding. Mothers often demonstrate a strong brand loyalty when choosing formula milk. Many formula milks for term infants, particularly the prestige or 'gold' versions, are supplemented with long chain polyunsaturated fatty acids, DHA and AA (Heird, 2007), to benefit brain growth and optimize the immune system. The source of these fatty acids is often algae rather than marine oils which may result in fishy odour.

Hydrolyzed protein formula milks are produced for infants with gastrointestinal or allergy problems; the hydrolysis of the bovine milk proteins into smaller protein fragments appears to facilitate absorption and the smaller particles are less allergenic. Soy-based formulas were originally designed for infants intolerant of cow's milk protein-based formula milks. The early problems of loose malodorous stools, nappy rash and stained clothing associated with soy milk have been remedied by the use of isolated soy protein rather than soy flour. Concerns have been raised about the high levels of aluminium and phytoestrogens in soy formula milk; phytoestrogens may affect sexual development, immune and thyroid functions and neurobehavioural development (Bhatia and Greer, 2008). Soy-based formula milks are suitable for infants with the rare inborn errors of metabolism such as galactosaemia and hereditary lactase deficiency or where a vegetarian diet is preferred. Many infants with diagnosed allergy to cows' milk protein also have an allergy to soy so the extensively hydrolyzed protein formula is unusually the preferred option (Hays, 2006). Soy-based formula milks are not appropriate for preterm infants.

Trace minerals and vitamins are added in line with legal limits. Taurine is added to formula milk and, more recently, nucleotides have been added; they probably act as growth factors and may have immune effects, strengthening responses to immunization and reducing diarrhoea. Carnitine may also be added to formula milks (Heird, 2007). Carnitine is required for oxidation of fatty acids; levels in unsupplemented soy-based and protein hydrolysate formula milks are particularly low. Packaging of formula feed is important. Anaerobic storage and copper supplementation help to reduce fatty acid oxidation. Scoop and granule size are carefully designed to optimize precision in reconstitution. Current research into the optimal (and most profitable) formulations includes adding specific proteins such as α-lactalbumin, adjusting the ratio of amino acids such as glycine, leucine, arginine, cysteine and tryptophan, and adding probiotics and prebiotics such as synthetic HMO.

Breastfed infants grow at a slightly slower rate and have a different body composition than formula-fed infants. They consume less milk (about 85% of that consumed by formula-fed infants) and have lower energy expenditure. Breastfed infants have a lower risk for later obesity and possibly insulin resistance, obesity and type II diabetes mellitus. Gastric emptying is faster in breastfed infants and there is less gastro-oesophageal reflux and loss of intake in breastfed infants. They also have less infectious disease (see below) and a lower rate of necrotizing colitis. Concerns have been raised about rapid rates of weight gain in infancy, particularly in formula fed infants, being associated with later obesity. Breastfed infants self-regulate their appetite whereas formula-fed infants are often encouraged to finish their bottle. In addition, there may be factors in breast milk which affect satiety. Breastfed infants are often introduced to complementary feeding at a slightly older age which seems to protect against later weight gain (Schack-Nielsen et al., 2010). Growth charts derived from data from formula-fed infants are not appropriate to assess growth in breastfed infants.

Table 16.4 Protective factors in milk

FACTOR	FUNCTION
Cells	
B lymphocytes	Produce antibodies against specific microbes
T lymphocytes	Kill infected cells
Macrophages	Produce lysozyme and activate parts of the immune system
Neutrophils	Phagocytose bacteria
Lacto bifidus factor	Promotes an acidic environment favourable for the growth of *Lactobacillus bifidus* and inhibits the growth of pathogenic microorganisms
Immunoglobulins (antibodies IgA, IgG, IgM, IgD and IgE)	Active against specific organisms, that is, poliomyelitis, salmonella
Immunoglobulin A (IgA)	Lines the gut to discourage adhesion of pathogenic microorganisms and limits allergen entry
Lactoferrin	Decreases iron available by binding to iron for bacterial growth Acts as a bacteriostatic agent
Lysozyme	Act in a non-specific way by damaging the cell walls of microorganisms
Lactoperoxidase	
Complement	
Lipids	Inhibit growth of staphylococcus and viruses by disrupting cell membranes
Fibronectin	Promotes macrophage activity and aids repair to damaged gut tissue
γ-Interferon	Promotes activity of immune cells
Mucins	Adhere to microorganisms inhibiting attachment to the gut wall
Oligosaccharides	Inhibit attachment of microorganisms to mucosal surfaces, promotion of optimal profile of microbiota in colon
Bile salt-stimulated lipase	Acts as an antiprotozoal
Bile salt-stimulated lipase	Promote fat and protein digestion
Lipoprotein lipase, α-amylase	
α_1-Antitrypsin	Prevent breakdown of protective factors
α_1-Antichymotrypsin	
Epidermal growth factor	Promotes maturation of the gut wall
Binding proteins	Increase absorption of nutrients and limit availability of nutrients utilized by bacteria
B_{12}-binding protein (haptocorrin)	
Lactoferrin	
Transferrin	
Folate-binding protein	
Somatomedin C	

WEANING

Weaning can be defined as the progressive transition from milk to a normal family diet. Before 4 months, it is considered unnecessary, being associated with increased incidence of diarrhoea and interference with the maintenance of breastfeeding (the nutritional value of most complementary foods is usually lower than that of breast milk). An increase in dietary cereals and vegetables tends to affect the absorption of iron, which can be delicately balanced in younger infants. By 6 months, many babies may require complementary feeding and will have sufficiently developed to cope with it. Deciduous teeth erupt at about 6 months. Incisors, which cut food, are the first teeth to appear, followed by molars at about 12 months, which allow grinding of food. Although it is not the current practice in many developed and developing countries, there is a call for meat to be introduced as an early complementary food as it provides essential micronutrients (Krebs, 2007).

Determination of the appropriate time to introduce foods other than milk is not just by age but should also take into consideration the food available, conditions to prepare it, the growth velocity and the neuromuscular development of the infant. It is not clear which pattern of growth is optimal. Growth charts are based on weight and height data from clinical surveillance. Ethnicity and both environmental and genetic factors affect growth. Practically, the high weight velocity, which is seen in the first 3 months of life, is not related to overfeeding. The deceleration of growth after 3 months is not in itself an indicator to wean. Early weaning is associated with an increased number of respiratory symptoms (Forsyth et al., 1993).

By 6 months, normal physiological development can support the introduction of alternative foods. The baby is able to hold its head erect and can control the movement of its hands to mouth. The tongue extrusion reflex is waning and can be overcome. Indeed, it is suggested that there is a critical window for introducing solid food, and if it is not done within this window, the baby tends to develop a preference for liquid feeds and may become a child with feeding problems. The kidneys are mature enough to cope with a solute load.

Although the health benefits of breastfeeding are not disputed, opinions and recommendations are divided on the optimal duration of exclusive breastfeeding. In March 2001, the World Health Organization convened an expert consultation committee to systematically review the evidence and make recommendations about the optimal duration of exclusive breastfeeding. The committee called for exclusive breastfeeding of infants until 6 months old and continued breastfeeding with appropriate complementary feeding until 2 years old. These recommendations would reduce deaths of children under 5 years by about 30% worldwide (Bryce et al., 2005). Despite this, many authorities argue that there is a lack of clear evidence to either support or refute recommendations for the age of introduction of complementary foods to the breastfed or formula-fed infant to be between 4 and 6 months. Although exclusive breastfeeding for the first 6 months of life can support growth and development in some infants, subgroups have been identified within certain populations who may require complementary feeding prior to this age, particularly larger, and often male, infants (Lanigan et al., 2001). To be confident that exclusive breastfeeding does not increase the risk of undernutrition (growth faltering) in healthy term infants, it may be necessary to make recommendations per infant weight rather than infant size.

Weaning is an important biological and social learning process as well as offering foods of higher nutrient and energy density than milk. Exposing different tastes to children has already begun in utero with amniotic fluid and is consolidated by breast milk feeding because compounds ingested by the mother are transported into the milk (Mennella, 2009). This develops the inherent taste variation of breastfed infants, affecting the development of food preferences; this important learning experience is not received by bottle-fed babies.

Key points

The physiological unit of the mammary gland is the alveolus. Prolactin, from the anterior pituitary, stimulates milk production from the alveolar cells. Oxytocin, from the posterior pituitary, stimulates contraction of the myoepithelial cells lining the alveoli and the ducts, resulting in milk ejection or 'let-down'.

Prolactin secretion slowly reaches a peak following stimulation at the nipple. Secretion is pulsatile and circadian and is controlled by the abrogation of tonic inhibition from dopamine produced by the hypothalamus. Prolactin inhibits ovulation thus suppressing fertility.

Oxytocin release is stimulated by nipple stimulation and by thinking about or hearing the baby. Secretion of oxytocin immediately follows stimulation and can be inhibited by stress.

The effects of prolactin are locally controlled by the production of FIL in the milk. Increased concentrations of FIL suppress the response to prolactin thus inhibiting milk production. This is important in mammary gland involution when breastfeeding is curtailed.

Continued

Key points—cont'd

Lactating women appear to have increased efficiency of energy utilization. The nutritional composition of the milk is not affected greatly by maternal diet unless the mother is extremely undernourished; however, concerns have been expressed about effects on maternal calcium balance and the tendency to develop obesity. Breastfeeding is associated with a reduced risk of maternal breast and ovarian cancer.

Human milk provides optimal nutrition for the human neonate, which has immature renal, hepatic and gastrointestinal functions and a rapidly developing nervous system. Breastfed babies have a lower incidence of infection.

Colostrum is the early secretion from the breast; it provides important anti-infective properties and promotes favourable colonization of the gut.

Protein requirements are relatively low as the human neonate has a relatively slow growth rate. Human milk has a high concentration of whey proteins and non-protein nitrogen components, which include growth factors. The amino acid composition of human milk protein compensates for the neonate's limited ability to convert essential amino acids to non-essential amino acids; the net protein utilization of human milk is high.

Fat is the main energy source in milk and the most variable constituent. The proportion of fat is higher in hindmilk. The fatty acid composition of human milk allows optimum absorption. Human milk fat is rich in polyunsaturated fatty acids required for development of the brain and nervous system.

Lactose is the major carbohydrate of milk; it provides energy, aids absorption of other nutrients and promotes an environment favourable to beneficial microorganisms.

Human milk has important immunological properties and is associated with a lower incidence of infections and a persistently more responsive immune system in breastfed babies.

Application to practice

It is consistently shown that breastfeeding is influential in the reduction of many disease states and thus should be encouraged. The midwife is uniquely placed to influence the overall health of the nation. Midwives must ensure women are aware of what the health benefits of breast feeding are for both them and their babies.

Knowledge of lactation and its benefits are important if the midwife is to promote breastfeeding in practice.

Following birth mother's should be encouraged to offer the breast as soon as possible after delivery. By placing the naked baby on the abdominal wall of the mother in close proximity of the breasts will enable the baby to spontaneously fix and suckle. This is important if the baby is cold following delivery and/or required initial resuscitation following birth. Cold, shocked babies are less likely to feed spontaneously and so skin to skin not only is efficient in warming babies up it also gives them comfort.

Women who have received pharmacological drugs during labour will need extra help and support as the baby's spontaneous urge to feed may be reduced.

If mother and baby are well and the mother has chosen to breast feed there are no reasons why exclusive breast feeding cannot be achieved.

If babies are drowsy or seem disinterested in the breast then the mother should be encouraged to keep offering the breast. The introduction of formula milk or bottles should be avoided as this will interfere with the establishment of lactation.

In the rare cases where the baby has difficulty latching on the mother should be encouraged to hand express and the expressed milk offered to the baby via a small cup or spoon.

The midwife must ensure that women who have chosen to bottle feed are aware of the need to ensure all equipment used is sterilized and milk made up is appropriately stored to minimize the risk of infection. The milk must be prepared as directed by the manufacturers as diluted or concentrated mixes are potentially harmful to the neonate.

ANNOTATED FURTHER READING

Fomon S: Infant feeding in the 20th century: formula and beikost, *J Nutr* 131(2):409S–420S, 2001.

A history of changing infant feeding practices in the 20th century, including the effects of sanitation, dairying practices and milk handling on home- and commercially prepared formulas.

Goldberg GR, Prentice A, Prentice A, Filteau S, Simondon K, editors: *Breast feeding: early influences on later health* (*advances in experimental medicine and biology*), 2008, Springer.

This book comprises several papers which examine early life programming of adult health, particularly the influence of infant feeding practices on early metabolism and behaviour and thus later function including risk of disease.

Howard BA, Gusterson BA: Human breast development, *J Mammary Gland Biol Neoplasia* 5:119–137, 2000.

A comprehensive well-illustrated review of physiological states of the human breast including prenatal, prepubertal and pubertal development, adult resting state, pregnancy, lactation and postinvolution.

Joeckel RJ, Phillips SK: Overview of infant and pediatric formulas, *Nutr Clin Pract* 24:356–362, 2009.

A clear summary of the differences between various types of infant and paediatric formula milks and their indications for use.

Levy O: Innate immunity of the newborn: basic mechanisms and clinical correlates, *Nat Rev Immunol* 7:379–390, 2007.

A beautifully written description of the complex immunological challenges faced by the fetus and neonate, particularly the demands of projection against infection, avoiding harmful inflammatory immune responses and balancing the transition from a sterile uterine environment to an extrauterine environment rich in foreign antigens.

Manuel R, Martens PJ, Walker M: *Core curriculum for lactation consultant practice (ICLA)*, ed 2, 2007, Jones and Bartlett.

This is essential reading for practitioners who want to extend their knowledge of breastfeeding and lactation and support women in the establishment of breastfeeding.

Newburg DS, Walker WA: Protection of the neonate by the innate immune system of developing gut and of human milk, *Pediatr Res* 61:2–8, 2007.

A well-balanced discussion of the neonatal innate immune system and its interaction with components of human milk which act to both protect the neonatal gut and compensate for the immature state of neonatal adaptive immunity.

Palmer G: *The politics of breastfeeding: when breasts are bad for business*, ed 3, 2009, Pinter & Martin Ltd.

This book explores the influence of artificial feeding on the population from a global perspective. It discusses social, historical and economic factors affecting a woman's decision to breastfeed and the implications of the type of infant feeding method on health, the environment and the global economy with a particular focus on the pressures put on parents to use alternatives to breastmilk.

Riordan J, Auerbach KG: *Breastfeeding and human lactation.* ed 4, London, 2008, Jones & Bartlett.

A comprehensive text on breastfeeding aimed at midwives, breastfeeding consultants, antenatal teachers, dietitians and nutritionists. Covers cultural aspects, anatomy and physiology, breastfeeding education and practical considerations such as breast pumps, donor milk and breastfeeding the ill child.

Rogers IS: Relactation, *Early Hum Dev* 49: S75–S81, 1997.

This article discusses the possibility of re-establishing lactation in certain situations and includes information on promoting lactation in women who have never been pregnant.

Sellen DW: Evolution of infant and young child feeding: implications for contemporary public health, *Annu Rev Nutr* 27:123–148, 2007.

A framework for understanding prehistoric, historic and contemporary variations in human lactation and infant feeding patterns which suggests complementary feeding evolved as a trade-off between the maternal cost of lactation and the risk of poor infant outcome.

West D, Marasco L: *The breastfeeding mother's guide to making more milk*, 2008, McGraw-Hill.

Written by lactation consultants, this book is aimed at mothers to help promote and establish breastfeeding but practitioners will also find this text useful.

Winberg J: Mother and newborn baby: mutual regulation of physiology and behavior – a selective review, *Dev Psychobiol* 47:217–229, 2005.

An interesting review of the interactions between the mother and newborn infant in the period just after delivery and how these influence the physiology and behaviour of both.

REFERENCES

Abou-Dakn M, Schafer-Graf U, Wöckel A: Psychological stress and breast diseases during lactation, *Breastfeed Rev* 17:19–26, 2009.

Adlercreutz H: Phytoestrogens – epidemiology and a possible role in cancer protection, *Environ Health Perspect* 103:103–112, 1995.

Amir LH, Donath SM: Does maternal smoking have a negative physiological effect on breastfeeding? The epidemiological evidence, *Breastfeed Rev* 11(2):19–29, 2003.

Amir LH, Donath S: A systematic review of maternal obesity and breastfeeding intention, initiation and duration, *MC Pregnancy Childbirth* 7:9, 2007.

Andersen AN, Ronn B, Tjonneland A, et al: Low maternal but normal fetal prolactin levels in cigarette smoking pregnant women, *Acta Obstet Gynecol Scand* 63:237–239, 1984.

Bartick M, Reinhold A: The burden of suboptimal breastfeeding in the United States: a pediatric cost analysis, *Pediatrics* 125:1048–1056, 2010.

Bayley TM, Alasmi M, Thorkelson T, et al: Influence of formula versus breast milk on cholesterol synthesis rates in four-month-old infants, *Pediatr Res* 44:60–67, 1998.

Ben-Jonathan N, Laudon M, Garris PA: Novel aspects of posterior pituitary function: regulation of prolactin secretion, *Front Neuroendocrinol* 12:231–277, 1991.

Bhatia J, Greer F: Use of soy protein-based formulas in infant feeding, *Pediatrics* 121:1062–1068, 2008.

Bode L: Recent advances on structure, metabolism, and function of human milk oligosaccharides, *J Nutrition* 136:2127–2130, 2006.

Bramson L, Lee JW, Moore E, et al: Effect of early skin-to-skin mother–infant contact during the first 3 hours following birth on exclusive breastfeeding during the maternity hospital stay, *J Hum Lact* 26:130–137, 2010.

Britton H: Mother–infant interaction: relationship to early infant nutrition and feeding. In Suskind RM, Lewinter-Suskind L, editors: *Textbook of pediatric nutrition*, New York, 1993, Raven Press, pp 43–48.

Broadhurst CL, Cunnane SC, Crawford MA: Rift Valley lake fish and shellfish provided brain-specific nutrition for early Homo, *Br J Nutr* 79:3–21, 1998.

Bryce J, Boschi-Pinto C, Shibuya K, et al: WHO estimates of the causes of death in children, *Lancet* 365:1147–1152, 2005.

Butte NF: Energy requirements during pregnancy and consequences of deviations from requirement on fetal outcome, *Nestle Nutr Workshop Ser Pediatr Program* 55:49–67, 2005.

Casey TM, Plaut K: The role of glucocorticoids in secretory activation and milk secretion, a historical perspective, *J Mammary Gland Biol Neoplasia* 12:293–304, 2007.

Chang S-J: Antimicrobial proteins of maternal and cord sera and human milk in relation to maternal nutritional status, *Am J Clin Nutr* 51:183–187, 1990.

Chin JR, Krause KM, Ostbye T, et al: Gestational weight gain in consecutive pregnancies, *Am J Obstet Gynecol* 203:279–286, 2010.

Chesney RW, Helms RA, Christensen M, et al: The role of taurine in infant nutrition, *Adv Exp Med Biol* 442:463–476, 1998.

Crawford MA: The role of essential fatty acids in neural development: implications for perinatal nutrition, *Am J Clin Nutr* 57(Suppl):S703–S710, 1993.

Dewar CS, Psych MR: Enhanced nutrition of offspring as a crucial factor for the evolution of intelligence on land, *Med Hypotheses* 62(5):802–807, 2004.

Dewey KG: Energy and protein requirements during lactation, *Annu Rev Nutr* 17:19–36, 1997.

Dewey KG: Is breastfeeding protective against child obesity? *J Hum Lact* 19 (1):9–18, 2003.

Dobbing J, Sands J: Comparative aspects of the brain growth spurt, *Early Hum Dev* 3:79–83, 1979.

Doucet S, Soussignan R, Sagot P, Schaal B: The secretion of areolar (Montgomery's) glands from lactating women elicits selective, unconditional responses in neonates, *PLoS One* 4:e7579, 2009.

Ebrahim GJ: The scientific contribution of breast feeding research, *Maternal Child Health March* 92–93, 1990.

Emmett PM, Rogers IS: Properties of human milk and their relationship with maternal nutrition, *Early Hum Dev* 49:S7–S28, 1997.

Flidel-Rimon O, Shinwell ES: Breast feeding twins and high multiples, *Arch Dis Child Fetal Neonatal Ed* 91: F377–F380, 2006.

Forsyth JS, Ogston SA, Clark A, et al: Relationship between early introduction of solid food to infants and their weight and illnesses during the first two years of life, *Br Med J* 306:1572–1576, 1993.

Fudge NJ, Kovacs CS: Pregnancy up-regulates intestinal calcium absorption and skeletal mineralization independently of the vitamin D receptor, *Endocrinology* 151:886–895, 2010.

Gabay MP: Galactogogues: medications that induce lactation, *J Hum Lact* 18:274–279, 2002.

Golding J: Unnatural constituents of breast milk: medication, lifestyle, pollutants, viruses, *Early Hum Dev* 49: S29–S43, 1997.

Golding J, Emmett PM, Rogers IS: Does breast feeding have any impact on non-infectious, non-allergic disorders? *Early Hum Dev* 49: S131–S142, 1997.

Goldman AS: Modulation of the gastrointestinal tract of infants by human milk. Interfaces and interactions. An evolutionary perspective, *J Nutr* 130:426S–431S, 2000.

Gordon I, Zagoory-Sharon O, Leckman JF, et al: Oxytocin and the development of parenting in humans, *Biol Psychiatry* 68:377–382, 2010.

Grattan DR: Behavioural significance of prolactin signalling in the central nervous system during pregnancy and lactation, *Reproduction* 123 (4):497–506, 2002.

Gunderson EP, Jacobs DR, Chiang V, et al: Duration of lactation and incidence of the metabolic syndrome in women of reproductive age according to gestational diabetes mellitus status: a 20-Year Prospective Study in CARDIA (Coronary Artery Risk Development in Young Adults), *Diabetes* 59:(2):495–504, 2010.

Hammond KA: Adaptation of the maternal intestine during lactation, *J Mammary Gland Biol Neoplasia* 2:243–252, 1997.

Hartmann PE, Sherriff JL, Mitoulas LR: Homeostatic mechanisms that regulate lactation during energetic stress, *J Nutr* 128:394S–399S, 1998.

Hays T: Infant formulas for primary allergy prevention, *J Allergy Clin Immunol* 117:471–472, 2006.

Heird WC: Progress in promoting breast-feeding, combating malnutrition, and composition and use of infant formula, 1981–2006, *J Nutr* 137:499S–502S, 2007.

Horne RS, Parslow PM, Ferens D, et al: Comparison of evoked arousability in breast and formula fed infants, *Arch Dis Childhood* 89:22–25, 2004.

Howie PW, McNeilly AS, McArdle T, et al: The relationship between suckling-induced prolactin response and lactogenesis, *J Clin Endocrinol Metab* 50:670–673, 1980.

Huang YY, Lee JT, Huang CM, et al: Factors related to maternal perception of milk supply while in the hospital, *J Nurs Res* 17:179–188, 2009.

Hytten F: *The clinical physiology of the puerperium*, 1995, London, Farrand Press.

Illingworth PJ, Jung RT, Howie PW, et al: Diminution in energy expenditure during lactation, *Br Med J* 292:437–442, 1986.

Innis SM: Human milk: maternal dietary lipids and infant development, *Proc Nutr Soc* 66:397–404, 2007.

Institute of Medicine: *Dietary reference values for energy, carbohydrates, fiber, fat, protein and amino acids (macronutrients). IOM Standing Committee on the Scientific Evaluation of Dietary Reference Intakes, Food and Nutrition*, Washington DC, 2002, National Academy of Sciences.

Jackson AA, Golden MHN: The human rumen, *Lancet* 1978:764–767, 1978.

Jensen CL, Lapillonne A: Docosahexaenoic acid and lactation, *Prostaglandins Leukot Essent Fatty Acids* 81:175–178, 2009.

Johnston JM, Amico JA: A prospective longitudinal study of the release of oxytocin and prolactin in response to infant suckling in long term lactation, *J Clin Endocrinol Metab* 62:653–657, 1986.

Jonas K, Johansson LM, Nissen E, et al: Effects of intrapartum oxytocin administration and epidural analgesia on the concentration of plasma oxytocin and prolactin, in response to suckling during the second day postpartum, *Breastfeed Med* 4:71–82, 2009.

Kalliomäki M, Isolauri E: Role of intestinal flora in the development of allergy, *Curr Opin Allergy Clin Immunol* 3:15–20, 2003.

Karjalainen J, Martin JM, Knip M, et al: A bovine albumin peptide as a possible trigger of insulin-dependent diabetes mellitus, *N Engl J Med* 327:302–307, 1992.

Keenan TW: Milk lipid globules and their surrounding membrane: a brief history and perspectives for future research, *J Mammary Gland Biol Neoplasia* 6(3):365–371, 2001.

Kent JC, Arthur PG, Mitoulas LR, et al: Why calcium in breastmilk is independent of maternal dietary calcium and vitamin D, *Breastfeed Rev* 17:5–11, 2009.

Krebs NF: Food choices to meet nutritional needs of breast-fed infants and toddlers on mixed diets, *J Nutr* 137:511S–517S, 2007.

Lanigan JA, Bishop J, Kimber AC, et al: Systematic review concerning the age of introduction of complementary foods to the healthy full-term infant, *Eur J Clin Nutr* 55 (5):309–320, 2001.

Labbok MH, Clark D, Goldman AS: Breastfeeding: maintaining an irreplaceable immunological resource, *Nat Rev Immunol* 4:565–572, 2004.

Lapillonne A, Jensen CL: Reevaluation of the DHA requirement for the premature infant, *Prostaglandins Leukot Essent Fatty Acids* 81:143–150, 2009.

Lau C: Effects of stress on lactation, *Pediatr Clin North Am* 48:221–234, 2001.

Lawrence RA: Maternal nutrition and supplements for mother and infant. In *Breastfeeding: a guide for the medical profession*, ed 7, St Louis, 2010, Mosby, pp 283–318.

Ledo A, Arduini A, Asensi MA, et al: Human milk enhances antioxidant defenses against hydroxyl radical aggression in preterm infants, *Am J Clin Nutr* 89:210–215, 2009.

Lönnerdal B: Trace element transport in the mammary gland, *Annu Rev Nutr* 27:165–177, 2007.

Lovelady CA, Stephenson KG, Kuppler KM, et al: The effects of dieting on food and nutrient intake of lactating women, *J Am Diet Assoc* 106:908–912, 2006.

Lucas A, Cole TJ: Breast milk and neonatal necrotising enterocolitis, *Lancet* 336:1519–1523, 1990.

Lucas A, Ewing G, Roberts SB, et al: How much energy does the breast fed infant consume and expend? *Br Med J* 295:75–77, 1987.

Lucas A, Morley R, Cole TJ, et al: Breast milk and subsequent intelligence quotient in children born preterm, *Lancet* 339:261–264, 1992.

Manuel R, Martens PJ, Walker M: *Core curriculum for lactation consultant practice*, Jones and Bartlett, 2007, International Lactation Consultant Association.

McJarrow P, Schnell N, Jumpsen J, et al: Influence of dietary gangliosides on neonatal brain development, *Nutr Rev* 67:451–463, 2009.

McManaman JL, Neville MC: Mammary physiology and milk secretion, *Adv Drug Rev* 55:629–641, 2003.

McNeilly AS: Lactational control of reproduction, *Reprod Fertil Dev* 13(7–8):583–590, 2001.

Mennella JA, Beauchamp GK: The transfer of alcohol to human milk: effects on flavor and the infant's behavior, *N Engl J Med.* 325:981–985, 1991.

Mennella JA, Jagnow CP, Beauchamp GK: Prenatal and postnatal flavor learning by human infants, *Pediatrics* 107(6):E88, 2001.

Mennella JA: Flavour programming during breast-feeding, *Adv Exp Med Biol* 639:113–120, 2009.

Mitoulas LR, Kent JC, Cox DB, et al: Variation in fat, lactose and protein in human milk over 24 h and throughout the first year of lactation, *Br J Nutr* 88:29–37, 2002.

Monte CS, Johnston CS, Roll LE: Bovine serum albumin detected in infant formula is a possible trigger for insulin dependence diabetes mellitus, *J Am Diet Assoc* 94:314–316, 1994.

Morelli L: Postnatal development of intestinal microflora as influenced by infant nutrition, *J Nutr* 138:1791S–1795S, 2008.

Neifert MR, McDonough SL, Neville MC: Failure of lactogenesis associated with placental retention, *Am J Obstet Gynecol* 140:477–478, 1981.

Neville MC, Morton J: Physiology and endocrine changes underlying human lactogenesis II, *J Nutr* 131:3005S–3008S, 2001.

Neville MC, McFadden TB, Forsyth I: Hormonal regulation of mammary differentiation and milk secretion, *J Mammary Gland Biol Neoplasia* 7:49–66, 2002.

Nickerson K: Environmental contaminants in breast milk, *J Midwifery Womens Health* 51:26–34, 2006.

Nommsen-Rivers LA, Dewey KG: Growth of breastfed infants, *Breastfeed Med* 4(Suppl 1):S45–S49, 2009.

Nommsen-Rivers LA, Cohen RJ, Chantry CJ, et al: Risk factors for delayed onset of lactogenesis among northern California primiparous women, *FASEB J* 23:344, 2009.

Oddy WH, Kendall GE, Li J, et al: The long-term effects of breastfeeding on child and adolescent mental health: a pregnancy cohort study followed for 14 years, *J pediatr* 156 (4):568–574, 2010.

Peaker M: Evolutionary strategies in lactation: nutritional implications, *Proc Nutr Soc* 48:53–57, 1989.

Pisacane A, Impagliazzo N, Russo M, et al: Breast feeding and multiple sclerosis, *Br Med J* 308:1411–1412, 1994.

Pond C, editor: *Reproductive physiology.* Milton Keynes, 1992, Open University, pp 197–200.

Porter TE, Grandy D, Bunzow J, et al: Evidence that stimulatory dopamine receptors may be involved in the regulation of prolactin secretion, *Endocrinology* 134:1263–1268, 1994.

Powe CE, Knott CD, Conklin-Brittain N: Infant sex predicts breast milk energy content, *Am J Hum Biol* 22:50–54, 2010.

Prentice A: Breast feeding increases concentration of IgA in infants' urine, *Arch Dis Child* 62:792–795, 1987.

Prentice A: Calcium in pregnancy and lactation, *Ann Rev Nutr* 20:249–272, 2000.

Prentice AM, Prentice A: Evolutionary and environmental influences on human lactation, *Proc Nutr Soc* 54:391–400, 1995.

Prentice A, Ewing G, Roberts SB, et al: The nutritional role of breast-milk IgA and lactoferrin, *Acta Paediatr Scand* 76:592–598, 1987.

Ramsay DT, Kent JC, Hartmann RL, et al: Anatomy of the lactating human breast redefined with ultrasound imaging, *J Anat* 206:525–534, 2005.

Rasmussen KM, Hilson JA, Kjolhede CL: Obesity may impair lactogenesis II, *J Nutr* 131(11):3009S–3011S, 2001.

Rogers IS: Lactation and fertility, *Early Hum Dev* 49(Suppl):S185–S190, 1997.

Saint L, Maggiore P, Hartmann PE: Yield and nutrient content of milk in eight women breast-feeding twins and one woman breast-feeding triplets, *Br J Nutr* 56:49–58, 1986.

Schack-Nielsen L, Michaelsen KF: Advances in our understanding of the biology of human milk and its effects on the offspring, *J Nutr* 137:503S–510S, 2007.

Schack-Nielsen L, Sorensen TI, Mortensen EL, et al: Late introduction of complementary feeding, rather than duration of breastfeeding, may protect against adult overweight, *Am J Clin Nutr* 91:619–627, 2010.

Sowers M: Pregnancy and lactation as risk factors for subsequent bone loss and osteoporosis, *J Bone Miner Res* 11:1052–1060, 1996.

Svensson M, Duringer C, Hallgren O, et al: Hamlet – a complex from human milk that induces apoptosis in tumor cells but spares healthy cells, *Adv Exp Med Biol* 503:125–132, 2002.

Turgeon-O'Brien H, Lachapelle D, Gagnon PF, et al: Nutritive and non-nutritive suckling habits, *J Dent Child* 63:321–327, 1996.

Van de Perre P: Postnatal transmission of human immunodeficiency virus type 1: the breast-feeding dilemma, *Am J Obstet Gynecol* 173:483–487, 1995.

Warner BB, Sapsford A: Misappropriated human milk: fantasy, fear and fact regarding infectious risk, *Newborn Infant Nurs Rev* 4(1):56–61, 2004.

Wharton BA, Balmer SE, Scott PH: Faecal flora in the newborn: effect of lactoferrin and related nutrients, *Adv Exp Med Biol* 357:91–98, 1994.

Wilde CJ, Prentice A, Peaker M: Breast-feeding: matching supply with demand in human lactation. *Proc Nutr Soc* 54:401–406, 1995.

Williams GL, McVey WR, Hunter JF: Mammary somatosensory pathways are not required for suckling-mediated inhibition of luteinizing hormone secretion and delay of ovulation in cows, *Biol Reprod* 49:1328–1337, 1993.

Wöckel A, Beggel A, Rucke M, et al: Predictors of inflammatory breast diseases during lactation –results of a cohort study, *Am J Reprod Immunol* 63:28–37, 2010.

Woolridge MW: Breastfeeding: physiology into practice. In Davies DP, editor: *Nutrition in child health*, London, 1996, RCOP, pp 13–31.

Woolridge MW, Fisher C: Colic, 'overfeeding', and symptoms of lactose malabsorption in the breast-fed baby: a possible artifact of feed management? *Lancet* ii:382–384, 1988.

Wysolmerski JJ: The evolutionary origins of maternal calcium and bone metabolism during lactation, *J Mammary Gland Biol Neoplasia* 7:267, 2002.

Zimmermann MB: Iodine deficiency in pregnancy and the effects of maternal iodine supplementation on the offspring: a review, *Am J Clin Nutr* 89:668S–672S, 2009.

Glossary

Aerobic metabolism The production of ATP requiring oxygen.

Aetiology The cause of.

Afferent Conducting or leading towards a target or centre.

Agonist A substance that interacts with a receptor molecule that initiates the same response as the hormone/transmitter usually binding to that site.

Aliphatic An organic compound that contains carbon atoms arranged in a chain rather than a ring formation.

Alkalosis An increase above that within the normal pH range of the body.

Allograph Implanted tissue that is of different genetic origin to the donor.

Alopecia The loss of body and scalp hair.

Amoeboid Appearing and behaving like the large single-celled organism called an amoeba.

Amplitude The difference between the highest and lowest measurement within a regular cycle.

Anabolic metabolism The synthesis of biological compounds involving the expenditure of energy.

Anaerobic metabolism The production of ATP in the absence of oxygen.

Anastomose The joining up of two tubes, vessels, etc., ensuring that the lumen remains patent between them.

Androsperm A sperm carrying a Y chromosome.

Aneuploidy Presence of an abnormal number of chromosomes.

Angiogenesis The formation of new blood vessels.

Anisogamy The existence of different forms of gametes related to sexual dimorphism.

Antagonist A substance that blocks receptor sites and then inhibits any further responses.

Anteflexed Curved inwards.

Anteverted Folded over.

Antibody (immunoglobulin) A 'Y'-shaped molecule that combines with an antigen (foreign protein) as part of the immune response, synthesized by white blood cells.

Antigen A molecule that initiates the immune response found within foreign tissue.

Antral A cavity within the body.

Apoptosis The genetic programming resulting in the death of a cell.

Aquatic Pertaining to an underwater environment.

Arborize To grow in a branch-like formation.

Asynclitism To be tilted laterally on either side of the anterior/posterior mid-plane.

Asphysia The death of a cell through a lack of oxygen.

Atresia The abnormal narrowing or closure of the lumen in a tube or vessel.

Atretic Having the characteristics of or pertaining to atresia; without an opening.

Atrophy Decreased functioning due to hypoplasia with increasing age.

Attenuated Modified to have less of an effect than normal.

Bactericidal Containing substances that can kill bacteria.

Bacteriostatic Containing substances that inhibit the reproduction of bacteria.

Basal metabolic rate The amount of energy expenditure required for the maintenance of essential body function only.

Behaviour The study of how organisms interact within the environment.

Biosynthesis The manufacture of body tissues and substances.

Breech Pertaining to the fetal rump.

Carotenoid Naturally occurring fat-soluble pigment that colours plants red, yellow, orange or brown.

Catabolic metabolism The breakdown of compounds requiring the expenditure of energy.

Cephalic Pertaining to the fetal head.

Chemoattractant A substance that acts as an attractant.

Chemostasis The maintenance of a chemical balance.

Chorioamnionitis Infection of the chorion and amnion during pregnancy.

Glossary

Circadian About one day.

Clonal expansion The ability of white blood cells to duplicate rapidly as part of the immune response.

Cloning Reproduction of an organism identical to an organism from which non-gamete genetic material is obtained.

Co-dominant Expression of both of two differing alleles in the phenotype when present in the genotype.

Coitus The act of sexual intercourse.

Colloid A protein suspended in a liquid.

Contraception Prevention of pregnancy by intervention.

Cortex The outer tissue layer or part of a structure.

Cranial Pertaining to the skull.

Cyanosis The bluish appearance of body tissues in situations of hypoxia.

Cyclical Repeated on a regular basis.

Cytoplasm The intercellular tissue contained within the cell membrane.

Decidualization The formation of the decidua of pregnancy.

Deletion The loss of part of a chromosome.

Dermatome Area of skin supplied by a single spinal nerve; derived from segmental development during embryonic stage.

Desquamation The loss of the outer layers of a continuously growing squamous tissue.

Detumescence The resolution of the inflammatory response.

Diapedesis The passage of blood cells through the blood vessel wall into the surrounding tissue.

Diastolic The period of relaxation of the ventricles of the heart.

Dichrotic A notch observed on the downstroke of the arterial pressure waveform that indicates the closure of the aortic valve.

Differentiation The division of cells resulting in the daughter cells becoming different owing to the activation of particular genes.

Dimorphism The existence of an organism in distinct forms such as male and female.

Diploid The normal number of paired chromosomes.

Discoid Disc-like.

Dorsal Pertaining to the back.

Dysgenesis Abnormal formation.

Dyspnoea Difficulty in breathing.

Ectopic pregnancy Implantation occurs outside the uterine cavity, usually in a uterine tube.

Efferent Carrying away from a centre (e.g. a blood vessel or nerve).

Endocytosis The process by which substances are transported into the cell within envelopes formed out of the outer cell membrane.

Endogenous Pertaining to the internal physiological environment.

Entrained Reset by an external factor.

Enzyme A protein that is able to speed up a chemical reaction without being structurally altered by the process itself.

Epitopes A cluster of antigens that evoke an immune response.

Ergometrine A drug derived from alkaloids of ergot that causes a sustained, strong contraction of the myometrium.

Erythropoietin A hormone produced chiefly by the kidneys (in the adult) and by the liver (in the fetus) that initiates red blood cell production.

Eugenics The science aimed at producing the perfect individual.

Euploidic Contains the normal number of chromosomes.

Evolution The study of genetic variation and change within generations of populations.

Exogenous Pertaining to the external environment.

Extended Tilted away from.

Flexed Tilted towards.

Follicle Tissue structure that is fluid-filled.

Free radical An oxygen molecule containing an unpaired electron.

Gametogenesis The formation of gametes.

Gastrulation The formation of the inner layers of the embryo by cell migration in a process of invagination.

Gene manipulation The science of artificially adding or removing genes to effect a change within an individual.

Gene pool The total number of genes within a population.

Genome The total number of genes within a single organism.

Gluconeogenesis The synthesis of glucose from non-carbohydrate sources.

Glycolytic The breakdown of glucose.

Graft rejection The rejection of donor tissue by the recipient's immune system.

Grey matter of brain Unmyelinated axons, nuclei and dendrites in the brain.

Gynosperm A sperm carrying an X chromosome.

Haemoptysis The presence of blood in sputum.

Half-life The time taken for the reduction by half of the quantity present.

Haploid Half of the normal chromosomal number (containing only one chromosome from the normal paired chromosomes).

Hermaphrodism The presence of male and female sex organs within the same individual.

Heterozygous Alleles at a particular locus of paired chromosomes each coding for a different phenotype.

Hirsutism The presence of excess body hair.

Homeothermic A warm-blooded animal (sometimes referred to as endothermic).

Homozygous Alleles at a particular locus of paired chromosomes both coding for the same phenotype.

Hydrolytic Dissolving in water.

Hyperaemia An excessive quantity of blood.

Hyper/hypoglycaemia Abnormally high/low level of glucose within the blood.

Hyperprolactinaemia Abnormally raised levels of the hormone prolactin.

Hyperventilation Overbreathing resulting in alkalosis.

Imprinting A behaviour pattern initiated by specific stimulation of a neural pathway that cannot be further influenced once it has occurred.

Incompatible Not tolerated and so initiating the immune response.

Inherent Having a genetic basis, hereditary, innate.

Innate Present from birth, congenital, e.g. a behaviour pattern that is not learnt but instinctive.

Invaginate To fold inwards to form a pouch.

Inversion The translocation of a portion of a chromosome comprising an upside-down switch.

Ischaemia The death of tissues due to a reduction or loss of the blood supply.

Keratinized Containing the protein keratin.

Ketotic Detectable amounts of ketone bodies present indicating that metabolism of fats is occurring.

Lipolysis The release of fatty acids from the breakdown of adipose tissue.

Lipophilic Having an affinity for fat.

Luteolysis The degradation of the corpus luteum.

Macromolecules Large organic compounds.

Macrosomic Larger than normal body size.

Maturation The achievement of full function following a period of growth and/or development.

Medulla The central tissue layer or part of a structure.

Menarche The commencement of the menstrual cycles.

Menopause The cessation of the menstrual cycles.

Menses The period of shedding of the endometrium during the menstrual cycle.

Mentum Pertaining to the fetal chin.

Methylation The addition of a methyl group ($-CH_3$) to a compound.

Micturition The voiding of urine.

Mitogen A substance that initiates the process of mitosis.

Morphogenesis The formation of body structure.

Morphology The development of form and size.

Necrotic The bacterial decomposition of dead tissue.

Neuronal Pertaining to the nervous system.

Neurotransmitter A chemical that crosses a synaptic gap to initiate an action potential in the receiving neuron.

Neurulation The embryonic formation of the neural tube from the neural plate.

Nidation The process of implantation of the blastocyst into the uterine endometrium.

Nocturia The need to void urine frequently at night.

Nomenclature Terminology describing systematic naming.

Occiput A bone at the posterior lower part of the skull.

Oedema Excess fluid in the extracellular compartments.

Opsonization The process by which bacteria and other cells are made susceptible to phagocytosis.

Oxidative The combination of oxygen with other molecules.

Pathogen A foreign organism that causes harm.

Penile Pertaining to the penis.

Perfusion The blood flow.

Peristaltic Coordinated contraction of smooth muscle around the lumen of a tube or vessel that facilitates the unidirectional movement of the contents within the lumen.

Phagocytic The ingestion of foreign material by phagocytes.

Phosphorylation The addition of an organic phosphate group to a molecule (often activating an enzyme).

Photoperiod The period of natural daylight exposure.

Placebo An inert/harmless substance that has no pharmacological effect, used in double-blind trials in comparison with drugs to assess their clinical effectiveness.

Placentation The formation of the fetal and maternal components of the placenta.

Placentome A lobe of the placenta.

Poikilothermic A cold-blooded animal (sometimes referred to as exothermic).

Polycythaemic An abnormally high number of red blood cells.

Polysperm Fertilization by more than one sperm.

Postprandial The period following the consumption of a meal.

Preantral Before the antral phase.

Precursor A substance that is altered into another substance.

Primordial Existing from the beginning.

Proliferative The ability to increase quickly in numbers.

Prophylaxis Treatment aimed at prevention rather than cure.

Pseudopodia A temporary protrusion in the cell membrane.

Psychogenic The development of the mind.

Pulsatile Released episodically rather than continuously.

Pyrexia An abnormally high body temperature.

Rate-limiting A process that proceeds in relation to the amount of precursor available.

Receptor A molecule that combines with a chemical signal that initiates a response within the cell.

Reticulocyte An immature red blood cell.

Sacrum The bony vestigial remains of the prehensile tail that forms the posterior part of the pelvis.

Senescence Old age.

Septum (pl. septa) A structure that divides the body or body area/organ.

Sinciput Pertaining to the fetal forehead.

Sinusoids An irregularly shaped blood vessel.

Specific gravity The relative density of a fluid in relation to pure water.

Sphincter A ring of muscle that can occlude a tube or vessel when contracted.

Steroidogenesis The production of steroid hormones.

Stroma The structural framework of a cell or organ.

Syncytium A mass of cells in which the cellular membranes have broken down forming a continuous mass.

Syntocinon A synthetic analogue of naturally occurring oxytocin used in obstetrics as a pharmacological method of augmenting uterine contractions via a controlled intravenous infusion.

Tactile Pertaining to touch.

Teratogen A chemical that interferes with the formation of the embryo.

Thermostasis The maintenance of a constant body temperature.

Totipotent A cell that has the capability of dividing to form a complete new individual.

Transcription The process of synthesizing mRNA from a DNA template.

Translation The process of forming an amino acid chain from a coded sequence of mRNA bases.

Transudation Blood plasma that collects within the interstitial space.

Unicellular Made up of one cell.

Uterotonins Substances that encourage the myometrium to contract.

Vascularization The growth of blood vessels into tissue.

Vascularized Perfused with blood vessels.

Vasoactive Has an effect on vascular smooth muscle.

Vasoconstriction Contraction of smooth muscle within the blood vessels.

Vasodilation Relaxation of the smooth muscle within blood vessels.

Ventral Pertaining to the front.

Vestigial A physical characteristic (structure) in evolutionary decline, i.e. remaining present but no longer necessary for survival.

Villus (pl. villi) A finger-like projection from a membrane surface.

Volatile Evaporates at ambient temperatures.

White matter of brain Bundles of myelinated axons within the brain.

Zygote A totipotent cell formed from the fusion of two gametes.

Index

Note: Page numbers followed by *b* indicate boxes, *f* indicate figures and *t* indicate tables.